Preparation for NCLEX-RN

FOURTH EDITION

SAUNDERS NURSING REVIEW and PRACTICE TESTS

Dee Ann Gillies, Ed.D., R.N.
Associate Professor
University of Illinois
College of Nursing

1987

W.B. Saunders Company
Philadelphia Sydney
London Tokyo
Toronto Hong Kong

W. B. Saunders Company: West Washington Square
Philadelphia, PA 19105

Library of Congress Cataloging-in-Publication Data

Gillies, Dee Ann

Preparation for NCLEX-RN.

Rev. ed. of: Saunders tests for self-evaluation of nursing competence. 3rd ed., rev. reprint. 1980. Includes bibliographies and index.

1. Nursing—Examinations, questions, etc. I. Gillies, Dee Ann. Saunders tests for self-evaluation of nursing competence. II. Title. [DNLM: 1. Educational Measurement. 2. Nursing—examination questions. WY 18 G481s]

RT55.G5 1987 610.73′076 86–26135

ISBN 0–7216–1454–X

Editor: Ilze Rader
Designer: Terri Siegel
Production Manager: Carolyn Naylor
Manuscript Editor: Mary Anne Folcher
Indexer: Alexander Weir

Preparation for NCLEX-RN: Nursing Review and Practice Tests ISBN 0–7216–1454–X

Last digit is the print number: 9 8 7 6 5 4 3 2 1

This book is lovingly dedicated
to the memory of

William Love Gillies,
Mary Griffiths Gillies,
and their remarkable *son, Rexford*

Contributors

CAROLE AUVIL, M.S.
Former Assistant Professor
University of Illinois
College of Nursing
Chicago, Illinois
Psychiatric Nursing

DEE ANN GILLIES, Ed.D., R.N.
Associate Professor
University of Illinois
College of Nursing
Chicago, Illinois
Medical Surgical Nursing

CAROL HOWLEY, M.S.N.
Assistant Professor of Maternal-Child Nursing
University of Illinois
College of Nursing
Chicago, Illinois
Maternal-Child Nursing

CHIEKO ONODA, M.S.
Associate Professor of Maternal-Child Nursing
University of Illinois
College of Nursing
Chicago, Illinois
Pediatric Nursing

Introduction To Preparation for NCLEX-RN

The purpose of the State Board Test Pool Examination is to protect the public. Therefore, the examination is designed to ensure that those individuals who are licensed to practice as registered nurses have demonstrated that they possess sufficient knowledge to practice safely.

ORGANIZATION OF THE EXAMINATION

The State Board Test Pool Examination consists of 4 tests of approximately 93 questions each. The tests are administered on 2 consecutive days, 1 in the morning and 1 in the afternoon of each day. The candidate is allowed 90 minutes to complete each of the 4 tests or approximately 1 minute to answer each test item. All 4 tests consist of situation-related multiple choice items that cover subject matter from all clinical nursing areas. Thus, in each test there are items that test *knowledge, understanding,* and *application of information* about the patient's needs and the nurse's interventions with patients of different ages, who have disorders of different types, and who receive care from different health agencies.

For each test item there is only 1 correct answer, and the candidate is not penalized for guessing.

The State Board Test Pool Examination items are written by nursing educators from diploma, associate degree, and baccalaureate nursing programs from all regions of the United States. Because the State Board Test Pool Examination is designed to assure minimum nursing competence and to reflect nursing practice throughout the nation, the items test for understanding of accepted, basic, safe nursing practice, rather than for knowledge of controversial, highly specialized, or experimental nursing approaches. The test items are designed to elicit cognitive activities at the levels of knowledge, comprehension, application, and analysis. Items are also designed to reflect the steps of the nursing process, *assessing, analyzing, planning, implementing,* and *evaluating.* These steps can be defined as follows:

1. **Assessing**—gathering information about the patient through taking a nursing history, performing a physical examination, reviewing laboratory test results and diagnostic test findings, consulting with other health professionals, and studying relevant scientific literature.

2. **Analyzing**—breaking down and scrutinizing patient data, drawing inferences from the data, establishing nursing diagnoses, developing a nursing problem list, and setting priorities for care.
3. **Planning**—determining the patient's needs, stating the patient's goals in behavioral terms, developing a plan of care to assure achievement of goals, securing personnel and material resources to support the care plan, and coordinating nursing care with the contributions of other health professionals.
4. **Implementing**—carrying out planned nursing interventions by writing nursing orders, assisting the patient with activities of daily living, administering care or directing others to do so, giving medications, performing ordered treatments, facilitating normal growth and development, teaching and motivating the patient for independence in self care and for directing others in his care, and referring patient and family to appropriate agencies for support.
5. **Evaluating**—establishing standards against which to judge the efficacy of the nursing care plan and the patient's progress under the established plan, recording and interpreting the patient's symptoms and responses to care measures, weighing the advantages and disadvantages of each nursing intervention, and modifying the care plan as necessary to maximize goal attainment.

In addition to testing for understanding of basic and safe nursing care, for different levels of cognitive ability, and for facility in the steps of the nursing process, the State Board Test Pool Examination items are designed to test the candidate's understanding of normal human growth and development, basic needs, coping techniques, and effects of age and culture on health.

The nursing behaviors that are tested by the State Board items are behaviors that were identified as pivotal to patient welfare in a study of critical nursing incidents.* In that study, analysis of 2000 critical incidents revealed that, to provide safe and effective care to patients, the nurse must be able to:

1. Exercise her professional prerogatives based on accurate clinical judgments.
2. Promote the patient's ability to cope with immediate, long range, and potential health related changes.
3. Help maintain patient comfort and normal body functions.
4. Initiate precautionary and preventive measures in administering patient care.
5. Check, compare, verify, monitor, and follow up effects of medications and treatment measures.
6. Interpret symptom complexes presented by the patient and intervene appropriately.
7. Respond appropriately to emergencies.
8. Obtain, record, and exchange information on behalf of the patient.
9. Employ patient care planning techniques.
10. Teach and supervise other staff members in provision of safe and effective patient care.

PREPARATION FOR THE EXAMINATION

Obviously, taking the State Board Test Pool Examination is an important event in a nurse's life, since the test serves both as the culmination of undergraduate nursing education and as a rite of passage into the world of work. Since passing the examination is important to the nurse's self esteem, employment opportunities and financial welfare, the nurse candidate should maximize chances for success by careful emotional, cognitive, and physical preparation.

The most important emotional preparation for taking the State Board Test Pool Examination is to approach the testing situation confidently, seeing the examination as a welcome, even enjoyable challenge to your abilities, rather than as a dreaded obstacle to desired status. One way to increase self-confidence in test performance is to repeatedly visualize yourself as a successful test taker, that is, to fantasize sitting comfortably in the examination room and answering the test items easily and accurately.

---

*Robey, M., Kingsbury, C. & Kane, J. (1979). Examining the Validity of the State Board Test Pool Examinations for Registered Nurse Licensure. Kansas City: American Nurses' Association.

While thus rehearsing the testing situation, you can imagine problems that could arise during the examination, together with actions that would resolve them. For example, you can mentally forecast actions to be taken in the event that any of the following develop during the examination: headache, urinary frequency, runny nose, feeling too hot, feeling too cold, breaking a pencil point, and distraction by surrounding noise. Such anticipatory problem solving will enable you to avoid some problems and minimize others. Remember to emphasize the positive aspect of solving problems.

Probably the greatest confidence in your ability for successful test performance can be achieved through "overlearning" the subject matter on which test items are based. In order to "overlearn" basic nursing knowledge, you should review the content of the major clinical nursing areas 2 or 3 times, approaching the content from a different viewpoint with each review.

This "overlearning" of subject matter, which contributes to emotional preparation for the State Board Test Pool Examination, is also the basic cognitive preparation for test taking. This book provides three mechanisms by which the candidate can effectively study the necessary knowledge base for nursing practice as follows: reviewing clinical nursing subject matter or content outlines, answering practice questions for each clinical nursing subject, and completing each of the 4 sections of the comprehensive examination that tests all clinical nursing subjects.

Subject Matter Outlines

Subject matter outlines are presented for Maternal-Child Nursing, Pediatric Nursing, Medical Surgical Nursing, and Psychiatric Nursing, each of which contains significant facts and pivotal principles underlying effective care of patients with common disorders and problems. Following each subject matter outline is a Bibliography, which indicates references to clarify and amplify major topics in the outline. Practice questions are provided following the content outlines.

Comprehensive Tests Simulating the State Board Test Pool Examination

Four comprehensive tests that simulate in length, subject matter, and item type the 4 tests that compose the State Board Test Pool Examination are provided. By working through these comprehensive tests under the conditions of the State Board Test Pool Examination, you can assess mastery of basic nursing knowledge and detect possible problems in taking the examination. *Allow 90 minutes for each test, taking 1 test each morning and each afternoon on two successive days.*

If you find that you cannot complete each comprehensive test in the allotted time period, you may need to use a different approach in identifying the problem proposed in the item's stem and in differentiating among clearly erroneous, partially accurate, and best possible answer to a question. If, while completing the comprehensive tests in this book, you become distracted by radio or TV noise from the next room or traffic noise from the street, you may need to wear ear plugs during the State Board Test Pool Examination. If hunger pangs impair your concentration during the comprehensive tests, you may need to eat a more substantial breakfast or lunch (higher carbohydrate and protein content than usual) on the 2 examination days.

After completing the four comprehensive tests in this book, you should compare your answers with the correct answers and rationales. It is a good idea to record on a file card the fact and principle underlying the correct answer of any item that was answered incorrectly and to look up additional information concerning the subject during remedial study.

By checking your answers with the test item grid that follows each comprehensive test, you can determine whether you missed more questions in 1 of the 5 steps of the nursing process than the others (assessment, analysis, planning, implementation, or evaluation). If this is the case, you can devote additional study time to material related to the step in question.

TAKING THE EXAMINATION

As the scheduled date for the State Board Test Pool Examination approaches, plan your daily activities so as to optimize physical health and strength. If you have studied diligently for several weeks, there will be no need to "cram" information during the 2 or 3 days preceding the examination. The majority of examination items test for *analysis* and *application*, rather than for recall and recognition. Since higher order cognitive processes, such as analysis and application, require a higher degree of mental alertness than do lower order processes, you should come to the examination well rested and relaxed, having obtained a full night's sleep each night for 2 to 3 nights before the examination. Not only is it a good idea to obtain extra sleep before the test, it is also advisable to avoid any unusually stimulating interpersonal encounters (both positive and negative) during the evening and morning before the examination. However, *it is not advisable to use chemical tranquilizers or stimulants to reduce nervousness or prevent drowsiness during the tests.* Use of a drug to which one is unaccustomed during a stressful testing situation would be likely to upset mental functioning rather than to improve it. Even increased coffee intake should be avoided during the testing period, as excess caffeine can cause insomnia, nervousness, or gastric upset.

On examination day you should arise early; dress in layered, loose fitting clothing (to be able to don and doff garments if the temperature of the examination room is uncomfortable); eat a well balanced breakfast in relaxed surroundings; and *allow plenty of time for the trip to the testing center*. A common anxiety relates to being late or missing the examination. To reduce the risk of unforeseen travel delays and parking or transfer problems, it is wise to make a "dry run" to the testing center during the week before the examination, taking care to travel at the same time of day, along the same route, and in the same vehicle (car, bus, or train) that will be used on the testing date.

You should take to the testing center a supply of sharpened number 2 pencils, handkerchiefs or tissues, ear plugs (if desired), aspirin (for headache or minor discomfort), candy (to relieve hunger pains or hypoglycemia), sanitary supplies (if menstruating or due to menstruate), money for transportation and meals, written directions to the testing center, and documents indicating that you are registered to take the examination.

After arriving at the testing center, the candidate should first use the rest room, if needed, enter the examination room, and select a seat that promises adequate lighting, comfortable temperature, and minimum noise. Since candidates will not be allowed to bring books or notes into the examination room, and the time between morning and afternoon testing sessions should be devoted to eating and relaxing, it is advisable to leave all study materials at home. Test monitors will examine the contents of purses and briefcases before admitting candidates to the room and will circulate through the room during the test session to prevent candidates from consulting "crib" notes or item responses of other candidates.

When examination booklets and answer sheets have been distributed, you should read the test directions carefully and follow them consistently in answering all questions. The candidate is expected to record her responses on the answer sheet by blacking in the space that corresponds with the answer selected for the number of the test item. The candidate should read and attempt to answer each test item, proceeding on the assumption that there are no "trick" questions and that each question can be answered correctly on the basis of information given in the patient situation that precedes the question and the problem that is posed in the item stem. In other words, in answering a question, the candidate should not infer any information about the situation that is not included in the patient situation or the item stem.

After reading the item stem, try to imagine the correct answer and then read the item distractors to find the one that most closely matches it. If none of the distractors coincides with the imagined answer, you should mentally recast the question into more simple terms, as such rephrasing may reveal that one of the distractors is more plausible than the others.

To improve chances for success, the candidate should *set time limits for completing various sections of the test*. For example, the candidate should aim to complete approximately 31 items within the first half hour of the test session, to complete 62 items by the end of the second half hour, and to complete all 93 items by the end of the third half hour. If an item seems especially difficult or confusing and no distractor seems more accurate than the others, it would be advisable *to flag the item for later consideration and move on to the next question*. In skipping an item, the candidate should be sure *to leave the corresponding space blank on the answer sheet* so as to ensure proper grading of test item answers. After answering the last test item, the candidate should *return to those items that were earlier flagged*, as thought processes provoked by later test questions may have activated logical connections that would reveal the answer to an earlier item. You should use all of the time allowed for completing each test. If time remains after all test questions have been answered, you should review those items whose answers you were unsure of to see whether, on reconsideration, the selected answer still seems the best choice.

Finally, when the 4th test of the State Board Test Pool Examination has been completed on the 2nd day of testing, you can relax, congratulate yourself on having met the test challenge bravely, and avoid post-mortem discussions of answers to particular test questions.

The passing score on the State Board Test Pool Examination is 1600. After an interval of several weeks, you will be notified in writing of your score. Should a candidate fail to pass the examination, she may apply to retake the examination at a later date. In preparing to repeat the examination the candidate should be aware that the tests are changed for each examination period, although the revised tests are designed to serve the same purpose, cover the same subject material, tap the same cognitive processes, contain the same type of item, and highlight the same concepts. Since individual states differ with regard to the number of times that a candidate is allowed to retake the State Board Test Pool Examination, the candidate who does not obtain a passing score should complete an intensive and well planned review of nursing information before taking the examination a 2nd time.

Contents

PART ONE
Nursing Review

UNIT I *Maternal-Child Nursing* 3

- Content Outline 3
- Practice Questions 31
- Answer Sheet 43
- Answers and Rationales for Practice Questions 45

UNIT II *Pediatric Nursing* 51

- Content Outline 51
- Practice Questions 83
- Answer Sheet 95
- Answers and Rationales for Practice Questions 97

UNIT III *Medical Surgical Nursing* 102

- Content Outline 102
- Practice Questions 190
- Answer Sheet 203
- Answers and Rationales for Practice Questions 205

UNIT IV *Psychiatric Nursing* 218

- Content Outline 218
- Practice Questions 247
- Answer Sheet 259
- Answers and Rationales for Practice Questions 261

PART TWO
Comprehensive Examination

SECTION 1 269

- Item Analysis 285
- Answer Sheet 287

SECTION 2 289

- Item Analysis 304
- Answer Sheet 305

SECTION 3 307

Item Analysis 322
Answer Sheet 323

SECTION 4 325

Item Analysis 340
Answer Sheet 341

ANSWERS AND RATIONALES 343

Section 1 343
Section 2 353
Section 3 364
Section 4 374

INDEX 383

PART ONE

Nursing Review

UNIT I

Maternal–Child Nursing

Section

MATERNAL–CHILD NURSING CONTENT OUTLINE

ANATOMY OF FEMALE REPRODUCTIVE ORGANS

A. External Genitalia

1. Mons veneris; mons pubis
2. Labia majora
3. Labia minora
4. Clitoris
5. Vestibule
6. Urinary meatus
7. Bartholin's glands; Skene's ducts
8. Hymen
9. Perineum

B. Internal Organs

1. Ovaries (2)

   Attached to uterus by ovarian ligaments; all eggs present at birth. Function is production of ova and estrogen and progesterone.

2. Fallopian tubes (2)

   Extend from cornu of uterus for 10 cm. Fertilization occurs in middle third of tube. Egg is transported through tube to uterus by peristaltic and ciliary actions.

3. Uterus

   Muscular organ; major functions include housing developing fetus and menstruation. Two distinct portions of uterus:

   a. Corpus (body)—3 layers
      (1.) Perimetrium—external layer
      (2.) Myometrium—middle layer
      (3.) Endometrium—inner layer

   b. Cervix—3 sections
      (1.) Internal os—opening into body of uterine cavity
      (2.) Cervical canal—portion between internal and external os
      (3.) External os—opening into vagina

4. Vagina

   Canal extending from external genitalia to cervix. Major functions include passageway for menstrual discharge, passageway for fetus and organ of copulation. Environment is acidic to protect against invasion of pathogens.

ANATOMY OF MALE REPRODUCTIVE ORGANS

A. External Genitalia

1. Penis
2. Scrotal sac—contains testes.

B. Internal Genitalia

1. Testes—descend into scrotum during 7th or 8th month of gestation.
2. Canal system—consists of seminiferous tubules, epididymis, vas deferens, ejaculatory duct, and urethra.

PHYSIOLOGY OF FEMALE REPRODUCTIVE ORGANS: MENSTRUATION AND MENSTRUAL CYCLE

A. Menstrual Cycle

Cycle begins on day 1 of onset of menstrual discharge and extends to onset of next cycle of bleeding; normal range varies from 20 to 45 days with majority of women around 28 days. Begins at puberty and ends at menopause. Ovulation occurs at midcycle or around the 14th day in majority of women.

B. Hormonal Control

Menstrual cycle is regulated through control of pituitary gland, ovaries, and uterus.

1. Proliferative Phase
   a. FSH (follicle stimulating hormone) released by anterior pituitary stimulates graafian follicle development.
   b. The developing graafian follicle produces estrogen containing fluid.
   c. Estrogen stimulates build-up of endometrium.
   d. Increasing amounts of estrogen in blood stream suppress FSH secretion and enhance LH (luteinizing hormone) secretion.
   e. LH stimulates ovulation and initiates development of corpus luteum.
2. Secretory Phase
   a. Follows ovulation; release of mature ovum from the ruptured graafian follicle.
   b. LH influences rapid changes in the ruptured follicle.
   c. Corpus luteum replaces graafian follicle; main function is to secrete progesterone and estrogen.
   d. Progesterone acts on endometrium to prepare it for pregnancy if it occurs. Also acts to maintain pregnancy in initial stages.
3. Menstrual Phase
   a. Unless fertilization occurs, corpus luteum degenerates.
   b. Decrease of progesterone and estrogen.
   c. Endometrium degenerates, leading to menstruation.
   d. New cycle begins as decreased levels of estrogen and progesterone stimulate production of FSH.

PHYSIOLOGY OF PREGNANCY

A. Fertilization and Implantation

1. Occurs with union of sperm and ovum.
2. Each carries 23 chromosomes.
3. Sperm carries X and Y sex chromosomes, which unite with female X chromosome. This determines fetal sex.
   a. Male child XY
   b. Female child XX
4. Fertilization occurs in distal portion of tube, and fertilized egg descends to uterus for implantation.
5. Implantation occurs between 6 and 9 days after fertilization.
6. Embryonic development begins; in 1st or blastocyte stage cells are arranged in 3 layers; ectoderm, mesoderm, and endoderm.

B. Fetal Membranes and Amniotic Fluid

1. Fetal membranes surrounding fetus in 2 layers.
   a. Amnion—inner membrane forms from the blastocyte about 2nd to 3rd week of embryonic development.
   b. Chorion—outer layer is developed from the trophoblast.

2. Amniotic fluid.
   a. Amount of fluid at term consists of 500 to 1000 ml.
   b. Function is to provide optimum environment and temperature for fetus and to act as a cushion against injury.

C. Fetal Circulation

Differs from adult owing to following structures:

1. Placenta—serves as organ providing exchange of nutrients and waste products between mother and fetus. Provides O_2 and removes CO_2 from fetal circulation. Fully functioning by 14th to 16th week of gestation.
2. Placenta's structure and function as follows:
   a. Formed by union of chorionic villi and decidua basalis.
   b. Fetal surface is smooth and shiny.
   c. Maternal surface is red and globular.
   d. Diffusion causes exchange of nutrients, wastes, and gases between mother and fetus.
   e. Hormones produced by placenta include estrogen, progesterone, ACTH, growth hormone, and gonadotropic hormones (HCG and HPL).
3. Umbilical Cord
   a. Attaches from central portion of placenta to fetus.
   b. Consists of 1 vein and 2 arteries; vein transports nourishment and arteries transport waste.
   c. Wharton's jelly—protective covering surrounding cord.
4. Foramen ovale—opening between right and left atria; bypasses fetal lungs; lungs nonfunctioning; need blood only for nourishment.
5. Ductus arteriosus—connects pulmonary trunk and aorta; bypasses fetal lungs.
6. Ductus venosus—connection between umbilical vein and ascending vena cava.

D. Fetal Growth and Development

Development proceeds in a cephalocaudal pattern.

1. End of 4 weeks' gestation
   a. No clearly defined features.
   b. Body systems very crude.
   c. Heart beating at about 14 days.
   d. Cardiovascular system functioning.
   e. Susceptible to teratogenic effects.
2. End of 8 weeks' gestation
   a. Head very large in comparison with body.
   b. Some fetal movements.
   c. Facial features becoming distinct.
   d. Chadwick's sign—cervix and vagina are blue.
   e. Hegar's sign—lower uterine segment soft.
   f. Goodell's sign—cervix soft.
   g. Ossification of skeleton begins.
3. End of 12 weeks' gestation
   a. Teeth forming under gums.
   b. Fingers and toes bear nails.
   c. Kidneys able to secrete.
   d. Eyelids fused until 6 months.
   e. Sex distinguishable.
   f. Takes on more human appearance.
   g. Bile present in intestines.
   h. FHT (fetal heart tone) may be detected by Doppler ultrasound method.
4. End of 16 weeks' gestation
   a. Lanugo appears over body.
   b. Human facial appearance.
   c. Fetal movements stronger; felt by mother.
   d. Size about 6″ long; weight about 3.5 oz
   e. About 200 ml of amniotic fluid; can do amniocentesis.
5. End of 20 weeks' gestation
   a. Vernix caseosa appears.
   b. Fetal heart rate (FHR) heard clearly with fetoscope.
   c. Size about 10″ long; weight about 11 oz.
6. End of 24 weeks' gestation
   a. Fat beginning to deposit beneath skin.
   b. Better proportion between head and body.
   c. Eyebrows and eyelashes appear.
   d. Size about 12″ long; weight about 1½ lb.
   e. Respiratory system is immature and will not sustain fetus.
7. End of 28 weeks' gestation
   a. Skin covered with vernix caseosa.
   b. Size about 14″ long; weight about 2½ lb.
   c. Although immature, fetus may be viable if delivered at this time.
8. End of 32 weeks' gestation
   a. Nails extend to ends of fingers.
   b. Lanugo begins to disappear.
   c. Size about 16″ long; weight about 4 lb.
9. End of 36 weeks' gestation
   a. Increased fat deposits under skin.
   b. Increased chances for survival.
   c. Size about 18″ long; weight about 5 lb.
10. End of 40 weeks' gestation
   a. Full term gestation.
   b. Little lanugo or vernix caseosa remains.
   c. Smooth skin.
   d. Size about 20″ long; weight 7 to 7½ lb.

11. Post term—over 42 weeks' gestation
    a. Vernix caseosa, lanugo absent.
    b. Breast tissue of about 10 mm.
    c. Skin thick, dry, deeply cracked, and wrinkled.
    d. Nails long.
    e. May have increased morbidity and mortality risks.

E. Maternal Changes During Pregnancy

Pregnancy is a normal physiological process that affects all body systems.

1. Endocrine System
   a. Enlarged pituitary gland
   b. Placental production of estrogen, progesterone, HCG, and HPL
   c. Increase in corticosteroids due to hyperplasia of adrenal cortex
   d. Increase in basal metabolic rate (BMR)
   e. Increase in thyroid function
   f. Increase in production of insulin by pancreas
2. Gastrointestinal (GI) System
   a. General decrease in smooth muscle tone causes delayed emptying time of stomach
   b. Relaxed cardiac sphincter
   c. Gingivae soft and enlarged
   d. Decreased gastric acid leads to flatulence and heartburn
   e. Decreased GI mobility leads to constipation
   f. Increased nausea and vomiting occur early in pregnancy
3. Urinary Tract System
   a. Increased pressure on bladder by uterus during the 1st and 3rd trimester leads to increased urinary frequency.
   b. Bladder tone reduced
   c. Bladder capacity increased
   d. Increased urinary output
   e. Increased excretion of glucose causes lowered renal threshold
   f. Presence of HCG in urine and blood is basis for pregnancy tests
4. Circulatory System
   a. Heart displaced; systolic murmurs are common.
   b. Increased cardiac volume (30%)
   c. Increased cardiac output (35%)
   d. Increased heart rate or beats per minute (5 to 10 bpm)
   e. HCT and HCB levels decrease by 10%
   f. No rise in blood pressure (BP); should remain stable.
   g. Stasis of blood causes edema late in pregnancy.
5. Respiratory System
   a. Increased ventilation with increased O_2 consumption.
   b. Respiratory rate unchanged (16 min).
   c. Vital capacity unchanged.
6. Integumentary System
   a. Increased pigmentation causes linea nigra, darkened genitalia, chloasma, darkened areolae in 2nd trimester.
   b. Spider nevi and palmar erythema due to increased estrogen.
   c. Striae gravidarum usually do not totally disappear after pregnancy.
   d. Increased sebaceous gland activity
7. Skeletal System
   a. Softening of all ligaments and joints caused by hormonal action of relaxin.
8. Nervous System
   a. No specific changes unless related to causes other than pregnancy.
9. Reproductive—Mammary System
   a. Uterine changes include
      (1.) Goodell's sign—softening of cervix detected by 6 to 8 weeks.
      (2.) Hegar's sign—softening of the lower uterine segment detected by 6 to 8 weeks.
      (3.) Chadwick's sign—purplish hue to vaginal mucosa due to increased vascularization. Detected by 6 to 8 weeks.
      (4.) Uterus rises out of pelvic cavity by about 12 weeks.
      (5.) Increased uterine secretions with high pH.
   b. Breast changes include
      (1.) Increased fullness, tingling, tenderness, and size.
      (2.) Areola darkens due to hormone levels.
      (3.) Montgomery's glands enlarge.
      (4.) Colostrum appears about 5th month.
      (5). Ductal system developed due to hormonal influences.

F. Emotional Changes of Pregnancy

Pregnancy is considered to be one of life's crises and produces a multitude of emotional changes. The major changes include the following:

1. Emotional lability
2. Ambivalence; common 1st trimester.
3. Acceptance occurs as obvious signs of pregnancy develop, such as lightening and quickening.
4. Passivity and introversion commonly occur late in 2nd trimester.
5. Fears and concerns are heightened for the woman herself and for the fetus.

6. Fantasies—woman may fantasize her role as mother before birth.
7. Letting go—woman experiences letting go of former role and lifestyle.

G. Diagnosis of Pregnancy

To validate pregnancy, diagnosis must be accurate.

1. Presumptive signs of pregnancy; these are subjective and include amenorrhea; breast changes, especially tenderness; nausea and vomiting (N & V); bladder irritability, especially urinary frequency; and fatigue.
2. Probable signs of pregnancy; these are objective and include abdominal enlargement, uterine changes, Braxton Hicks' contractions, ballottement, Hegar's sign, Chadwick's sign, and sensation of fetal movement.
3. Positive signs of pregnancy; these are fetus' heart rate heard and counted separately from mother's, fetal activity felt by examiner, and ultrasonographic diagnosis.
4. Course of Pregnancy; calculating estimated date of confinement (EDC) by Nagele's rule—count back 3 months from the 1st day of the last normal menstrual period and add 7 days.
5. Estimating gestational age; noninvasive techniques include measuring fundal height and correlating with EDC and measuring estriol levels in maternal urine.
6. Estimating gestational age using invasive techniques includes the following:
   a. Amniocentesis—measurement of fetal lung maturity and the ability of the fetus to survive in extrauterine environment; lecithin/sphingomyelin (L/S) ratio of greater than 2 indicates lung maturity.
   b. Radiography/x-rays should not be done until after the 3rd month of pregnancy; at about 36 weeks' gestation the presence of distal femoral ossification centers can be detected.
   c. Ultrasound—measurement of a biparietal diameter of greater than 9.8 cm indicates term gestation.

H. Prenatal Instructions

1. Nutritional guidelines during pregnancy and lactation are as follows:
   a. Consider prepregnancy nutritional state of mother.
   b. Monitor weight with regard to amount and pattern of gain.
   c. Never recommend weight reduction or severe caloric restriction.
   d. Restriction of sodium is no longer recommended unless medical problems occur.
   e. Increased fluids to combat constipation.
   f. Increased caloric intake needed to meet basal metabolic demands and to support weight gain (25 to 30 lb).
   g. Increased protein needed for growth demands (74 to 76 gm/day).
   h. Increased vitamins needed, especially folic acid which aids in preventing anemia.
   i. Increased iron intake aids in blood formation, preventing anemia and increasing resistance to infection (normal pregnant female should increase iron intake by 3 to 6 mg/day).
   j. Increased carbohydrate demands provide protective substances and bulk (approximately 9 mg/day).
   k. Caloric intake should be between 2300 and 2500 calories/day.
   l. Lactating mothers have extra caloric and fluid demands.
   m. Dietary instruction is a vital part of prenatal instruction and must take into account cultural, ethnic, and economic differences.
2. Use of drugs, as follows:
   a. All drugs can be expected to cross placenta and affect fetus.
   b. Greatest danger during 1st trimester.
   c. Omit or restrict use of nicotine and ingestion of alcohol throughout pregnancy.

PRENATAL CARE REGIMEN

A. Initial examination includes complete history; general health and past obstetrical history; physical examination includes adequacy of pelvis, laboratory tests, and diet and health instructions.

B. Subsequent examination is usually monthly until 32 weeks, then more frequently. Each examination includes evaluation of BP, weight gain, urine, fundal height, FHT, observation for any abnormal physical symptoms and continuing health instructions.

COMPLICATIONS OF PREGNANCY

A. Common Discomforts of Pregnancy and Relief Measures

1. Nausea and vomiting (1st trimester); small frequent meals, avoid causative foods.

2. Frequency of urination (1st and 3rd trimester); continue adequate fluid intake.
3. Heartburn (2nd and 3rd trimester); small frequent feedings; avoid spicy, fatty foods.
4. Flatulence (2nd and 3rd trimester); daily bowel elimination, avoid gas-forming foods.
5. Constipation (2nd and 3rd trimester); increase fluids, eat fruits and foods high in roughage.
6. Hemorrhoids (3rd trimester); avoid constipation, elevate legs several times daily.
7. Insomnia (3rd trimester); promote relaxation.
8. Backaches (3rd trimester); improve posture, wear comfortable shoes.
9. Cramping in legs (3rd trimester); increase calcium intake; extend toes toward knee of affected leg.
10. Shortness of breath (3rd trimester); maintain sitting position as much as possible to aid respiration.

B. Danger Signals During Pregnancy

1. Bleeding from vagina.
2. Escape of amniotic fluid, denoting premature rupture of membranes
3. Abdominal pain
4. Dizziness or blurring of vision
5. Persistent headache
6. Edema of face and fingers
7. Persistent and severe vomiting
8. Chills and elevated temperature

C. Abortion

Abortion is the expulsion of the fetus before it is viable; abortion may be spontaneous or induced.

1. Categories of Abortion (Spontaneous and Induced)
   a. *Threatened abortion*—some blood loss and pain without loss of products of conception. No cervical dilatation.
   b. *Imminent*—bleeding profuse, contractions severe, bearing down sensation. Without intervention, products of conception will be lost.
   c. *Inevitable*—bleeding, contractions, ruptured membranes, and cervical dilatation.
   d. *Incomplete*—portion of products of conception remain in uterine cavity.
   e. *Complete*—all products of conception expelled.
   f. *Habitual*—abortion in 3 or more succeeding pregnancies.
   g. *Therapeutic*—medically terminated for mother's physical or emotional health.
   h. *Criminal*—termination of pregnancy outside medical or approved facilities.
2. Etiology of Abortion
   a. Abnormalities of fetus
   b. Abnormalities of reproductive tract
   c. Injuries—physical and emotional shocks
   d. Endocrine disturbances
   e. Acute maternal infectious diseases
   f. Other maternal diseases
   g. Psychogenic problems
3. Clinical Manifestations of Abortion
   a. Vaginal bleeding.
   b. Intermittent contractions and pain, usually beginning in the small of the back; abdominal cramping.
4. Treatment of Threatened and Inevitable Abortions
   a. Notify physician immediately, save all perineal pads.
   b. Endocrine therapy, usually progesterone if deficient.
   c. Correction of abnormalities or disturbances of reproductive tract.
   d. Avoidance of stress and exertion during early pregnancy
   e. Bed rest and sedation; avoid climbing stairs and coitus until bleeding stops.
   f. Oxytoxic drug may be given to hasten process of abortion, if it is inevitable, and to promote contraction of uterus after abortion.
   g. Medication for pain, if necessary.
   h. Blood available for transfusion, if necessary.
   i. Dilatation and curettage may be necessary in an incomplete abortion.
   j. Administration of RhoGAM (immune globulin) to Rh-negative mothers who abort.
   k. Maintain sterile technique in all examinations and treatments.
5. Nursing Management of Abortion
   a. Offer emotional support and comfort.
   b. Save all perineal pads and expelled tissue for examination.
   c. Observe for signs of shock, and institute emergency measures for treatment, if necessary.
   d. In criminal abortions, observe for serious complications, such as septic shock, thrombophlebitis, and renal failure.

D. Hydatidiform Mole

Hydatidiform mole is a benign neoplasm of the chorion, in which chorionic villi degenerate, become filled with a clear viscous fluid, and assume the appearance of grape-like clusters, involving all or part of the decidual lining of the uterus.

1. Incidence
   a. Rare; occurs in 1 of every 2000 pregnancies, except in the Orient where it is more common; increased incidence in older women.
   b. Usually no fetus is found.
2. Etiology
   a. May be pathological ova
   b. High incidence in the Orient may be due to dietary protein deficiency.
3. Clinical Manifestations
   a. Pregnancy appears normal at first.
   b. Bleeding varies from "spotting" to profuse.
   c. Rapid enlargement of the uterus.
   d. Nausea and vomiting appear earlier and are usually more severe and last longer.
   e. Severe preeclampsia may develop in the early part of the 2nd trimester.
   f. Hypertension may occur with the rapid expansion of the uterus.
   g. Characteristic vesicles may be passed.
4. Diagnosis
   a. Test for increased titer of chorionic gonadotropin. It is best to collect a 24-hour urine specimen for the total output.
   b. Sonography—gives positive diagnosis in the 1st trimester.
   c. Amniography—x-ray following injection with contrast dye
5. Treatment
   a. Evacuation of uterus by dilatation and curettage or vacuum curettage suction, as soon as positive diagnosis is made.
   b. Follow-up visits to physician for examination, because hydatidiform mole may lead to carcinoma. Usually HCG levels must be followed for a period of 1 year.
6. Nursing Management
   a. Observe for hemorrhage.
   b. Provide emotional support; patient may have a fear of malignancy, or patient may feel the loss of the anticipated birth.
   c. Encourage follow-up treatment.

E. Ectopic Pregnancy

Ectopic pregnancy is a pregnancy that implants and begins developing outside of the uterus.

1. Process of Pregnancy
   a. Although the fertilized ovum usually attaches to the uterine lining, it may become implanted at any point between the graafian follicle and the uterus.
   b. Tubal pregnancy is the most common form (95%), but the ovum may attach to an ovary, the abdomen, or interligaments.
   c. Implantation
      (1.) Ovum attaches to fallopian tube and erodes into mucosal lining of the tube, as it would to the endometrial lining of the uterus.
      (2.) Tube increases in size and stretches.
      (3.) Pregnancy usually terminates during the 1st 3 months by the following:
         (a.) Spontaneous tubal abortion
         (b.) Tubal rupture
         (c.) Death and disintegration of products of conception within the tube.
2. Etiology
   a. Progress of ovum through tube is delayed for some reason.
   b. Tubal deformities—congenital or due to disease, such as gonorrhea.
   c. Tumors pressing against the tube
   d. Adhesion from previous surgery
   e. Tubal spasms
   f. Migration of ovum to opposite tube
   g. Use of IUDs
3. Clinical Manifestations
   a. Woman may or may not know she is pregnant.
   b. Many have history of missed periods and "spotting."
   c. Many have slight abdominal pain.
   d. Early signs of pregnancy may be absent.
   e. Uterus enlarges and decidua develops due to hormonal influence.
   f. Often 1st symptom is a sudden excruciating pain in lower abdomen.
   g. May feel faint and have signs of shock as a result of hemorrhage into the peritoneal cavity.
   h. May have external bleeding.
4. Treatment
   a. Immediate removal of the affected tube.
   b. Blood transfusions may be necessary.
5. Nursing Management
   a. Observe for signs of shock, and give treatment for shock as necessary.
   b. Protect patient against exertion.
   c. Provide emotional support; patient may be frightened and feel the loss of pregnancy.

F. Placenta Previa

Placenta previa occurs when the ovum implants low in the uterus, toward the cervix; the placenta develops so that it partially or completely covers the internal os; occurs in 1 of every 150 deliveries.

1. Types
   a. Complete—internal os entirely covered.
   b. Partial—only part of internal os covered.
   c. Marginal—portion of placenta approaches the internal os.
2. Etiology
   a. Occurs more often in multiparas.
   b. Occurs more often with increased age of mother.
3. Clinical Manifestations
   a. Painless vaginal bleeding after the 7th month without precipitating cause.
   b. Bleeding may be intermittent.
   c. As internal os begins to dilate, the part of placenta that overlies the os separates and leaves gaping vessels, so that bleeding occurs.
   d. Uterus remains soft.
4. Diagnosis
   a. History of painless bleeding begins late in pregnancy.
   b. Localization of placenta by ultrasonography.
   c. Sterile vaginal and pelvic examinations are usually not done as part of diagnosis until adequate preparation has been made.
      (1.) Have blood available for transfusion.
      (2.) Set up for possible emergency cesarean section.
      (3.) Determine whether fetal age is adequate for survival.
5. Treatment
   a. Hospitalize immediately.
   b. Usually, place on bed rest.
   c. Type and cross match blood for possible transfusion.
   d. Treatment depends upon type of placenta previa, condition of mother, and viability of baby.
      (1.) Mechanical pressure applied to placental site by bringing down baby's head and occluding blood vessels; usually accomplished by the rupture of membranes.
      (2.) Delivery by cesarean section.
   e. If baby is small and bleeding stops, delivery is usually postponed.
6. Nursing Management
   a. Maintain patient on bed rest and provide quiet restful atmosphere.
   b. Count perineal pads.
   c. Observe for hemorrhage.
   d. Give emotional support, explain procedures, and help allay fears.
   e. Do not perform vaginal examinations.
   f. Have emergency setup for cesarean section availabile.
   g. Carefully monitor FHT.

G. Abruptio Placentae

Abruptio placentae occurs when the placenta separates from the normal implantation site in the upper segment of the uterus before birth of baby; occurs in 1 in 500 deliveries.

1. Types
   a. Complete separation—placenta becomes completely detached from uterine wall.
   b. Partial separation—portion of placenta adheres to uterine wall.
   c. External—blood escapes from the vagina.
   d. Concealed—blood is retained in uterine cavity.
2. Etiology
   a. Trauma
   b. Chronic renal vascular disease
   c. High parity
3. Clinical Manifestations
   a. External—chief symptom is vaginal bleeding accompanied by abdominal pain.
   b. Concealed
      (1.) Intense, cramp-like uterine pain.
      (2.) Uterine tenderness and rigidity.
      (3.) Lack of alternate contraction-relaxation of uterus.
      (4.) FHT—bradycardia or absent.
4. Treatment
   a. Depends upon severity and extent of labor.
   b. Moderate bleeding—rupture membranes to hasten delivery and help control bleeding.
   c. Severe bleeding—immediate cesarean section.
   d. Treat for blood loss and shock.
   e. Draw blood for coagulation studies.
5. Nursing Management
   a. Keep patient on bed rest.
   b. Observe for signs of shock.
   c. Carefully monitor contractions, FHT, and vital signs.
   d. Type and cross match blood for possible transfusion.
   e. Maintain record of intake and output.
   f. Nursing interventions after delivery are as follows:
      (1.) Observe closely for hemorrhage.
      (2.) Carefully record intake and output, and observe for anuria or oliguria.

6. Complications of Abruptio Placentae
   a. Disseminated intravascular disease
      (1.) Thromboplastin from placental tissue and clots enters the blood stream through open vessels at the placental site and initiates an exaggeration of the normal clotting process.
      (2.) As more thromboplastin is introduced into circulation, more fibrinogen and clotting factors are used up.
      (3.) In addition, a fibrinolytic process that disintegrates fibrin is initiated, resulting in fibrin degradation products, which in turn further interfere with the clotting process.
   b. Treatment
      (1.) Treat for hypovolemic shock—fluid and blood.
      (2.) May administer heparin solution—prevents clot formation and increases available fibrinogen, coagulation factors, and platelets.
      (3.) Remove source of triggering mechanism.
      (4.) Monitor circulatory and renal functions.

H. Pregnancy Induced Hypertension (PIH)

Pregnancy induced hypertension is a group of conditions that have similar symptoms. The incidence is approximately 7 to 10% of all pregnancies. Clients at risk to develop PIH are adolescents and older primigravidas. Those with conditions of multiple pregnancy, polyhydramnios and diabetes are also considered to be at risk.

Preeclampsia

Preeclampsia is an acute, hypertensive disease peculiar to pregnancy that may be mild or severe.

1. Clinical Manifestations
   a. Usually appears after the 24th week
   b. Major symptoms are hypertension, proteinuria, and edema. Two of the 3 abovementioned symptoms are usually needed for diagnosis.
   c. Mild preeclampsia
      (1.) Blood pressure above 140/90 mmHg, or systolic of 30 mmHg and diastolic of 15 mmHg above baseline on 2 occasions at least 6 hours apart.
      (2.) Weight gain greater than 3 lb/month during 2nd trimester.
      (3.) Proteinuria—1 gm in 24 hours; + 1 or + 2 on "dipstick."
      (4.) Edema—slight, generalized in body.
   d. Severe preeclampsia
      (1.) Blood pressure 160/110 mmHg or more on 2 separate occasions 6 hours apart with the patient on bed rest.
      (2.) Massive edema—excessive weight gain.
      (3.) Proteinuria—5 gm or more in 24 hours; +3 or +4 on "dipstick."
      (4.) Oliguria—400 ml or less in 24 hours.
      (5.) Visual disturbances
      (6.) Headache
      (7.) Vasospasms
      (8.) Hemoconcentration causes an increase in hematocrit values.
      (9.) Epigastric pain (usually a late sign) tends to precede convulsions.
2. Treatment
   a. Mild preeclampsia
      (1.) Patient usually remains at home.
      (2.) Extra rest is prescribed.
      (3.) Adequate fluid intake is maintained.
      (4.) Highly salted food is avoided; diet includes high protein foods.
      (5.) Weight is checked daily.
      (6.) Further symptoms are watched for.
      (7.) Physician may order antihypertensive drug therapy.
   b. Severe preeclampsia
      (1.) Medications may include antihypertensive drugs, such as hydralazine (Apresoline) and anticonvulsive drugs, such as magnesium sulfate.
      (2.) Increase protein intake; sodium intake is usually not restricted, but patient should avoid use of highly salted foods. (Note: This is a recent trend. The use of low sodium diet may still be included on state board examinations).
      (3.) Bed rest—left lateral recumbent position to increase O_2 to fetus and aid in diuresis.
      (4.) Efforts to increase diuresis—diuretics may or may not be given.
      (5.) Sedatives may be ordered by physician.
      (6.) Observe for signs of central nervous system irritability and hyperactivity.
3. Nursing Management
   a. Maintain patient on bed rest and plan care to promote rest.
   b. Provide adequate diet.
   c. Carefully assess vital signs, including maternal reflexes.

d. Record intake and output.
e. Observe for increase in signs and symptoms and report to physician immediately.
f. Check weight at the same time each day.
g. Examine urine for increased protein.
h. Examine for visual changes; blurred vision, headaches, and ataxia.
i. Limit visitors for patient with severe pre-eclampsia.
j. Maintain seizure precautions.
k. Provide diversional activities.
l. Check for increased edema.

ECLAMPSIA

Eclampsia is the most severe form of toxemia and is always accompanied by convulsions and even coma. Eclampsia means a convulsion has occurred and may be accompanied by a coma.

1. Clinical Manifestations
   a. Severe edema—tremendous weight gain.
   b. Scanty urine output
   c. Urine may contain red blood cells, varied casts, and protein.
   d. Blood pressure may rise to 200/110 mmHg.
   e. There may be visual disturbances, blurring, or even blindness caused by edema of the retina.
   f. Severe epigastric pain.
   g. Convulsions—both tonic and clonic.
   h. Labor may begin, and fetus may be born prematurely or die.
2. Treatment
   a. Control convulsions.
   b. Promote vasodilation to combat vasospasms.
   c. Promote diuresis.
   d. Control blood pressure.
   e. Physician may elect to terminate pregnancy at a carefully chosen time.
3. Nursing Management
   a. Provide a quiet, darkened room with a constant attendant.
   b. Emergency measures include preparing a padded tongue blade and having emergency medications available.
   c. Suction, if necessary.
   d. Provide O_2 as necessary.
   e. Keep record of vital signs.
   f. Keep patient NPO (nothing by mouth).
   g. Main I.V., and give medications.
   h. Monitor FHT.
   i. Observe carefully after delivery for anuria and convulsions.

HIGH RISK PREGNANCY

High risk pregnancy refers to any condition that may interfere with the normal development or delivery of the fetus or any preexisting maternal disease that may increase the risk of pregnancy.

1. Factors that increase risk
   a. Age and economic status—under 17 years or over 35 years; lower socio-economic status.
   b. Parity—5 or more pregnancies.
   c. Previous conditions that increase risk
      (1.) Previous infant death, premature birth, or congenital malformations.
      (2.) History of cardiac disease, diabetes, renal disease, or other maternal condition.
      (3.) Difficulty in conceiving.
      (4.) Narcotic or alcohol addiction.
      (5.) Less than a year since last pregnancy.
      (6.) RH incompatibility and sensitization.
2. Conditions that increase risk
   a. Infection
   b. Chronic vaginal bleeding
   c. Toxemia syndrome
3. Intrapartum conditions that increase risk
   a. Premature labor
   b. Malpresentation
   c. Premature rupture of membranes

A. Cardiovascular Disease During Pregnancy

1. Classification
   a. Class I—no alteration of activity.
   b. Class II—slight limitation of activity.
   c. Class III—marked limitation of activity.
   d. Class IV—symptoms present at rest.
2. Considerations
   a. Pregnancy expands plasma volume, increasing cardiac output and load on heart.
   b. Most deaths are caused by cardiac failure, when blood volume is increased to the peak at approximately 28 weeks' gestation.
   c. Heart failure occurs infrequently in labor; however, the greatest threat is during the 2nd stage.
   d. Over age 35 years, there is an increase in the incidence of heart failure and death.
3. Nursing Management During Pregnancy
   a. With proper management, mortality is minimal.
   b. Patient should avoid sources of acute infections, especially respiratory infections.
   c. Patient should rest frequently, with head elevated to aid in oxygenation.

d. Strenuous activities, such as stair climbing and heavy cleaning, should be avoided.
e. Patients in Class III and over may be hospitalized before labor for controlled rest and diet.
f. If patient decompensates or has distress symptoms with exertion, she should remain in bed or in a chair.
g. Salt intake is usually not restricted nor are diuretics prescribed unless heart failure occurs, although use of highly salted foods may be discouraged.
h. Iron supplementation is important to aid in preventing anemia.
i. Digitalis treatment prescribed when indicated.
j. Emotional stress should be avoided.

4. Management During Labor
   a. Observe for signs that cardiac function is deteriorating, such as pulse rate over 110 or respiratory rate over 24.
   b. Relieve pain and anxiety.
   c. Vaginal delivery usually preferred.
   d. Patient may decompensate in early postpartum period, presenting the greatest mortality risk.
   e. Monitor fetal status.
5. Nursing Management
   a. Provide education of special needs during pregnancy and of danger signals.
   b. Be alert for signs of decompensation during pregnancy, especially in the 2nd trimester.
   c. During labor
      (1.) Check vital signs every 15 minutes or more often as needed.
      (2.) Keep patient in bed, preferably lying on one side, or in a semirecumbent position.
      (3.) Administer O_2 as necessary.
      (4.) Provide calm atmosphere and emotional support to alleviate fears.
      (5.) Administer pain alleviating medications as ordered to reduce discomfort during labor.
      (6.) Be alert for signs of impending heart failure.
      (7.) Monitor FHT.
   d. Careful observation during postpartum period or until circulatory volume has decreased.

B. Diabetes in Pregnancy

1. White's Classification
   a. Class A—abnormal glucose tolerance test results, indicative of latent or gestational diabetes.
   b. Class B—diabetes beginning after age 20 years.
   c. Class C—diabetes at ages 10 to 19 years or beginning in adolescence after age 10.
   d. Class D—diabetes of long duration or onset in childhood before the age of 10 years.
   e. Class E—evidence of pelvic vascular disease.
   f. Class F—nephropathy, including capillary glomerulosclerosis.
2. Implications
   a. Patient has tendency to develop acidosis and diabetic coma.
   b. Patient has increased susceptibility to infection.
   c. Toxemia, dystocia, hemorrhage, and polyhydramnios are more likely to develop.
   d. Latent diabetes may develop into fullblown diabetes.
   e. Insulin requirements are raised.
   f. Premature labor and delivery are more frequent.
   g. Infant may be large for gestational age (LGA) but have functions related to actual gestational age rather than size.
   h. Infant is subject to hypoglycemia, hyperbilirubinemia, respiratory distress syndrome, and congenital anomalies.
   i. Stillborn and neonatal mortality rates are increased.
3. Medical Management
   a. Keep blood glucose level near normal through diet, and use insulin to avoid complications such as acidosis.
   b. Observe for signs of acidosis or insulin reaction.
   c. Instruct patient in nutrition and regulation of diabetes.
   d. Be alert for signs of infection, toxemia.
   e. Check urine frequently for glucose and acetone.
   f. Patient may be hospitalized at 36 to 37 weeks' gestation for evaluation and possible termination of pregnancy.
      (1.) Placental function may be evaluated; placental insufficiency (pathological process in placenta resulting in inefficient exchange of waste and gases between mother and fetus) is common in diabetics due to vascular changes.
      (2.) Assessment of fetal growth and maturity should early delivery be indicated.
      (3.) Strict control of diabetes.
4. Nursing Management
   a. Teaching the effects of diabetes on the mother and fetus during pregnancy and the reasons

for frequent testing of blood glucose level and urine for glucose and acetone levels.

b. Teaching good nutrition and health practices.
   (1.) Maintain insulin on a regular schedule.
   (2.) Test urine for glucose and acetone levels as ordered.
   (3.) Provide adequate diet for diabetic as prescribed by physician.
   (4.) Provide activities for diversion.
   (5.) Monitor FHT at each prenatal visit.
   (6.) Check vital signs, especially blood pressure q.i.d. and p.r.n.
   (7.) Weigh daily at the same time each day.
   (8.) Keep accurate records of intake and output.
   (9.) Provide support and explanations to help allay fears and anxieties.

LABOR AND DELIVERY

Labor is the process by which the products of conception are expelled from the body. Delivery refers to the actual birth.

A. Terms

1. Attitude—refers to the posture the fetus assumes in utero.
2. Fetal lie–refers to the relationship of the long axis of the baby to the long axis of the mother.
3. Presentation—refers to the part of the fetus that lies closest to the true pelvis.
   a. Cephalic (head)—vertex, brow, or face.
   b. Breech—frank, complete, single, or double footling.
   c. Transverse—shoulder presentation.
4. Position—refers to the relationship of the fetal presenting part to the maternal bony pelvis. (Letters L and R signify left and right, letters A and P signify anterior and posterior, letter O signifies occiput, letter M signifies mentum or face, and letter S signifies sacrum.)
   a. L.O.A.—left occiput anterior; occiput on left side of maternal pelvis and toward front, face down, favorable for delivery.
   b. L.O.P.—left occiput posterior; occiput on left side of maternal pelvis and toward rear or face up.
      (1.) Usually causes severe back pain during labor.
      (2.) May slow the progress of labor.
      (3.) Fetus usually rotates before delivery to anterior position.
      (4.) Fetus may be rotated in delivery room by physician.
   c. R.O.A.—right occiput anterior; occiput on right of maternal pelvis, toward front, face down, and favorable for delivery.
   d. R.O.P.—right occiput posterior; occiput on right side of maternal pelvis, face up; same problems as L.O.P.
   e. Assessing fetal position
      (1.) Leopold's maneuver
      (2.) Vaginal examination
      (3.) Rectal examination may be done.
      (4.) Ultrasonography
5. Engagement usually occurs 2 to 4 weeks prior to onset of labor with primigravidas; refers to the occurrence of the largest diameter of the fetal presenting part passing into the inlet of the true maternal pelvis.
6. Station—the term that refers to the degree to which the presenting part has descended into the pelvis.
   a. Assessed by vaginal examination.
   b. 0 station—at level of ischial spine.
   c. +1, +2, +3—below level of ischial spine.
   d. −1, −2, −3—above level of ischia spine.

B. Signs of Impending Labor

1. Lightening—descent of the uterus downward and forward, which takes place as the fetal presenting part descends into the pelvis.
   a. Time in which it takes place varies from a few weeks to a few days before labor. In multigravidas, it may coincide with the onset of labor.
   b. Sensations
      (1.) Relief of pressure on diaphragm, and breathing is easier.
      (2.) Increased pelvic pressure leading to leg cramps, frequent micturition, and pressure on rectum.
2. Braxton Hicks' contractions
   a. May become quite regular but do not effectively dilate cervix.
   b. Usually are more pronounced at night.
   c. May play a part in ripening the cervix.
3. Decrease in weight; usually a decrease in water retention due to hormonal influences.
4. Cervical changes—usually becomes softer, shorter, and somewhat dilated; may be dilated 1 to 2 cm by the time labor begins.

5. Bloody show
   a. Tenacious mucous vaginal discharge, usually pinkish or streaked with blood, which is expelled from the cervix as it shortens and begins to dilate.
   b. Labor usually begins within 24 to 48 hours.
6. Rupture of membranes
   a. May break at any time before labor or during labor. Occasionally, they remain intact and are ruptured by the physician during labor (amniotomy).
   b. May gush or trickle; color should be clear.
   c. Patient usually advised to come to the hospital, as labor may begin within 24 hours.
   d. If labor does not begin spontaneously, it is induced to avoid intrauterine infections.
   e. FHT should be taken after rupture of membranes.

C. Signs of True Labor

1. Uterine contractions increase in frequency, strength, and duration.
2. Bloody show

D. Stages and Phases of Labor and Delivery

1. First stage—period from onset of true labor to complete dilatation and effacement.
   a. Latent phase—dilatation from 0 to 4 cm.
   b. Active phase—dilatation from 4 to 7 cm.
   c. Transition—dilatation from 7 to 10 cm.
2. Second stage—stage of expulsion from time of complete dilatation to delivery of infant.
3. Third stage—from time infant is delivered to time placenta is delivered.
   a. Shultz—shiny fetal side of placenta presents.
   b. Matthews, Duncan—maternal side of placenta presents.
4. Fourth stage—stage of maternal stabilization.

E. Mechanism of Labor and Delivery

1. Sequence of movements of presenting part through birth canal; head usually enters transverse and must rotate L.O.A. or R.O.A. for birth.
2. Engagement—widest part of fetus enters the pelvis, usually at station 0.
3. Descent—movement that occurs simultaneously with passage of head through pelvis.
4. Flexion—occurs as head descends and meets with resistance. In extreme flexion, the smallest diameter of the head presents.
5. Internal rotation—head usually enters with long diameter of inlet (usually transverse position) and must rotate before it can emerge from outlet; head rotates so that smallest diameter presents to conform to pelvis.
6. Extension—follows internal rotation. The head, which is flexed as it passes through birth canal, must extend for birth.
7. External rotation—soon after birth, the head rotates to either mother's right or left side; fetal position before birth.
8. Expulsion—with delivery of shoulders, rest of body is expelled spontaneously.

F. Nursing Care During Labor and Delivery

1. Emotional support by husband, nurse, or significant others.
2. Maintenance of asepsis.
3. Timing of frequency, duration, and strength of contractions.
4. Auscultation or monitoring of fetal heart sounds as to rate, regularity, and tone.
5. Frequent observation of perineum for show, rupture of membranes, and presenting part.
6. Check vital signs at least every hour.
7. Emergency equipment available for the safety and care of mother and baby, such as O_2, blood, and drugs.
8. Assessment of basic needs, such as body fluids, and bladder and bowel function.
9. Assist mother with breathing techniques throughout labor.

G. Induction and Control of Uterine Contractions by Pharmacological Agents

1. Oxytocin (Pitocin, Syntocinon)
   a. Used to induce labor by stimulation of characteristic rhythmic contraction and relaxation of uterine muscles
   b. Administered I.M. after delivery of the anterior shoulder or I.V. after delivery of the baby to provide uterine contractions that complete expulsion of uterine contents and decrease bleeding from endometrial sites.

H. Danger Signs and Symptoms During Labor

1. Tonic, strong, continuous contractions with sharp abdominal pain and, on palpation, abdomen taut and board like.
2. Variations in rate, regularity, and tone of fetal heart sounds.
3. Meconium stained or excessive amount of amniotic fluid.
4. Elevation or drop in blood pressure.
5. Increase in pulse rate or temperature.
6. Sudden excessive fetal movements.
7. Bleeding, protrusion of umbilical cord or placenta.

I. Nursing Care Immediately Following Delivery

MOTHER

1. Palpate fundus every 15 minutes (×4) for firmness and height in relation to umbilicus.
2. Keep airway open if inhalation anesthesia has been given.
3. Monitor blood pressure, pulse, and respirations every fifteen minutes (× 4) or until stable and report fluctuations.
4. Check perineum for vaginal and suture line bleeding.
5. Administer oxytocic drug as ordered.
6. Administer lactogenic inhibitor as ordered, if bottle feeding preferred.
7. Administer immune globulin (RhoGAM) as ordered if mother is RH-negative within 72 hours.
8. Assess for distended bladder; encourage voiding, as necessary.

BABY

1. Clear airway of mucus.
2. Observe frequently.
3. Use Apgar scoring to determine respiratory effort.
4. Maintain body heat; dry baby immediately.
5. Assess the newborn for visible anomalies.
6. Instill silver nitrate or other medication into each eye to prevent ophthalmia neonatorum. May be done later in nursery rather than in delivery room to facilitate bonding via eye-to-eye contact.
7. Identify mother and baby prior to leaving delivery room by use of prints and application of bands.

ASSESSMENT OF FETUS DURING LABOR AND DELIVERY

A. Signs of Fetal Distress

1. FHT above 160 or below 120 bpm (beats per minute)
2. Meconium-stained fluid; during hypoxia, bowel peristalsis increases, and meconium is likely to be passed.
3. Fetal hyperactivity
4. If labor is monitored:
   a. Prolonged variable deceleration pattern
   b. Late deceleration pattern
   c. Fetal pH below 7.2
   d. Decreased beat-to-beat variability

B. Immediate Nursing Interventions

1. Turn patient to left side; if no improvement turn to right side. This procedure relieves pressure on umbilical cord during contractions and pressure of uterus on the inferior vena cava, preventing vena cava syndrome.
2. Administer O_2 via mask up to 10 L/min.
3. Discontinue oxytocin if infusing.
4. Correction of hypotension—elevate legs, and increase perfusion of clear I.V. fluids.
5. Prepare for delivery.

C. Observations of Fetal Heart Rate

1. Normal fetal heart rate—120 to 160 bpm.
   a. *Early deceleration*—10 to 20 bpm drop in rate, usually within normal range of 120 to 160 bpm.
      (1.) Occurs before peak or early contracting phase. Recovery as soon as acme of contraction has passed.
      (2.) Uniform wave shape of the heart rate tracing reflects shape of the contraction.
      (3.) Indicates head compression—vagal stimulation results in decreased heart rate.
      (4.) V-shaped appearance
      (5.) Not considered ominous; no intervention necessary except to inform parents of reason for deceleration.
   b. *Late deceleration*—decrease in FHT of 10 to 20 bpm.
      (1.) Occurs after peak or late contracting phase.

(2.) Uniform wave shape of the heart rate tracing may reflect shape of the contraction; occurs at different time than the early deceleration pattern.
(3.) Indicates fetal distress.
(4.) Likely to appear in any situation where fetal-maternal exchange in placenta is reduced, resulting in hypoxia.
(5.) Interventions necessary, such as reposition on left side, begin O_2, notify physician.

c. *Variable deceleration* — decrease in FHR occurring any time during contracting phase, usually below 120 bpm.
(1.) Indicates cord compression.
(2.) Frequently occurs when mother is pushing.
(3.) Must be evaluated carefully; may or may not indicate fetal difficulty.

d. *Fetal blood analysis*
(1.) Procedure—A few drops of capillary blood are obtained from the baby's scalp under sterile technique (membranes must be ruptured).
(2.) pH of blood immediately determined.
(3.) pH less than 7.2 indicates fetal distress.
(4.) Immediate delivery by cesarean section may be indicated.

e. *Signs of complication of labor*
(1.) Fetal distress
(2.) Fetal tachycardia—persistent FHR above 160 bpm or an increase in basal rate of 20 to 30 bpm.
(3.) Bradycardia: FHR below 120 bpm.
(4.) Absent, minimal, or irregular FHR.
(5.) Meconium-stained amniotic fluid (MSAF)
(6.) Fetal hyperactivity
(7.) Elevated maternal temperature
(8.) Maternal dehydration
(9.) Maternal hemorrhage
(10.) Uterine hyperactivity

COMPLICATIONS OF LABOR AND DELIVERY

A. Dystocia

Dystocia is defined as prolonged or difficult delivery, due to mechanical factors stemming from the fetus, the mother's pelvis or inadequate uterine activity. Labor is considered prolonged when it extends for 24 hours or more after the onset of regular contractions.

1. Classification

Dystocia may be classified in several ways:

a. Dysfunctions of powers or forces with respect to the uterus and abdominal muscles.
b. Abnormalities of the passengers—fetus and placenta.
c. Abnormalities of the passages—bony and soft tissue.
d. May be a combination of 2 or more dysfunctions and abnormalities.

2. Dysfunctional Labor

Prolonged latent phase—primipara over 20 hours; multipara, 14 hours; time required to dilate cervix to 4 cm is prolonged.

a. Causes or contributing conditions
(1.) Oversedation
(2.) "Unripe" cervix
(3.) False labor
(4.) Uterine dysfunction or abnormalities

b. Medical treatment
(1.) Patient is usually exhausted and will benefit from rest.
(2.) Vaginal examination is made to determine fetal position and station.
(3.) X-ray pelvimetry is made to determine the disorder. Amniotomy can be carried out (artificial rupture of membranes), if conditions are favorable for vaginal delivery. (Fetus must be at station 0.) Oxytocin can be given as a stimulant. Labor usually progresses normally after rest and stimulation by oxytocin.

Prolonged active phase—primigravida, dilatation slower than 1.2 cm/hr; and multigravida, dilatation slower than 0.25 cm/hr

a. Causes include cephalopelvic disproportion (CPD); malpositions; excessive sedation or anesthesia; and unknown causes.
b. Usually no active medical treatment is given, if prolonged. Cesarean section may be indicated.
c. Abnormal presentations and positions

3. Abnormal Presentations and Positions

a. Occiput posterior—baby must rotate greater distance to reach symphysis.

b. Treatment—if head does not rotate spontaneously with contractions, physician may rotate manually or with forceps.
c. Breech presentation; prolongs labor because soft tissue does not aid dilatation effectively. Cesarean delivery may be indicated.
d. Face presentation is rare; results in increased perinatal mortality rate.
e. Transverse lie; cesarean section is usual mode of delivery.

4. Abnormalities of Passage

a. Cephalopelvic disproportion; trial labor may be done in borderline cases; can be diagnosed with x-ray or pelvic examination. Cesarean delivery generally recommended.

5. Premature Labor and Delivery

Premature labor and delivery occur when the pregnancy terminates after the period of viability and usually before the end of the 36th week.
a. Treatment is bed rest.
b. Medications such as isoxsuprine (Vasodilan), ritodrine or terbutaline may be used to stop labor. These medications are used for their inhibitory effects on smooth muscle. They produce significant relaxation in the uterus.
c. Attempts to arrest premature labor are contraindicated when the pregnancy is greater than 37 weeks' gestation, membranes are ruptured, cervix is dilated to 4 cm, or the gestation is prior to 20 weeks.

6. Prolonged Pregnancy

Refers to a pregnancy greater than 42 weeks' gestation.
a. Complications lie in a greater fetal morbidity and mortality due to decreased amniotic fluid and decreased placental perfusion.
b. Stress and nonstress tests can be used to determine fetal ability to withstand labor and mode of delivery.
c. Ultrasonography can be done to determine gestation.

7. Prolapsed Umbilical Cord

Prolapsed cord descends through cervical canal alongside presenting part.
a. Causes include rupture of membrane prior to engagement, abnormal presentation, premature infant, and polyhydramnios.
b. Complications of fetal asphyxia.
c. Treatment—elevate presenting part of cord; place mother in knee-chest position; administer O_2 to mother; monitor FHT; remain with mother; prepare for delivery.

8. Ruptured Uterus

Usually occurs after fetal viability.
a. Causes include perforation during abortions, rupture of previous uterine scar, and rapid labor induction.
b. Treatment—relieve symptoms of shock from hemorrhage; *surgical* intervention may be necessary, such as hysterectomy.

POSTPARTUM PERIOD

The puerperium is a 6-week period following delivery in which the reproductive system returns to the nonpregnant state by a process called involution. Major changes occurring in the reproductive system include the following:

A. Physiology

1. Reproductive System
   a. Uterus; rapid involution in size through contracting processes; occurs more rapidly if breast-feeding.
   b. Lochia flow—vaginal discharge after delivery; changes from rubra to serosa to alba, as healing occurs at the site of placental detachment.
   c. Vagina returns to nonpregnant state as estrogen production begins.
   d. Cervix remains soft and flabby for a few days after delivery, then becomes firm as internal os closes.
   e. Breasts; colostrum usually is first secretion for 2 to 3 days after delivery. Pituitary stimulates secretion of prolactin after delivery of placenta. Engorgement may occur. Milk produced in response to breast stimulation.

B. Nursing Management of the Postpartum Patient

1. Check vital signs every 8 hours and p.r.n. Decreased blood pressure, increased pulse, or temperature over 100.4°F may indicate problems with infection or bleeding.
2. Check fundus for consistency and height. Massage fundus lightly with fingers if it is relaxed.
3. Check lochia for amount, color, consistency, and odor. Watch for hemorrhage.
4. Check perineum for redness, discoloration, or swelling.
5. Check episiotomy for healing; check for drainage.
6. Check breasts for engorgement and cracking of nipples.
7. Check emotional status of new mother for depression or withdrawal.
8. Check for problems with flatus or elimination and bladder or bowel retention; encourage early voiding.
9. Administer drug to inhibit lactation if not breast-feeding.
10. Administer immune globulin (RhoGAM) as ordered within 72 hours postpartum to Rh-negative mother who is not sensitized and who has an Rh-positive infant. Assess the need for rubella vaccine.
11. Monitor intake and output until patient is voiding a sufficient quantity of urine without difficulty; usually the first 2 voids are measured (voids should be at least 150 ml each).
12. Teach mother perineal care and give perineal care until mother is able to do so. Sitz baths as ordered.
13. Encourage ambulation as soon as ordered and as patient is able to tolerate it, giving assistance the first time.
14. Encourage verbalization of mother's feelings about labor, delivery, and baby.
15. Encourage early and sustained mother-baby contact to foster bonding process. Encourage rooming-in.
16. Encourage mother's efforts to breast-feed.

C. Emotional Care of the Postpartum Patient

Observe for signs that restorative process is progressing.

1. *Taking-in phase*—the first 2 to 3 days.
   a. Mother s concern is for herself.
   b. Mother usually is quite talkative. She wants to discuss labor and delivery. She is absorbing the experience and making it a part of herself.
   c. Nurse's role is to listen and help the patient interpret events to make it more meaningful.
2. *Taking-hold phase*—from the 3rd postpartum day to about 2 weeks. The phase varies with each individual.
   a. Emphasis is on present.
   b. Mother is impatient and wants to organize herself.
   c. Mother is less passive and more in control of situation.
   d. Begins to take hold of tasks of mothering, which takes priority over all else.
   e. May be unsure of herself. It is important for nurse to reassure mother.
   f. Success at this time is important to future mother and child relationship.
   g. Important time for teaching without making mother feel inadequate.
3. *Letting-go phase*—may begin by the end of the lst week postpartum. The phase varies with each individual.
   a. Mother may feel a deep loss over the separation of the baby from part of her body and may grieve over this loss.
   b. Mother may be caught in dependent and independent roles.
   c. Woman may have difficulty adjusting to the mothering role.
   d. Woman may feel conflict between the roles of mother and wife.
   e. Mother may feel upset and depressed at times, i.e., postpartum "blues."
   f. Allow mother time to further verbalize about labor and delivery. Assess attitude regarding infant.

D. Deviations from Normal Postpartum Period

1. Postpartum Hemorrhage—the loss of 500 ml or more of blood during or after delivery.
   a. Causes
      (1.) Uterine atony—exhaustion of muscle. Uterine atony may be due to the following:
         (a.) Prolonged labor
         (b.) Overdistention from multiple pregnancies, polyhydramnios.
         (c.) Sluggish muscle multiparity, and uterine inertia in labor.
         (d.) Overmassage of fundus
         (e.) Presence of fibroid tumors
         (f.) Deep inhalation anesthesia may inhibit uterine activity.
         (g). Conduction anesthesia (epidural or spinal).

(2.) Lacerations of the reproductive tract.
   (a.) Cervix or the high vaginal walls.
   (b.) Oozing from blood vessels.
   (c.) Hematomas
(3.) Retained placental tissue or incomplete separation of the placenta, which is the most frequent cause of late postpartum hemorrhage.

b. Clinical Manifestations
   (1.) Uterine atony
      (a.) Boggy, relaxed uterus
      (b.) Dark bleeding
      (c.) Passage of clots
   (2.) Lacerations
      (a.) Firm fundus
      (b.) Oozing of bright red blood
   (3.) Retained placental tissue
      (a.) Boggy, relaxed uterus
      (b.) Dark bleeding
   (4.) Signs and symptoms of shock
      (a.) Air hunger; difficulty in breathing.
      (b.) Restlessness
      (c.) Weak rapid pulse
      (d.) Rapid respirations
      (e.) Decrease in blood pressure

c. Nursing Management
   (1.) Remain with the patient.
   (2.) Monitor vital signs every 15 minutes or p.r.n. until stable; report any deviations from normal to physician.
   (3.) Palpate fundus every 15 minutes or p.r.n. while bleeding continues; then every 2 to 4 hours.
   (4.) Gently massage fundus until firm; be careful not to overmassage.
   (5.) Have physician notified.
   (6.) Weigh pads and linen, or count pads as ordered.
   (7.) Provide for warmth.
   (8.) Measure intake and output. Administer fluids and blood as ordered.
   (9.) Explain problem carefully to patient and family to help allay anxiety.

2. Puerperal Infection—an infection of the genitals as a consequence of abortion or labor and delivery. *General considerations are as follows:*
   a. Cause
      (1.) Organisms that were introduced during labor and delivery.
      (2.) Bacteria normally present in vaginal tract.
   b. Predisposing factors
      (1.) Weakened resistance due to prolonged labor and dehydration.
      (2.) Traumatic delivery
      (3.) Excessive vaginal examination during labor
      (4.) Premature rupture of membranes
      (5.) Excessive blood loss
      (6.) Anemia
      (7.) Intrauterine manipulation
      (8.) Retained placental fragments
   c. Clinical Manifestations
      (1.) Elevated temperature of 100.4°F or more
      (2.) Discomfort in abdomen and tenderness
      (3.) Burning on urination
      (4.) Foul-smelling lochia or discharge
      (5.) Pelvic pain
      (6.) Chills
      (7.) Rapid pulse
      (8.) Malaise

3. Endometritis—an inflammation of the lining of the uterus.
   a. General Considerations
      (1.) Most frequent site of infection
      (2.) Uterus may be boggy, relaxed, and tender.
      (3.) If untreated, infection may spread through lymphatic system to whole body causing septicemia.
      (4.) May have pelvic examination.
   b. Treatment
      (1.) Antibiotics
      (2.) Laboratory studies of blood and urine.
      (3.) Establish adequate drainage of uterus.
      (4.) Blood transfusion, if anemic.
      (5.) Fluids 3000 to 4000 ml daily, oral or parenteral.
   c. Nursing Management
      (1.) Administer I.V. fluids or blood as ordered.
      (2.) Encourage fluid intake of 3000 to 4000 ml if not contraindicated.
      (3.) Administer medications as ordered.
      (4.) Provide high-calorie nutritious diet.
      (5.) Place patient in Fowler's or semi-Fowler's position as ordered.
      (6.) Provide emotional support to mother, who may be in isolation and unable to see baby.

4. Thrombophlebitis—one form occurs when the placental site becomes infected, causing inflammation of the deep pelvic veins. Thrombophlebitis may be confined to blood vessels in the uterine wall, or it may extend to ovarian, hypogastric, or femoral veins. Femoral thrombophlebitis, commonly called "milk leg," usually originates in a leg vein and is more common. The incidence has been reduced with early ambulation.

a. Clinical Manifestations
   (1.) Discomfort in abdomen and pelvis.
   (2.) Tenderness localized on one side of the pelvis.
   (3.) Femoral symptoms usually don't appear until the 2nd week or later.
      (a.) Edema and pain in affected leg, i.e., positive Homan's sign.
      (b.) Chills and fever.

b. Treatment
   (1.) Antibiotics until temperature is stable.
   (2.) Anticoagulents may be ordered.
   (3.) Bed rest
   (4.) Warm compresses and heat
   (5.) Bed cradle—keep bed clothes off leg.
   (6.) Anti-embolic stockings

c. Nursing Management
   (1.) Maintain bed rest.
   (2.) Administer medications as ordered.
   (3.) Apply warm compresses as ordered for 15 to 20 minutes.
   (4.) Elevate affected leg.
   (5.) Apply bed cradle.
   (6.) Never massage leg, and teach mother not to do so.
   (7.) Teach mother to watch for signs of excessive bleeding.
   (8.) Allow mother to express fears and concerns.
   (9.) Watch for signs of pulmonary embolism.

5. Mastitis—an infection in breast tissue due to invading organisms, usually *Staphylococcus*.
   a. Causes
      (1.) Infected hands of mother or attendants
      (2.) Bacteria normally present in lactiferous glands
      (3.) Fissure in nipples
      (4.) Bruising of breast tissue
      (5.) Stasis of milk or overdistention may injure tissue but does not cause infection in itself.
   b. Clinical Manifestations
      (1.) Chills
      (2.) Fever of 103°F or above
      (3.) Elevated pulse rate
      (4.) Lobe may become hard to touch, red, and painful.
      (5.) May progress to abscess if untreated.
   c. Treatment
      (1.) Provide support for breast.
      (2.) Antibiotics
      (3.) Apply ice pack to breast.
      (4.) May require incision and drainage if abscess develops.
      (5.) Some physicians recommend breastfeeding be stopped, or they favor temporary discontinuance with artificial removal of milk for a few days.
   d. Nursing Management
      (1.) Administer medications as ordered.
      (2.) Apply ice pack as ordered.
      (3.) Make sure mother is wearing snug-fitting, supportive brassiere.
      (4.) Teach mother to empty breast if breastfeeding is to be continued.
      (5.) Wash hands before touching patient's breast.
      (6.) Teach mother careful handwashing and care of the breast.

6. Subinvolution—the uterus does not return to usual size as rapidly as normal following delivery.
   a. Causes
      (1.) Retained placental tissue or fetal membranes
      (2.) Endometritis
   b. Clinical manifestations
      (1.) Uterus enlarged and boggy
      (2.) Profuse red lochia
   c. Nursing Management
      (1.) Administer medications as ordered; medications may include ergot products.
      (2.) Explanation of problem to patient.
      (3.) Continue to monitor height and consistency of uterus.
      (4.) Monitor lochia flow; watch for presence of clots.
      (5.) If subinvolution due to retained placenta tissue, dilatation and curettage will be done.

NORMAL NEWBORN

A. Maintain Body Temperature

1. Place infant in a heated incubator or a crib with radiant heat.
2. Wipe off fluid, mucus, and excessive vernix caseosa.
3. Avoid excessive exposure.
4. Wrap infant in warm blankets.
5. Transfer to the nursery after parents have seen and held infant, and early bonding has been initiated.

B. Maintain Respiration

1. Place infant on side, in modified Trendelenburg position, to facilitate drainage of mucus.
2. Aspirate mucus as needed with bulb or suction catheter attached to a mucous trap.
3. Provide O_2 as needed.

C. Prevent Infection

1. Eye care—usually 2 drops of 1% silver nitrate in conjunctival sacs; may flush eyes with water in about 2 minutes, or apply antibiotic ointment to prevent eye infection in the infant if the mother was infected with gonorrhea. Prophylactic eye care may also include other medications, such as erythromycin products.
2. Cord care—use sterile scissors and clamp; wash area with an agent that aids drying process.
3. Carry out proper hand washing before receiving baby, or wear sterile gloves.

D. General Observations

1. Apgar scoring, 1 and 5 minutes

Apgar Scoring

Sign	0	1	2
Heart rate	Absent	Slow (less than 100)	More than 100
Respiratory effort	Absent	Slow, irregular	Good cry
Muscle tone	Flaccid	Some flexion of extremities	Active motion
Reflex irritability	No response	Cry	Vigorous cry
Color	Blue, pale	Body pink, extremities blue	Completely pink

2. Congenital malformations
3. Umbilical cord—2 arteries and 1 vein.
4. Meconium staining—skin and nails.
5. Abnormal cry or no cry
6. Injuries caused by birth trauma—dislocated shoulder, edema of scalp, and lacerations.
7. Respiratory—nasal flaring, retractions, and expiratory grunt.
8. Neurological status—reflexes, tremors, and twitching.
9. Assess for gestational age.

E. Nursing Management

1. Clamp the cord if the physician does not do so; it should be clamped 1 inch from the base, or left longer if the mother is Rh negative (in case of possible blood exchange).
2. Identify the baby with bands and footprints.
3. Show the baby to the parents and allow them to hold the infant (if not contraindicated).
4. Observe the mother's reactions to baby.
5. Transfer the baby to the admitting nursery with appropriate data.

F. Care in the Nursery

1. Steps at admission and during the first 12 hours.
   a. Check rectal temperature.
   b. Weigh and measure total length and head circumference.
   c. Place in heated crib.
   d. Check respiratory rates every hour for 4 to 5 hours and p.r.n.
   e. Check for nasal flaring, retractions, expiratory grunt, and breath sounds.
   f. Check apical pulse every hour for 2 to 3 hours; watch for rate above 180 or below 100.
   g. Keep bulb syringe available, and aspirate as needed.
   h. Administer vitamin K as ordered.
   i. Bathe and dress baby when his temperature is stable.
   j. Place in an open crib when his temperature is stable.
   k. Administer feeding as ordered; usually sterile water or glucose water is given every 4 to 6 hours.
   l. Assess baby for congenital defects, tremors, color, acrocyanosis. (Acrocyanosis is normal for 1 to 2 hours after birth, because of sluggish peripheral circulation.)

G. Routine Nursing Management

1. Assessment
   a. Observe for jaundice—check general skin color, blanching, and sclerae of the eyes.
   b. Check for respiratory difficulty—mucus, flaring of nostrils, grunting, and so forth.
   c. Note tremors, twitching, muscle tone, and reflexes.

d. Take baby's temperature (axillary) during each shift.
e. Check baby's weight daily.
f. Note amount of urine voided and number of stools.
g. Check for signs of infection on the skin and cord.
2. Apply alcohol to cord daily or p.r.n.
3. Circumcision Care
a. Observe for bleeding.
b. Change petroleum jelly and gauze as necessary.
c. Keep area clean to prevent infection.
4. Check to see if the phenylketonuria test has been done.
5. Provide for nutrition and hydration either with formula (20 cal/oz) or breast-feeding.
6. Teach mother how to hold and burp the baby.
7. Use proper hand washing between babies to prevent spreading of infections.
8. Isolate babies with known or suspected infections.
9. Be sure that the mother understands the doctor's orders regarding care of the infant before she goes home and plan follow-up visits for the mother with the physician.

PHYSICAL CHARACTERISTICS OF THE NEWBORN

A. Respiratory Status

1. Infant's respiratory system must function immediately after loss of placental function; adequate maturation at birth is necessary.
2. From 80 to 100 ml of fluid are present in the lungs at birth. Approximately one third is removed as a result of compression of the chest during delivery. The remainder is carried off through pulmonary circulation and by the lymph system.
3. Surfactant (a phospholipid found in the lungs) reduces surface tension in alveoli and keeps them from collapsing. Surfactant is necessary to maintain lung expansion and to prevent respiratory distress syndrome.
4. Normal respiration is about 30 to 40; above 60 or below 30 may indicate a problem. Respiration may be slightly elevated during crying episodes or shortly afterward.

B. Circulatory Status

1. Ductus arteriosus, ductus venosus, and foramen ovale should close but closure may not be complete for 1 or 2 days.
2. Peripheral circulation may be sluggish: there may be mottling, acrocyanosis.
3. Pulse may be variable, normal is 120 to 160; it may be as high as 170 when crying or below 120 when resting.
4. Anemia is common in early months because of decrease in erythropoiesis and breakdown of red blood cells. Baby may need an iron supplemented formula.
5. Physiologic juandice; average bilirubin level 6 mg/dl at 3rd day of life.
a. Jaundice visible in the skin, sclerae.
b. Jaundice does not become visible until the 2nd or 3rd day after birth. This differentiates physiological from pathological jaundice.
c. Caused by impairment in the removal of bilirubin—deficiency in the production of glucuronyl transferase, which is needed to convert indirect insoluble bilirubin to direct water soluble bilirubin that is excreted.
d. Jaundice begins to decrease by the 6th or 7th day.
e. Jaundice may require treatment, although it usually does not if watched carefully.
f. Usual treatment is phototherapy. If indirect bilirubin level (13 mg/100 ml blood) continues to go up, a cause other than physiological jaundice is searched for.
g. Infant may be placed on forced fluids between feedings to aid in excretion of bilirubin, as it is broken down.

C. Ability to Maintain Body Heat

1. The baby suffers a large loss of heat because he is wet at birth and because of the coolness of the delivery room. The infant should be placed immediately in a warmer and dried off.
2. Means of heat production in the newborn are as follows:
a. Increasing metabolism
b. Metabolism of brown fat
3. Effects of chilling are as follows:
a. Increased consumption of O_2.
b. Use of glucose stored as glycogen.
c. May become hypoglycemic.
d. May develop metabolic acidosis; products of incomplete metabolism accumulate along with fatty acids from breakdown of brown fat.

D. Weight

1. Infants usually lose between 5 to 10% of their body weight the first few days, because of low fluid intake and loss of excess fluid from tissue.
2. They usually regain weight loss at birth within 7 to 14 days.

E. Head

1. Head or face may be asymmetrical due to birth trauma.
2. Molding of head (elongation of head as it passes through birth canal to accommodate pelvis) may be present; usually disappears in about a week.
3. Caput succedaneum—diffuse swelling of soft tissues of scalp, caused by an arrest in circulation in those tissues present over the cervix as it dilates.
4. Cephalhematoma—extravasation of blood beneath periosteum of one of the cranial bones because of a ruptured blood vessel during the trauma of labor and delivery.
5. Anterior and posterior fontanel
   (a.) Should be open.
   (b.) Should neither bulge (may indicate intracranial pressure) nor be depressed (may indicate dehydration).
6. Ears should be well formed, and cartilage should be present.

F. Gastrointestinal System

1. Salivary glands are immature.
2. May have Epstein's pearls—white raised areas on palate caused by an accumulation of epithelial cells.
3. May have transient circumoral cyanosis.
4. Sucking pads—fatty tissue deposits in each cheek that aid sucking. They usually disappear when no longer needed.
5. Infant Stools
   a. Meconium plug—thick, gray-white mucus passed before meconium.
   b. Meconium—sticky, black, tarry looking stools, consisting of mucus, digestive secretions, vernix caseosa, and lanugo; usually passed during the 1st 24-hours after birth.
   c. Transitional stool, 2nd to 5th day, greenish-yellow color and loose (partly meconium and partly milk).
   d. Number of bowel movements varies. Breast-fed infants usually have more bowel movements.
   e. Stools should be observed for color, frequency, and consistency.

G. Genitourinary System

1. Urinary Functions
   a. Observe ability to concentrate urine, and check to see if specific gravity is elevated.
   b. Uric acid crystals (pink or reddish spots) may appear on diaper owing to high uric acid secretion.
2. Genitalia
   a. Female
      (1.) May have heavy coating of vernix caseosa between labia.
      (2.) Usually has mucous discharge. Mucus may be blood-tinged due to elevated hormone levels in mother.
   b. Male
      (1.) Size of penis and scrotum varies.
      (2.) Testicles should be descended or in the inguinal canal.
      (3.) Circumcision—surgical removal of foreskin of penis by physician.
         (a.) Usually performed by the 2nd or 3rd day.
         (b.) Observe for bleeding from post-operative site.

H. Skin

1. Should be pinkish in color.
2. Acrocyanosis (cyanosis of extremities) may be present for the 1st hour or 2 after birth. Persistent "blueness" may indicate complications, such as heart disease.
3. Lanugo and vernix caseosa may be present.
4. Petechiae may be present because of the trauma of birth.
5. Milia (secretions of sebaceous materials in obstructed sebaceous glands) may be present and will disappear.
6. Erythema toxicum neonatorum (small harmless eruptions on the skin) are transient in nature.
7. Hemangiomas may be present on nape of neck or upper eyelids.
8. Skin may appear dry or cracked.
9. Mongolian spots—bluish pigmented areas present on the buttocks of babies of Oriental, Negro, or Mediterranean heritage.
10. Mottling may occur if the infant is chilled.

I. Neurological System

1. Reflexes (Moro's, Babinski's, suck, swallow, grasp, and tonic neck) present and intact at birth.
2. Muscle Tone
   a. Fist usually kept clenched.
   b. Baby should offer resistance when change in position is attempted.
   c. Head should be supported when baby is lifted.
   d. Muscles should not be limp.

DISEASES AFFECTING THE NEWBORN

A. Respiratory Distress Syndrome

Respiratory distress syndrome refers to a group of clinical symptoms signifying that the infant is experiencing problems with the respiratory system.

1. Etiology
   a. Symptoms are the result of a decrease in the amount of surfactant in the infant's lungs, as a result of one of the following conditions:
      (1.) Prematurity—immaturity of lungs and inability to produce surfactant.
      (2.) Hypoxia and acidosis
      (3.) Hypothermia
      (4.) High concentration of oxygen
   b. Respiratory distress syndrome is the most common cause of death in infants.
2. Clinical Manifestations
   a. Increased respirations of 60/min
   b. Retractions; subcostal followed by intercostal.
   c. Cyanosis
   d. Expiratory grunting
   e. Lack of activity
   f. Inability to take in sufficient O_2 leading to hypoxemia.
   g. Hypercarbia due to elevated levels of CO_2.
   h. Respiratory acidosis due to retention of CO_2 owing to inadequate pulmonary ventilation.
   i. Metabolic acidosis due to increased production of lactic acid.
   j. X-ray examination reveals
      (1.) Atelectasis—collapsed portions of lung.
      (2.) Fibrinous membrane that lines alveolar ducts and terminal bronchioles; membrane is formed by transudation of fluid from pulmonary tissue.
3. Nursing Management
   a. Primarily supportive
   b. Maintain warmth; infant usually placed in Isolette or open crib with overhead warmer. Skin temperature is maintained at 97.6°F.
   c. Provide for nutrition and hydration; usually give glucose in fluids I.V. during acute periods, then gradually increase feedings as tolerated.
   d. Careful monitoring of blood gas and electrolyte levels.
   e. Administration of O_2, warmed and humidified in lowest concentration possible via hood, nasal prongs, endotracheal tubes, or bag and mask. O_2 may be given at atmospheric or increased airway pressure.
   f. Continuous positive pressure applied to lungs during spontaneous breathing.
   g. Positive pressure applied to lungs during expiratory cycle when using the mechanical ventilator.
   h. When nasal prongs are being used, they should be checked and changed frequently.
   i. When an endotracheal tube is being used, it should be loosely taped and checked frequently for correct placement and connection at adaptor site.
   j. Aspirating infant with endotracheal tube, as follows:
      (1.) Disconnect from respirator at site of adaptor.
      (2.) Instill few minims to 0.5 ml of sterile normal saline into tube to loosen secretions.
      (3.) Aspirate no longer than 5 seconds using sterile catheter.
      (4.) Ventilate infant as needed during procedure.
      (5.) Reconnect tube to respirator; be sure it is in place and adaptor is secure.
      (6.) Auscultate chest for breath sounds.
   k. Postural drainage, percussion, and suction as ordered.
   l. Analyze O_2 concentration.
   m. Keep parents informed of infant's progress.
   n. Allow parents to visit child as much as possible.

B. Hyperbilirubinemia

Hyperbilirubinemia is an abnormal elevation of the bilirubin level in the newborn (above 13 to 15 mg/100 ml).

1. Etiology
   a. Functional immaturity of the liver; usually appears after 24 hours and disappears after 10 days.
   b. Bacterial infections
   c. ABO, B, and Rh incompatibilities usually show up in the first 24 hours and may be severe.
   d. Enclosed bleeding, such as hematoma, from trauma of delivery.
   e. Pregnanediol hormone present in mother's breast milk may contribute to jaundice. (It inhibits conjugation of bilirubin to a water soluble form (direct).
2. Clinical Manifestations
   a. Jaundice appears, progressing from head to extremities.
   b. Pallor appears.
   c. Infant is lethargic and feeds poorly.
   d. Urine is concentrated, and stools are light in color.
   e. If untreated, infant may progress to muscular rigidity or flaccidity, increased lethargy, high-pitched cry, respiratory distress, decreased Moro's reflex, and spasms.
   f. Blood tests
      (1.) Hemoglobin concentration
      (2.) Bilirubin level—important to measure amount of indirect bilirubin in blood, since unbound bilirubin is free to deposit in body tissues, such as skin, cardiac muscle, brain, and kidney. Unconjugated bilirubin deposited in the brain determines the extent of kernicterus.
3. Nursing Management
   a. Careful observation of infant for signs of increased jaundice.
   b. Careful observations for and prevention of acidosis (hypoxia) and hypoglycemia, which decrease binding of bilirubin to albumin and contribute to jaundice.
   c. Maintain adequate hydration, and offer fluids between feedings as ordered.
   d. Maintain temperature at 97.6° to avoid cold stress.
   e. Careful avoidance of infection.
   f. Phototherapy—fluorescent light breaks down bilirubin into water soluble products.
      (1.) Do not clothe infant.
      (2.) Cover infant's eyes to prevent retinal damage.
      (3.) Change baby's position every 2 hours to ensure adequate exposure.
      (4.) Remove infant from light, and remove eye patches during feedings.
      (5.) Carefully examine eyes for signs of irritation from eye patches.
      (6.) Keep an accurate record of hours spent under fluorescent lights.
   g. Meet emotional needs of infant.
   h. Reinforce physician's teaching to parents, and allow parents to express concerns and feelings.
   i. Exchange transfusion; considered only when bilirubin reaches extremely high levels (20 mg/ml in full term infant and 16 mg/ml in premature infant).

C. Hemolytic Disease of the Newborn

Hemolysis is the alteration, dissolution, or destruction of red blood cells.

1. Etiology
   a. Rh incompatibility—Rh antigens from the baby's blood enter the maternal blood stream through the placenta. The mother's blood does not contain Rh factor, so she produces anti-Rh antibodies. These antibodies are harmless to the mother but in future pregnancies can cross the placental barrier and attach to the erythrocytes in the fetus and cause hemolysis.
      (1.) Problem may begin in early pregnancy; it may be mild to severe and can cause the death of the fetus.
      (2.) Sensitization usually does not occur with the first pregnancy.
      (3.) Diagnosis of Rh incompatibility
         (a.) Begins in pregnancy, with discovery of antibodies in an Rh-negative mother's blood by means of indirect Coombs' test.
         (b.) Titration is used to determine the extent to which antibodies are present.
         (c.) Analysis of amniotic fluid for bilirubin level determines the severity of the disease; the higher the bilirubin content, the more severe the disease.
         (d.) Testing the cord blood (direct Coombs' test)—determines the presence of maternal antibodies attached to the baby's blood cells.
         (e.) Intrauterine transfusion with Rh-negative blood may be done.
   b. ABO incompatibility is usually less severe.
2. Clinical Manifestations
   a. Anemia—caused by destruction of red blood cells.
   b. Jaundice—develops rapidly after birth.

c. Edema—usually seen in stillborn infants or those who die shortly after birth, most likely due to cardiac failure.

D. Sepsis in the Neonate

1. Predisposing Factors
   a. Prolonged rupture of membranes—over 24 hours.
   b. Long difficult labor or prolonged resuscitation after birth
   c. Maternal infection
   d. Aspiration of amniotic fluids or vaginal secretions during birth
   e. Aspiration of formula after birth
   f. Infection within nursery or among nursery personnel
   g. Usually appears within the first 48 hours after birth
   h. May quickly lead to septicemia or meningitis if not treated promptly.
2. Clinical Manifestations
   a. May be vague.
   b. Neonate may feed poorly and have poor sucking reflex.
   c. May regurgitate feedings.
   d. May have diarrhea.
   e. Periods of apnea or irregular respirations.
   f. Jaundice may appear.
   g. May have a low-grade fever.
   h. Lethargy
   i. Irritability
3. Diagnosis
   a. Aspiration of gastric contents; examined for polymorphonuclear cells.
   b. Cultures taken of the blood, urine, spinal fluids, throat, skin lesions, and umbilical area.
4. Nursing Management
   a. Antibiotics; observe carefully for toxicity because of liver and kidney immaturity.
   b. Maintain warmth; usually in an Isolette.
   c. Administer O_2 as necessary.
   d. I.V. fluids may be ordered; otherwise, give fluids as ordered to maintain hydration, electrolyte levels, and calories.
   e. Maintain isolation and proper hand washing techniques.
   f. Check respiratory rate and apical pulse frequently.
   g. If apnea is present, stimulate by gently rubbing chest or foot.
   h. Maintain record of intake and output.
   i. Check temperature.
   j. Weigh daily.
   k. Keep parents informed of infant's progress.
   l. Allow parents to visit child as much as possible.
   m. Talk to infant and gently stroke him while giving care.

E. Infants of Diabetic Mothers

1. General Considerations
   a. May be delivered early to prevent intrauterine death; usually delivered after 36 weeks.
   b. Often delivered by cesarean section.
   c. Higher incidence of congenital anomalies than the general population.
   d. High incidence of hypoglycemia, respiratory distress, hypocalcemia, and hyperbilirubinemia.
2. Clinical Manifestations
   a. Baby is usually excessive in size and weight owing to more fat and glycogen in tissues.
      (1.) High blood glucose levels in mother cross the placenta and enter the baby's blood stream, elevating blood glucose levels in baby.
      (2.) High blood glucose level stimulates infant's metabolic system to store glycogen and fat and increase the production of insulin.
   b. May have puffy appearance of face and cheeks.
   c. Enlarged heart, liver, and spleen.
   d. Lethargy
   e. Irregular respiration
3. Nursing Management
   a. Observe for signs of hypoglycemia—twitching, difficulty feeding, lethargy, apnea, seizures, and cyanosis.
   b. Observe for signs of respiratory distress—tachypnea, cyanosis, retractions, grunting, and nasal flaring.
   c. Care is the same as for a premature infant.

FAMILY PLANNING

A. General Concepts Related to Family Planning

1. Dealing with individuals with particular ideas regarding contraception.
2. No perfect method of birth control.
3. Method must be suited to individuals.

4. Both individuals involved must be thoroughly counseled on all available methods and how they work, including advantages and disadvantages. This counseling includes not only the woman but also her sexual partner when possible.
5. Once a method is chosen, both partners should be thoroughly instructed in its use and how it works.
6. Individuals involved must be motivated to use the method successfully.
7. Effectiveness depends upon the following:
   (a.) Method chosen
   (b.) Degree to which couple follow prescribed regimen.
   (c.) Thorough understanding of method.
   (d.) Motivation on part of individuals concerned.

B. Contraceptive Methods

Rhythm

1. Based upon 3 principles, as follow:
   a. Ovulation usually occurs 14 days before menstrual period begins.
   b. An ovum may be fertilized 12 to 24 hours after release from ovary.
   c. Sperm usually will last up to 72 hours in the uterine environment.
2. Based on these principles, if coitus is avoided during the fertile period, pregnancy should not occur.

Chemical Agent

1. Agent acts by killing or paralyzing sperm.
2. Combined with a compound that coats the vagina; agent acts as a vehicle for spermicide as well as a mechanical barrier through which sperm cannot swim.
3. Available forms are foams, creams, and jellies.

Diaphragm

1. Functions by blocking external os and closing access to cervical canal by sperm. It is a mechanical barrier.
2. Must be used in conjunction with vaginal cream or jelly to be effective.

Condom

1. Acts as a mechanical barrier by collecting sperm and not allowing contact with vaginal area.
2. It is relatively inexpensive and may be easily purchased in a drugstore.

Coitus Interruptus

1. Early form of contraception.
2. Requires withdrawal of penis before ejaculation.

Oral Contraceptives

1. Contraceptive effect occurs as follows:
   a. Artificially raises the blood levels of estrogen and progesterone, thereby preventing the release of FSH from the anterior pituitary. Without FSH the follicle does not mature, and ovulation fails to take place.
   b. Endometrial changes
   c. Alteration in cervical mucus making it hostile to sperm.
   d. Altered tubal function
2. Minor side effects; usually diminish within a few months.
   a. Breast fullness and tenderness
   b. Edema, weight gain
   c. Nausea and vomiting
   d. Chloasma
   e. "Breakthrough" bleeding
3. More serious side effects
   (a.) Thrombophlebitis
   (b.) Pulmonary embolism
   (c.) Hypertension

Intra-uterine Devices (IUD)

1. Methods of action not completely clear.
   a. More rapid transport of ovum through tube, reaching endometrium before it is "ready" for implantation.
   b. IUD may cause substances to accumulate in uterus and interfere with implantation.
   c. IUD may stimulate production of cellular exudate, which interferes with the ability of sperm to migrate to fallopian tubes.
2. Usually made of soft plastic or nickel-chromium alloy.

3. Some types of intra-uterine device are still available on market.
4. Complications
   a. Perforation of uterus
   b. Infection
   c. "Spotting" between menstrual periods
   d. Heavy menstrual flow or prolonged flow
   e. Cramping during menstruation

STERILIZATION

1. General considerations
   a. Should be considered permanent; no guarantee that fertility can be restored.
   b. Requires written consent of responsible, fully informed individual.
2. Male sterilization (vasectomy)—severing of sperm duct from each testicle, making it impossible for sperm to pass from testes.
3. Female sterilization—accomplished by the removal of the uterus and the ovaries or the destruction of ovum conducting ability of fallopian tubes.

ROLE OF NURSE IN FAMILY PLANNING

A. Education of client in various methods available, their effectiveness and side effects.
B. Help clients explore their feelings regarding birth control and what they find acceptable and not acceptable.
C. Create open relaxed atmosphere, allowing clients to express concerns and feelings about birth control.
D. Thorough explanation of how method works and client's role, such as insertion, checking, and so forth.
E. Instruction of client in possible complications and side effects.

Maternal–Child Nursing Bibliography

Adamkiewicz, V. W. (1976). What are the bonds between the fetus and the uterus? *Nurse*, 72:26–28.

American College of Obstetricians and Gynecologists, Committee on Mental Health (1970). *National Study of Maternity Care.* Chicago: American College of Obstetricians and Gynecologists.

Anthony, E. J. & Benedek, T. (eds.) (1970). *Parenthood: Its Psychology and Psychopathology.* Boston: Little, Brown and Company.

Applebaum, R. M. (1970). The modern management of successful breast feeding. *Pediatric Clinics of North America*, 17:203.

Arey, L. B. (1974). *Developmental Anatomy*, 7th ed. Philadelphia: W. B. Saunders.

Avery, G. B. (1975). *Neonatology: Pathophysiology and Management of the Newborn.* Philadelphia: J. B. Lippincott.

Auger, J. R. (1976). *Behavioral Systems and Nursing.* Englewood Cliffs, New Jersey: Prentice-Hall.

Bardwick, J. M. (1971). Psychology of Woman: A Study of Biocultural Conflicts. New York, Harper and Row.

Benson, L. (1968). Fatherhood. A Sociological Perspective. New York, Random House.

Bergersen, B. & Krug, E. (1976). *Pharmacology in Nursing*, 13th ed. St. Louis: C. V. Mosby Co.

Billingsley, A., et al. (1970). *Illegitimacy: Changing Services for Changing Times.* New York: National Council on Illegitimacy.

Bonovich, L. (1970). Participation: the key to learning for patients in antepartal clinics. *Journal of Obstetric, Gynecologic, and Neonatal Nursing*, 9:75–79.

Bretschneider, J. W. & Minetola, A. C. (1983). Another look at early pregancy classes. *The American Journal of Maternal-Child Nursing*, 8:268–273.

Carter, A. B. (1971). Hypertension: its causes and treatment. *Nursing Times*, 67:531–533.

Chesley, L. C. (1977). Hypertensive disorders in pregnancy. *Drug Therapy*, 7:10–16.

Claypool, J. M. (1981). Rubella protection for maternal-child health care providers. *The American Journal of Maternal-Child Nursing*, 6:53–56.

Cochran, L. (ed.) (1971). Symposium on care of the newborn. *Nursing Clinics of North America*, 6:1–112.

Colman, A. L. (1971). *Pregnancy: The Psychological Experience.* New York: Herder and Herder.

Dawkins, V. E. (1975). *The Effects of a Planned Program of Nutritional Counseling on the Nutritional Status of a Group of Pregnant Methadone Maintained Narcotic Addicts and Their Infants.* University of Illinois: Master's Thesis.

Deibel, D. (1980). Effects of cigarette smoking on maternal nutrition and the fetus. *Journal of Obstetric, Gynecologic, and Neonatal Nursing*, 9:333–336.

Deskins, B. & Laska, M. (1982). The community health nurses' nutrition guidelines: A trimester approach for expectant mothers. *The American Journal of Maternal-Child Nursing*, 7:202–205.

Franz, I. D. (1981). Report on the status of glucocorticoids to hasten fetal lung maturation. *Contemporary OB/GYN*, 17:79–81.

Hammer, R. M. & Bower, I. M. (1984). The prenatal use of RHO_0 (D) immune globulin. *The American Journal of Maternal-Child Nursing*, 9:29–31.

Howley, C. (1981). The older primipara: Implications for nurses. *Journal of Obstetric, Gynecologic, and Neonatal Nursing*, 10:182–185.

Jones, M. B. (1979). Hypertensive disorders of pregnancy. *Journal of Obstetric, Gynecologic, and Neonatal Nursing*, 8:92–96.

McKay, S. R. (1980). Smoking during the childbearing year. *The American Journal of Maternal-Child Nursing*, 5:46–50.

Leonard, L. (1982). Twin pregnancy: Maternal-fetal nutrition. *The American Journal of Maternal-Child Nursing*, 7:139–145.

Lieber, M. T. (1980). Nonstress antepartal monitoring. *The American Journal of Maternal-Child Nursing*, 5:335–339.

Luke, B. (1977). Understanding pica in pregnancy. *The American Journal of Maternal-Child Nursing*, 2:97–100.

Moore, D. S., Bingham, P. R. & Keesling, O. (1981). Nursing care of the pregnant woman with diabetes mellitis. *Journal of Obstetric, Gynecologic, and Neonatal*, 10:188–194.

Norr, K. L., Block, C. R., Charles, A. G. & Meyering, S. (1980). The second time around: Parity and birth experience. *Journal of Obstetric, Gynecologic, and Neonatal Nursing*, 9:30–36.

Oliver, C. & Oliver, G. (1978). Gentle Birth: Its Safety and Its

Effect on Neonatal Behavior. *Journal of Obstetric, Gynecologic, and Neonatal Nursing*, 7:35–40.

Oxorn, H. & Foote, W. (1975). *Human Labor and Birth*. New York: Appleton-Century-Crofts.

Penny, K. S. (1979). Postpartum perceptions of touch received during labor. *Research in Nursing and Health*, 2:9–16.

Perez, P. (1979). Nursing children who attend the birth of a sibling. *Journal of Maternal-Child Nursing*, 4:215–217.

Pridham, K. F. & Schutz, M. E. (1983). Parental goals and the birthing experience. *Journal of Obstetric, Gynecologic, and Neonatal Nursing*, 12:50–55.

Roberts, J. E. (1979). Maternal positions for childbirth. A historical review of nursing care practices. *Journal of Obstetric, Gynecologic, and Neonatal Nursing*, 8:24–32.

Shannon-Babitz, M. (1979). Addressing the needs of fathers during labor and delivery. *Journal of Maternal-Child Nursing*, 4:378–382.

Standely, K. & Nicholson, J. (1980). Observing the childbirth environment: A research model. *Birth and the Family Journal*, 7:15–20.

Taubenheim, A. M. (1981). Paternal-infant bonding in the first-time father. *Journal of Obstetric, Gynecologic, and Neonatal Nursing*, 10:261–264.

Worthington, E., Martin, G. & Shumate, M. (1982). Which prepared childbirth coping strategies are effective? *Journal of Obstetric, Gynecologic, and Neonatal Nursing*, 11:45–51.

Wright, B. (1982). Understanding fetal monitoring. *Perinatology/Neonatology*, 6:27–30.

Section

MATERNAL–CHILD NURSING PRACTICE QUESTIONS

1 • The cyclic activities of the ovaries and uterine endometrium are regulated by the:

1. Cerebral cortex and the adrenal gland.
2. Hypothalamus and the anterior pituitary gland.
3. Cerebellum and the posterior pituitary gland.
4. Medulla oblongata and the thyroid gland.

2 • The hormone that enhances ovarian production of estrogen during the first half of the menstrual cycle is the:

1. Growth hormone.
2. Follicle stimulating hormone.
3. Luteinizing hormone.
4. Adrenocorticotrophic hormone.

3 • How many chromosomes does the mature human ovum contain?

1. 46
2. 35
3. 23
4. 11

4 • The chromosomes of the human ovum are composed of:

1. Amino acids.
2. Ribonucleic acids.
3. Branched-chain fatty acids.
4. Deoxyribonucleic acid.

5 • At which of the following points in the normal menstrual cycle is the serum level of estrogen highest?

1. 3rd day.
2. 8th day.
3. 13th day.
4. 23rd day.

6 • At which of the following points in the normal menstrual cycle is the serum level of estrogen lowest?

1. 3rd day.
2. 8th day.
3. 13th day.
4. 23rd day.

7 • The anterior pituitary hormone that stimulates production of progesterone during the latter half of the menstrual cycle is the:

1. Growth hormone.
2. Follicle-stimulating hormone.
3. Luteinizing hormone.
4. Adrenocorticotrophic hormone.

8 • During the latter half of the menstrual period progesterone is secreted by the:

1. Posterior pituitary gland.
2. Ovarian follicle.
3. Corpus luteum.
4. Endometrial glands.

9 • Conception is most likely to occur during which interval of time?

1. The 1st day of the menstrual period.
2. 12 hours following cessation of menstruation.
2. 12 to 24 hours following ovulation.
4. The day or two preceding menstruation.

10 • In human beings fertilization of the ovum usually occurs in the:

1. Ovarian follicle.
2. Fallopian tube.
3. Uterine fundus.
4. Uterine corpus.

11 • Implantation or attachment of the fertilized ovum to the endometrium usually occurs about which day of the normal menstrual cycle?

1. 15th day.
2. 20th day.
3. 25th day.
4. 1st day.

12 • The principal source of progesterone and estrogen during the 1st 6 to 8 weeks of pregnancy is the:

1. Pituitary gland.
2. Embryonic chorion.
3. Corpus luteum.
4. Adrenal cortex.

13 • In addition to amenorrhea, which of the following presumptive signs of pregnancy might a woman experience before consulting her doctor?

1. Morning sickness.
2. Fetal movement.
3. Ankle swelling.
4. Pigment changes.

14 • The nurse should instruct the pregnant woman that which of the following would be most apt to relieve her morning sickness?

1. Eliminating breakfast and eating a slightly larger than normal lunch.
2. Eating some dry, absorbent food such as crackers before arising.
3. Drinking copious amounts of clear fluids with and between meals.
4. Avoiding foods that are high in roughage or acidic in nature.

15 • Morning sickness of pregnancy usually disappears by the end of the:

1. First month.
2. Third month.
3. Fifth month.
4. Seventh month.

16 • Chadwick's sign, or the purplish discoloration of the vulvar, vaginal, and cervical mucosa, is thought to be caused by:

1. Circulatory changes produced by increased amounts of ovarian hormones.
2. Rapid growth of microorganisms in the increased vaginal secretions.
3. Decreased O_2 tension of maternal blood produced by fetal metabolism.
4. Obstruction of venous flow caused by pressure of the enlarged uterus.

17 • If the woman's last normal menstrual period began on December 15 and the last episode of vaginal bleeding on January 12, her expected confinement date would be:

1. September 15.
2. September 22.
3. October 12.
4. October 19.

18 • The VDRL test is used to diagnose:

1. Syphilis.
2. Choriocarcinoma.
3. Gonorrhea.
4. Erythroblastosis.

19 • Pregnant women should be advised that which of the following foods is the best source of vitamin A?

1. Radish.
2. Turnip.
3. Cucumber.
4. Spinach.

20 • Which of the following foods is the best source of vitamin B_1 (thiamine)?

1. Pork.
2. Pear.
3. Milk.
4. Carrot.

21 • A particularly good source of vitamin C is:

1. Peach.
2. Broccoli.
3. Apple.
4. Carrot.

22 • Anticipatory nutritional guidance should include that, in addition to milk, which of the following is highest in calcium content?

1. Turnip greens.
2. Green peppers.
3. Sweet corn.
4. White potatoes.

23 • Which of the following foods is a good source of iron?

1. Corn oil.
2. Beef liver.
3. Bran flakes.
4. Tangerines.

24 • During pregnancy varicose veins of the lower extremities or vulva might develop as a result of:

1. Systemic circulation of microorganisms harbored in vaginal secretions.
2. Compression of the abdominal veins by the progressively enlarging uterus.
3. Increased cardiac load imposed by the O_2 needs of the growing fetus.
4. Increased venous blood volume due to return of blood from the fetus.

25 • During pregnancy heartburn may develop as a result of:

1. Excessive secretion of hydrochloric acid by the gastric mucosal glands in response to appetite increase.
2. Tendency of acid contents of the compressed and upward displaced stomach to reflux into the lower esophagus.
3. Friction of the parietal pericardium against the dome of the diaphragm elevated by the enlarging uterus.
4. Gastritis due to hyperacidity and hyperperistalsis provoked by emotional stresses of impending motherhood.

26 • The pregnant woman is most apt to first perceive quickening or "feel life" between her:

1. 10th and 12th weeks of pregnancy.
2. 16th and 20th weeks of pregnancy.
3. 26th and 28th weeks of pregnancy.
4. 34th and 36th weeks of pregnancy.

27 • The umbilical cord is composed of:

1. Two arteries and a vein embedded in a gelatinous substance.
2. An artery, a vein, and a nerve surrounded by smooth muscle.
3. An artery and 2 veins encased in a sheath of skin and mucosa.
4. A network of arterioles, capillaries, and venules enclosed in fascia.

28 • Ferrous sulfate supplements should be administered:

1. Midway between meals.
2. Immediately before meals.
3. Immediately after meals.
4. Separately from other medications.

29 • The pregnant uterus can usually be palpated at the level of the umbilicus at about the:

1. 14th week of pregnancy.
2. 20th week of pregnancy.
3. 26th week of pregnancy.
4. 32nd week of pregnancy.

30 • Fetal heart tones are rarely audible before which point in pregnancy?

1. 6th week.
2. 12th week.
3. 18th week.
4. 24th week.

31 • The fetal heart rate normally lies within which range?

1. 80 to 120 beats per minute.
2. 120 to 160 beats per minute.
3. 160 to 200 beats per minute.
4. 200 to 240 beats per minute.

32 • How frequently should the nurse take fetal heart tones during the latent phase of a normal labor?

1. Every 15 minutes.
2. Every 30 minutes.
3. Every 60 minutes.
4. Every 90 minutes.

33 • The nurse should be aware that which of the following variations in fetal heart tones may be considered normal?

1. Decrease in volume during the 2nd stage of labor.
2. Decrease in rate during the midportion of contraction.
3. Increase in rate following rupture of the membranes.
4. Increase in volume during internal rotation of the head.

34 • During the transitional phase of the 1st stage of labor the pregnant woman may seem somewhat confused, discouraged, and irritable. Which of the following comments by the nurse would be most supportive at this time?

1. "This phase of your labor will last only 1 hour. Since you've already weathered 9 hours of pain, you can surely hang on for a little longer."
2. "These are the hardest pains you will have. Before long you'll be able to bear down with your contractions and it will be much easier for you."
3. "I know that you're feeling great pain, but I'm sure that you can withstand this discomfort in a way that you can retain your self control."
4. "You have no reason to be discouraged. Your doctor is here, the nurses are all ready to help you, and the finest obstetrical equipment is available."

35 • The physician should wait until the fetal head is well engaged before he ruptures the bag of waters in order to:

1. Enable the bag of waters to rupture spontaneously if possible, thus avoiding difficult and painful instrumentation.
2. Prevent prolapse of the umbilical cord during the forceful expulsion of amniotic fluid from the sac.
3. Ensure that a small amount of amniotic fluid would be left in the upper portion of the amniotic sac.
4. Have the amniotic sac in a dependent enough position that it could be reached without difficulty.

36 • The 1st stage of labor is considered to have terminated when:

1. Regular 3 minute contractions have been established.
2. The bag of waters has ruptured.
3. The cervix has been completely effaced and dilated.
4. The presenting part is visible during contractions.

37 • The cervix is considered to be completely dilated when the diameter of the os is:

1. 6 cm.
2. 8 cm.
3. 10 cm.
4. 12 cm.

38 • In timing contractions the nurse should notify the physician if she detects a contraction lasting longer than:

1. 30 seconds.
2. 60 seconds.
3. 90 seconds.
4. 120 seconds.

39 • The mechanics of the 2nd stage of labor differ from those of the 1st in that during the 2nd stage:

1. The lower uterine segment contracts more than the fundus.
2. The abdominal muscles assist in the expulsion of the fetus.
3. The joints of the pelvis are stretched and dislocated.
4. All muscles involved in fetal propulsion undergo tetany.

40 • The fetal head is engaged when:

1. The vertex of the skull is level with the symphysis pubis.
2. The biparietal diameter has passed the pelvic inlet.
3. The head rotates from the transverse to the anteroposterior position.
4. The head has descended beyond the external cervical os.

41 • Fetal position during labor refers to the:

1. First body part of the fetus felt by the examiner upon vaginal examination.
2. Relationship of a fixed point of the fetus to the quadrants of the maternal pelvis.
3. Relationship of the furthermost fetal part to the ischial spines of the maternal pelvis.
4. Relationship of the long axis of the fetus to the long axis of the mother's body.

42 • The nurse should expect to observe which of the following changes in maternal vital signs during the 2nd stage of labor?

1. Decrease in temperature.
2. Increase in blood pressure.
3. Decrease in pulse rate.
4. Increase in urinary output.

43 • During the early 2nd stage of labor fetal heart tones should be taken at least every:

1. 2 to 4 minutes.
2. 5 to 10 minutes.
3. 10 to 20 minutes.
4. 20 to 30 minutes.

44 • The changes in shape of the infant's head that occur owing to pressure from the walls of the birth canal are called:

1. Molding.
2. Cephalhematoma.
3. Microcephaly.
4. Caput succedaneum.

45 • If crowning occurs while the nurse is alone with the patient, she should:

1. Place a sterile towel over the infant's head and apply manual pressure until a physician arrives.
2. Place a mask over the woman's face and administer a few drops of ether to delay delivery.
3. Call for help, stay with the patient and guide the slow delivery of the head between contractions.
4. Instruct the woman to hold her knees together and leave to obtain help from an experienced nurse.

46 • The most common position for the fetus at birth is the:

1. Right occiput anterior.
2. Left occiput anterior.
3. Right occiput posterior.
4. Left occiput posterior.

47 • The 2nd stage of labor ends with:

1. Complete cervical dilation.
2. Bulging of the perineum.
3. Delivery of the baby.
4. Removal of the placenta.

48 • Baby Smith, an 8 lb 6 oz girl was born at 8:30 AM by normal spontaneous vaginal delivery. Apgar scores were 9 at 1 min and 9 at 5 min, and no abnormalities were noted. Cord was clamped, and the baby was placed in a warming crib in a Trendelenburg position. After being dried thoroughly and identified with bands, eye care was given using a silver nitrate solution. Baby Smith was then placed with her parents who were apparently very pleased with their new daughter. Immediate status of the infant showed FHR 120, vigorous cry, blue extremities, and flexed extremities. The Apgar score is determined at 1 min and 5 min:

1. To determine the sex of the baby.
2. To appraise the infant for anomalies.
3. To give an immediate appraisal of the infant's cardiac and respiratory status.
4. To give an immediate appraisal of the infant's Rh status.

49 • Baby Smith was given an Apgar score of 9 at 1 min after delivery. One point was deducted because:

1. Her heart rate was over 100.
2. Her cry was loud and strong.
3. She demonstrated flexed extremities.
4. She demonstrated acrocyanosis of her extremities.

50 • The infant was placed in the warming crib in the Trendelenburg position after her initial care to:

1. Prevent loss of heat and facilitate drainage.
2. Increase O_2 use.
3. Allow the parents time to recover.
4. Place the infant in an environment similar to that of the uterus.

51 • Silver nitrate (1%) is inserted into the newborn's eyes to prevent:

1. Spirochete infection.
2. Gonococcal infection.
3. Toxoplasmosis.
4. Thrush.

52 • An injection of vitamin K was given to Baby Smith in the nursery. Vitamin K is given to:

1. Help conjugate bilirubin.
2. Prevent Rh sensitization.
3. Reduce the possibility of hemorrhage.
4. Increase the resistance to infection.

53 • Baby Smith had a large caput succedaneum on her head. The mother is concerned and asks what the swelling is. You would tell her:

1. It is extravasion of blood into the tissue caused by trauma from delivery.
2. It will take a couple of months to disappear on its own.
3. The infant may suffer brain damage as a result of the caput.
4. It is a swelling of the soft tissues of the scalp due to pressure on the cervix during dilatation.

54 • The normal respiratory rate in the newborn is between:

1. 16 and 20.
2. 60 and 80.
3. 80 to 100.
4. 30 and 50.

55 • The normal apical pulse rate in the newborn is between:

1. 120 and 160.
2. 60 and 80.
3. 80 and 100.
4. 180 and 200.

56 • Baby Smith showed signs of jaundice, and her laboratory values for bilirubin showed a total bilirubin of 15.0, direct bilirubin of 1.7, and indirect bilirubin of 13.3. The physician ordered continuous "bile" light and forced fluids between feedings. Physiological jaundice is due to:

1. Rh incompatibility with the mother.
2. Presence of *Staphylococcus* infection within the newborn.
3. ABO incompatibility.
4. Inability of the newborn to conjugate bilirubin.

57 • An important principle to consider with an infant receiving phototherapy would be to:

1. Cover the eyes with eye patches to prevent retinal damage.
2. Dress the infant to prevent chilling.
3. Isolate the infant to prevent cross-contamination.
4. Avoid handling the infant because it interferes with the treatment.

58 • Baby Smith's laboratory test results showed a steady decline in the level of indirect bilirubin after 2 days' treatment with phototherapy. She was discharged, and the physician prescribed a formula of Similac 20 on a demand feeding schedule. Physiological jaundice usually appears:

1. Within the 1st 24 hours and disappears after 3 days.
2. Within the 1st 24 hours and lasts 6 to 7 days.
3. On the 2nd or 3rd day and lasts 48 hours.
4. On the 2nd or 3rd day and begins to decrease on the 6th or 7th day.

59 • Which of the following is true regarding the newborn's weight after birth?

1. Weight usually remains constant the first few days, then drops when infant goes home.
2. Infant usually loses between 5 and 10% of body weight during the first few days after birth, and then begins to increase in weight after the 4th day.
3. Infant usually begins to gain weight the 1st day after birth, when put on bottle or breast.
4. Infant normally loses between 15 and 20% of body weight after birth but regains it rapidly.

60 • Of the following conditions which one is *not* a result of metabolic error in the fetus?

1. Phenylketonuria.
2. Maple syrup urine disease.
3. Galactosemia.
4. Pyloric stenosis.

Mrs. Sampson is a Rh-negative woman with an Rh-positive husband. Mrs. Sampson had 2 abortions before she was married. She is now 24 years of age and anxiously expecting a child at any moment. Mrs. Sampson was watched carefully during her pregnancy. Her Rh-antibody titer and indirect Coombs' test results showed signs of slight elevations during her pregnancy. During her last trimester, an amniocentesis was done and the spectrophotometric analysis showed a relatively low titer and was not repeated at 40 weeks. Mrs. Sampson delivered a 7 lb 6 oz baby boy. Laboratory tests on cord blood indicated the infant was Rh positive. The Coombs' test was positive, and the serum bilirubin level was 5.9.

61 • Nursing care of the infant diagnosed as having hyperbilirubinemia includes all *but which one* of the following?

1. Pallor
2. Flushing
3. Progressive jaundice
4. Lethargy

62 • Hyperbilirubinemia occurs in Rh incompatibility between mother and fetus because:

1. The mother's blood does not contain the Rh factor, and so she produces anti-Rh antibodies that cross the placental barrier and cause hemolysis of red blood cells in the infant.
2. The mother's blood contains the Rh factor, and the infant's blood does not; antibodies are formed in the fetus that destroy red blood cells.
3. The mother has a history of previous "yellow" jaundice caused by a blood transfusion, which was passed to the fetus through the placenta.
4. The infant develops a congenital defect shortly after birth that causes the destruction of red blood cells.

63 • ABO incompatability differs from Rh incompatability in that it:

1. Is less severe.
2. Is more severe.
3. Is more difficult to diagnose.
4. Always requires an in utero *transfusion.*

64 • Baby Sampson's condition continues to worsen, and he is given an exchange transfusion. Nursing care of the infant following the transfusion would include all *but which one* of the following?

1. Observe for bleeding from the umbilical cord.
2. Take vital signs frequently.
3. Give IPPB therapy.
4. Observe for signs of hypoglycemia and sepsis.

65 • The development of anti-Rh antibodies within the mother could have been prevented with the administration of RhoGAM (immune globulin) post abortions. Which of the following is true about RhoGAM?

1. It must be given on the 6th day post delivery.
2. It should be given after each pregnancy or abortion.
3. It may be given even after sensitization occurs.
4. It may be given to the infant.

---

66 • Signs of sepsis in the newborn would include all *but which one* of the following?

1. Periods of apnea or irregular respiration.
2. Poor sucking reflex and feeding.
3. Constipation.
4. Irritability.

67 • Mrs. Johnson, who delivered a baby boy the previous evening, is crying when you enter her room. When you ask her what is wrong, she tells you that the doctor told her that her baby has a functional heart murmur. The best nursing response in this situation would be to:

1. Tell her to ask the doctor what it means.
2. Tell her everything will work out all right.
3. Tell her that a functional murmur is normal and will last a few weeks.
4. Tell her that this type of murmur may indicate heart damage, but the baby will certainly survive.

68 • Baby Jackson, an 11 lb 6 oz girl, was delivered by cesarean section to a diabetic mother. Apgar score was 7/9. The infant was aspirated and placed in the intermediate care nursery for observation. Problems in the infant of a diabetic mother could include all *but which one* of the following?

1. Hypoglycemia.
2. Sepsis.
3. Respiratory distress.
4. Hypocalcemia.

69 • Infants of diabetic mothers are often of excessive weight because:

1. High blood glucose levels in the mother stimulate the infant's metabolic system to store glycogen and fat.
2. The infant also is diabetic and stores fat.
3. The infant is suffering from excessive edema.
4. Inactivity in the infant caused by elevated blood glucose levels results in weight gain.

70 • Signs of hypoglycemia in the infant include all *but which one* of the following?

1. Twitching or jitteriness.
2. Increased respiratory rate.
3. Apathy and poor muscle tone.
4. Weak, soft cry.

71 • Nursing care of the infant with hypoglycemia would include which of the following?

1. Administer whole blood.
2. Administer glucose I.V. or orally if infant is able to suck and swallow.
3. Place infant on respirator.
4. Give calcium gluconate I.V.

72 • Nursing care of the "drug addicted" infant includes all *but which one* of the following?

1. Frequent handling of infant.
2. Frequent monitoring of cardiac and respiratory rates.
3. Padding side of crib to protect from injury.
4. Cleansing buttocks carefully to avoid skin breakdown from diarrhea.

73 • RhoGAM (immune globulin) is given to Mrs. Bade, who delivered a healthy baby 24 hours ago. In order for it to be effective, which of the following conditions should *not* be present?

1. Mrs. Bade is Rh negative.
2. The baby is Rh positive.
3. Mrs. Bade has no titer in her blood.
4. Mrs. Bade has some titer in her blood.

On April 16 at 3:45 PM, Baby Jones (a 34 week, 1550 gm female) was delivered to a 17-year-old unmarried primigravida. The infant demonstrated nasal flaring, intercostal retractions, expiratory grunt, and slight cyanosis. An umbilical catheter was inserted with I.V. infusion of 5% dextrose and water, 30 ml, to run over a 10-hour period. Blood gas values and electrolyte studies were ordered immediately.

74 • The nurse would place baby Jones in a heated Isolette immediately after delivery because:

1. The premature infant has a small body surface for her weight.
2. Heat decreases oxygen use by tissues.
3. Temperature control mechanism is immature.
4. Heat within the Isolette facilitates drainage of mucus.

75 • The temperature of the infant in the heated Isolette should be taken regularly to observe for *all but which* sign?

1. Dehydration.
2. Cold stress.
3. Increased need for oxygen.
4. Elevated glucose levels.

76 • Immediate assessment of the premature infant in the nursery by the nurse would include all *but which one* of the following?

1. Hunger status.
2. Cardiac status.
3. Respiratory status.
4. Congenital abnormalities.

77 • An infant with respiratory distress will show all *but which one* of the following?

1. Respiratory rate between 30 and 40.
2. Cyanosis.
3. Expiratory grunt.
4. Pco_2 between 35 and 45.

78 • Blood gas values and electrolyte studies were ordered immediately on Baby Jones to assess:

1. The infant's leukocyte count.
2. The infant's O_2 and CO_2 levels and pH.
3. The infant's antibody titer for Rh.
4. The infant's blood glucose level.

79 • Baby Van was diagnosed as having respiratory distress syndrome. Premature infants are likely to develop respiratory distress. Which one of the following conditions is *not* considered a possible cause?

1. Alveoli are immature and produce inadequate amounts of surfactant.
2. The premature infant has not received adequate numbers of antibodies from his mother before birth.
3. Nerves and respiratory center are immature.
4. The premature infant's thoracic cage and respiratory muscles are weak.

80 • The air in Baby Van's Isolette is humidified to:

1. Improve cardiac rhythm.
2. Prevent hyperbilirubinemia.
3. Increase the infant's temperature.
4. Prevent drying of bronchial secretions.

81 • The physician will carefully regulate the concentration of O_2 Baby Van receives, based upon the infant's PO_2 and PCO_2 levels, because high blood levels of O_2 can cause:

1. Kernicterus.
2. Retinal spasms leading to the development of retrolental fibroplasia.
3. Peripheral circulatory collapse.
4. Temporary cardiac dysfunction.

82 • The nurses caring for Baby Van use careful hand washing techniques while caring for him because they know premature infants are more susceptible to infection than full term infants. Which of the following does *not* explain why premature infants are more likely to develop infection?

1. Liver enzymes are immature.
2. Antibody formation is immature.
3. Premature infants receive few antibodies from the mother, because antibodies pass across the placenta during the last month of pregnancy.
4. Cellular and white blood cell defense may be ineffective.

83 • Nursing care of the premature infant in preventing infection includes all *but which one* of the following interventions?

1. Cover I.V. sites and keep dressings clean.
2. Avoid caring for the infant if you have an infection.
3. Use tap water for aspiration.
4. Prevent skin breakdown with careful skin cleansing and little use of tape.

84 • The premature infant has a tendency toward hemorrhage and anemia; therefore, nursing care of Baby Van would include all *but which one* of the following?

1. Administer vitamin C shortly after birth.
2. Record all blood loss including blood test samples.
3. Use care in handling the infant.
4. Secure all I.V. connections, and look for backflow of blood in tubing.

85 • One of the most important principles in providing nutrition to Baby Van would involve:

1. Using a regular nipple for bottle feeding.
2. Gavage feeding the infant.
3. Using "premie" soft nipple for bottle feeding.
4. Using milk high in fat.

86 • The premature infant has difficulty concentrating urine and may have large amounts of fluid loss. The nurse caring for Baby Van would:

1. Force fluids every half hour.
2. Observe color and amounts of urine and check its specific gravity.
3. Administer only high protein fluids.
4. Warm fluids before administering them.

Mrs. Gibson, a 32-year-old housewife with a 3-year-old child, had been trying to get pregnant for several months. She had trouble with spotting between periods and excessive bleeding at menstruation. She consulted her physician, who administered a pelvic examination and a PAP smear. The results of her PAP smear were Class V. Her physician scheduled her for an immediate hysterectomy.

87 • Mrs. Gibson was admitted to the hospital and scheduled for a total abdominal hysterectomy and bilateral salpingo-oophorectomy. While passing her room the evening before surgery, the nurse heard her crying. The nurse went into the room and sat on the chair beside the bed. Mrs. Gibson said, "I wanted another baby so badly, and now I will never have another child." Which of the following statements by the nurse would be most helpful to Mrs. Gibson?

1. "It is all right to cry. I know how difficult it must be to know you will never be able to have another child. I'll sit here with you for a while."
2. "No, you won't be able to have another child, but you can always adopt a child."
3. "Maybe you could talk to your doctor about postponing surgery until you have another child."
4. "At least you were lucky enough to have one child before the surgery."

88 • Preoperative care of Mrs. Gibson would include all *but which one* of the following?

1. Insertion of an indwelling catheter.
2. Forcing fluids after midnight.
3. Teaching the patient to support her incisional area and to deep breathe and cough.
4. Administration of a cleansing enema.

89 • Mrs. Gibson is worried about her relationship with her husband and says, "Will I ever be able to have sexual relations with my husband again?" You could best respond by saying:

1. "Yes, but it will be at least a year before you can resume sexual relations."
2. "No, unfortunately the nature of your surgery makes it impossible for you to ever have sexual relations again."
3. "Yes, you will be able to resume normal sexual relations with your husband about 6 weeks after surgery."
4. "Since you cannot have children, there is no need for you to continue sexual relations with your husband."

90 • Convalescent care of Mrs.Gibson would include all *but which one* of the following?

1. Observe for signs of infection.
2. Listen for breath sounds.
3. Involve significant others in patient's care.
4. Daily vaginal irrigations.

---

91 • Barbara, a 21-year-old patient, who is 18-weeks pregnant, is admitted to the hospital for a saline abortion. Care of the patient during the saline infusion would include which of the following?

1. Check urine for glucose and acetone.
2. Ask the patient to deep breathe at appropriate times.
3. Observe for signs of saline leakage within the mother's circulatory system.
4. Massage the fundus of the uterus.

92 • Nursing management of the patient after a saline abortion would include all *but which one* of the following?

1. Administration of RhoGAM (immune globulin) to Rh-negative mothers.
2. Check vital signs frequently.
3. Teach the patient careful perineal care.
4. Explain to the patient that she will probably have bright red bleeding for about 3 weeks.

93 • After the abortion, Barbara begins to cry and says, "I feel so guilty. I should never have killed my baby." You could be most supportive to Barbara by saying:

1. "You should be more careful in the future and use a method of birth control."
2. "It's natural to feel sad, but you'll be back to normal in a short time."
3. "You are feeling very sad right now, Barbara. I'll sit with you for a while; it may help to talk about it."
4. "Your friend will be here soon to pick you up. Why don't you tell her about it when she comes."

94 • Of the following, which one is a known teratogen?

1. Scarlet fever.
2. Rubella.
3. Coronary heart disease.
4. Dental x-rays.

95 • Which of the following conditions might precipitate acidosis in a pregnant diabetic woman?

1. Decreased salt diet.
2. Decreased activity.
3. Diarrhea.
4. High protein diet.

96 • In an emergency delivery which of the following principles best explains why the nurse would not cut the cord?

1. It is the physician's responsibility to cut the cord.
2. Cutting the cord under emergency conditions might lead to hemorrhage.
3. Cutting the cord under emergency conditions might lead to infection.
4. The nurse was never trained in the proper procedure.

97 • Which of the following is *not* a rationale for doing an amniocentesis on a woman who is 30-weeks pregnant?

1. To determine fetal maturity.
2. To determine presence of Tay-Sachs disease.
3. To determine L/S ratio.
4. To determine placental sufficiency.

98 • In explaining the side effects of the pill to your client you would tell her that:

1. There are no known side effects.
2. The pill is so effective that she need not be concerned with the side effects.
3. If side effects show up, she should skip the pill for a few days.
4. Side effects such as weight gain, nausea, and vomiting may appear but these usually clear up within the 1st to 3rd cycle.

99 • In preparing a patient for an IUD, you would:

1. Explain how an IUD functions and where it is placed.
2. Tell the patient that the IUD will probably interfere with coitus.
3. Tell the patient she will no longer be able to wear tampons.
4. Explain that it is impossible to expel the IUD once it is in place.

100 • When discussing family planning methods, the nurse should:

1. Include only the female in the discussion.
2. Help the couple to have a thorough understanding of the method they choose.
3. Choose the method she feels would best suit the couple.
4. Point out that all methods are 99.9% effective, so it makes no difference which method they choose.

Answer Sheet for Maternal–Child Practice Questions

1. 1 2 3 4
2. 1 2 3 4
3. 1 2 3 4
4. 1 2 3 4
5. 1 2 3 4
6. 1 2 3 4
7. 1 2 3 4
8. 1 2 3 4
9. 1 2 3 4
10. 1 2 3 4
11. 1 2 3 4
12. 1 2 3 4
13. 1 2 3 4
14. 1 2 3 4
15. 1 2 3 4
16. 1 2 3 4
17. 1 2 3 4
18. 1 2 3 4
19. 1 2 3 4
20. 1 2 3 4
21. 1 2 3 4
22. 1 2 3 4
23. 1 2 3 4
24. 1 2 3 4
25. 1 2 3 4
26. 1 2 3 4
27. 1 2 3 4
28. 1 2 3 4
29. 1 2 3 4
30. 1 2 3 4
31. 1 2 3 4
32. 1 2 3 4
33. 1 2 3 4
34. 1 2 3 4
35. 1 2 3 4
36. 1 2 3 4
37. 1 2 3 4
38. 1 2 3 4
39. 1 2 3 4
40. 1 2 3 4
41. 1 2 3 4
42. 1 2 3 4
43. 1 2 3 4
44. 1 2 3 4
45. 1 2 3 4
46. 1 2 3 4
47. 1 2 3 4
48. 1 2 3 4
49. 1 2 3 4
50. 1 2 3 4
51. 1 2 3 4
52. 1 2 3 4
53. 1 2 3 4
54. 1 2 3 4
55. 1 2 3 4
56. 1 2 3 4
57. 1 2 3 4
58. 1 2 3 4
59. 1 2 3 4
60. 1 2 3 4
61. 1 2 3 4
62. 1 2 3 4
63. 1 2 3 4
64. 1 2 3 4
65. 1 2 3 4
66. 1 2 3 4
67. 1 2 3 4
68. 1 2 3 4
69. 1 2 3 4
70. 1 2 3 4
71. 1 2 3 4
72. 1 2 3 4
73. 1 2 3 4
74. 1 2 3 4
75. 1 2 3 4
76. 1 2 3 4
77. 1 2 3 4
78. 1 2 3 4
79. 1 2 3 4
80. 1 2 3 4
81. 1 2 3 4
82. 1 2 3 4
83. 1 2 3 4
84. 1 2 3 4
85. 1 2 3 4
86. 1 2 3 4
87. 1 2 3 4
88. 1 2 3 4
89. 1 2 3 4
90. 1 2 3 4
91. 1 2 3 4
92. 1 2 3 4
93. 1 2 3 4
94. 1 2 3 4
95. 1 2 3 4
96. 1 2 3 4
97. 1 2 3 4
98. 1 2 3 4
99. 1 2 3 4
100. 1 2 3 4

Section

ANSWERS AND RATIONALES FOR MATERNAL–CHILD NURSING PRACTICE QUESTIONS

1. (2) Under the influence of follicle stimulating hormone (FSH) and luteinizing hormone (LH), endometrium changes and ovarian development occur. The source of FSH and LH is the anterior pituitary gland. It receives messages regarding the secretion rate of FSH and LH from the hypothalamus. Thus, the anterior pituitary and the hypothalamus are responsible for uterine and ovarian development.

2. (2) Release of FSH acts on the ovaries to develop an ovum from the surrounding follicular cells. As the follicular cells develop, more estrogen is secreted; thus, plasma estrogen increases and circulates back to the hypothalamus.

3. (3) The mature human ovum contains 23 chromosomes.

4. (4) Chromosomes are made up of molecules of deoxyribonucleic acid (DNA). They carry the genetic information that determines the characteristics of an individual.

5. (3) Estrogen secretion is highest during the pre-ovulatory or follicular phase. Its maximal secretion occurs at about day 13.

6. (1) Serum estrogen levels are lowest at the beginning of the menstrual cycle.

7. (3) During the last half of the menstrual cycle, LH is released from the anterior pituitary. Anterior putuitary hormones are transported via the circulatory system to their target organs.

8. (3) During the luteal phase of ovarian function, progesterone is secreted in substantial amounts by the corpus luteum.

9. (3) Conception is most likely to occur within 24 hours of ovulation.

10. (2) Fertilization usually occurs in the distal portion of the fallopian tube.

11. (2) Implantation occurs at the blastocyst stage, or at 6 to 7 days after fertilization. This would be approximately 20 to 21 days since the last menstrual period.

12. (3) The corpus luteum secretes levels of estrogen and progesterone sufficient to maintain the pregnancy until the placenta is able to function as an endocrine gland.

13. (1) Presumptive signs of pregnancy are subjective and recognized by the woman. They include amenorrhea, nausea and vomiting, breast changes (tenderness and pigmentation), urinary frequency, quickening, pigmentation of the skin, and fatigue.

14. (2) Nausea and vomiting during pregnancy have been attributed to hormonal changes, gastrointestinal alterations, and hypoglycemia. Small, frequent carbohydrate-rich meals have been found to be effective in combating morning sickness.

15. (2) By the end of the 3rd month the maternal system has adapted to the body changes evoked by pregnancy, and nausea and vomiting have disappeared.

16. (1) Chadwick's sign is attributed to the intense congestion of the pelvic vessels due to the presence of ovarian hormones.

17. (2) EDC is calculated using Nagele's rule: take the 1st day of the last menstrual period, add 7 days, and then subtract 3 months, changing to the appropriate year.

LMP =	12 (December)	15
	− 3	+ 7
EDC =	9 (September)	22

18. (1) VDRL is a serological test used to detect the presence of syphilis.

19. (4) Dark green and yellow vegetables provide high sources of vitamin A. Spinach per half-cup serving provides 6000 IUs of vitamin A.

20. (1) Lean pork is especially high in thiamine concentration. Thiamine functions in the release of energy from the metabolism of carbohydrate.

21. (2) Good sources of ascorbic acid (vitamin C) include citrus fruits, greens, broccoli, and Brussels sprouts.

22. (1) Good sources of calcium include cheese, spinach, greens, and oysters.

23. (2) Iron is necessary for maternal and fetal well-being. Good sources are liver, beans, raisins, lean pork, and beef.

24. (2) Varicosities occur in about 20% of all pregnant women and tend to become more prominent with each successive pregnancy. The gravid uterus causes pressure on the vessels of the vulva and lower extremities, thus obstructing venous return.

25. (2) Heartburn is probably due to relaxation of the cardiac sphincter (at the junction of the eosphagus and the stomach) and relaxation of the lower end of the esophagus. Pressure of the gravid uterus on the stomach and decreased gastric motility facilitate regurgitation of the stomach contents into the esophagus.

26. (2) Sensation of fetal movements may be experienced as early as 16 weeks by most women. This is viewed as a presumptive sign of pregnancy, since it can be confused with intestinal peristalsis.

27. (1) The umbilical cord consists of 3 vessels: an umbilical vein that carries oxygenated blood from placenta to fetus and 2 umbilical arteries that carry deoxygenated blood from fetus to placenta. The vessels are enclosed in a gelatinous substance.

28. (3) Ferrous sulfate can produce side effects of gastrointestinal upset, with possible nausea and vomiting. These can be minimized if the drug is taken on a full stomach, and therefore ingestion after meals is most appropriate.

29. (2) By 13 weeks of pregnancy the fundus of the uterus rises out of the pelvis and can be palpated just above the symphysis pubis. The fundus reaches the lower border of the umbilicus at 20 weeks and the xiphoid process at 36 weeks.

30. (3) Fetal heart tones can be auscultated with a fetoscope by 20 weeks of gestation. If ultrasonic Doppler technique is used, they can be heard as early as 16 weeks.

31. (2) The rhythm of the fetal heart rate is regular at 120 to 160 beats per minute. Very slow or accelerated heart rates are usually indicative of fetal distress.

32. (3) Assessments of the fetal heart rate pattern should increase proportionately with the progress of labor in the 1st stage. Suggested minimal intervals in the various phases are latent—minimum every hour; active—minimum every half hour; transitional—minimum every 15 minutes.

33. (2) Early deceleration of the fetal heart rate produces a uniform pattern, the shape of which reflects the uterine pressure curve. The pattern is thought to be due to application of mechanical forces of uterine contractions to the fetal head by the dilating cervix. This pattern is not associated with fetal distress.

34. (2) During transition the woman needs to be reminded that this is the hardest but also the shortest period of labor. It is time limited, and relief occurs with complete dilation.

35. (2) Engagement of the fetal head eliminates a space for the umbilical cord to slip downward.

36. (3) The 1st stage of labor, the stage of dilation, begins with the onset of regular uterine contractions and ends with the complete dilation of the cervix.

37. (3) Cervical dilation is measured in centimeters, from 0 to 10. The completely dilated cervix is 10 cm.

38. (3) Contractions of prolonged duration (over 90 seconds), constant with no interval or relaxation phase, or of extreme tonus are abnormal and should be reported to the physician.

39. (2) During the 2nd stage the woman bears down with uterine contractions to provide intra-abdominal pressure to aid in the expulsion process.

40. (2) Engagement indicates that the fetal presenting part has traversed the pelvic inlet and has settled into the midpelvis.

41. (2) Position refers to the more specific relationship of the presenting part to the maternal pelvis. This relationship is the point on the presenting part that is being directed to the front, back, or left and right sides of the maternal passage.

42. (2) In addition to an increase in blood pressure, respiratory rate is altered and usually increased between contractions.

43. (3) Fetal heart rate must be carefully monitored during the 2nd stage. During the early 2nd stage, auscultation should occur at least every 15 minutes. As the 2nd stage advances, fetal heart rate should be assessed after every contraction.

44. (1) Molding is the overlapping of the bones of the skull and the narrowing of sutures caused by normal compression during delivery to accomodate passage through the birth canal.

45. (3) The mother should not be left unattended if delivery is near. The nurse should call for help, instruct the patient not to push, and slowly deliver the head between contractions.

46. (2) The occiput anterior position occurs most often, since 97% of presentations are vertex, and the left occiput anterior position is more common than the right.

47. (3) The stage of expulsion or delivery begins with the complete dilation of the cervix and ends with the birth of the baby.

48. (3) Apgar scoring indicates whether or not resuscitative measures are required. A score of 7 to 10 is vigorous, and the babies usually cry soon after birth; a score of 4 to 6 is depressed, some resuscitative measures are required; 0 to 3, severely depressed, resuscitative measures are required.

49. (4) Apgar scoring is the evaluation of 5 vital signs; heart rate, respiratory rate, muscle tone, reflex irritability, and color. Scores of 0, 1, or 2 are given to each vital sign for a total of 10. Since the infant showed acrocyanosis, a score of 1 not 2 was given for color, for a total score of 9.

50. (1) The infant is wet, and delivery rooms are usually cool, resulting in heat loss from the infant through conduction, convection, and radiation. Placing her in a heated crib decreases heat loss, and the Trendelenburg position is used to facilitate drainage.

51. (2) Silver nitrate is an anti-infective agent and is used to prevent development of gonorrheal conjunctivitis in the newborn.

52. (3) Vitamin K is necessary for blood coagulation. The newborn has a transitory deficiency in the ability of the blood to clot. Bacteria are necessary for the production of vitamin K in the intestines, and bacteria are not present in sufficient numbers in the newborn until several days after birth.

53. (4) Caput succedaneum is edema of the soft tissues of the scalp due to the difference in pressure on the scalp between those tissues directly against cervix and those that lie on the dilated portion of cervix.

54. (4) Normal respiratory rate in infants is between 30 and 50. Above or below that rate indicates respiratory distress.

55. (1) Normal cardiac rate in an infant is between 120 and 160. It may drop down to 100 when the child is resting and up to 180 when he is crying. Above or below that rate indictes a cardiac or circulatory problem.

56. (4) The newborn's liver is immature; consequently, it cannot conjugate bilirubin (bind it to glucuronic acid), in order to excrete it from the body.

57. (1) The eyes of the infant are covered with patches during treatment because of the possibility of damage to the retina.

58. (4) Physiological jaundice appears as the bilirubin level in the blood rises. As liver function increases, bilirubin is excreted, and blood levels of bilirubin go down.

59. (2) The infant usually loses 5 to 10% of his weight after birth due to excess loss of fluids from body tissues and relatively low fluid intake. Infant usually regains weight in 10 to 14 days.

60. (4) This is an example of a congenital abnormality and does not fall into the category of a disorder of protein (abnormal or missing enzyme that interferes with metabolism).

61. (2) The infant with hyperbilirubinemia usually has an excessive breakdown of red blood cells, resulting in pallor. Flushing is usually not observed as part of this syndrome.

62. (1) Rh antigens from the fetus enter the blood stream of the mother, inducing the production of anti-Rh antibodies in the mother. These anti-Rh antibodies cross the placenta, enter the fetal circulation, and cause hemolysis. The red blood cells are destroyed and broken down faster than the products of hemolysis, including bilirubin, can be excreted. Serum bilirubin level rises quickly.

63. (1) ABO incompatibility occurs more frequently and is always considered less severe for the neonate than Rh incompatibility.

64. (3) Intermittent positive-pressure breathing (IPPB) therapy is prescribed in respiratory conditions when the infant is having difficulty with O_2-CO_2 exchange.

65. (2) RhoGAM (immune Globulin) should be given after an abortion, since fetal blood may enter the mother's circulation and set up a sensitization process.

66. (3) Constipation is rarely a problem in the newborn. Diarrhea would more likely be the result of sepsis.

67. (3) Your responsibility is to clarify her understanding of the meaning of the term functional heart murmur and to allay her fears.

68. (2) The infant of a diabetic mother may develop sepsis, but usually from a cause unrelated to the diabetes itself. Infants of diabetic mothers are prone to develop hypoglycemia, respiratory distress, and hypocalcemia. Hyperbilirubinemia is also fairly common in these infants.

69. (1) Glucose of the diabetic mother passes into the baby's blood stream keeping the blood glucose level high. The elevated blood glucose level in the infant exaggerates certain metabolic functions, resulting in increased storage of glycogen and fat.

70. (4) Infants with signs and symptoms of hypoglycemia usually have a high-pitched cry, not a weak soft cry.

71. (2) Administration of glucose usually establishes normal glucose blood levels in the newborn.

72. (1) Infants born to mothers with drug addictions are hyperirritable, and care should be planned so as not to constantly stimulate the infants. When held, the infants should be wrapped snugly in blankets and held close to the body.

73. (4) RhoGAM (immune globulin) will not work if there is any titer in the mother's blood; thus, it is important to administer it within 72 hours after delivery or abortion if the mother shows no evidence of antibody production.

74. (3) The premature infant has poor control of temperature and needs immediate attention to keep from losing heat. Reasons for heat loss include little subcutaneous fat and poor insulation, large body surface for weight, immaturity of temperature control, and lack of activity.

75. (4) If temperature in Isolette is too high, the infant will have an elevated temperature and may have periods of apnea and may have increased need for oxygen or become dehydrated. If temperature in the Isolette is too cool the infant's temperature will drop, and the infant may have periods of apnea and he will develop cold stress and increased need for oxygen. Cold stress will increase metabolism and deplete glucose levels, not elevate glucose levels.

76. (1) It is important to provide nutrients to the infant and not deplete glucose stores, but other factors are more important in immediate assessment—cardiac, respiratory, temperature, and neurological status, and the presence of congenital abnormalities.

77. (1) An infant with respiratory distress will have an elevated respiratory rate to try to increase the intake of O_2 by his damaged lungs, which are not functioning properly. A respiratory rate between 30 and 40 is within the normal range. Cyanosis, expiratory grunt, and PCO_2 between 35 and 45 are all signs of respiratory distress.

78. (2) Blood samples are drawn to determine if the O_2 and CO_2 levels and pH are within normal range. The treatment given to the infant depends to a great extent upon these results. For example, if the blood PO_2 level is down and the PCO_2 is elevated, the concentration of PO_2 the infant is receiving will be increased, and the infant may be placed on CPAP or PEEP to increase re-

sidual capacity and improve oxygenation. Drugs such as sodium bicarbonate may be given to correct acidosis or a low pH. Normal values are pH, 7.35 to 7.45: Po_2, 40 to 60; Po_2, 35 to 45.

79. (2) Premature infants are prone to respiratory distress, because they are unable to produce surfactant, which leads to atelectasis. The alveoli and the thoracic cage and respiratory muscles are weak, so the infant cannot take in enough air on inspiration. Antibodies from the mother are not related to respiratory distress.

80. (4) The infant has a weak cough and gag reflex and has difficulty removing mucus. Should the bronchial secretions become dry, they become tenacious, almost impossible for the baby to bring up, and difficult to remove by aspiration. O_2 is very drying to the mucous membranes and should always be humidified while being given (whether to an infant or adult).

81. (2) High blood levels of O_2 cause spasms of the retinal vessels, and the destruction of these vessels can cause retrolental fibroplasia and blindness.

82. (1) Immaturity of the liver is responsible for hyperbilirubinemia but is not directly related to the infant acquiring an infection.

83. (3) Tap water is not used for aspiration. Sterile water should be used and changed at least once during each shift.

84. (1) *Vitamin K* (not Vitamin C) is administered after birth to aid in the clotting process.

85. (3) A regular nipple is too hard and will make it difficult for the infant to suck, causing unnecessary fatigue. A premie soft nipple should be used.

86. (2) It is important for the nurse to note the amount and color of urine excreted and to check its specific gravity when there is any question about the concentration. Fluids are usually administered at room temperature and include glucose (carbohydrate) as well as protein. The premature infant does not absorb fat well. Fluids are usually given routinely, but not on a forced fluid basis because it would be too fatiguing.

87. (1) At this time the nursing intervention that would be most helpful to Mrs. Gibson would be to be supportive by letting her cry and express her feelings about having the operation and being unable to have another child.

88. (2) Patients about to have surgery are usually kept NPO after midnight the day of surgery to prevent emesis and aspiration while under anesthesia and while recovering from anesthesia.

89. (3) After a hysterectomy, a patient is usually able to resume normal sexual relationships after 6 weeks provided healing has taken place and the physician says it is all right.

90. (4) Daily vaginal irrigations after a hysterectomy are usually contraindicated because of the danger of introducing microorganisms and infection into a new surgical area.

91. (3) A major complication of saline abortion is the introduction of the hypertonic solution into the patient's blood stream during the infusion. The symptoms to watch for are thirst, flushed face, headache, tachycardia, numbness, and tingling in extremities.

92. (4) After an abortion, there should be slight bleeding (about the same as for a menstrual period) for about 7 days. Any bright red bleeding after this time would indicate that the products of conception were probably not completely expelled.

93. (3) Following an abortion the patient may have feelings of remorse and guilt. It is important for the nurse to allow the patient to express these feelings openly. The nurse should be an active listener and not pass judgment.

94. (2) Teratogen is a term denoting "monster former" and rubella in the first trimester is known to produce "monster" babies. X-rays are also considered teratogens, but dental x-rays would not deliver a high roentgen dose.

95. (3) Diarrhea would cause excessive loss of fixed base from the body, which would lead to acidosis.

96. (3) Since the Warton's jelly expands as it contacts air, ligating blood vessels, there is no danger of hemorrhage. Cutting the cord under emergency conditions could lead to infection.

97. (2) Thirty weeks is past the legal time period to perform an abortion. The procedure should be done before 20 weeks so the fetus with Tay-Sachs disease can be aborted if the mother chooses to do so.

98. (4) Side effects may appear during the 1st few months while taking birth control pills owing to the hormonal influence. These side effects usually disappear after the 3rd month, as the body adjusts.

99. (1) Since the IUD may cause cramping and heavy bleeding the 1st few months after insertion, it is important that the client be thoroughly instructed in where the IUD is inserted, how it works, and common discomforts following its insertion. The client should also be instructed in how to feel the strings to determine if it is in place and that these strings will in no way interfere with intercourse.

100. (2) Contraceptive methods must be thoroughly understood if they are to be used properly and prevent pregnancy; both partners should be instructed.

UNIT II

Pediatric Nursing

Section

PEDIATRIC NURSING CONTENT OUTLINE

BASIC CONCEPTS

A. The child is an open system with the ability to adapt to change. The dynamics of nature and nurture influence that open system into a unique individual.
B. Each child has his own genetic potential for growth and development that can be modified at any stage.
C. The family bears primary responsibility for meeting the child's basic physiological needs. In addition, the family provides the means for socialization to enable the child to experience personal growth.
D. Maintenance of optimum physical, psychological, and social well-being is of prime importance during the child's growth.

THE FAMILY

A. The family functions as a unit within a society.
B. The functions and roles of families differ depending upon their structure, i.e., nuclear families, extended families, communal families, single-parent families, and dual-career families.
C. The function of the family is to provide protection, socialization, economic well-being, affection, recreation, religious values, and social placement.
D. All families have sets of norms and expectations that specify the behaviors of all its members.

PRINCIPLES OF GROWTH AND DEVELOPMENT

A. Growth and development are influenced by genetic and environmental factors.
B. Growth and development occur in an organized, predictable, and sequential manner that is largely determined by maturation and individual variation.
C. Physical development of the body occurs in a cephalocaudal pattern and in a proximodistal pattern.
D. Children are expected to perform certain age-appropriate developmental tasks during specific periods of growth. Innate temperamental char-

acteristics and family and environmental influences can affect the emergence of developmental tasks.

E. Developmental tasks must be completed or mastered before the child can proceed to the next stage.

THE INFANT

A. Physical Growth and Development

1. Infants can be expected to triple their weight and grow 10 in by the end of the 1st year of life.
2. The infant's head is larger in proportion to the rest of his body than that of the adult.
3. The infant's brain grows rapidly until about 2 years of age, at which time it is about ⅔ the adult size.
4. Eruption of 1st teeth takes place at about 6 or 7 months of age.
5. The muscles grow rapidly during the 1st year; the rate is about twice that of bones.
6. The infant's posterior soft palate is longer than that of the older child. This specific anatomy accommodates the infant's sucking and breathing activity.
7. Although the taste buds are developed at birth, taste discrimination is not fully developed until about 3 months of age.
8. At birth the infant responds to loud noise by startle reflex, but starting at approximately 3 months, the infant locates sound by turning the head toward the source of the sound.
9. Abdominal respirations continue throughout infancy (and through the preschool years), and the respirations slow down somewhat and become relatively stable.
10. Due to the anatomical structure of the infant's respiratory tract, the infant needs to breathe about twice as fast as the adult to provide the body with the required amount of O_2.
11. The chest circumference approximately equals head circumference by the end of the 1st year.
12. The heart rate slows down steadily throughout infancy, and the rhythm remains irregular. (This condition is normal among infants, whose cardiac rhythm is affected by respiration).
13. Digestive processes do not start functioning well until about the 3rd month; therefore, many solid foods are passed incompletely digested. By the end of the 1st year, the infant's stomach has sufficiently enlarged to permit 3 meals a day.
14. The entire immune capacity of the infant is immature, and in particular the gastrointestinal tract is immature, which predisposes the system to increased risk of infection and inflammation.
15. The kidneys do not reach complete maturity until the end of the 2nd year, predisposing the infant to dehydration.

B. Psychosocial Development

1. The degree to which infants are able to accomplish initial developmental tasks depends to a great degree upon how their needs have been met by caregivers.
2. Erikson's 1st stage of trust versus mistrust requires an infant to develop a sense of trust. Mistrust develops when trust-developing experiences are deficient or lacking.
3. Freud's oral dependent stage is described as the infant's getting pleasure from oral activities, such as sucking, eating, and rooting.
4. Play during infancy primarily revolves around the body, starting with the infant's fingers and hands at about 2 months of age and proceeding to his feet at about 6 months of age. An infant is a responsive social being, and as early as 6 to 8 weeks a social smile is present. By 3 months of age, he is ready to engage in active social "play" by showing excitement with a toy, demonstrating this excitement and happiness by squealing.
5. At around 8 to 9 months of age, the infant acquires mobility through crawling and gains his 1st experience of independence.
6. Infants are born with a preference for the human face, and by 6 months of age, they respond to facial expressions and can distinguish between familiar and strange faces.

C. Cognitive Development

1. Piaget's sensorimotor stage is seen first in the infant's cognitive development when the infant progresses from reflex behavior to simple repetitive acts to imitate activity.
2. The major milestone of infancy is the development of object permanence at approximately 4 months of age.

D. Health Maintenance and Promotion

1. Infants require regular appointments with health care providers for evaluation of physical growth, nutrition, sleep habits, elimination patterns, and parent-child interaction.
2. The first series of immunizations are completed during this period.
3. The nurse should make parents aware of sources of home accidents and the use of car seats.

THE TODDLER

A. Physical Growth and Development

1. Physiological growth and development slows considerably. Weight gain is 4 to 6 lb/year, and the increase in height is approximately 3 in. Head circumference is equal to chest circumference by 1 to 2 years of age.
2. Ordinarily, primary dentition should be completed by no later than 2½ years. Retarded eruption, however, is more common than accelerated eruption and may be caused by heredity or may indicate health problems, such as endocrine disturbances, nutritional factors, or malposition of teeth.
3. Although the normal heart rate for a toddler is around 110 beats per minute, fluctuation of heart rate during this period of perpetual activity is considered normal.
4. There is a steady increase in blood volume, and chemical components of the blood become stabilized at around 1 year of age.
5. Sensory apparatuses have now become increasingly well developed.
6. Maturation of the respiratory system lessens the risk of frequent infection experienced during infancy.
7. Stomach capacity and maturation of digestive processes now permit 3 meals a day, consisting of usual table foods.
8. With the proportional growth of the lower extremities and the slowing down of head circumference growth, the toddler begins to assume more adult-like proportions.
9. Motor control is still immature due to incomplete myelination of the spinal cord.
10. Toilet training has now become a possibility due to voluntary control of elimination.
11. The toddler experiences a great improvement in his immune system. His defense mechanisms, particularly phagocytosis, are much more efficient, and the production of antibodies is well established.

B. Psychosocial Development

1. According to Erikson, this is the stage of autonomy versus shame and doubt. Although the child strives for autonomy, he experiences a fear of separation.
2. Freud's anal stage includes the period from 18 months to 3 years of age. The anal zone becomes a source of pleasure to the toddler; consequently, he gains satisfaction from moving his bowels.
3. Increasing large and small muscle development enables toddlers to become relatively self sufficient in such tasks as eating, washing, dressing, and toileting.
4. The child learns the extent to which the environment can be influenced by direct manipulation.
5. Children between the ages of 1 and 3 years involve themselves in solitary or parallel play. All children engage in solitary play, and in parallel play there is psychological closeness, but there is still no direct interaction between children.

C. Cognitive Development

1. The toddler is completing the latter phase of the sensorimotor phase and entering the preconceptual phase. The child has acquired minimal ability to conceptualize and can begin to solve problems by mental trial and error as well as by being able to attend to more than one aspect of a situation at a time.
2. The child's thinking remains egocentric; he cannot see things from the point of view of others and thinks that all people think and feel the same way he thinks and feels.
3. There is magical thinking—the inability to distinguish fantasy from reality and the belief that he can cause things to happen.
4. Level of the child's language is closely associated with his cognitive development. Although language develops markedly during this period, toddlers differ in the speed of language acquisition.

5. Toddlers understand more words than they express; by 2 years of age, the child is able to use sentences of 2 to 3 words, and at 3 years of age, the child uses about 900 words.

D. Health Maintenance and Promotion

1. Accident prevention is critically important since accidents are the leading cause of death among toddlers.
2. The MMR (Measles, Mumps, Rubella) immunization is administered at 15 months of age.
3. Sleep disturbance is quite common owing to the high activity level, and if treated as a normal occurrence, the problem will resolve itself.
4. Toddlers generally have a full set of teeth by the time they are 2½ years old; dental examinations should begin at this time.

THE PRESCHOOLER

A. Physical Growth and Development

1. Height increases remain steady at 2½ to 3 in/year, and the average weight gain remains at 5 lb/year.
2. The child is usually slender with erect posture.
3. The face has a growth spurt downward and forward, giving the child a more mature appearance. By the age of 3 years, the child has 20 primary teeth; by the age of 5 years, the child has mixed dentition with 24 teeth.
4. The preschooler is capable of cooperation during dental examination; the majority of preschoolers have no cavities.
5. The chest becomes broader and flatter; there is a great increase in the child's respiratory ability and endurance.
6. Although the position of the heart now approximates that of the adult, arrhythmias are still normal.
7. Marked improvement is seen in the ability to control and coordinate the small and large voluntary muscles and to maintain visual attention. During the preschool years, the child begins to show a clear preference for the right or left hand.
8. Immunity to various microorganisms is developing due to the child's increasing exposure to a variety of illnesses. The lymph nodes, tonsils, adenoids, spleen, and thymus all increase in size in response to infection.
9. Because of the relatively small size of the bladder, the preschooler needs to empty his bladder 6 to 8 times a day; the total daily urine output is 600 to 750 ml.

B. Psychosocial Development

1. The child is in the period of initiative versus guilt. The child acquires a sense of initiative through work and play, but the child experiences a sense of guilt if he feels he has not acted appropriately.
2. The development of a conscience, or the understanding of right and wrong, is also acquired at this time.
3. Freud considers preschoolers to be in the oedipal stage. The child competes with the parent of the same sex for the attention of the parent of the opposite sex.
4. Peer group membership is loosely organized and changes frequently.
5. Although preschoolers vary in their reactions to separations from parents, most preschoolers have sufficient inner resources to enjoy activities with other caretakers.
6. Sometime around 4 years of age, most children stop napping on a regular basis. However, preschoolers who do not take naps still require 8 to 12 hours of sleep at night.
7. Although parallel play persists in preschoolers, the primary mode of play is dramatic play. Usually the dramatic play is based upon the child's actual experience, but sometimes the play is an attempt by the child to understand adult activities. Other typical preschooler plays are cooperative (or group play), associative, solitary independent, and onlooker.

C. Cognitive Development

1. According to Piaget, the preschooler is in the preoperational stage of cognitive development. This stage is divided into 2 phases: between 2 to 4 years, the preconceptual phase and between 4 to 7 years, the intuitive phase. The elements of the preconceptual phase are symbolism, ego-

centrism, transductive reasoning, and reality distortion. The elements of the intuitive phase are centration and the static and irreversible quality of thought.

2. The preschooler increases his vocabulary by about 600 words a year. These children talk constantly, exaggerate, and tend to boast. They constantly ask "why, what, when, where, and how" in order to understand the world around them.
3. A 4-year-old has some conception of time of day, and the 5-year-old usually knows the day, month, and year, in addition to having a sense of time.

D. Health Maintenance and Promotion

1. This preschool period is one of numerous acute illnesses, particularly upper respiratory infections (URI) and accidents. Parents need to be aware of prodromal signs of illnesses because children are too busy to complain of not feeling well.
2. The child should have an annual physical examination and immunization updating. Vision, dental, and developmental screenings should also be done.
3. Accidents continue to be the leading cause of death in this preschool age group. Parents must be made aware that most of these accidents are due to poor adult supervision.
4. The preschooler's appetite fluctuates from overeating to refusing to eat entirely. Parents need to avoid conflict with the child in regard to this fluctuation
5. Preschoolers generally "don't know when to quit" and expend huge amounts of energy. These periods of great activity should be alternated with periods of rest.
6. This age group varies in the amount of sleep needed from 8 hours a night to as much as 14 hours. Preschoolers are ritualistic about bedtime. Sticking to a routine and a specific hour for bedtime will promote better sleep patterns.
7. Because of improved motor skills, balance, and coordination, preschoolers experience fewer accidents while engaging in physical activities. On the other hand, preschoolers must now be taught safety procedures in regard to crossing the street, riding their tricycles, using playground equipment, and playing in the street.

THE SCHOOL-AGE CHILD

A. Physical Growth and Development

1. Physical growth in this group continues steadily and slowly. The average increase in height is 2½ to 3 in/year, and the average weight gain is 5 to 7 lb/year.
2. The child is now better coordinated, looks slimmer, and moves about with more control and precision.
3. Motor coordination is being continually refined and expanded, and although his muscle strength is not yet that of an adult, the child now has the stamina to remain active for a long period of time.
4. This period is an active time for dentition; the child should be seen regularly by a dentist.
5. Owing to increase in lung size, the school-age child tires much less easily.
6. The size of the heart increases, resulting in a more efficient transportation system within the body. The blood pressure slowly rises during childhood.
7. The immunoglobulin values gradually rise during this period, with the immunological functions reaching their peak.
8. The digestive process is almost fully mature by 6 years of age, with the stomach retaining food for a much longer period of time.
9. Children of both sexes begin to display many of the secondary sex characteristics.
10. The kidneys will mature completely during this time with average urinary output of 700 to 1500 ml/day.

B. Psychosocial Development

1. According to Erikson, the child at this age enters the stage of industry versus inferiority. The child tries to resolve feelings of inferiority by taking advantage of all opportunities to learn by doing. Tremendous amounts of time and energy are devoted to every conceivable type of activity, with a constant drive to succeed.
2. Self awareness, self worth, and self concept are now viewed by the child from a different perspective. Rather than from a self-centered focus, these concepts of self are perceived by seeing

himself as others see him. Peer groups have tremendous influence on the child in relation to the development of these concepts.

3. The child is now aware that he has control over his environment and is aware of different options available to him.
4. By 7 or 8 years of age, most children have communication skills close to an adult level.
5. During this school-age period, any new role or situation is experienced in a very rigid, precise way in order to successfully master any feelings of inferiority.
6. Bedtime rituals still continue, and unless the child becomes so obsessed that he is unable to sleep without them, these rituals are considered normal.
7. Play for the school-age child means he is a member of a group. The children interact through cooperative play in which the child learns to relinquish his own needs for the overall good of the team. Competitiveness, however, is decidedly strong among this group. Since children of school age generally feel that "winning is everything," tremendous amounts of energy are invested competing against each other.
8. Although the child now spends as much time in school as he does at home, he still periodically retreats to his family for emotional and moral support.
9. School-age children's consciences are puritanical and unbending; they actually judge themselves and one another more stringently than adults do, and the punishments they suggest are extremely severe.

C. Cognitive Development

1. The school-age child is in Piaget's phase of concrete operations; the child no longer has to touch or see an object in order to experience it. He is now able to understand and use principles of relationships between things and ideas; he can classify, use symbols, apply rules, and understand cause and effect. He is also beginning to use logic and is able to consider several points of view simultaneously.
2. Between 6 and 12 years of age, vocabulary doubles and articulation increases, with sentences becoming longer and more complex. Socialized speech becomes more frequent, as the child interacts more with other individuals.

D. Health Maintenance and Promotion

1. Motor vehicle accidents, both as a passenger and a pedestrian, are the most common cause of accidental injury and death among children between the ages of 6 and 12 years.
2. With the acquisition of the concept of death, school-age children commonly experience nightmares and sleep disturbances.
3. Tooth decay is a commonly neglected health problem among school-age children. Extra effort must be directed toward regular use of the toothbrush and periodic dental checkups.
4. With a decrease in rate of growth, caloric requirements per unit of body weight also decrease. Some children in this age group require careful food intake monitoring to prevent them from becoming overweight.
5. School-age children are generally agreeable about being responsible for their personal hygiene. Encouragement and praise for a good job in this regard will promote development of long range beneficial health habits.
6. Use of harmful drugs and cigarettes is a problem among school-age children in many parts of the United States. The dangers of indulging in these activities need to be stressed in the homes as well as in the schools.

THE ADOLESCENT

A. Physical Growth and Development

1. The physical growth spurt begins about 2 years prior to the maturing of the reproductive system. Growth spurts begin approximately 2 years earlier in girls than in boys: in girls, 8½ to 11½ years of age; and in boys, 10 to 15 years of age. During this growth spurt, the girl's average gain is 3 in and the boy's average gain is 8 in.
2. Dramatic musculoskeletal changes take place during adolescence; almost every part of the body is affected. The facial bones grow forward and lengthen, the shoulders broaden, the trunk lengthens, the legs lengthen, and the thighs widen. Amount of muscle mass and fat doubles,

with the female averaging twice as much fat as the male.

3. All of the organs of the body increase in size during this period, while the tissues of the immune system decrease in size.
4. Other adult norms reached by adolescence are visual and auditory acuities and the vital signs, such as pulse, respirations, and blood pressure.
5. Primary and secondary sex characteristics will have reached near maturation by 18 years of age (the entire process is not complete until about 21 years of age).

B. Psychosocial Development

1. According to Erikson, the adolescent has the task of establishing his identity or he will experience role diffusion. The adolescent has to determine a self identity that is personally acceptable to him; if he is not able to accomplish this task, he will experience role confusion and remain uncertain as to who he really is.
2. The adolescent's age mates or peers now exert strong influence upon his views, his thinking processes, and his ultimate decisions. Although parents remain the primary influence in his life, the adolescent feels compelled to free himself from family domination.
3. He is developing emotional independence from family members and is becoming socially responsible.
4. The adolescent is beginning to achieve mature sexual identity, i.e., understanding and acceptance of himself as a sexual individual.
5. The adolescent is gradually developing his own system of moral and ethical beliefs.
6. He is beginning to make career choices; many adolescents start to work part-time to gain some semblance of financial independence.

C. Cognitive Development

1. The adolescent acquires adult cognitive capacities as he enters Piaget's stage of formal operations. The adolescent is now capable of thinking hypothetically as well as thinking abstractly.
2. This ability to think abstractly enables him to view his role in life and the world in general in new ways. He can conceptualize various possibilities as well as project these possibilities into future experiences. These thought processes are based on logical principles; in other words, adolescents are dealing more with the realities of life.

D. Health Maintenance and Promotion

1. Mortality rates reach their lowest level during adolescence.
2. Accidents are the leading cause of death among adolescents; car accidents are the most common cause, with drowning the 2nd most common cause. Homicides and suicides are also responsible for a number of deaths among adolescents each year.
3. Although morbidity rates among adolescents are low, this group engages in practices that are detrimental to health. Drinking, smoking, eating junk food, and using controlled drugs are a few examples.
4. Dental care is notoriously neglected during adolescence despite the fact that this period constitutes the peak years for dental caries.
5. Adolescents need comprehensive sex education; both the number of sexually active teenagers and of teenage pregnancies have increased in recent years.

DISRUPTION OF REGULATORY INTEGRATIVE PROCESSES IN THE CHILD

Fluid and Electrolyte Disturbances

A. General Principles

1. Stress in itself can cause (and contribute to) fluid and electrolyte imbalance.
2. Total body water is separated into intracellular fluid and extracellular fluid; all fluids not contained in cells are extracellular.
3. There is a continual replacement and exchange of fluid and electrolytes between the intracellular and extracellular fluids.
4. Infants and young children have a greater need

for water and are more vulnerable to alterations in fluid and electrolyte balance for the following reasons:
   a. The infant's relatively greater surface area allows larger quantities of fluid to be lost in insensible perspiration through the skin.
   b. Rate of metabolism in infancy is significantly higher because of the larger surface area in relation to the mass of active tissue.
   c. Kidneys of the infant are functionally immature at birth and are, therefore, inefficient in excreting waste products of metabolism.
5. The need for fluid decreases proportionately throughout life.
6. Inter-relationships of many organ systems are involved in the regulation of fluid and electrolyte balance; the cardiovascular system, the respiratory system, the gastrointestinal system, the renal system, and the endocrine system are all involved.
7. In older children, a deficit in one system can be compensated for by a reserve capacity in another system. But in infants and young children, the malfunction of one system usually places such a strain on other organs that their reserve capacity is exceeded and homeostasis is impaired.
8. With the exception of newborns, under normal conditions the amount of water ingested closely approximates the amount lost by the body.
9. Water is normally lost through urine, feces, lungs, sweat, and insensible perspiration.
10. All the factors that contribute to the shift of fluids between plasma and interstitial fluids are referred to as "capillary dynamics."
11. Edema is essentially a problem in exchange of fluid between the plasma and the interstitial space, i.e., the capillary dynamics have become unbalanced.
12. The 3 main lines of defense against changes in pH of body fluids are as follows:
    a. The buffers present in the blood, such as carbonic acid, carbonates, bicarbonates, phosphates, and proteins.
    b. The respiratory system.
    c. The kidneys.
13. Laboratory data are absolutely essential to determine the nature and extent of acid-base disturbances.
14. The organ system that is most vulnerable to pH disturbance is the nervous system.
15. Infants through 2 years of age show lowered values for plasma bicarbonate, making them prone to development of acidosis.
16. Because electrolyte imbalances produce notably nonspecific symptoms, they can only be confirmed with laboratory data.
17. Serum electrolyte levels may vary from moment to moment and are therefore only rough indications of the total body concentration of ions.
18. The primary purposes for I.V. infusions are as follows:
    a. To keep the patient hydrated.
    b. To meet electrolyte needs.
    c. To modify pH.
    d. To meet basic nutritional needs.
19. The initial treatment of fluid and electrolyte imbalance should be most vigorous in the most severe imbalances. However, too rapid correction of an imbalance can produce new symptoms, which may be more devastating than the original ones.

B. Sources for Assessment Data

1. Skin and mucous membranes; level of hydration, color.
2. Urine output
3. Laboratory values
4. Vital signs and blood pressure
5. Weight comparison
6. Level of consciousness; behavior.

C. Clinical Manifestations

1. Dehydration
   a. Poor skin turgor and dry mucous membranes
   b. Depressed fontanelles in infants
   c. Decreased urine output
   d. Increased specific gravity, hematocrit value, serum osmolality concentration, and blood urea nitrogen (BUN) level.
   e. Increased pulse and respirations
   f. Weight loss
2. Extracellular Volume Excess
   a. Weight gain
   b. Increased blood pressure
   c. Edema, particularly periorbital.
   d. Pulmonary edema
   e. Tachycardia

Burns

A. General Information

1. Burns are tissue trauma caused by thermal, chemical, electrical, or radioactive agents. Most burns are caused by thermal agents.

2. The majority of burns among the pediatric population occur when adult supervision is lacking; approximately 75% of these cases are preventable.
3. In case of severe burns, every organ system of the body becomes involved.
4. The severity of the burn is assessed on the basis of the location of the burn, the depth, and the percentage of body surface involved.
5. Other factors influencing therapy and prognosis are as follows:
   a. Causative agent
   b. Age of child
   c. General health of child
   d. Respiratory involvement
   e. Other associated injury or condition
6. There are 2 ways of describing the characteristics of burns:
   a. 1st, 2nd, or 3rd degree
   b. Partial thickness or full thickness.
7. First degree or epidermal partial thickness involves the epidermis only. Although the burn can cause pain, no scars are left on the skin.
8. Second degree or partial thickness superficial burn involves all epidermal layers and some of the dermis; there is much pain as well as edema, but the burn leaves minimal or no scarring.
9. Second degree or partial thickness deep dermal burn extends deep into the dermis. The patient experiences little pain 1 or 2 days after injury; however, this type of burn heals more slowly, and scarring is common.
10. Third degree or full thickness burn destroys the entire skin and all its structures. Although there is little pain, skin grafting is necessary, and severe scarring (due to destruction of nerve endings), results.

B. Sources for Assessment Data

1. Skin—characteristics of burn, location, and percentage of body involved; subsequent infection.
2. Vital signs
3. Physical examination
4. Health history
5. Circulatory system—changes in plasma volume, hypertension.
6. Renal—decrease in urine output.
7. Laboratory reports—hematuria, elevated BUN levels, elevated creatinine and blood glucose levels.
8. Weight—gain with fluid shift immediately after burn.
9. Respiratory—possibility of smoke irritation, resulting in edema of respiratory tract.
10. Gastrointestinal system—stress ulcers and paralytic ileus.
11. Level of consciousness—seizures, personality changes, hallucinations, delirium, or coma.

C. Nursing Activities

1. For 1st and 2nd degree burns covering less than 10% of the body, the immediate treatment is to immerse the burn area into cold water until pain subsides. After cleansing with mild soap, use over-the-counter burn ointment with light bandaging. However, if the burn involves more than 10% of total body surface, a physician should be consulted regarding medication to be used.
2. All children under 2 years of age who suffer burns and all children who suffer burns that cover more than 10% of the body should receive immediate medical attention; hospitalization may be necessary
3. For major burns, 3 immediate interventions are as follows:
   a. Maintain adequate airway.
   b. Start fluid therapy.
   c. Institute burn care.
4. Maintain isolation techniques to prevent local as well as systemic infections.
5. Monitor child's diet to make certain adequate protein and calories are provided.
6. Be alert for complications
   a. Renal and cardiac failure
   b. Fluid overload
   c. Stress ulcers and paralytic ileus
   d. Respiratory failure
7. Offer psychological support to child and family.
8. Prepare for discharge planning
   a. Multidisciplinary support
   b. Teaching
   c. Clinic visits
   d. Rehabilitative follow-up care
   e. Community support groups
   f. Possible visiting nurse arrangnements

Renal Disorders

A. General Information

1. The primary function of the kidney is to maintain the volume and composition of the body fluids at a constant level, i.e., to excrete urine and to help regulate the water, electrolyte, and acid-base content of the blood.

2. Normal kidneys are able to adjust the urine and solute excretion in response to the requirements for body water and electrolyte balance. They excrete or conserve both water and most electrolytes in addition to excreting end products of protein metabolism, primarily urea.
3. The blood supply to the kidneys constitutes about ⅕ of the total cardiac output.
4. Filtration of the kidneys takes place as long as the hydrostatic pressure within the glomerular capillaries exceeds the opposing colloidal osmotic pressure of the plasma protein.
5. Glomerular filtration rate reaches adult values at about 2 years of age, and the concentrating ability reaches adult values at about 3 months of age. Specifically, the normal range for urine specific gravity for newborns and infants is 1.001 to 1.020. Thereafter, the normal range is between 1.001 and 1.030.
6. Kidney or urinary tract problems change with the age and maturation of the child.
7. The majority of causes of glomerular kidney dysfunction in childhood are the following:
   a. Acute post-streptococcal glomerulonephritis
   b. Idiopathic nephrotic syndrome
8. Approximately 80% of minimal change nephrotic syndrome cases in children are idiopathic; the peak age of onset is between 2 and 3 years of age.
9. The precise pathophysiology of nephrotic syndrome is unknown, but there is an increased permeability of the glomerular membrane, resulting in proteinuria. Loss of protein in the urine decreases the colloidal osmotic pressure in the capillaries, resulting in increased hydrostatic pressure that in turn forces plasma into the interstitial spaces and body cavities.
10. Nephrotic syndrome is characterized as congenital, secondary, or idiopathic.
    a. Congenital—autosomal recessive. Infants are usually small for gestational age (SGA). Proteinuria with edema manifests early, and there is an uncertainty regarding possible mortality within the 1st year or 2.
    b. Secondary—secondary to glomerular damage caused by various insults to the kidneys, such as acute or chronic glomerulonephritis, collagen diseases, and drug toxicity.
    c. Idiopathic or minimal change nephrotic syndrome; usually preceded by a viral URI.
11. Diagnosis of nephrotic syndrome is based upon consistent history, proteinuria, and typical clinical manifestations.
12. In the majority of cases, etiology can be established for acute glomerulonephritis, i.e., an immune complex disease following a *Streptococcus* infection with a latent period of about 10 days.
13. In acute glomerulonephritis, glomerular function is impaired by swelling and appearance of immune complex nodules on the basement membrane of the glomeruli, resulting in both water and sodium retention causing generalized edema.
14. Hypertensive encephalopathy and acute cardiac and renal failures are the major complications during the acute phase of glomerulonephritis.

B. Sources for Assessment Data

1. Physical examination
2. Health history
3. Laboratory reports
   a. Urine quality and output
      (1.) Decreased, dark and frothy, proteinuria with hyaline casts, oval fat bodies, and red blood cells.
      (2.) High specific gravity
   b. Blood—elevated serum cholesterol level with lowered serum sodium level.
4. Weight—increased owing to systemic edema.
5. Edema—progressive on face, eyelids, abdomen, lower extremities, labia, and scrotum.
6. Respiratory—dyspnea with pleural effusion.
7. Gastrointestinal—edema of gastrointestinal system causes diarrhea, anorexia, and disruption of intestinal absorption.
8. Hair—poor quality due to malnourishment.
9. Integument—skin pallor and tendency toward breakdown.
10. Disposition—irritable, fatigable, and lethargic.
11. X-rays—enlarged kidney or bladder or both reported.
12. Renal biopsy report.
13. Input and output.
14. Appetite—anorexic, vomiting.

C. Nursing Activities

1. Monitor input and output closely along with daily weight to evaluate fluid retention closely; assess degree of edema daily.
2. Watch for and prevent skin breakdown during edematous stage by encouraging frequent position changes.
3. Because of susceptibility to infection during edematous stage and during steroid treatment, maintain extra protection against any type of infection.

4. Offer nutritious and attractive diet that is high in protein.
5. Encourage appropriate play and recreational activities, depending on child's fatigue level.
6. Institute discharge planning, which is primarily teaching patient and family about medication and its side effects, urinalysis, prevention of infection, signs of relapse, and clinic or physician follow-up visits.

Sickle Cell Anemia

A. General Information

1. Sickle cell anemia is a chronic, genetically transmitted, hemolytic anemia in which normal hemoglobin A is replaced by an abnormal hemoglobin. The basic defect occurs in the hemoglobin molecule. The amino acid glutamine is replaced by another amino acid, valine, in the beta-polypeptide chain.
2. Sickle cell anemia is found predominantly, but not exclusively, in the black race. In the United States, 1 of 450 to 500 black babies are born with sickle cell anemia, and 1 of 8 to 10 black babies are born with sickle cell trait.
3. In the homozygous state (the child inherits hemoglobin S [HbS] from both parents), the child has sickle cell disease; in the heterozygous state (the child inherits HbS from only one parent), the child will be a trait carrier. The child with sickle cell anemia may experience varying degrees of vaso-occlusive crisis; the child who is a trait carrier may experience minimal symptoms to no symptoms during his lifetime. In addition to vaso-occlusive crisis, other crises, although infrequent, are seen in children with sickle cell disease. The other types of crises are splenic sequestration, aplastic crisis, and hyperhemolytic crisis.
4. Symptoms of vaso-occlusive crisis usually appear around the 1st birthday, as there is a rapid decrease in the amount of HbF and a reciprocal increase in the amount of HbS. These crises occur when O_2 in the blood decreases, and the abnormal hemoglobin forms crystalline-like structures, deforming the cells into the characteristic sickle shape. As the sickling progresses, the blood flow becomes sluggish owing to the "log-jamming" caused by deformed red blood cells. The occlusion causes further anoxia and more sickling. The resulting ischemia produces infarction in the surrounding organs and tissues, swelling, and extreme pain.
5. Sickling usually affects the joints, extremities, spleen, liver, lungs, kidneys, and bones.
6. Although a mild crisis can be managed at home, a severe crisis requires hospitalization. Treatment consists chiefly of supportive care—rest, I.V. fluids, and analgesics.
7. There is no cure for sickle cell anemia at this time.

B. Sources for Assessment Data

1. Physical examination—many children with sickle cell anemia are described as having barrel-shaped chests, enlarged protruding abdomens, and thin extremities. As a group, these children weigh less, are shorter with thinner body build, and experience delayed sexual maturity.
2. Medical history—both parents carry the sickle gene. The child could have experienced his first sickle cell crisis, "the hand and foot syndrome," when he was between 6 months and 1 year of age.
3. The older child may have other complaints such as back, abdominal, and joint pain, fever, weakness, and anorexia.
4. Laboratory reports
   a. Hemoglobin electrophoresis is a specific test that detects the homozygous and heterozygous forms of the disease as well as the percentage of the various hemoglobins.
   b. Sickledex—with the presence of HbS, the solution becomes turbid. However, it is not specific for the disease or the trait but is frequently used as a screening tool.

C. Nursing Activities

1. During acute phases of crisis, monitor I.V. administration and support appropriate maximum hydration.
2. Recognize the severity of pain, and give analgesics promptly.
3. Institute all protection measures to prevent further infection.
4. Give emotional support to child and family. Because of its genetic etiology, many parents react to their production of a child with sickle cell anemia with anger, guilt, and frustration.
5. Teach steps to prevent the further occurrence of crisis. On the other hand, support the child's desire for a "normal life."

β-Thalassemia

A. General Information

1. β-Thalassemia is a severe hemolytic anemia that is associated with impaired production of β-chains in the hemoglobin molecule. The homozygous state or thalassemia major is a serious life-threatening disease, but in the heterozygous state or thalassemia minor, the child could either be asymptomatic or experience mild anemia.
2. This disorder is found primarily in persons of Mediterranean descent, especially Italians, Sicilians, and Greeks, but cases occur in most racial groups. In the United States, there are approximately 650 to 700 thalassemic patients; β-thalassemia is found in up to 1% of black Americans.
3. Transmission of the defective hemoglobin is through the autosomal recessive mode.
4. Treatment—a program of routine red blood cell transfusion is instituted to maintain hemoglobin levels above 9 gm/dl.
   a. At these levels, the children show normal prepubertal growth, decreased enlargement of spleen and liver, and do not develop disfiguring facies.
   b. Older children reach a peak requirement of 500 ml of packed cells every 2 to 3 weeks.
   c. Although this program enables children to experience fairly normal lifestyles, the incidence of transfusion complications increases with the frequency of transfusions.
5. Even in the case in which the child is routinely transfused, splenomegaly is the usual finding in thalassemia major. Often the transfusion requirement increases as the spleen enlarges. Eventually, a splenectomy may be necessary, resulting in the child's being highly susceptible to overwhelming infection, especially from pneumococcus, *Haemophilus influenzae*, and meningococcus.
6. Ultimately, the resulting toxicities of chronic iron overload are the cause of death for most of these patients. Hemochromatosis or excess iron stored in body tissues results from the increased hemolysis of transfused erythrocytes.
7. There is no cure for β-thalassemia at this time.

B. Sources for Assessment Data

1. Physical examination
   a. In an untreated child, as a response to hypertrophy of erythropoietic tissue, there will be an overgrowth of the facial bones and the upper jaw, resulting in Cooley's facies.
   b. There will be hepatosplenomegaly and a brownish bronze hue to the skin from the systemic iron overload.
   c. There will be cardiac decompensation and poor growth.
2. Medical History
   a. Racial descent is from some country adjacent to or near to the Mediterranean Sea, with a possible history of thalassemia in the family.
   b. The child is usually irritable, anorexic, and weak.
3. Laboratory report
   a. The untransfused child with thalassemia major usually has a hemoglobin level of less than 5 gm/dl by the end of the 2nd year of life.
   b. The red blood cells reflect severe microcytosis (small in size) and hypochromia (reduced hemoglobin content).
   c. The peripheral blood smear shows many bizarre shaped cells (poikilocytosis).

C. Nursing Activities

1. Encourage out-patient treatment for transfusions to decrease necessity for hospitalization.
2. Observe for complications of blood transfusion; carry out transfusion protocol meticulously.
3. Give emotional support to child and family to deal with a disorder that, in all probability, will end in death.

Hemophilia

A. General Information

1. The term hemophilia is used to describe coagulation disorders of the blood. The 2 most common are hemophilia A in which factor VIII is present but is defective, and hemophilia B in which factor IX is defective or deficient.
2. Hemophilia is characterized by greatly prolonged coagulation time; the blood fails to clot owing to deficiencies of the factors in plasma necessary for coagulation.
3. Hemophilia is caused by a sex-linked hereditary trait, being transmitted by normal heterozygous females who carry the recessive gene. It occurs almost exclusively in males.
4. The degree of factor deficiency is directly related to the tendency to bleed.

5. The classic sign of the disorder, besides a prolonged coagulation time, is the tendency to bleed into joints, muscles, and body cavities. Bleeding is characterized as a prolonged oozing, occurring spontaneously in severe cases or after surgery or trauma.
6. Although the clinical manifestations are similar in hemophilia A and B, different factor deficiencies require treatment with those specific missing factors. The primary therapy for hemophilia is preventing spontaneous bleeding by replacing missing factors.
7. Once the child becomes ambulatory, his play activities have to be carefully supervised because of the possibility of bleeding with any trauma.
8. Initial symptoms of hemorrhage into the joint or muscle are pain and stiffness. Immediate factor injection should stop the hemorrhage. With extensive hemorrhage into a joint, aspiration may be necessary.

B. Sources for Assessment Data

1. History
   a. A male predecessor with hemophilia may be identified in the family.
   b. The mother may be aware that she is a hemophilia carrier.
2. History and physical examination
   a. A child with mild factor deficiency may have essentially little or no difference in findings from that of a normal child with the exception of, perhaps, a slightly longer period of time necessary for bleeding to stop.
   b. A child with moderate factor deficiency may have had several episodes of mild subcutaneous, intramuscular, and joint hemorrhages but no residual deformities.
   c. A child with severe factor deficiency may have numerous episodes of subcutaneous, intramuscular, and joint hemorrhages from traumas and spontaneous bleedings.
   d. There are various degrees of joint deformities.
   e. Periodic hematuria.
3. Laboratory findings
   a. All platelet function test results are normal.
   b. In blood clotting mechanism tests, those that depend upon specific factors for reactions show deficiencies.

C. Nursing Activities

1. In case of bleeding
   a. For superficial abrasions and cuts, apply firm pressure for several minutes to stop bleeding.
   b. For larger injuries or spontaneous bleeds, administer deficient factor.
   c. Apply ice pack, raise affected area, splint area involved, and institute bed rest.
   d. After all swelling has subsided, exercise of the affected joints should follow in order to prevent stiffness and contractures.
2. Teach older children and family members factor replacement procedures. Remind them of absolute necessity for observing sterile technique and total compliance.
3. Older children should be encouraged to become independent and responsible for their own care. They should be encouraged to engage in noncontact sports; well-programmed physical activities are encouraged in order to strengthen muscles and joints.
4. Assist the child as well as family members to cope with a life-long problem that, although incurable, is controllable.
5. Introduce child and family to various support groups in the community.

Leukemia

A. General Information

1. Leukemia is a primary disorder of bone marrow, a blood forming tissue, in which normal blood cells in the marrow are replaced by immature cells (blast cells) as a result of an unrestricted proliferation of leukocytes. These immature blast cells accumulate in the marrow, inhibiting the production of other cells such as the erythrocytes or platelets. The inconsistency here is that in the acute form, the leukocyte count is low. The low count results from immaturity of these cells. These leukocytes are identified as "blasts" rather than as mature leukocytes, owing to their immaturity.
2. The 2 most common leukemias in pediatrics are acute lymphocytic leukemia (ALL) and acute myelocytic leukemia (AML). The peak age for ALL is between 2 and 5 years, and AML usually occurs in older children.
3. Clinical manifestation depends upon the amount of bone marrow compromise and the extent of infiltration. Diagnosis is sometimes difficult because symptoms are frequently non-specific and suggestive of other childhood diseases.
4. The 3 main consequences of bone marrow suppression are anemia from decreased erythrocytes, secondary infections from leukopenia (abnormal decrease of white corpuscles), and bleeding tendencies from thrombocytopenia (abnormal decrease in the number of blood platelets). These

3 problems are the basis of nursing care in leukemia:
   a. Anemia—priority nursing responsibility for anemia is to minimize tissue O_2 needs. The nurse anticipates activities that are physically tiring to the child and allows for conservation of energy by assisting the child as needed. The most sensible approach would be to permit the child to regulate his activity with reasonable supervision by the nurse.
   b. Secondary infection—the most effective action against infection is prevention. During hospitalization, the child is placed in a private room, if not in protective isolation. Potential sites of infection, such as mucosal ulcerations, minor abrasions, and needle punctures, are carefully examined. Exposure to all individuals with active infections is restricted, meticulous hand washing is observed, and adequate nutrition is maintained.
   c. Bleeding tendencies—the nurse's primary responsibility in this regard is to monitor the child's susceptibility to bleeding. The child should be examined periodically for bruising and petechiae, his platelet count should be followed, and his urine and stools should be regularly checked for blood. In addition, a soft bristle toothbrush or a sponge should be used for cleaning teeth, and forceful nose blowing should be avoided. Any product that contains aspirin should be avoided, since aspirin destroys platelets.
5. The 3 most important factors that could determine the survival period are the patient's age at diagnosis, the initial white blood cell count, and the predominant cell type of the disease.
6. The goal of treatment through radiation and chemotherapy is to reduce the number of leukemia cells and allow the return of normal bone marrow productivity. It usually takes about 4 weeks for a remission to occur. Children can remain in remission for an indefinite period of time.
7. The most frequently used drugs for treatment are prednisone and vincristine. Medications are usually discontinued after 2 or 2½ years of remission.
8. Relapse occurs when the drugs being used are no longer effective and abnormal cells reappear. After each relapse, each remission becomes shorter and shorter until death occurs.
9. In addition to radiation and chemotherapy, transfusion of packed red blood cells may be necessary for the treatment of anemia, and transfusion of platelets may be necessary for the treatment of thrombocytopenia.
10. The majority of leukemic deaths are due to massive infections and hemorrhage as the result of depressed bone marrow and thrombocytopenia.

B. Sources for Assessment Data

1. Medical history
   a. Complaints of headache, vomiting, irritability, and lethargy could result from increased intracranial pressure due to invasion of arachnoid by proliferating cells.
   b. Complaints of bone and joint pain are caused by pressure of leukemic cells invading periosteum.
   c. Frequent epistaxis due to inhibition of platelets in marrow.
   d. Abdominal pain due to immunosuppression; normal flora causes inflammation of intestinal tract.
2. Physical examination
   a. Petechiae and bruising due to decreased platelet production.
   b. Anemia with pallor due to decreased erythrocyte production in marrow.
   c. Weakness in lower extremities caused by infiltration of spinal nerve.
   d. Hepatosplenomegaly results from infiltration and damage caused by chemotherapeutic agents.
   e. Muscle wasting, weight loss, and fatigue from tremendous increase in metabolic need of the body, which is attempting to resist leukemic cell proliferation.
3. Laboratory findings
   a. Hemoglobin level and hematocrit value decrease owing to inhibition of erythrocyte production.
   b. Complete blood count and platelet count are decreased owing to inhibition of all normal cells in marrow.
   c. Peripheral blood smear shows immature leukocytes.
   d. Bone marrow aspiration—product is hypercellular with greatly elevated number of blast cells. Differentiation can be made between ALL and AML. Definitive diagnosis is based on bone marrow aspiration.
   e. Lumbar puncture is performed to examine cerebral spinal fluid for leukemic cells.
   f. I.V. pyelogram is done to assess function of the kidneys before starting chemotherapy.
   g. Long bone surveys are made to determine degree of leukemic cell proliferation.
   h. Uric acid output is increased in leukemia; reflects status of disease.

C. Nursing Activities

1. Upon admission to the hospital, carefully explain to patient and family the tests and treatment procedures planned.
2. Explain protocols of chemotherapy to child and family and some of the side effects, i.e., alopecia, oral lesions, nausea, and so forth.
3. During chemotherapy
   a. Give careful oral hygiene, especially if there are oral lesions and gingival bleeding.
   b. Make certain child is encouraged to take high protein, high caloric diet.
   c. Assess anal area frequently to detect first signs of lesion.
   d. No rectal temperatures taken or suppositories inserted.
   e. If child is on vincristine, take measures to prevent constipation.
   f. Change child's position frequently; use sheep skin blanket to avoid skin breakdown.
   g. Protect child from infection by
      (1.) Placing him in a private room.
      (2.) Thorough and frequent hand washing
      (3.) Avoiding contact with individuals with colds.
   h. Examine entire body frequently for signs of hemorrhage, ecchymosis, and petechiae.
4. Provide emotional support to child and family who are going through an extremely stressful experience.

Meningitis

A. General Information

1. Meningitis is an infection of the meninges, which include the pia mater, the arachnoid, and the dura mater.
2. Meningitis is caused by bacteria, viruses, fungi, yeasts, or any other organisms that reach the meninges. Meningitis is usually secondary to another infection; from a limited condition, such as sinusitis or otitis media; or from a more significant infection involving the heart or lungs. Pathogens can also be introduced into the meninges through head trauma, lumbar puncture, or surgical procedures.
3. Acute bacterial meningitis is an emergency that requires early recognition and prompt medical management to prevent death and avoid residual neurological disabilities.
4. The majority of cases of meningitis occur in children under 15 years of age, and of those who recover, 15 to 20% experience some degree of neurological damage.
5. Analysis of cerebral spinal fluid is essential for a definitive diagnosis. All children with suspected meningitis should be isolated until the pathogen is identified since *Haemophilus influenzae* and meningococcus are contagious at this time. If either of these is identified as the pathogen, family members should receive chemoprophylaxis.
6. Because of the possibility of serious neurological damage, all cases of meningitis are immediately treated with antibiotics until the exact pathogen is identified. Drugs chosen for intravenous therapy are ampicillin and gentamycin for newborns, and ampicillin or penicillin G for all other children. These drugs are continued for 10 days or until the cerebral spinal fluid findings are normal.

B. Sources for Assessment Data

1. Medical history
   a. Newborns and premature infants—irritability, poor feeding, and possible diarrhea and vomiting.
   b. Infants and young children—irritability, poor feeding, vomiting, fever, and high pitched cry; possibility of seizures.
   c. Older children and adolescents—abrupt onset of illness with chills, fever, headache, vomiting, and confusion. Could be irritable and agitated or drowsy and stuporous. History of mild URI or GI symptoms.
2. Physical examination
   a. Newborns and premature infants—several days after birth, display lack of movement, poor muscle tone, and weak cry. There are respiratory irregularities or apnea, jaundice or cyanosis, and there may or may not be a bulging fontanelle; the neck is supple.
   b. Infants and young children—nuchal rigidity may or may not be present; bulging fontanelle is significant finding.
   c. Older children and adolescents—nuchal rigidity progressing to opisthotonos. Positive Brudzinski's and Kernig's signs; reflex responses are usually hyperactive. With meningococcal infection, petechial or purpuric rashes (or both) and arthralgia.
   d. Cranial nerve function—extension of infection to areas of cranial nerve may cause blindness, deafness, and weakness or paralysis of facial or other muscles of head and neck.

e. Other signs of increased intracranial pressure—papilledema, slowed pulse rate, altered respiratory pattern, and increased blood pressure.
f. Sensorium—aggressive behavior, seizures, or coma due to meningeal irritation, which affects normal neurological functioning.
3. Laboratory findings
   a. Cerebral spinal fluid
      (1.) Usually shows an elevated white blood cell count.
      (2.) Glucose level, is reduced (amount of reduction reflects severity of infection).
      (3.) Can determine the presence and type of bacteria within 24 to 48 hours.
      (4.) Virus identification takes several weeks.
   b. Blood culture (before administration of medication)—occasionally results prove positive when cerebral spinal fluid culture results prove negative.
   c. Nose and throat cultures (before medication) may provide helpful information in some cases.

C. Nursing Activities

1. In all probability, a lumbar puncture will be done soon after admission if one was not done in the emergency room.
   a. Explain procedure and the necessity for the test to family and patient, if appropriate.
   b. Restrain child properly to prevent trauma.
   c. Maintain child in prone position for 2 to 3 hours to prevent leakage of fluid into the subarachnoid space.
2. Place child in isolation until specific pathogen is identified; if the pathogen is meningococcus, the child will remain in isolation.
3. Support parents and give them as much information as possible at this time. The child is critically ill, possibly comatose or suffering seizures.
4. Continual neurological assessment, including pupillary reaction and level of consciousness, is essential to identify increased intracranial pressure.
5. Monitor respiratory status frequently, and observe for signs of impending septic shock. Anticipate respiratory irregularity due to cerebral edema.
6. Precise monitoring of input and output—although maintenance of hydration is of prime concern, cerebral edema with increased intracranial pressure is a definite possibility; therefore, fluid intake has to be measured meticulously to prevent overhydration.
7. Take temperature every 4 hours to monitor effectiveness of antibiotics; temperature should return to normal within 24 to 48 hours.
8. Take seizure precautions at bedside, since seizure activities occur in 30% of meningitis cases due to cerebral edema or subdural effusion.
9. As child's condition improves, special attention will have to be paid to immobilization of I.V. site; I.V. medication continues for 10 days or more, and a young child will find it difficult to be restrained for this long a period. Plan bedside games and other appropriate diversional activities. Encourage parents to continue support of child.
10. Prepare for discharge. Teach parent about possible long-term neurological impairment; the child's growth and development should be evaluated periodically.
11. Make referrals to an outreach team or a public health agency.

Brain Tumors

A. General Information

1. A brain tumor is a spontaneous new growth of tissue forming an abnormal mass; the growth develops independent of and unrestrained by normal laws of growth and morphogenesis.
2. Although brain tumors are found at any age, the peak incidence is during the early school-age years.
3. About ⅔ of brain tumors in infants and children occur in the infratentorial area, primarily in the cerebellum and brain stem. The remaining ⅓ are located mainly in the cerebrum.
4. Brain tumors are not easy to diagnose in children because the early symptoms are associated with other childhood problems.
5. A CAT scan has major advantages over other tests because it is noninvasive and indicates the exact location of tumors. With the development of the CAT scan, invasive tests, such as the brain scan, cerebral angiography, and dye injection, are now rarely used.
6. Definitive diagnosis is based on tissue reports from the laboratory.
7. The ideal treatment for brain tumor is surgical excision without residual neurological damage. Surgery is frequently followed by chemotherapy when the tumor proves to be malignant.

8. Despite surgery and radiation therapy, most childhood brain tumors will regrow and eventually become fatal.

B. Sources for Initial Assessment Data

1. Medical history
   a. Headache—more profound in the morning and may be accompanied by vomiting, with or without nausea; improves during the day.
   b. Vomiting—upon awakening in the morning and could become projectile with increasing intracranial pressure.
   c. Disposition—becomes increasingly irritable and restless.
   d. Seizures—may be the first indication of a brain tumor when it is localized in the cerebrum.
2. Physical examination
   a. Enlarging head size in infants, papilledema, increased blood pressure, and decreased pulse rate are all signs of increased intracranial pressure.
   b. Impaired vision, nystagmus, and strabismus may be present with infratentorial involvement, due to pressure on cranial nerves III, IV, VI, and VII, and the cerebellum.
   c. Other cranial nerve involvement—any of the cranial nerves can be involved, depending upon the location of tumor, i.e., head tilt due to involvement of cranial nerve IV.
   d. Ataxia and hypotonia, positive Romberg's test results—common findings with cerebellar tumors.
   e. Lower extremities weakness, positive Babinski's sign, and spasticity—cerebral lesions may produce these signs.

C. Nursing Activities

1. During diagnostic phase
   a. Explain anticipated procedures and the necessity for them.
   b. Give emotional support to child and family who are under tremendous stress while waiting for the diagnosis.
2. Pre-operative phase; teaching patient and family.
   a. Explain tumor involvement, location, and symptoms.
   b. Indicate approximate location of incision and the inevitable shaving off of hair. (Hair can be saved for parents if they wish.)
   c. A stay in the intensive care unit is needed for I.V. infusion and probable cardiopulmonary monitoring, suctioning, and various other procedures requiring tubes.
   d. Arrangements will be made for parents and child to tour the ICU.
   e. Parents will be given as much information as possible and as soon as possible.
3. Post-operative phase; massive cerebral edema.
   a. Observe for changes in neurological status.
   b. Regularly arouse patient to evaluate level of consciousness.
   c. Check pupils and eye movements—should respond bilaterally to direct and indirect light; watch for vertical and horizontal nystagmus.
   d. Motor function of extremities—check for bilateral strength and appropriate movements.
   e. Frequent checking of vital signs, including blood pressure; watch for indications of increasing intracranial pressure.
   f. Positioning—generally the head is elevated to promote drainage and prevent further edema; patient should be turned to side to prevent aspiration of emesis. Keep pressure off head dressing, i.e., keep child on nonoperative side, and always turn child without flexing his neck.
   g. Care of face and eyes—the face is usually swollen, and the eyes are swollen shut; use ice packs to lessen edema.
   h. Seizure precautions—seizures can be expected due to insult to brain during surgery.
   i. Input and output—monitor carefully to prevent overhydration that could worsen intracranial pressure.
   j. Begin implementing plans for patient's eventual discharge. Rehabilitative care, such as exercises, should be started as soon as possible. Teach parents home care of child and necessity for follow-up evaluation of neurological development.

Seizure Disorders

A. General Information

1. Epilepsy, a convulsive disorder, is a chronic condition of recurring seizures. A seizure is characterized as a temporary, uncontrolled alteration in perception and thought processes caused by abnormal electrical discharges initiated by a group of hyperexcitable cells in the brain. Mobility can also be impaired during seizures.

2. These discharges in the brain could be focal or diffuse, and the origin of the discharge determines the clinical manifestations observed during the attack.
3. Approximately ⅓ of convulsive disorders appear during the 1st 5 years of life, ⅓ during elementary school age, and ⅓ during adolescence and young adulthood.
4. Seizures have been classified according to their etiology and site of origin in the brain. Under the 2 main categories of idiopathic (unknown) and symptomatic (acquired) seizures, there are 4 main classifications:
   a. Generalized seizures are bilaterally symmetrical and may arise from central areas of the brain, particularly the midbrain and the reticular formation, that affect consciousness immediately.
      (1.) These seizures occur at any time, and the intervals between attacks vary from person to person.
      (2.) Rapid succession of epileptic attacks without regaining consciousness during intervals is called status epilepticus, and this condition requires emergency intervention.
   b. Partial seizures begin locally, producing manifestations characteristic of that particular anatomical focus; these may or may not generalize.
      (1.) The frontal, temporal, and parietal lobes are the ones most often affected.
      (2.) The 2 primary forms of partial seizures are those with elementary symptoms and those with complex symptoms.
   c. Unilateral seizures are usually seen in children.
   d. Unclassified epileptic seizures, e.g., febrile seizure.
5. Treatment of seizures is symptomatic unless the etiological agent is remediable. The most effective treatment for epilepsy is anticonvulsant therapy. Anticonvulsant agents raise the seizure threshold, thereby preventing the spread of abnormal electrical discharges through the brain.
6. Drug therapy is begun using 1 medication until the therapeutic blood level is reached. If the seizure is controlled, the dose is increased until toxic side effects appear. The dose then is decreased until the toxic effects disappear. If control is not obtained by using 1 drug, another will be used or added to the 1st one. Signs of toxicity include drowsiness, diplopia, ataxia, and mental dullness.
7. Some of the most commonly used drugs for epilepsy are as follows:
   a. Phenobarbital—PO, maintenance dosages for infants, 5 to 8 mg/kg/24 hr, and for children, 3 to 5 mg/kg/24 hr.
   b. Phenytoin (Dilantin)—PO, infants and children, 4 to 7 mg/kg/24 hr.
   c. Primidone (Mysoline)—PO, maintenance dosage under 8 years of age, 10 to 25 mg/kg/24 hr, over 8 years of age, 750 to 1500 mg/24 hr.
   d. Valproic Acid (Depakene)—PO, 10 to 30 mg/kg/24 hr (children under 8 years of age may need higher dosage of 40 to 50 mg/kg/24 hr).
   e. Carbamazepine (Tegretol)—PO, maintenance dosage for 6 to 12 years of age, 20 to 30 mg/kg/24 hr, over 12 years of age, 600 to 1200 mg/24 hr.
8. Patients and families need to be reminded that it will probably take months to establish an individualized therapeutic drug program.
9. Drug therapy will need reevaluation during periods of growth spurts and during periods of physical or emotional stress and when the patient is free of seizures for 2 to 3 years.

B. Sources for Initial Assessment Data

1. Medical history
   a. Family history—in cases of idiopathic epilepsy, hereditary electroencephalographic abnormalities have been found in some families. There is a higher incidence of seizures among relatives of children with idiopathic convulsive disorders.
   b. Brain injuries during prenatal, perinatal, or postnatal periods.
   c. Other head traumas; this is found particularly in the pre-adolescent years
   d. Systemic infections with neurological impairments, such as meningitis and encephalitis; complications of some of the communicable diseases.
   e. Other causative factors of seizures—fatigue, stress, hormonal or metabolic changes, photostimulation, and dehydration.
3. Physical examination includes a detailed neurological examination and a complete developmental assessment.
4. Laboratory findings
   a. Various blood tests to identify abnormal amounts of lead, thallium, copper, and so forth.
   b. White blood cell count for signs of infection.
   c. Studies of electrolyte levels to detect metabolic disturbances.
   d. Lumbar puncture to detect cerebral spinal fluid infections.

C. Nursing Activities

1. Prepare for seizures with precautions such as padded side rails, suction equipment, and a soft rubber airway at the bedside. A child with uncontrolled seizures should be wearing a helmet so that he will be free to engage in play activities.
2. In case of a seizure
   a. Prevent child from falling; ease him to floor and loosen any tight clothing.
   b. Quickly survey child's immediate surroundings to make certain child will not injure himself, particularly if he is having clonic type convulsions.
      (1.) Note time of onset.
      (2.) Do not leave child alone.
   c. As convulsions subside, turn child's face to side to prevent aspiration of emesis or secretions.
   d. Document with a clear description of what occurred during seizure.
      (1.) Type and length of seizure
      (2.) Respiratory patterns
      (3.) Pupil change
      (4.) Level of consciousness
      (5.) Incontinence
3. As part of discharge planning, stress to both patient and family that compliance is the key to success of the drug therapy program.
   a. If drugs should be discontinued, seizures may occur.
   b. Parents should know the side effects of the drugs prescribed; remind them to report any unusual reactions.
4. Encourage parents to notify child's school nurse and teacher about his condition, and the medication he is taking. The child should participate in all normal activity of his age mates; safety factors and any restrictions have to be individualized.

Mental Retardation

A. General Information

1. Mental retardation refers to significant subaverage intellectual functioning that exists concurrently with deficit in adaptive behavior and is manifested during the developmental period.
   a. "Significant subaverage functioning" falls 2 standard deviation below the mean, or at an I.Q. of approximately 70.
   b. Adaptive behavior provides a more functional definition in that it is a measure of the degree to which an individual meets his social responsibilities at a given age within a specific culture.
   c. Mental retardation manifests itself during the developmental period, which is between birth and 18 years of age.
2. In 1983 the American Association of Mental Deficiency revised their earlier description of mental retardation. The revised I.Q. range is as follows:
   a. Mild retardation—I.Q. of 50–55 to approximately 70.
   b. Moderate retardation—I.Q. of 30–40 to 50–55.
   c. Severe retardation—I.Q. of 20–25 to 35–40.
   d. Profound retardation—I.Q. of below 20 or 25.
   e. The category of borderline intelligence of 70 to 84 I.Q. was formerly included but has been eliminated in the newer category.
3. This definition recognizes that self help skills, living independently, and the ability to get around independently have direct bearing on the learning and potential of the child. This definition also implies that a child's classification may change with improvement in adaptive behavior.
   a. Mild retardation or I.Q. of 50–55 to approximately 70.
      (1.) Could have normal physical development but is slow or clumsy with some motor skills.
      (2.) Child is placed in educable class.
      (3.) Achieves 3rd to 6th grade level skills.
      (4.) Can become independent and self supportive but usually remains on lower end of economic scale because of limitation in cognitive abilities.
   b. Moderate retardation or I.Q. of 35–40 to 50–55.
      (1.) Delay in growth and development with noticeable delay in motor development, particularly speech.
      (2.) Assigned to trainable class and some reach 1st or 2nd grade level.
      (3.) Cannot maintain independent life as an adult but is able to care for himself with supervision.
   c. Severe retardation or I.Q. of 20–25 to 35–40.
      (1.) Functions on the level of a 2 to 3-year-old toddler.
      (2.) Severe motor development delays.
      (3.) Little or no communication skill but may understand simple sentences.
      (4.) Needs protective environment with constant supervision.
   d. Profound retardation or I.Q. below 20 or 25.
      (1.) Functions on level of infant.
      (2.) Requires complete custodial care with all needs met.

4. In 75 to 90% of the cases, the cause of the retardation is unknown or is based on multifactorial genetic and environmental factors. As the symptom of the retardation becomes more severe (the I.Q. decreases), the number of known causes increase.

B. Sources for Initial Assessment Data

1. Medical history
   a. Prenatal
      (1.) Maternal health
      (2.) Maternal weight gain
      (3.) Maternal use of drugs, alcohol, or cigarettes.
   b. Perinatal
      (1.) Record of fetal monitoring
      (2.) Gestation
      (3.) Abnormal presentation
      (4.) Delivery method
      (5.) Prolapsed cord
      (6.) Meconium staining
      (7.) Apgar score
      (8.) Infant's need for resuscitation
      (9.) Neurological state
   c. Postnatal
      (1.) Neonatal suck, muscle tone, apnea, and seizures.
      (2.) Developmental milestones in fine and gross motor, personal-social, and language-cognitive skills.
      (3.) Psychosocial deprivation
      (4.) Accidents with head trauma
      (5.) Infections such as meningitis, encephalitis; complications of immunizations resulting in encephalopathies.
      (6.) Lead and other poisonous metal toxicities.
2. Physical examination
   a. General appearance—observe dysgenetic features; 45% of infants whose birth weights are 1500 gm or less and who are dysgenetic frequently have low I.Q.s.
   b. Height and weight—growth failure is frequent in children with chromosomal abnormalities or in those who are small for gestational age.
   c. Head—the most commonly found major malformation is that of the central nervous system, including primarily microcephaly, hydrocephaly, and anencephaly.
   d. Eyes
      (1.) Chorioretinitis of toxoplasmosis
      (2.) Cherry red spot on fundus of Tay-Sachs disease
3. Audiometry test (or other hearing test) results—hearing difficulties occur in approximately 10% of moderately to severely retarded children.
4. CAT scan is helpful in identifying cerebral dysgenesis or atrophy, central nervous system bleeding, and hydrocephalus.
5. Laboratory findings—blood tests needed to detect metabolic defects.

C. Nursing Activities

1. In prevention during pregnancy
   a. Encourage early prenatal care.
   b. Genetic counseling, when appropriate.
   c. Advise women concerning adequate nutrition.
   d. Advise women to stop smoking and drinking alcohol.
2. In prevention in neonates and infants
   a. Refer infant with or at risk for developmental delay for assessment.
   b. Keep up with immunizations.
   c. Carefully monitor acute illnesses and high fevers.
   d. Prevent accidents, particularly those involving the child's head.
3. Care of hospitalized child
   a. Identify existing self-help skills and functional level for dressing, eating, toileting, sleeping, and communicating needs.
   b. Give parent specific information on child's condition and treatments that are planned.
   c. Do not isolate child; speak with him; involve him in as much of his own care as possible.
   d. Facilitate growth promoting activities for child; allow him to interact with other children in playroom.
4. Long-term care
   a. Assist parents in setting realistic goals for child and for themselves.
   b. Encourage parents to investigate community programs and resources in order to acquire maximum professional assistance in the care of their child.
   c. Emphasize that their child has the same needs as other children related to feeling loved, needing praise and encouragement, and feeling part of the family.
   d. As the child matures, discuss vocational training, sheltered workshops, and other options to home care.

GASTROINTESTINAL DISORDERS

Gastrointestinal Anomalies

A. General Information

1. Gastrointestinal tract disorder is one of the largest categories of illnesses that occur among infants and children. Problems can be structural, inflammatory, malabsorptive, or maldigestive.
2. Gastrointestinal tract anomalies can affect both the absorptive surfaces and the time during which the intestinal substances come in contact with the digestive juices.

Cleft Lip and Palate

A. General Information

1. Cleft lip is the result of incomplete fusion of the nasomedial or intermaxillary process with the more laterally placed maxillary process.
2. Types of cleft lip are as follows:
   a. Unilateral cleft—caused by failure of the maxillary process to fuse with median nasal process. Cleft may vary from slight notch to complete separation, extending into the nostril.
   b. Bilateral cleft—caused by failure of both maxillary processes to fuse with the medial nasal process, which then remains as a central flap.
   c. Oblique facial cleft—caused by the failure of the maxillary process to fuse with the lateral and median nasal process.
   d. Medial cleft of upper lip—caused by the failure of fusion of the globular processes of the median nasal process.
   e. Cleft of lower lip—caused by incomplete fusion of the mandibular process.
3. Cleft palate is the result of failure of the palatal processes of the maxilla to fuse with each other in the midline and in severe cases of failure of these processes also to fuse with the premaxilla.
4. Types of cleft palate are as follows:
   a. Cleft uvula
   b. Ununited palatal process
   c. Ununited palatal process with cleft on one side of the premaxilla.
5. Treatment for cleft lip and cleft palate is surgical repair.
6. Problems resulting from cleft lip and palate are the inability to suck, mild to severe facial malformation, hearing loss from repeated ear infections, and speech disturbances.
7. Parents experience severe emotional trauma upon learning of their child's defect, for it is a very obvious defect.
8. Intellectual deficits and other congenital malformations are commonly associated with cleft lip and palate.

B. Sources for Assessment Data

1. Examination of the mouth—cleft lip is immediately obvious, but inspect palate with fingers to determine presence of cleft and whether or not the uvula is involved.
2. Sucking and swallowing ability—clefts of the hard palate form a continuous opening between the mouth and the nasal cavity, which prevents the infant from effectively sucking and swallowing.
3. Parental response to defect—when a child is born who is less than perfect because of a congenital anomaly, the parents experience tremendous emotional setbacks. The parents go through the adaptive processes of shock, denial, sadness and anger, disequilibrium, and reorganization.

C. Nursing Activities

1. Pre-operative care includes the following:
   a. Preventing aspiration of feedings.
   b. Preventing infection around cleft.
   c. Using special nipple for feeding followed by frequent burping.
   d. Facilitating the parent-child attachment process.
2. Post-operative care for cleft lip repair includes the following:
   a. Observe carefully for respiratory distress from swelling of lips, nostrils, and tongue.
   b. Use arm restraints to prevent damage to the suture line.
   c. Make certain Logan's bow or butterfly closure is taped securely to cheeks.
   d. Hold and cuddle infant to prevent excessive crying.
   e. Keep suture line clean with mixture of ½ hydrogen peroxide and ½ water or saline; remove crusts gently.
   f. Start feeding with clear liquids and resume formula when tolerated, using Asepto syringe or medicine dropper; discourage sucking during this time.

g. May keep infant in a misted tent to keep mucous membranes moist.
h. Remove arm restraints one at a time at least every 4 hours to allow range of motion and inspection of skin condition.
i. Position infant on the back or in an infant seat, making certain he is not left in one position for any length of time; never place infant on his abdomen.
j. Plan for discharge of infant and teaching of parents pertaining to appropriate feeding techniques, restraints, positioning, lip care, and future surgeries.
k. Refer to a public health agency or a cleft lip clinic for continuity of care.

3. Post-operative care for cleft palate repair includes the following:
   a. Use arm restraints.
   b. Hold and cuddle infant to prevent excessive crying.
   c. May position infant on his abdomen for first few hours after surgery to facilitate drainage of excess mucus.
   d. Avoid inserting anything in infant's mouth; this may damage suture line.
   e. Feed from side of spoon; use cup for fluids.
   f. May keep in misted tent.
   g. Remove restraints one at a time to exercise arms.
   h. Plan for discharge; caution parents against feeding infant anything hard, which could damage newly repaired palate.
   i. Refer to a public health agency or a cleft palate clinic for continuity of care.

Pyloric Stenosis

A. General Information

1. Pyloric stenosis is caused by hypertrophy and hyperplasia of the muscle adjacent to the pyloric region, resulting in the narrowing of the lumen of the pylorus; therefore, food cannot pass through the pyloric sphincter to the duodenum.
2. First-born children are more commonly affected, and male infants acquire this defect 5 times more frequently than female infants.
3. This is a relatively minor defect that is easily corrected.
4. Effective treatment for pyloric stenosis is a surgical procedure; the enlarged muscle fibers are split without entering the duodenum.

B. Sources for Assessment Data

1. Physical examination—if the condition has persisted for some time, the infant could appear thin and emaciated, with loss of subcutaneous fat.
   a. Hard, nontender, mobile, olive-shaped mass is palpable in the right epigastrium, with visible peristalsis moving from left to right in the upper quadrant. The infant is irritable and extremely hungry.
2. Medical history—child was healthy with no outstanding problems, gaining weight normally. Suddenly, there was persistent vomiting, often projectile, of non-bilious material. The infant continued to nurse hungrily, but the vomiting continued and the stool decreased in size and quantity.
3. Laboratory reports—blood will show decreases in levels of potassium, chloride, and sodium and increase in pH from the persistent vomiting.
4. Integument—dehydration from the persistent vomiting.

C. Nursing Activities

1. Pre-operatively, acquire data base for vital signs.
2. Explain operative procedure to parents and support them during surgery.
3. A few hours after surgery, small clear liquid feedings may be given; if there is no resumption of vomiting, regular formula or breast milk may be given. Normal feeding amounts should be accomplished within 2 days. Hold infant in sitting position, feed slowly, and burp frequently.
4. Inspect incision site for drainage and infection.
5. Place infant on right side with head elevated to promote emptying of stomach.
6. Teach parents care and feeding of infant to prepare for discharge.

Hirschsprung's Disease (Megacolon)

A. General Information

1. Hirschsprung's disease is caused by the congenital absence of parasympathetic nerve ganglion cells in an area extending from the internal anal sphincter through varying lengths of rectum and colon. The area most frequently affected is the rectosigmoid area.

2. There is a 4 to 1 ratio of affected boys to girls, and a familial tendency in a small number of cases.
3. The primary problem is a mechanical obstruction caused by inadequate motility in a particular part of the intestine.
4. The obstruction is caused by accumulation of fecal material secondary to lack of innervation, and the failure of the internal rectal sphincter to relax, resulting in the distention of the intestine proximal to the defect.
5. Delay in passage of meconium in a newborn may be the first sign of Hirschsprung's disease.
6. Treatment for this disease is surgery; a colostomy is performed first for elimination. The second surgery is performed when the infant is 6 months of age or older; this procedure involves resecting the distended portion of the bowel and bringing the normal bowel down to form an anastomosis, creating a new rectum.

B. Sources for Assessment Data

1. Physical examination
   a. Neonate
      (1.) Complete intestinal obstruction or intermittent abdominal distention
      (2.) Bile stained vomitus
      (3.) Irritability
   b. Infants and children
      (1.) Failure to thrive
      (2.) Protuberant abdomen
      (3.) Visible peristalsis
      (4.) Muscle wasting
      (5.) Foul smelling stools
2. Medical history
   a. Neonate
      (1.) Failure to pass meconium
      (2.) Constipation or diarrhea
3. Barium enema aids in the diagnosis by outlining the dilated bowel segment.
4. Abdominal x-ray will show a distended colon that ends at the rectum.
5. Rectal biopsy tissue will be free of ganglionic nerve cells.

C. Nursing Activities

1. Pre-operative
   a. Explain surgical procedures to parents.
   b. Maintain optimum hydration and nutrition.
   c. Schedule several days for careful colonic irrigations using either saline or milk.
   d. For older children, explain colostomy.
2. Post-operative
   a. Take frequent vital signs.
   b. Carefully monitor I.V. fluids, nasogastric tube, and catheter.
   c. Keep perineal area meticulously clean.
   d. Carefully watch for signs and symptoms of anastomosis breakdown or leakage.
   e. Assess for return of bowel sounds.
   f. Start with clear liquid diet and gradually advance to normal diet.
   g. Prepare for discharge planning.
      (1.) Indicate to parents that there may be occasional staining and constipation.
      (2.) There may be a delay in toilet training.

Neonatal Necrotizing Enterocolitis (NEC)

A. General Information

1. This disease is characterized by developing necrosis of the intestine, usually the ileum and colon. The bowel becomes hemorrhagic, edematous, and engorged. The necrosis could lead to perforation.
2. NEC occurs in approximately 3 to 8% of all premature infants but has occurred in some full term infants as well.
3. The exact cause of this problem has not been identified, but nasogastric tube feeding, sepsis, exchange transfusion, and the use of umbilical catheters all have been related to the incidence of this problem.
4. Clinical signs usually develop insidiously; first signs may be as follows:
   a. Poor feeding
   b. Vomiting
   c. Gastric distention
   d. Reduced or absent bowel sounds
   e. Blood in the stool
   f. Frequent diarrhea
5. If infant's condition does not improve or if there is perforation, surgery is done, often intestinal resection and a colostomy or an ileostomy.

B. Sources for Assessment Data

1. Physical examination
   a. Abdominal distention
   b. Reduced or absent bowel sounds
   c. Lethargy
   d. Irritability

e. Thin
f. Wrinkled skin
2. Medical history
a. Poor feeding
b. Blood tinged stools
c. Bile containing vomitus
d. Highly irritable
3. Diagnosis is usually confirmed by x-ray demonstration of presence of free abdominal air.

C. Nursing Activities

1. Discontinue feedings and start I.V.
2. Avoid abdominal pressure; observe abdomen for degree of distention.
3. Give anal area extra care to avoid excoriation; avoid taking rectal temperature.
4. Frequently monitor vital signs, including blood pressure, for changes that may indicate sepsis or shock. Pay particular attention to fluid input and output, and the infant's hydration status.
5. If surgery is required, observe usual nursing procedures involved.

Pneumonia

A. General Information

1. Pneumonia is seen in children of all ages but occurs more frequently during infancy and early childhood.
2. Infants and young children are more vulnerable to respiratory problems because:
a. They have less alveolar surface for gas exchange.
b. The narrow branching peripheral airways become easily obstructed.
c. The lack of collateral pathways inhibits ventilation beyond obstructed units.
3. Pneumonia is caused by bacteria, viruses, *Mycoplasma*, or by aspiration of a foreign object.
4. It is characterized by a general inflammation and infection of lung tissue. The infection could be localized or could involve the entire lung. Generally, the clinical manifestations vary greatly depending upon the etiological agent, child's age, and child's reaction to infection.
5. Types of pneumonia and treatment are as follows:
a. Bacterial pneumonia (pneumococcus, *Streptococcus, Staphylococcus, Haemophilus influenzae*)
(1.) Sudden onset
(2.) High fever
(3.) Respiratory distress
(4.) Child appears very ill
(5.) Child could have circumoral cyanosis, retraction, tachypnea, or tachycardia.
b. Treatment for bacterial pneumonia consists of
(1.) Antibiotics
(2.) Fluids
(3.) Antipyretics
(4.) Rest
c. Viral pneumonia (respiratory syncytial virus, adenoviruses) and *Mycoplasma pneumoniae*
(1.) Gradual onset with dry, hacking, nonproductive cough
(2.) Child appears mildly ill, but condition can be potentially serious for infant.
d. Treatment is usually symptomatic. Pneumonia is self limiting and resolves spontaneously.
6. Older children and adolescents are usually treated at home, but infants and very young children are usually treated in the hospital for closer monitoring.

B. Sources for Initial Assessment Data

1. Medical history
a. Previous URI—pneumonia is frequently preceded by URI.
b. Malaise, fatigue, anorexia, chills, and feverishness.
c. Productive or non-productive cough.
2. Physical examination
a. Nasal passageway and oropharynx may be inflamed.
b. Cervical lymph nodes may be affected.
c. There may be slight wheezing on expiration.
d. Breath sounds—rales or rhonchi over involved areas, diminished breath sounds, or general dullness.
e. Temperature between 100° and 104° F.
3. Laboratory reports
a. White blood cell count could be elevated.
b. Trachea culture and blood culture; etiological organism can be identified.
c. Chest x-ray—characteristic infiltration will be seen.

C. Nursing Activities

1. Place child in "respiratory" isolation (if at home, keep child isolated from other children).

2. Promote bed rest; needs to conserve energy.
3. Position—lying on affected side splints area and reduces pain of pleural friction.
4. Assess breath sounds; assess progress of disease and identify further lung involvement.
5. Aspirate; if child is unable to manage pharyngeal secretions, aspirate to keep airway open. Child may have to remain NPO, and fluids provided I.V., if danger of aspirating remains.
6. Chest physical therapy—carry out every 4 hours, or as needed.
7. Keep in cool misted tent; moistens airway, helps mobilize secretions, reduces bronchial edema, and promotes temperature reduction.

Asthma

A. General Information

1. Asthma, a reversible allergic response to specific antigens, is the episodic wheezy dyspnea produced by a narrowing of the bronchioles. Narrowing is due to:
   a. Increased mucus in the airways.
   b. Edema of the airway lining
   c. Bronchospasm
   d. All 3 aforementioned combined.
2. Asthma is the most severe of the respiratory allergic disorders, and among school-age children, this disorder is the major cause of absenteeism.
3. It usually starts between 2 and 3 years of age; etiology of asthma is multifactoral. Heredity, infection, allergy, and psychological stress all play an important role.
4. An asthma attack, which is a sudden and rapid manifestation of symptoms, may be triggered by a variety of causes:
   a. A common cold
   b. Rapid change in temperature or humidity
   c. Laughing
   d. Exercise
   e. Exposure to allergens, such as animals and plants.
5. Symptoms vary from a mild cough to severe dyspnea with hypoxemia and respiratory acidosis.
6. Some asthma attacks will subside when the allergen is removed, but most cases require treatment.
7. Long-term treatment is preceded by identification of allergens through skin testing and trial and error. It is possible to undergo hyposensitization treatment.

B. Sources for Initial Assessment Data

1. Medical history
   a. Family—in approximately 75% of children with asthma, there is a positive family history of allergy.
   b. Eczema as an infant.
   c. Experiences of other signs of allergy, such as allergic rhinitis and skin reactions to allergens (food, soap, and so forth).
2. Physical examination
   a. Appearance of child is anxious or frightened and restless.
   b. Respiration
      (1.) Dyspneic with rapid and shallow breathing.
      (2.) Accessory muscles (shoulder, sternal, and abdominal muscles) are used for breathing.
   c. Chest and lungs
      (1.) Whistling sounds are produced in chest on expiration due to air being forced through narrowed bronchioles.
      (2.) Barrel chest due to air becoming trapped in alveoli.
      (3.) Percussion reveals hyperresonance.
      (4.) Child needs to take a breath between every few words spoken.
3. Laboratory reports
   a. pH falls with respiratory acidosis.
   b. Hematocrit value and hemoglobin level could be above average owing to chronic hypoxemia with dehydration.
   c. Sputum demonstrates large numbers of eosinophils.

C. Nursing Activities

1. Short-term care during an asthmatic attack is as follows:
   a. Take steps to get immediate medication for child.
      (1.) The standard emergency treatment is 1:1000 aqueous epinephrine (0.01 mg/kg) given subcutaneously.
      (2.) After 20 minutes if airway has not cleared, the dose is repeated.
      (3.) Children who do not respond to epinephrine will be given I.V. aminophylline, very slowly, and over a 15-minute period.
   b. Reassure child that treatment will work.
   c. Prevent any type of exertion; distract him, if possible.

d. Keep child in sitting position, leaning forward on his hands.
e. Administer
   (1.) Bronchodilator
   (2.) Anti-inflammatory agents
   (3.) Expectorant
   (4.) O_2
f. Encourage child to breathe slowly.
g. Chest percussion, vibration, and deep breathing facilitate removal of secretions.
h. Postural drainage and frequent turning also facilitate removal of secretions to open airway.
i. Hydration—hyperventilation, decreased oral intake, and some bronchodilators may cause dehydration; adequate hydration is necessary to keep body fluid volume to level necessary to liquify secretions.

2. Long-term care or maintenance is as follows:
   a. Teach child and parents related drug information.
      (1.) Proper name
      (2.) Dose
      (3.) Administration method
      (4.) Frequency
      (5.) Side effects
      (6.) Safe usage (drugs for asthma are generally all potent).
   b. Teach child and family the pathophysiology as well as the psychodynamics of asthma and the various measures of keeping this problem of asthma under control.
   c. Encourage family to allow child to try new experiences to develop independence and confidence in himself.
   d. Be a good listener to parents' dialogue; caring for a child with a chronic illness is extremely stressful for the entire family.
   e. Identify various community resources as well as support groups that the family can contact.

Cerebral Palsy

A. General Information

1. Cerebral palsy is the most common permanent physical disability of childhood.
   a. The disorder is non-progressive.
   b. The clinical features are variable.
2. This dysfunction is characterized by the following:
   a. Muscle weakness and spasticity
   b. Abnormal superficial reflexes
   c. Increased deep tendon reflexes
   d. Although the primary problem is abnormal muscle tone and coordination, often other central nervous system impairments occur such as the following:
      (1.) Seizures
      (2.) Cognitive impairment
      (3.) Learning disabilities
3. There are numerous etiologies of cerebral palsy that could be prenatal, perinatal, or postnatal. Whatever the factors contributing to the etiology, there is some type of insult to the brain, from hypoxia to gross malformation.
4. It is often difficult to make a definitive diagnosis of cerebral palsy until the child is approximately 6 months of age. As the neurological system matures, deficits become more apparent.
5. Children with cerebral palsy vary in the severity of their condition; 30% have normal intelligence, 50 to 70% have some degree of mental retardation, and 33% have seizures. Some are affected in such a mild way that their disability may go undetected for a long time.
6. The 3 types of cerebral palsy are as follows:
   a. Spastic
      (1.) Exaggerated reflexes
      (2.) Exaggerated movements of one or more limbs
      (3.) Muscle groups become tight, short, and contracted
      (4.) Head and neck muscle involvement results in poor speech, difficulty in swallowing, and drooling.
   b. Athetoid
      (1.) Writhing uncontrolled movements of the head, face, and all extremities
      (2.) Decreased muscle tone but hypertrophied muscles due to constant motion.
   c. Ataxic
      (1.) Poor balance
      (2.) Uncoordinated arms
      (3.) Hypoactive reflexes

B. Sources for Initial Assessment Data

1. Medical history of child
   a. Low birth weight—a large percentage of children with cerebral palsy weigh less than 2500 gm at birth.
   b. Prematurity
   c. Low Apgar score
   d. Trauma during birth process.
   e. Metabolic or electrolyte disturbances after birth.

2. Medical history of mother
   a. Complications of pregnancy with risk of anoxia.
   b. Maternal metabolic disease.
   c. Maternal anemia during pregnancy.
   d. Drugs taken during pregnancy.
   e. Radiation during pregnancy.
3. Physical examination of child
   a. Emphasis on neurological examination; this will determine quality of motor and sensory responses.
   b. Look for the following:
      (1.) Delayed gross motor development
      (2.) Abnormal motor performance
      (3.) Alterations of muscle tone
      (4.) Abnormal posture
      (5.) Abnormal reflexes
4. Vision and hearing tests
   a. Deficits are common.
   b. Early identification of deficits will enhance training and education.
5. Electromyogram (EMG)—measures electrical activities in individual muscles.
6. Laboratory tests—measurement of serum enzyme levels found primarily in muscles and to a lesser degree in other organs of the body helps diagnosis and also reflects course of muscular disease.

C. Nursing Activities

1. Recognize that the multifaceted problems faced by the child and family require a multidisciplinary approach to care; the nurse cannot do an adequate job unassisted.
2. Be prepared to give long-term assistance to the child and family to cope with the numerous problems and to facilitate the child's attaining maximum potential
3. Feeding process—child has poor sucking and swallowing reflexes, a hyperactive gag reflex, and poor control of tongue movements.
   a. Feed slowly and in small amounts.
   b. The feeding environment must be quiet.
   c. Use special feeding utensils, such as a large-bowled spoon.
   d. Provide extra calories to meet extra energy demands due to constant movement. Special care must be taken, however, to balance caloric intake with child's activity level to prevent excess weight gain.
   e. Offer new foods periodically and promote chewing for muscle development.
4. Mobility—neuromuscular dysfunction prevents normal ambulation as well as normal body and limb movements.
   a. Prevent contractures through passive and active stretching exercises.
   b. Use braces and splints and other adaptive devices to maintain correct positioning.
   c. Orthopedic surgery, such as heel cord lengthening, may be required to decrease spastic muscle imbalance.
   d. Meticulous care of skin; watch for redness, cyanosis, and blisters.
   e. Provide incentives to ambulate.
   f. Provide safe environment; use helmet on child who falls.
   g. Maintain regular schedule to prevent fatigue.
5. Speech—communication problems are usually severe due to involvement of head and neck muscles.
   a. Be patient and attentive.
   b. Teach use of speech aids, such as sign language, picture boards, and typewriters.
   c. Begin speech therapy early.
6. Independence—acquisition of self help skills promotes feeling of independence.
   a. In fostering independence, the occupational therapist assists the child and family by developing a training program to increase manual skills and activities of daily living. Frequently, special adaptive devices are customized for the child to enable him to eat, button clothes, and groom himself.
   b. Physical therapists are primarily responsible for developing individualized programs for children to achieve their maximum functional goals. Rehabilitation programs are multidisciplinary, involving the physical therapist, the family, the nurse, and other health personnel.
   c. Assess the child's skills; then encourage him to help in his own care, based on age and capabilities.
   d. Teach the parents the principle of breaking down skills into small steps in order to teach the child.
   e. Set realistic goals for child.
7. Support of family
   a. Be aware of and offer support during grieving process after parents learn of diagnosis. Recognize processes of chronic and periodic sorrow.
   b. Allow for expression of strong negative feelings regarding diagnosis, physicians, nurses, treatments, and other concerns.
   c. Encourage early participation in treatment program but recognize that there may be many obstacles to parent participation.

d. Refer family to counseling services, various community support groups, and organizations with special services, such as the United Cerebral Palsy Foundation.

Cystic Fibrosis

A. General Information

1. Cystic fibrosis, which is found primarily among whites, is a dysfunction of the mucus producing glands.
2. These dysfunctional glands produce abnormally viscous secretions (this mucus is 100 times thicker than normal mucus), which obstruct organ passages precipitating the various pathological changes and clinical symptoms. These pathological changes result in chronic obstructive lung disease, progressive pulmonary infection, pancreatic deficiency, chronic malabsorptive syndromes, hepatic cirrhosis, and intestinal obstruction. It is, however, the inability to utilize O_2 that ultimately determines prognosis and quality of life.
3. This is the most common genetic disease among pediatric patients in which the prognosis is invariably grave; it is transmitted as an autosomal recessive trait.
4. Diagnosis is usually established by symptoms of chronic obstructive lung disease, gastrointestinal dysfunction, and elevated levels of electrolytes in sweat.
5. There is no successful treatment for cystic fibrosis since the precise etiology remains unknown. However, life expectancies for these patients have greatly increased with early diagnosis and early treatment. Since patients are ill from complications of this disease, treatment is focused on control and prevention of these complications. The 3 outstanding complications are as follows:
   a. Pulmonary obstructive process
   b. Pulmonary infection
   c. Nutritional deficiencies
6. At the present time, the mean age of survival is 19 years; many persons do, however, survive longer into adulthood.

B. Sources for Initial Assessment Data

1. Medical history
   a. Positive family history; this disease is genetically determined.
   b. Meconium ileus as newborn; earliest sign of disease in 10 to 15% of affected babies.
   c. Poor weight gain despite good food intake; malabsorption of food.
   d. Large amount of foul smelling, fatty appearing stool; lack of digestive enzymes into the duodenum prevents digestion of food, resulting in the excretion of undigested food that is large in amount, frothy, and foul smelling.
   e. Rectal prolapse may initially occur approximately between 6 months and 3 years and may result from poor control of steatorrhea (abnormal stools).
   f. Frequent abdominal pains could result from any number of problems occurring in the abdomen, such as undigested food, intussusception usually in the ileocecal area, gallstones, and subacute or chronic pancreatitis.
   g. Pulmonary problems increase gradually.
   h. Frequent productive cough, bronchitis, and pneumonia.
   i. Tires easily; faulty O_2 utilization.
   j. Menstrual irregularities due to poor nutritional status.
   k. Diabetes due to pancreatic destruction.
   l. Salty taste to skin; sweat production is normal; there is an abnormally high level of electrolytes in the sweat.
2. Physical examination
   a. Appearance
      (1.) The child is poorly nourished with delay in growth and development.
      (2.) Dyspneic with barrel chest.
      (3.) Cyanotic with clubbing of fingers and toes.
      (4.) Protruding belly
      (5.) Thin extremities
      (6.) Poor muscle mass
      (7.) Delayed secondary sex characteristics
      (8.) Increased respiratory rate
      (9.) Uses accessory muscles for respiration.
   b. Ears, nose, and throat
      (1.) Thick, sticky mucus.
      (2.) Nasal polyps (There is thought to be a relationship between the prolonged use of antibiotics and the development of nasal polyps.)
      (3.) Chronic otitis media.
   c. Rectal prolapse is due to the large amounts of bowel movements.
   d. Cardiac hypertrophy; right ventricular hypertrophy due to the increase in pulmonary vascular resistance.
3. Laboratory reports
   a. Sweat test
      (1.) Sweat is analyzed for sodium and chloride.

(2.) Children with cystic fibrosis will have chloride levels 2 to 5 times higher than normal; this is seen at birth and throughout their lives.

b. Liver function—abnormal levels of gamma-guanosine triphosphate (GTP) transaminase.
c. Rectal biopsy—fissure from the gastrointestinal tract found.
d. Urine—glycosuria; possible diabetes.
e. Blood may show glucose intolerance.
f. Chest x-ray, in more advanced cases, may show atelectasis, bronchiectasis, or pneumothorax.

C. Nursing Activities

1. Pulmonary therapy; pulmonary complications account for the majority of cases of disability and death in cystic fibrosis.
   a. Misted tent helps thin mucus secretions (usefulness of this treatment is now controversial).
   b. Aerosol inhalation thins and liquefies bronchial secretions; use prior to postural drainage (this treatment is also controversial).
   c. Postural drainage—with percussion and vibration, moves thick secretions toward larger airway, permitting child to cough mucus out; increases sputum expectoration.
   d. Antibiotics (usually sulfa drugs)—treatment and control of infection.
   e. Exercise strengthens respiratory muscles; improves pulmonary function; loosens and removes mucus from lungs; helps maintain normal patterns of breathing.
2. Well-balanced diet; the child will be given a well-balanced diet supplemented with pancreatic enzymes. There should be a 50 to 100% increase in calories, and protein content should be approximately 2 to 2½ times normal requirement. Vitamin supplements are also used to meet vitamin deficiency due to malabsorption.
3. Support of family
   a. Upon hearing the diagnosis of this inevitably fatal disease, most parents are overwhelmed with guilt, anger, and anxiety. Nursing activity at this time would be to offer complete emotional support and understanding.
   b. As soon as the initial shock wears off, the parents will have to deal with the sudden change in lifestyle, the stress of daily therapy, the financial burden, and the constant evidence of the potential death of their child.
   c. The nurse may be able to lessen the family's anxiety by eliminating many of the unknowns by providing a clear description of the illness, of the different treatment modalities, and of how parents can be responsible for the child's care.
   d. The parents should be informed immediately that the care of a child with cystic fibrosis is enormous; however, there are means of acquiring help through friends, relatives, and various support groups in the community; refer them to the National Cystic Fibrosis Foundation.

Hydrocephalus

A. General Information

1. Hydrocephalus is an abnormal accumulation of cerebrospinal fluid in the brain caused by excessive production, inadequate reabsorption, or obstruction of circulation of cerebral spinal fluid through the ventricles.
2. The major causes of hydrocephalus are as follows:
   a. Congenital abnormalities
   b. Trauma
   c. Postinflammatory lesions
   d. Tumors
3. Clinical manifestations depend primarily upon the site of obstruction, the age at which the obstruction develops, and pre-existing structural lesions.
4. The 3 types of hydrocephalus are as follows:
   a. Non-communicating (internal, obstructive, intraventricular) is due to circulation of fluid blocked within the ventricles preventing the cerebral spinal fluid from flowing to the subarachnoid spaces where it is absorbed.
   b. Communicating—cerebral spinal fluid is not absorbed by the arachnoid villi. Nonabsorption caused by fibrosis of the villi is often the result of hemorrhage or infection. This type is the most common.
   c. Overproduction of cerebral spinal fluid is due to tumors of the choroid plexus.
5. Rapid enlargement of the head is an important clue to the progression and prognosis of hydrocephalus.
6. Treatment for hydrocephalus is almost always surgical whereby a shunt is introduced into the ventricular system to reroute cerebral spinal fluid.
7. Infection, kinking of shunt, clogging of shunt, and separation of tubings are common, serious complications necessitating frequent revisions and replacements of shunts.

B. Sources for Initial Assessment Data

1. History—medical history will depend on whether the etiology of this deformity was congenital, infectious, traumatic, or a result of a preexisting structural defect.
2. Physical examination
   a. Infants before closure of fontanelles and sutures
      (1.) Bulging and tense fontanelle
      (2.) Enlarging head, producing Macewen's sign ("cracked pot" sign).
      (3.) Prominent scalp veins
      (4.) "Sunset" eyes
      (5.) Eventual thinning of scalp
      (6.) Lethargy alternating with irritability
      (7.) Frequent vomiting
   b. Older infants and children—after closure of sutures, clinical manifestations are the result of pressure on adjacent structures caused by lesions.
      (1.) Ultrasound scan is not too reliable.
      (2.) Transillumination
      (3.) Neurological evaluation
      (4.) CAT scan is most reliable.
      (5.) Head circumference

C. Nursing Activities

1. Pre-operative care of child with increased intracranial pressure
   a. Measure head circumference every morning at the same level using the same non-stretchable paper tape.
   b. Assess fontanelles and suture—palpate for size, tenseness, and separation.
   c. Handle child's enlarged head carefully; take measures to avoid skin breakdown.
   d. Take extra time to feed; infants are usually irritable and anorexic; arrange time to avoid excessive handling after feeding.
2. Older children (in addition to aforementioned steps a to d)
   a. Evaluate level of consciousness and present behavior compared with usual pattern of behavior.
   b. Prepare him for procedures and surgery.
3. Post-operative care
   a. Position on unoperated side; handle very gently to avoid sudden reduction in intracranial pressure.
   b. Child's head is flat on bed or elevated, depending upon surgical procedure.
   c. Monitor neurological status every 15 minutes; watch for signs of increasing pressure.
   d. Monitor input and output.
   e. Give prophylactic antibiotic.
4. Long-term care
   a. Parental support—assess knowledge pertaining to the following:
      (1.) Deformity
      (2.) Medication used
      (3.) Procedures and surgery
      (4.) Information parent has acquired; reinforce and update.
   b. Teach parents the following:
      (1.) To recognize signs of increasing intracranial pressure, infection, or other signs indicating shunt malfunction.
      (2.) Teach child to avoid contact sports, but to engage in other activities.
      (3.) Have child assessed periodically for intellectual functioning
      (4.) Contact the Spina Bifida Association of America for information and support.

Tetralogy of Fallot

A. General Information

1. Among the many types of congenital heart defects, some abnormalities may be so minor that the child is almost asymptomatic. In other affected children, the defect may be so extensive that other body systems must compensate for the defective structures. The severity of the defect directly influences the symptoms exhibited and the overall prognosis.
2. The causes of congenital heart defects are known in only about 5% of the cases. The known causes are rubella and other viruses, chromosomal abnormalities, and maternal drug and alcohol use during pregnancy.
3. Congenital heart defects are commonly classified as acyanotic or cyanotic. In acyanotic disease there is usually left to right shunting, with only O_2 enriched blood entering the systemic circulation. In cyanotic disease there is usually right to left shunt, which permits the deoxygenated systemic blood to reenter the systemic circulation.
4. Tetralogy of Fallot causes severe cyanosis, consists of 4 abnormalities:
   a. Stenosis of the pulmonary artery
   b. A large ventral septal defect

c. Overriding of the ventral septal defect by the aorta
d. Right ventricular hypertrophy

5. The prognosis for an infant born with tetralogy of Fallot depends upon the severity of the pulmonary stenosis. If the stenosis is mild, left to right shunt occurs and the infant may not be cyanotic, but if the stenosis is severe, right to left shunting occurs and the infant is cyanotic.
6. Total surgical correction of this defect during infancy is possible; this surgery is based on the size of the pulmonary artery rather than on the age of the child.

B. Sources for Initial Assessment Data

1. History
   a. Infant extremely mobile.
   b. Poor sucking ability.
   c. Poor weight gain.
   d. Poor eating pattern.
   e. Frequent respiratory infections.
   f. Evidence of exercise intolerance.
   g. In older children, unusual posturing (squatting).
2. Physical examination
   a. Integument—pallor, cyanotic.
   b. Poor growth and development.
   c. Fingers and toes—clubbing.
   d. Cardiac—pansystolic murmur at middle to lower left sternal border.
   e. Dyspneic, especially after crying or exertion.
3. Laboratory reports
   a. Cardiac catherization—evaluates severity of cardiac defects and changes.
   b. Blood; polycythemia; the tissue hypoxia relative to cyanosis.
      (1.) Stimulates bone marrow to increase red blood cell production.
      (2.) Hemoglobin level and hematocrit value are elevated.
      (3.) Arterial O_2 quantifies saturation.
   c. Chest x-ray will show right ventricular hypertrophy; left ventricles may be small because of decrease in pulmonary venous return.

C. Nursing Activities

1. Support parents when they first learn of this defect in their child; allow ample time for the grieving process.
2. Assess parents' knowledge of the defect; teach information needed.
3. Prepare child and parents for the various procedures to be done.
4. Develop overall nursing care that will conserve maximum energy for child.
5. Institute usual pre-operative and post-operative instructions, precautions, and care.
6. Refer child and family to appropriate support groups and other community agencies.

Pediatric Nursing Bibliography

Infants

Nelms, B. & Mullins, R. (1982). *Growth and Development.* Englewood Cliffs, New Jersey: Prentice-Hall, Infants, 257–360.

Whaley, L. F. & Wong, D. L. (1983). *Nursing Care of Infants and Children.* St. Louis: C. V. Mosby Co., Infants, 422–423, 430–458.

Toddlers

Nelms, B. & Mullins, R. (1982). *Growth and Development.* Englewood Cliffs, New Jersey: Prentice-Hall, Toddlers, 363–378, 380–400, 416–425.

Whaley, L. F. & Wong, D. L. (1983). *Nursing Care of Infants and Children.* St. Louis: C. V. Mosby Co., Toddlers, 449–522.

Preschoolers

Nelms, B. & Mullins R. (1982). *Growth and Development.* Englewood Cliffs, New Jersey: Prentice-Hall, Preschooler, 429–443, 495, 520–523.

Whaley, L. F. & Wong, D. L. (1983). *Nursing Care of Infants and Children.* St. Louis: C. V. Mosby Co., Preschool, 525–541.

School-age Children

Nelms, B. & Mullins, R. (1982). *Growth and Development.* Englewood Cliffs, New Jersey: Prentice-Hall, School age, 520–522, 537–540, 570–575.

Whaley, L. F. & Wong, D. L. (1983). *Nursing Care of Infants and Children.* St. Louis: C. V. Mosby Co., School age, 595–625.

Adolescents

Nelms, B. & Mullins, R. (1982). *Growth and Development.* Englewood Cliffs, New Jersey: Prentice-Hall, Adolescent, 521–522, 585–608.

Whaley, L. F. & Wong, D. L. (1983). *Nursing Care of Infants and Children.* St. Louis: C. V. Mosby Co., Adolescent, 671–701.

Common Health Problems

Chow, M. P., Durand, B. A., Feldman, M. N. & Mills, M. A. (1979). *Handbook of Pediatric Primary Care*. New York: John Wiley & Sons.

Whaley, L. F. & Wong, D. L. (1983). *Nursing Care of Infants and Children*. St. Louis: C. V. Mosby Co., Common Health Problems, 130.

Fluid and Electrolyte Disturbances

Metheny, N. M. & Snivelyn, W. G. (1980). *Nurses' Handbook of Fluid Balance*, 2nd ed. Philadelphia: J. B. Lippincott.

Finberg, L. (1980). Fluid, electrolyte, and acid-base abnormalities in pediatrics. *In* Maxwell, M. & Kleeman, C. (eds.). *Clinical Disorders of Fluid and Electrolyte Mechanism*. New York: McGraw-Hill Book Co.

Burns

Lushbaugh, M. A. (1981). Critical care of the child with burns. *Nursing Clinics of North America, 16*:635–645.

Quay, N. & Steele, S. (1983). Health promotion of the child with an acquired disability: *In* Burns, W. S. (ed.). *Health Promotion of The Child With Long-Term Illness*. Norwald, Connecticut: Appleton-Century-Crofts, 235–256.

Renal Disorders

Topor, M. (1981). Symposium on chronic renal failure: Chronic renal disease in children. *Nursing Clinics of North America, 16*:587–597.

Whaley, L. F. & Wong, D. L. (1983). *Nursing Care of Infants and Children*. St. Louis: C. V. Mosby Co.

Congenital Cardiac Problems

Graham, G. & Rossi, E. (eds.) (1980). *Heart Disease in Infants and Children*. Chicago: Year Book Medical Publishers.

Whaley, L. F. & Wong, D. L. (1983). *Nursing Care of Infants and Children*. St. Louis: C. V. Mosby Co.

Sickle Cell Anemia

Beck, W. S. (ed.). *Hematology*. Cambridge: The MIT Press.

Whaley, L. F. & Wong, D. L. (1983). *Nursing Care of Infants and Children*. St. Louis: C. V. Mosby Co.

Thalassemia, Hemophilia

Beck, W. S. (ed.) (1981). Hematology. Cambridge: The MIT Press.

Dressler, D. (1980). Understanding and treating hemophilia. *Nursing, 10*:72–73.

Ohene-Frenpong, K. & Schwartz, E. (1980). Clinical features of thalassemia. *Pediatric Clinics of North America*, 27:403–420.

Leukemia

Brown, M. H. & Kiss, M. E. (1984). Standards of clinical nursing practice for leukemia: anorexia, nausea and vomiting, and fluid volume deficit. *Cancer Nursing*, 7:62–66.

Whaley, L. F. & Wong, D. L. (1983). *Nursing Care of Infants and Children*. St. Louis: C. V. Mosby Co.

Acute Respiratory Disorders

Whaley, L. F. & Wong, D. L. (1983). *Nursing Care of Infants and Children*. St. Louis: C. V. Mosby Co., 56.

Respiratory Problems

Whaley, L. F. & Wong, D. L. (1983). *Nursing Care of Infants and Children*. St. Louis: C. V. Mosby Co., 328–329, 1213–1235.

Voyles, J. B. (1981). Bronchopulmonary dysplasia. *American Journal of Nursing, 81*:510–514.

Meningitis

Wink, D. (1984). Bacterial meningitis in children. *American Journal of Nursing, 84*:456–461.

Whaley, L. F. & Wong, D. L. (1983). *Nursing Care of Infants and Children*. St. Louis: C. V. Mosby, Co.

Neural Tube Defects, Cerebral Palsy, Hydrocephalus

Whaley, L. F. & Wong, D. L. (1983). *Nursing Care of Infants and Children*. St. Louis: C. V. Mosby Co.

Steele, S. (1985). Young children with cerebral palsy. *The American Journal of Maternal-Child Nursing, 11*:259–267.

Seizure Disorders

Barry, K. (1983). The role of the nurse in the diagnosis, classification, and management of epileptic seizures. *Journal of Neurosurgical Nursing, 15*:243–249.

Whaley, L. F. & Wong, D. L. (1983). *Nursing Care of Infants and Children*. St. Louis: C. V. Mosby Co.

Mental Retardation

Roberts, J. J. (1980). Behavior modification with a mentally retarded child. *American Journal of Nursing, 80*:679.

Whaley, L. F. & Wong, D. L. (1983). *Nursing Care of Infants and Children*. St. Louis: C. V. Mosby Co.

Brain Tumors, Neuroblastomas

Maul, S. K. (1984). Childhood brain tumors: A special nursing challenge. *The American Journal of Maternal-Child Nursing*, 9:123–129.

Whaley, L. F. & Wong, D. L. (1983). *Nursing Care of Infants and Children*. St. Louis: C. V. Mosby Co.

Immobilization and Orthopedic Problems

Ibrahim, K. (1984). An overview of childhood fractures. *Pediatric Nursing, 10*:57–65.

Whaley, L. F. & Wong, D. L. (1983). *Nursing Care of Infants and Children*. St. Louis: C. V. Mosby Co.

Gastrointestinal Anomalies

Sugar, E. C. (1981). Hirschsprung's disease. *American Journal of Nursing, 81*:2065–2067.

Whaley, D. F. & Wong, D. L. (1983). *Nursing Care of Infants and Children*. St. Louis: C. V. Mosby Co.

Failure to Thrive

Mira, M. & Cairns, G. (1981). Intervention in the interaction of a mother and child with non-organic failure to thrive. *Pediatric Nursing*, 7:41–45.

Rosenn, D. W., Loeb, L. S. & Jura, M. B. (1980). Differentiation of organic from non-organic failure to thrive syndrome in infancy. *Pediatrics, 66*:698–704.

Section

PEDIATRIC NURSING PRACTICE QUESTIONS

1 • Nicholas James is 4 months old. In teaching his mother, Mrs. James, about adding solid foods to Nicholas' diet, you would include which of the following?

1. Solid foods should be offered by 2 months of age to ensure a well-balanced diet.
2. Adding seasoning to baby food will make them more "acceptable" to the baby.
3. Loose stools or skin rash may mean that the baby is not tolerating new food.
4. If the infant refuses spoon feeding, add solid foods to his bottle.

2 • Part of the nurse's anticipatory guidance includes a discussion of safety. Considering Nicholas' developmental level, it would be most important to teach Mrs. James the following:

1. Never leave Nicholas alone in a room.
2. Fence stairways at the top and bottom.
3. Raise crib safety rails to full height.
4. Place all medication in a locked cabinet.

3 • When Nicholas is 6 months old, you should be able to normally elicit the following reflex:

1. Dance or step.
2. Startle.
3. Extrusion.
4. Sucking.

4 • When Nicholas becomes 9 months old, the following would be an abnormal finding:

1. Posterior fontanel is closed.
2. He rolls over.
3. He sits only with support.
4. He shows fear toward strangers.

5 • A 2-month-old infant has just received his 1st immunizations. You will tell the mother that the following could occur as a common result of the immunization:

1. Increased irritability.
2. Appearance of a mild rash 5 days after injection.
3. Symptoms of an upper respiratory infection.
4. Excessive drooling.

6 • Mrs. James occasionally substitutes Nicholas' breast-feeding with formula. She wants to know the difference in the stools' appearance between breast-feeding and formula feeding. Formula feeding results in the following type of stools:

1. Very pale yellow, usually formed.
2. Light beige color, very soft.
3. Dark brown color, very soft with white curd-like pieces.
4. Pale green, usually formed.

7 • The nurse discussed the normal infant's head circumference compared with the chest circumference with Nicholas' mother several months ago. The mother is now able to tell you that *after* a certain age, the chest circumference will exceed the head circumference. That age is:

1. 3 months.
2. 6 months.
3. 9 months.
4. 12 months.

8 • The following statement is correct pertaining to tooth eruption:

1. Most infants get their 1st teeth at about 3 months of age.
2. By the age of 12 months, the average infant has 8 teeth.
3. Upper teeth appear first.
4. Lower teeth appear first.

9 • When Nicholas is around 8 months of age, he will be expected to be able to play peek-a-boo. Which critical event of the sensorimotor phase of cognitive develpment does this demonstrate?

1. Egocentrism.
2. Use of symbols.
3. Object permanency.
4. Separation of self from environment.

10 • A 6-month-old infant is getting his checkup. Which of the following should be true of the infant if he is normal?

1. He should have tripled his birth weight.
2. His anterior fontanelle is closed.
3. He laughs and squeals.
4. He pulls himself to a stand.

11 • Changes in physical development occurring during the toddler period include the following:

1. Increase in caloric needs due to an increase in growth rate.
2. Atrophy of the lymphoid tissue of the tonsils and adenoids.
3. Increase in stomach capacity with slower passage of food through the gastrointestinal tract.
4. 75% completion of deciduous dentition.

12 • Language development during the toddler years is characterized by all of the following EXCEPT:

1. Acquisition of intelligible speech by 3 years of age.
2. Greater receptive vocabulary than expressive vocabulary.
3. Speech and motor skills develop concurrently at the same speed.
4. Delayed development when the child is not encouraged to express his wants.

13 • The nurse knows that a 30-month-old toddler has entered the pre-operational stage of cognitive thought because he does the following:

1. Uses 2-word phrases.
2. Says "No" whenever she asks him to do something.
3. His conception of time is now similar to that of an older child.
4. Has improved concept of space.

14 • Because toddlers engage in parallel play, they enjoy doing the following:

1. Playing games such as tag.
2. Playing alongside other children but not with them.
3. Dramatic play.
4. Sharing toys with other children.

15 • If a 30-month-old toddler's cognitive development is normal, he should be able to do the following:

1. Remember events that occurred the day before.
2. Understand why his mother is angry.
3. Understand the terms "above" and "below."
4. Understand why he cannot eat candy just before dinner.

16 • In counseling the toddler's parents about accidents, the nurse should do the following:

1. Strongly encourage parents to never let the child out of their sight.
2. Discourage exploration until the child is older.
3. Provide information about "child proofing" their home.
4. Remind parents to speak slowly and firmly so that their toddler will better understand their warnings about accidents.

17 • Interventions that help to decrease separation anxiety in the hospitalized toddler include all of the following EXCEPT:

1. Bringing a favorite blanket or toy from home.
2. Keeping parental visiting to a minimum.
3. Keeping the child distracted with suitable play activities.
4. Providing pictures of his family in his room.

18 • The following response to hospitalization is typically seen during the toddler years:

1. He may begin soiling himself, although he has been recently toilet trained.
2. He quickly adjusts to the new schedule of the hospital setting.
3. He responds positively to those staff persons who do not hurt him.
4. He will transfer trust to another adult.

19 • All of the following are stressors for the hospitalized toddler EXCEPT:

1. Separation from parents.
2. Disruption of daily routines.
3. Loss of independence.
4. Disturbance in body image.

20 • In assessing a 28-month-old child, which of the following should cause the nurse to be concerned about his developmental progress?

1. The child uses "No" even when agreeing to a request.
2. He has not achieved bowel and bladder control.
3. His vocalizations are unintelligible to his parents.
4. He refuses to share his toys with others.

21 • In counseling parents about the development of fears during the preschool period, the nurse should advise them of the following:

1. Fears are the result of *elementary logical conclusions*.
2. Fears are best dealt with by ignoring them.
3. Professional help is always required to adequately help the child.
4. Fears are best handled by actively involving the child in dealing with them directly.

22 • Cognitive development during the preschool period is characterized by the ability to do the following:

1. Understand time concepts such as tomorrow and yesterday.
2. Think of only one idea at a time.
3. Understand another person's thoughts and feelings.
4. Define elementary abstract terms.

23 • A mother of a preschooler is concerned because her child is constantly talking to an imaginary friend. You will advise the mother about this behavior in the following way:

1. This is most often seen in emotionally disturbed children.
2. This is abnormal and should be discouraged.
3. This is normal and satisfies emotional needs.
4. This is most often associated with retarded children.

24 • According to Freud, the genital (oedipal) stage of development in the preschooler is characterized by the following:

1. The fear of castration in boys.
2. The increased use of masturbation to decrease sexual tension.
3. An increase in modesty among both sexes.
4. Stronger attachment to the parent of the opposite sex.

25 • In advising the father of a preschooler weighing 35 lb, you will give him the following information about automobile safety:

1. The child needs a restraining belt, but keep it loose to permit mobility.
2. The child should be seated on a firm pillow wearing a lap belt.
3. The child must wear both lap and shoulder belts.
4. The child must use an approved car seat properly secured.

26 • All of the following are true of the language development of preschoolers EXCEPT:

1. Grammatical and pronunciation errors are common.
2. Experimentation with words and sounds is common.
3. Words are interpreted literally.
4. Single words and short phrases are used rather than complete sentences.

27 • From 3 through 5 years of age, all of the following characteristics and behaviors are commonly seen EXCEPT:

1. Negativism.
2. Fantasy.
3. Socialized speech.
4. Refinement of fine motor skills.

28 • The mother of a 3 year old is asking what immunization her child should be getting soon. Assuming that her child is up to date with prior immunizations, the child should now receive the following:

1. DPT
2. MMR
3. OPV
4. None

29 • Hospitalization and surgical procedures are difficult for the preschooler for all of the following reasons EXCEPT:

1. This is the period when separation anxiety is at its peak.
2. Even the healthy preschooler has many concerns about body integrity.
3. His fantasies about what is going to be done are often worse than reality.
4. He feels out of control.

30 • All of the following behaviors may be displayed by the preschooler experiencing pain EXCEPT:

1. Aggression.
2. Dependency.
3. Clenching of fists or teeth.
4. Anxiety.

31 • All of the following are true of children between the ages of 6 and 12 years EXCEPT:

1. Tonsils, adenoids, and thymus and lymph nodes reach their maximum size during this period.
2. The final 20 to 25% of linear growth is achieved.
3. The tissues of the gastrointestinal and respiratory systems have fully developed.
4. Immunological functions have matured.

32 • The school-age child's relationship with his family gradually changes. The following characteristic reflects the change in the relationship:

1. Increasing respect for siblings.
2. Dependency on family to help develop self image.
3. Comparison of family with social contacts.
4. Idolizing of parents and siblings.

33 • During the school-age years, the child's peer group accomplishes all of the following EXCEPT:

1. Helps him choose his vocation.
2. Provides him with a more realistic appraisal of his abilities.
3. Serves as his socializing agent.
4. Helps him form attitudes and values.

34 • According to Erikson, the school-age child may feel "inferior" if he experiences the following:

1. He is expected to assume some household chores.
2. He is encouraged to attempt projects beyond his abilities.
3. He has parents who provide consistent discipline.
4. He has 3 younger siblings.

35 • Cognitive operations during the school-age period is restricted by the following factor:

1. Failure to achieve reversibility.
2. Egocentrism.
3. Use of animism.
4. Inability to deal with abstractions.

36 • In selecting activities for the school-age child, the nurse should keep the following in mind:

1. Self control often may be accompanied by compulsive practices such as touching objects and stepping over cracks.
2. Most school-age children are "good losers."
3. School-age children start many projects but seldom complete them.
4. School-age children are relatively lenient about bending the rules of the game.

37 • The following statement is true about hospitalized school-age children:

1. They have the capacity to adequately rationalize about missing out on special events at their school or in their family.
2. Young school-age children may still experience separation anxiety.
3. This age group depends primarily upon their peer group for support.
4. Both boys and girls tolerate painful procedures relatively well.

38 • Practices common to school-age children include all of the following EXCEPT:

1. Talking in code.
2. Starting collections.
3. Telling jokes.
4. Participating mostly in activities with both boys and girls.

39 • The school-age child demonstrates he has reached the stage of "concrete operations" when he does all of the following EXCEPT:

1. Collects stamps from various countries.
2. Takes into consideration his playmate's ideas before making his response.
3. Depends to a great extent upon sensory stimulation.
4. Conceptualizes that when a measuring cup of water is poured into a tall beaker the amount of water in the beaker remains the same.

40 • Physical development in the school-age child may be characterized by the following:

1. An increase in height of approximately 1 to 2 in/year.
2. Development and full maturation of muscle fibers.
3. Eruption of the last permanent teeth.
4. A marked decrease in pulse rate.

41 • According to Erikson, role diffusion could occur in an adolescent for the following reason:

1. He fails to achieve emotional independence from his parents.
2. He is physically impaired.
3. He is unable to formulate a satisfactory identification from his uncertainties and confusions related to roles, identifications, and aspirations.
4. He is unable to complete a project he started.

42 • According to developmental authorities, the tasks of adolescence include all of the following EXCEPT:

1. Development of strong family ties.
2. Acquiring a set of values and ethics.
3. Acceptance of a new body image.
4. Achieving a masculine or feminine social role.

43 • The period of "formal operations" is characterized by the following:

1. Use of transductive reasoning.
2. Ability to deal with hypothetical situations that could occur in the future.
3. Achievement of conservation.
4. Thoughts influenced more by perceptions and experiences.

44 • In doing the physical assessment, the nurse should realize that increased estrogen levels in adolescent females could cause the following:

1. Reactivation of the sebaceous glands.
2. Development of body hair.
3. Epiphyseal closure.
4. A rise in hemoglobin level and hematocrit value.

45 • The numerous physical changes that adolescents experience often cause all of the following responses EXCEPT:

1. Increased awkwardness in movement.
2. Exaggerated response to bodily sensations.
3. Concern about normality.
4. Development of self confidence and pride.

46 • Legally, an adolescent can consent to some or all medical care (without parental consent) if he is in the following category:

1. He is considered an "emancipated" individual.
2. He is able to pay for his own medical services.
3. His medical care involves only minor surgery.
4. He has 2 peers who will vouch for his financial reliability.

47 • Nutritional problems during adolescence are caused by all of the following EXCEPT:

1. Increased concern about their developing body image.
2. Greater variability in caloric needs due to variability in activity patterns and growth requirements.
3. Peer group influence.
4. A lower basal metabolism.

48 • In working with adolescents in an out-patient clinic, the nurse should understand that her clients generally evidence the following characteristic:

1. Highly receptive to health care teaching.
2. Require help to learn how to use the health care system.
3. Easily establish relationships with health care workers.
4. Often seek help for minor physical problems that actually are caused by psychosocial stresses.

49 • Accidents are the greatest single cause of death in the adolescent age group. All of the following are reasons for the high incidence of accidents during adolescence EXCEPT:

1. Adolescents have an attitude of "It won't happen to me" about the possibility of dying.
2. The loss of parental control over their behavior makes them more vulnerable.
3. Poor judgment and disregard for sound, defensive driving principles are characteristic of many teenage drivers.
4. The use of drugs and alcohol has increased in recent years.

50 • Which of the following is *not* the reason why adolescents have difficulty coping with hospitalization?

1. Loss of independence.
2. Loss of self control over pain.
3. Increased preoccupation with bodily sensations.
4. Separation from peer group.

51 • In most cultures and societies, families have principal functions in relation to children. All of the following are functions EXCEPT:

1. To provide physical care for children.
2. To maintain children's emotional and psychological welfare.
3. To teach them to challenge societal institutions.
4. To educate them to adjust to their own culture.

52 • One of the main functions of the family is to socialize children into their culture. The following is one of the effective ways in which the family does this:

1. Make certain mother is home when the children return from school.
2. Enable them to watch television programs.
3. Help them with school homework.
4. Teach them the value system of the culture.

53 • Family structure consists of individuals, and this structure is altered from time to time. One of the factors that could alter this structure is:

1. Oldest child starts school.
2. A birth in the family.
3. Father gets a raise in wages.
4. Grandparents come to visit for the weekend.

54 • Small families tend to influence children differently compared with larger families. The following describes a typical activity occurring in a small family:

1. Parenting is extensive rather than intensive.
2. Less democratic participation by the children.
3. Adolescents identify more strongly with their parents.
4. Older siblings tend to discipline the younger ones.

55 • Lately, an increasing number of mothers have joined the work force, and the mothers' absence from home affects children in various ways. The following is *not* one of the factors that affect children of working mothers:

1. Age of child.
2. Attitude of father toward mother's work.
3. Regularity of mother's work.
4. Amount of money mother is able to contribute toward household expenses.

56 • A child has hypotonic dehydration. In this form of dehydration, the following occurs:

1. Primarily a loss of sodium exceeding extracellular fluid loss.
2. An equally proportionate loss of extracellular fluid and sodium.
3. Primarily a loss of extracellular fluid exceeding sodium loss.
4. Primarily a loss of intracellular fluid exceeding extracellular fluid loss.

57 • The following physical sign would be evident in severe extracellular fluid loss in an infant.

1. Hypertonicity of extremities.
2. Generalized edema.
3. Decreased pulse rate.
4. Sunken anterior fontanelle.

58 • Fluid replacement is begun on the child who is hospitalized for dehydration. The following is the 1st phase of fluid replacement in dehydration:

1. Restoration of circulation.
2. Restoration of intracellular fluid volume.
3. Restoration of calories and protein.
4. Restoration of intracellular potassium.

59 • Persistent vomiting can lead to metabolic alkalosis. The following is a sign of metabolic alkalosis:

1. Tachycardia.
2. Increased urinary output.
3. Decreased urinary output.
4. Hypertonicity of muscles.

60 • Fluid expenditure by the body is dependent upon 3 factors. The following are all correct EXCEPT:

1. Temperature, intrinsic and environmental.
2. Type of food eaten in last 24 hours.
3. Activity of patient.
4. Rate of respiration.

61 • Correct analysis of electrolyte laboratory test reports is an important aspect of nursing intervention. The nurse should know that with *one exception*, all of the following are in need of exact control for fluid and electrolyte balance. The *one exception* is:

1. Iron.
2. Sodium.
3. Potassium.
4. Calcium.

62 • Incidences of burns in children may be related to:

1. Position in family structure.
2. Amount of adult supervision.
3. Size of the child.
4. The distance to the closest fire station.

63 • A child is hospitalized with 2nd and 3rd degree burns covering most of his body. The prime objective of the child's treatment in the 1st 48 hours would be:

1. Providing emotional support.
2. Preventing infection.
3. Restoring and maintaining adequate intravascular fluid volume.
4. Cleansing and débriding the wound.

64 • Which of the following is *not* a symptom of prolonged smoke inhalation?

1. Dyspnea.
2. Stridor.
3. Frothy sputum.
4. Charcoal-colored sputum.

65 • The fluid shift occurring during the emergent phase of burn injury is caused primarily by the following:

1. Interstitial fluid from injured tissues leaking into the wound.
2. Severe red blood cell damage due to the injury.
3. Intracellular fluid leaking into the interstitial spaces.
4. Serum from the blood stream leaking into injured tissues.

66 • A 0.5% solution of silver nitrate is used topically as a treatment for burns. An important disadvantage to this treatment method is the following:

1. Antibacterial action is weak.
2. Serum electrolyte loss can result.
3. Skin grafting must be delayed until the drug is absorbed.
4. Hypertension is associated with prolonged use.

67 • The edema fluid resulting from the burn accumulates rapidly in the 1st 18 hours, and it reaches the maximum in approximately 48 hours. After the 1st 48 hours, the nurse can anticipate all of the following EXCEPT:

1. A marked decrease in blood pressure.
2. Increased urinary output.
3. A decrease in edema.
4. A decrease in fluid requirements.

68 • You are teaching burn first aid to a group of mothers. Which of the following is the most beneficial for a burn immediately after the injury:

1. Applying a small amount of polyunsaturated cooking oil to the burn.
2. Spraying the burn with an antiseptic spray.
3. Immersing in cold water.
4. Applying ice to the burn.

69 • Severity of the burn is assessed *immediately* after the injury on the basis of all the following EXCEPT:

1. Laboratory reports.
2. Location of the burn.
3. Depth of the burn.
4. Age of the child.

70 • A 3-year-old child has been hospitalized with nephrotic syndrome. You will most likely observe the following manifestation:

1. Elevated blood pressure.
2. Hematuria.
3. Ascites.
4. Low urine specific gravity.

71 • The child's mother is upset and wants to know what caused her child's nephrotic syndrome. You explain to her that there are several known etiologies and the following is one of them:

1. A previous β-hemolytic *Streptococcus*.
2. A recessive gene on an autosome.
3. Anomalous embryonic development of the glomeruli.
4. An acute allergic reaction to a protein substance.

72 • The most important developmentally related concern of this 3-year-old child would most likely be the following:

1. Fear of separation from parents.
2. Change in body image.
3. Compliance with treatments.
4. Fear of dying.

73 • The physician has ordered prednisone by mouth. All of the following actions are indicated EXCEPT:

1. Giving the prednisone when food is in the stomach.
2. Withholding the prednisone if the child's blood pressure becomes elevated.
3. Observing the child closely for signs of infection.
4. Providing foods high in potassium.

74 • The most effective way to assess the therapeutic effects of a diuretic given to a young child is to do the following:

1. Weigh the child immediately before and 4 hours after the medication is given.
2. Measure all of the child's output, including emesis.
3. Weigh the child at the same time every day, using the same scale.
4. Take the child's blood pressure every 4 hours.

75 • The following position would be best during the child's acute phase of illness.

1. On his left side.
2. On his back.
3. On his right side.
4. Semi-Fowler's.

76 • Laboratory test results from the child with nephrotic syndrome will usually show the following:

1. Increased serum cholesterol level.
2. Gross hematuria.
3. Low urine specific gravity.
4. Elevated serum protein concentrations.

77 • The following snack would be the best choice for this child.

1. Cheese and crackers, celery.
2. Fruit yogurt and raisins.
3. Buttered popcorn and 7-UP.
4. Chicken McNuggets and french fries.

78 • The nurse is discussing home care with the parents. One of the most important ways for the parents to detect relapse of nephrotic syndrome early is to do the following:

1. Bring the child to the clinic for monthly blood tests.
2. Perform daily urine tests.
3. Determine daily vital signs.
4. Examine for presence of edema.

79 • Prior to discharge, the nurse discusses with the parents their management of the child at home and what they can expect pertaining to the course of the illness. The nurse indicates the following to them:

1. The relapsing form of this disease is usually short.
2. The relapsing form of this disease is usually long.
3. There will be a sudden and remarkable improvement in the child's condition after 2 weeks or so.
4. There will be a steady course toward recovery.

80 • Tom, a 6 year old, has been admitted to the hospital with a diagnosis of hemophilia A. In collecting family data, you would expect to find the following:

1. His father is a defective gene carrier, and his mother is normal.
2. Both parents are normal, but his maternal grandfather is a defective gene carrier.
3. His father, paternal grandfather, and paternal great-grandfather are all hemophiliacs.
4. His mother is a defective gene carrier, and his father is normal.

81 • Tom's laboratory results, which would corroborate this diagnosis, would show the following:

1. Decreased platelet count.
2. Slow clotting time.
3. Deficiency in generation of thromboplastin.
4. Lack of Factor IX.

82 • The following is a classic symptom shown by Tom.

1. Purpura and bruises on his trunk and extremities.
2. Petechiae over his entire body.
3. Lumpy subcutaneous bruises and intramuscular hematomas.
4. Severe abdominal cramps with nausea and vomiting.

83 • Tom's mother heard about von Willebrand's disease, and she asks you to describe the disease. You will give her the following information about von Willebrand's disease:

1. Hemarthrosis is also common.
2. Mucous membrane bleeding hardly ever occurs.
3. Transmission from parent to child is autosomal recessive.
4. Platelet function is abnormal.

84 • Treatment for Tom's hemophilia A consists of the administration of the following:

1. An individualized mixture of coagulation factors determined by a blood assay.
2. Factor VIII, antihemophilic factor.
3. Equal amounts of factors VIII and IX.
4. The plasma thromboplastin antecedent.

85 • The following statement regarding bleeding episodes is correct:

1. If bleeding episodes are frequent, he may be placed on a prophylactic infusion program.
2. Gastrointestinal bleeding is the most frequent complication.
3. Replacement therapy is not initiated until a bleeding episode has ended.
4. When bleeding into a joint occurs, immobilization for 3 weeks is necessary.

86 • The nursing care of Tom during the period of hemarthrosis would include all of the following EXCEPT:

1. Immobilization of afflicted joint.
2. Application of heat to the joint.
3. Analgesia as prescribed for pain.
4. Bed rest or limited activity in a wheelchair.

87 • The following describes thalassemia major:

1. Inheritance is sex-linked recessive.
2. It is secondary to a qualitative defect of the hemoglobin chain.
3. It is secondary to a quantitative deficit of the hemoglobin chain.
4. It is primarily found in people of Far Eastern origins.

88 • In thalassemia major, keeping the child's hemoglobin level above 9 to 10 gm/dl does all of the following EXCEPT:

1. Permits normal activity with comfort.
2. Prevents progressive marrow expansion associated with bone changes.
3. Minimizes cardiac dilatation and osteoporosis.
4. Allows eventual recovery from the disease.

89 • All of the following statements are true regarding iron accumulation in thalassemia major EXCEPT:

1. The heart, pancreas, and liver are involved.
2. It frequently causes anuria.
3. The major source of iron comes from frequent transfusions.
4. It could cause cardiac failure.

90 • A child with thalassemia major is receiving a blood transfusion. He begins to complain of headache and develops shaking chills. The nurse would take the following step:

1. Check the child's temperature every 30 minutes, and if elevated, administer Tylenol.
2. Discuss the next course of action with a qualified colleague.
3. Stop the transfusion, notify the physician.
4. Slow down the transfusion and administer antihistamine p.r.n.

91 • The primary treatment for thalassemia major is the following:

1. Iron therapy.
2. Blood transfusion.
3. Vitamin B_{12}.
4. Vitamin E.

92 • Nine-year-old Nicholas, who has β-thalassemia, is recovering from splenectomy. The most important nursing intervention after splenectomy is the following:

1. Take measures to prevent any kind of infection.
2. Encourage fluids to maintain fluid and electrolyte balance.
3. Position him in such a way as to promote rapid healing of the surgical wound.
4. Watch his laboratory reports closely for results indicating severe anemia.

93 • In providing emotional support to Nicholas and his family, the nurse should keep the following in mind:

1. Recovery can be expected sometime during the adolescent years.
2. The chief cause of death is renal shutdown.
3. Few patients survive beyond the 3rd decade.
4. If splenectomy is not successful in alleviating symptoms, radiation treatments will most likely be tried.

94 • Nursing care of a newborn with a cleft lip and cleft palate would include all of the following EXCEPT:

1. Feeding newborn with a large, soft nipple with an enlarged hole.
2. Feeding newborn in a supine position.
3. Burping newborn frequently.
4. Supporting parents in accepting a child with a congenital anomaly.

95 • The infant will be taken home until surgical correction can be done. Teaching plan for the mother should include all of the following EXCEPT:

1. Follow each feeding with water.
2. Watch for signs of respiratory distress.
3. Train the infant to lie on his back.
4. Keep the infant's arms restrained at all times.

96 • Cleft palate surgery is frequently postponed to await further palatal development. The parent needs to be cautioned about protecting the infant from infections. The following is one of the most frequently seen complications of a palatal defect:

1. Recurrent otitis media.
2. Aspiration pneumonia.
3. Gastroenteritis.
4. Sinusitis.

97 • The parents ask the nurse about the causes of their infant's deformity. The following response would be the best:

1. The defects occurred because of hereditary factors.
2. The defects occurred because the mother contracted flu during her 5th month of pregnancy.
3. The actual cause is unknown but believed to be of multifactorial origin based on inheritance.
4. The defects occurred because the father had been on megavitamin therapy when conception occurred.

98 • The infant has now been admitted to the hospital for closure of the cleft lip. His postoperative care could include all of the following EXCEPT:

1. Position infant lying on side, flat in bed.
2. High humidity, misted tent.
3. Give only clear fluids, initially.
4. Elbow restraint, release periodically.

99 • Following surgery for cleft lip, it is essential that the infant does not cry. The following step would be most effective to keep his crying to a minimum:

1. Give the infant a pacifier, since he will be NPO for a while.
2. Allow the infant to lie on his abdomen, as most babies prefer this position.
3. Ask the mother to stay so she can console the infant.
4. Request a special nurse, as it is unrealistic to expect the regular staff to keep him from crying.

100 • After surgical repair of cleft lip, the suture line is kept meticulously clean. The following procedure should be carried out:

1. Wash suture line with soap and water 4 times a day.
2. Very gently swab area with hydrogen peroxide, and apply a thin coat of antibiotic ointment.
3. Apply baby lotion to the suture line 4 times a day.
4. Use lemon and glycerin swabs, and follow with antibiotic ointment.

Answer Sheet for Pediatric Nursing Practice Questions

1. 1 2 3 4	26. 1 2 3 4	51. 1 2 3 4	76. 1 2 3 4
2. 1 2 3 4	27. 1 2 3 4	52. 1 2 3 4	77. 1 2 3 4
3. 1 2 3 4	28. 1 2 3 4	53. 1 2 3 4	78. 1 2 3 4
4. 1 2 3 4	29. 1 2 3 4	54. 1 2 3 4	79. 1 2 3 4
5. 1 2 3 4	30. 1 2 3 4	55. 1 2 3 4	80. 1 2 3 4
6. 1 2 3 4	31. 1 2 3 4	56. 1 2 3 4	81. 1 2 3 4
7. 1 2 3 4	32. 1 2 3 4	57. 1 2 3 4	82. 1 2 3 4
8. 1 2 3 4	33. 1 2 3 4	58. 1 2 3 4	83. 1 2 3 4
9. 1 2 3 4	34. 1 2 3 4	59. 1 2 3 4	84. 1 2 3 4
10. 1 2 3 4	35. 1 2 3 4	60. 1 2 3 4	85. 1 2 3 4
11. 1 2 3 4	36. 1 2 3 4	61. 1 2 3 4	86. 1 2 3 4
12. 1 2 3 4	37. 1 2 3 4	62. 1 2 3 4	87. 1 2 3 4
13. 1 2 3 4	38. 1 2 3 4	63. 1 2 3 4	88. 1 2 3 4
14. 1 2 3 4	39. 1 2 3 4	64. 1 2 3 4	89. 1 2 3 4
15. 1 2 3 4	40. 1 2 3 4	65. 1 2 3 4	90. 1 2 3 4
16. 1 2 3 4	41. 1 2 3 4	66. 1 2 3 4	91. 1 2 3 4
17. 1 2 3 4	42. 1 2 3 4	67. 1 2 3 4	92. 1 2 3 4
18. 1 2 3 4	43. 1 2 3 4	68. 1 2 3 4	93. 1 2 3 4
19. 1 2 3 4	44. 1 2 3 4	69. 1 2 3 4	94. 1 2 3 4
20. 1 2 3 4	45. 1 2 3 4	70. 1 2 3 4	95. 1 2 3 4
21. 1 2 3 4	46. 1 2 3 4	71. 1 2 3 4	96. 1 2 3 4
22. 1 2 3 4	47. 1 2 3 4	72. 1 2 3 4	97. 1 2 3 4
23. 1 2 3 4	48. 1 2 3 4	73. 1 2 3 4	98. 1 2 3 4
24. 1 2 3 4	49. 1 2 3 4	74. 1 2 3 4	99. 1 2 3 4
25. 1 2 3 4	50. 1 2 3 4	75. 1 2 3 4	100. 1 2 3 4

Section

ANSWERS AND RATIONALES FOR PEDIATRIC NURSING PRACTICE QUESTIONS

1. (3) Developmentally and physiologically, infants are not ready for solid food before 5 to 6 months of age. Not only is their extrusion reflex so strong that most of the food is pushed out, but their gastrointestinal tract has not reached the maturity to handle solid foods. Food should not be mixed in the formula and added to the bottle because it deprives the infant of learning the taste and texture of new food, and it also deprives him of learning how to chew.

2. (3) Falls are most common after 4 months of age; the mother should make it a habit to never place a child on a raised surface that has no safety rails while the child is unattended.

3. (4) The sucking reflex does not disappear until 10 to 12 months; the other reflexes disappear before 6 months.

4. (3) Normally, most infants are sitting without support before 8 months of age. The remaining findings are all normal for a 9-month-old child.

5. (1) After immunizations, most infants are irritable owing to tenderness and swelling at the site of the injection and a mild temperature elevation. Excessive drooling at the time of immunization could be a coincidence if the child is teething. Upper respiratory infection is not in any way related to immunization. Rashes may occur with measles or rubella vaccine, but DPT does not cause rashes.

6. (1) Stools from breast-fed infants are bright yellow, very soft, and almost liquid. Formula-fed infants have stools that are paler yellow, usually formed, with a more offensive odor than those of breast-fed infants.

7. (4) After the 1st year of life, the chest circumference exceeds that of the head.

8. (4) Most infants get their 1st tooth at about 6 months of age. The lower central incisors are the 1st teeth to erupt. By the age of 12 months, the average infant has 4 teeth.

9. (3) By the time a normal infant is 8 months of age, he is able to realize that objects that leave one's visual field (hiding one's face in peek-a-boo) still exist.

10. (4) Most normal infants laugh and squeal by the time they are 4½ months old.

11. (3) During toddler years, transit time of ingested food slows, and stomach capacity increases to allow for the usual schedule of 3 meals a day.

12. (3) There is a slowing in the development of speech while the child's motor skills are being attained.

13. (1) The main cognitive achievement of early childhood is the acquisition of language; the toddler is able to use 2- to 3-word phrases.

14. (2) In parallel play of toddlers, play takes place alongside, but not with, other children.

15. (1) The conception of time is still developing in the toddler, but he does have some sense of time in terms of memory.

16. (3) Due to the toddler's cognitive level, he is unaware of danger within the environment. Temporarily "child proofing" the home to eliminate sources of accidents is the best possible action to take with a toddler in the home.

17. (2) Keeping parental visiting to a minimum when a toddler is going through separation anxiety merely begins the destructive cycle of exacerbating the child's unmet needs. It would be more beneficial to show the toddler that although separation has to take place, the parents will return.

18. (1) Regression is common in toddlers because almost any additional stress, such as separation from parents, lessens their ability to master present developmental tasks. In addition, stress can cause regression of recently acquired skills.

19. (4) Based on the toddler's cognitive level, he is yet unable to conceptualize body image; hence, altered body image would not be one of the toddler's stresses with hospitalization.

20. (3) By the time a child is 2 years old, about 66% of his speech is understandable.

21. (4) By actively dealing with fear directly, the experience that created the fear can be reconstructed without involving the child. If the child is afraid of dogs, for example, he can watch other children happily play with dogs. Exposing the child to the feared object in a safe situation provides a type of desensitization.

22. (2) During preschool years, the child's cognitive skills are developing rapidly. Despite this, he can still only think of one idea at a time. Preschoolers are involved in prelogical thinking; therefore, they do not understand the concept of time or anything else that is abstract.

23. (3) Playing with imaginary playmates is a normal and useful activity. Indulging in this type of play will enable the preschooler to differentiate between what is imaginary and what is real.

24. (1) According to Freud's concept of oedipal complex, every small boy's wish is to marry his mother and get rid of his father. However, he develops a feeling of guilt for wanting to get rid of his father, resulting in a fear of punishment by castration.

25. (4) Many states now have laws mandating car seats for children. This law is based on the fact that car accidents are one of the leading causes of death. Studies have shown that safety belts and harnesses are not sufficient for children to prevent serious injuries.

26. (4) Three and 4 year olds are able to form sentences of 3 to 4 words, and 4 and 5 year olds form longer sentences of 4 to 5 words.

27. (1) Negativism is a characteristic of a toddler in his quest for autonomy; a normal preschooler should have resolved this behavior.

28. (4) If a child is up to date with prior immunizations at 3 years of age, he will not be getting a booster until 4 years of age.

29. (1) Separation anxiety is at its peak during infancy, usually around 4 to 6 months.

30. (3) Preschoolers react to pain with aggression, dependency, and anxiety. Clenching of fists or teeth is a passive method of dealing with discomfort, and a preschooler has not yet learned this method of dealing with pain. A school-age child, around 9 or 10 years of age, generally learns and uses this method.

31. (2) Physical growth and change continue during the school-age period, but final linear growth does not occur until the adolescent period.

32. (3) Before the school-age period, the child idolizes his parents and older siblings, but as the child moves away from his family into the world of his peers, he begins to compare his family and his family's values with that of her peers. Eventually, the child will stand solidly with his peer group.

33. (1) School-age children normally do not preoccupy themselves with future vocational choices; this process usually begins taking place during adolescence.

34. (2) Through a sense of accomplishment, the school-age child avoids the feeling of inferiority. Should this child attempt projects beyond his abilities and fail, he will suffer frustration and experience a sense of inferiority.

35. (4) The normal school-age child increases his capacity for logical thinking; however, consistent application of abstraction does not occur until adolescence.

36. (1) Although school-age children have gained tremendous amounts of control compared with earlier years, this control is still far from being absolute; therefore, they indulge in compulsive practices involving motor activities, such as touching objects and stepping over cracks.

37. (2) Although school-age children are better able to cope with separation in general, the stress imposed by illness or hospitalization may generate separation anxiety.

38. (4) During school-age years, boys associate with boys, and girls with girls, each pursuing their own interests, with communication between sexes confined to only that which is necessary.

39. (3) The school-age child no longer relies heavily on sensory stimulation to experience events and actions; he is now able to use his thought processes.

40. (1) During the school-age years, growth in height and weight assumes a slower but steady pace as compared with the earlier years. Between ages 6 and 12 years, children will grow an average of 1 to 2 in/year.

41. (3) The process of evolving an identification is a period of confusion, discouragement, and depression for the adolescent. Role diffusion could be the result if the adolescent fails to develop a satisfactory identity for himself.

42. (1) During adolescence, the teenager is striving to break away from his strong family ties and to align himself with a peer group.

43. (2) Adolescents are able to live in the nonpresent (future) as well as the present; they are also able to think in the future.

44. (3) Although the estrogen secretion effect on bone growth is much stronger in females than in males, this bone growth stops sooner in females owing to epiphyseal closure.

45. (4) Rather than giving the adolescent a sense of pride and self confidence, the sudden physical changes are a source of embarrassment, self consciousness, and feelings of inadequacy.

46. (1) Adolescents who are no longer under parental control have legal authority over the conduct of their medical care. These are adolescents who are living alone, are married, are economically self sufficient, and understand the process of receiving informed consent.

47. (4) Although basal heat production does decrease in the adolescent years, this is not one of the reasons adolescents encounter nutritional problems.

48. (2) Adolescents in general have very little information pertaining to the health care system. Not only are they usually reluctant to take the initiative to seek health care, many have no idea how to proceed in this search. The nurse is in a position to introduce the adolescent to the essential health services available to him.

49. (2) Loss of parental control over adolescent behavior does not necessarily make the adolescent more vulnerable to accidents. Accidents are closely related to the developmental characteristics associated with the adolescents' growth and maturation.

50. (2) Adolescents react to pain with much self control. Therefore, the prospect of experiencing pain is not one of the reasons adolescents have difficulty coping with hospitalization.

51. (3) Generally families do not teach their children to challenge what they themselves accept—their societal institutions. Adolescents go through a period when they question and challenge societal institutions and norms, but this behavior is generally not taught to them by their parents.

52. (4) Families socialize their children by teaching them the language, the appropriate role behavior, and the value system and ethical standards of the culture.

53. (2) The family structure is altered when members are gained or lost through marriage, divorce, birth, death, and so on.

54. (3) Compared to adolescents from large families, adolescents from small families tend to identify more strongly with their parents and rely more on their parents for advice.

55. (4) The factors that are related to the effect that a mother's absence has on a child tend to be psychosocial in nature, such as the age of the child, the regularity with which she is away from home, and the father's attitude concerning the mother's employment.

56. (1) Hypotonic dehydration occurs when the electrolyte (sodium) deficit exceeds the water deficit.

57. (4) In severe depletion of extracellular fluid volume, skin and mucous membranes are dry, skin is gray, respirations are rapid, and the anterior fontanelle becomes depressed.

58. (1) Since disruption of adequate circulation constitutes the greatest threat to life, the first priority is restoration of circulation.

59. (4) Immediate effects of calcium imbalance associated with metabolic alkalosis are seen in the hypertonicity of muscles (tetany).

60. (2) Fluid expenditure by the body is dependent upon metabolic rate, and the *type* of food eaten has practically no bearing on fluid expenditure.

61. (1) Sodium is the primary cation found in the extracellular fluid; potassium is the primary cation found in the intracellular fluid. Calcium is the 3rd cation that needs exact control because of the severe effect it has on the body both in increased and decreased amounts. Iron, which is a part of the hemoglobin molecule, is only incidentally related to fluid and electrolyte balance.

62. (2) Adult supervision relates directly to incidences of burns in children. Most accidents are preventable and tend to occur when children have minimal adult supervision.

63. (3) Fluid replacement is essential because of water and sodium lost to traumatized areas and interstitial spaces. Owing to imminent danger of burn shock, the intravascular fluid volume must be kept balanced.

64. (3) Frothy sputum is not a manifestation of smoke inhalation; the sputum is usually a charcoal color.

65. (4) The increased capillary permeability causes loss of water, protein, and electrolytes from the intravascular compartment into the interstitial spaces.

66. (2) The hypotonicity pulls electrolytes from the wound causing depletion of sodium, chloride, potassium, and magnesium.

67. (1) A significant amount of diuresis takes place after 48 hours or so; generally the blood pressure stabilizes; under normal conditions, there is no marked decrease in the blood pressure.

68. (3) The most beneficial intervention immediately after a burn is slow immersion in cold water, which helps to relieve the pain and reduce the edema.

69. (1) Therapy is based on the severity of the wound, and assessment must be done *immediately* after the burn to determine management. During this period immediately after the burn, there would be no laboratory reports available.

70. (3) The clinical manifestations usually present are abdominal swelling from ascites, respiratory difficulty, and labial or scrotal swelling.

71. (2) There is a hereditary form of nephrotic syndrome that is caused by autosomal inheritance.

72. (1) From a developmental point of view, a 3-year-old hospitalized child's primary concern would be that of separation from his parents. The stress of illness renders him less able to cope with separation.

73. (2) An order for prednisone is never withheld. The dose must be tapered, or adrenal crisis could result.

74. (3) Diuretics that decrease sodium retention will cause diuresis with attendant loss of weight. Weighing the child at the same time of day, using the same scale, with the same amount of clothing is the most effective way to assess the amount of fluid lost.

75. (4) The Semi-Fowler's position makes breathing easier when ascites is present during the acute phase.

76. (1) Serum cholesterol level may be as high as 450 to 1500 mg/dl. Normal level is 120 to 200 mg/dl.

77. (2) The goal in nutrition for this child is to provide sufficient calories and protein for growth while limiting the excretory demands made on the kidney. Salt is usually restricted but not eliminated. A general protein intake is desirable.

78. (2) Massive proteinuria is one of the clinical manifestations of this disease, and urine tests can be easily done by the parents at home.

79. (2) The relapsing form of nephrotic syndrome is prolonged, with an up-and-down course of remissions and exacerbations.

80. (4) The most frequent pattern of transmission of hemophilia is between an unaffected male and a trait carrier female.

81. (3) The tests specific for hemophilia are those that depend upon specific factors for a reaction to occur, such as the thromboplastin generation test. Tests that measure platelet function, such as bleeding time, tourniquet test, and clotting time, are all normal in persons with hemophilia A.

82. (3) In hemophilia A, hemorrhages occur in subcutaneous and intramuscular areas. Purpura, bruises, and petechiae are rare because platelet function is not affected.

83. (4) In von Willebrand's disease, platelet adhesion to vascular subendolithium is reduced, resulting in prolonged bleeding because the platelets fail to form a plug. Although there is increased tendency to bleed from the mucous membanes, hemarthrosis is not seen. Von Willebrand's disease is dependent upon both parents being affected; therefore, this disease is not nearly as prevalent as hemophilia, which is an x-linked recessive disorder.

84. (2) The primary therapy for hemophilia is the replacement of the missing factor, and in Tom's case, factor VIII.

85. (1) Bleeding episodes particularly in the joints could cause bone and muscle changes, resulting in permanent disability. In order to avoid this, the child is placed on scheduled infusions of the missing factor.

86. (2) Heat to the joint would be contraindicated; cold is applied to promote vasoconstriction.

87. (3) The basic problem with thalassemia is a quantitative deficit in the polypeptide chain of the hemoglobin molecule.

88. (4) Thalassemia major is an inherited condition, and there is no cure for this disease at this time.

89. (2) Hemochromatosis results in tissue injury in various parts of the body, but anuria would not be a result of this process.

90. (3) Any reaction from blood transfusion could be life threatening. Immediately stop the transfusion and notify the physician.

91. (2) Since there is no cure for thalassemia major, the objective of therapeutic management is to maintain sufficient hemoglobin levels to permit the child some semblance of normal life.

92. (1) With splenectomy, the child is deprived of the organ that functioned to remove bacteria from the circulation, thus making him extremely susceptible to various infections.

93. (3) Many children with the severe form of thalassemia major die before puberty, and few patients survive beyond the 3rd decade.

94. (2) When feeding, hold the newborn's head in an upright position to facilitate swallowing and to prevent the liquid from coming back out through the cleft.

95. (4) It is helpful to *periodically* put the infant's arms in a restraint so that resistance associated with any change in routine after surgery will be minmized with these "practice" sessions.

96. (1) A palatal defect causes improper drainage of the middle ear, resulting in inefficient function of the eustachian tube. This problem in turn causes increased pressure in the middle ear and contributes to recurrent otitis media.

97. (3) Most cases of cleft lip and cleft palate appear to be of a multifactorial origin based on inheritance.

98. (1) A side-lying or partial side-lying position is used, but the head should be elevated to prevent aspiration of secretions.

99. (3) In most instances, the mother does the best job of comforting the infant.

100. (2) Hydrogen peroxide is usually the choice for cleansing the suture line, followed by a thin coat of antibiotic ointment after feedings and as needed. Avoid using substances that will irritate the suture line, such as baby lotion, soap, and lemon and glycerin.

UNIT III

Medical Surgical Nursing

Section

MEDICAL SURGICAL NURSING CONTENT OUTLINE

CARE OF THE PATIENT DURING THE PERI-OPERATIVE PERIOD

The patient may be subjected to a surgical procedure for any of several reasons:

A. **Diagnosis**—example, biopsy; a small piece of tissue is excised and sent to the laboratory for histological study in order to make a definitive diagnosis.
B. **Exploration**—example, laparotomy; the abdomen is opened so the surgeon can explore the contents in order to determine the nature and degree of disease or injury.
C. **Cure**—the procedure is performed to remove or repair diseased or damaged tissues or organs.
D. **Palliation**—the procedure is undertaken to relieve symptoms when cure of disease is not possible.

THE EFFECT OF SURGERY ON THE PATIENT

A. Provokes a generalized stress response (general adaptation syndrome) with release of pituitary and adrenal hormones.
B. Lowers body's resistance to infection; an intact skin is the body's first line of defense against microbial invasion.
C. Disrupts vascular system and depletes body

fluids; the surgical incision disrupts blood vessels and causes loss of blood and serum.

D. Disrupts normal functioning of body systems; handling of body organs and tissues during surgery causes pressure or torsion injury to sensitive tissues, disrupting circulatory and neuromuscular functions for a variable period of time. Surgical removal of secretory tissue, e.g., stomach, pancreas, and small bowel, diminishes the quantity of endocrine and exocrine secretions. Surgical removal or displacement of tubular structures, e.g., blood vessels, lymph vessels, and intestine, interferes with transmission of fluids or semisolids.

PRE-OPERATIVE NURSING CARE

A. Ideally, the nurse who will care for the patient throughout his hospital stay should admit him to the surgical unit.
   1. Health history
      a. Determine patient's previous experience with illness, hospitalization, and surgery.
      b. Identify patient's understanding of his current health problem and the type of surgery to be performed.
      c. Identify patient's use of prescription or non-prescription drugs to determine whether he has been taking any drugs that would interact significantly with proposed anesthetic or surgical procedure:
         (1.) Anticoagulants
         (2.) Antihypertensives
         (3.) Steroids
         (4.) Aspirin
         (5.) Anti-arthritics
         (6.) Diuretics
         (7.) Antidepressants
         (8.) Anticonvulsants
         (9.) Antibiotics
         (10.) Tranquilizers
         (11.) Hormones
         (12.) Narcotics
      d. Identify any allergies to drugs, foods, or contactants.
      e. Determine level of the patient's anxiety concerning his condition, forthcoming surgery, or both.
      f. Identify patient's support systems and coping methods.
   2. Physical examination—to assess patient's physical condition and to identify any factors that would increase the degree of his risk from surgery.
      a. Age
      b. Weight
      c. Nutritional status
      d. Cardiovascular function
      e. Respiratory function
      f. Neurological status
      g. Skin condition
      h. Any chronic diseases or disabilities

B. Orient patient to physical surroundings, to hospital rules, and to routines and procedures to be followed in his care.

C. Schedule ordered laboratory and diagnostic tests, informing the patient of the purpose and the procedure for each test and preparing the patient as necessary for particular tests.
   1. X-rays
   2. Laboratory tests
   3. Endoscopic procedures
   4. Scanning procedures

D. Facilitate patient's informed consent for surgery.
   1. The surgeon should give the patient a full explanation of the disease, the proposed surgical procedure, the possible complications from the surgery, and the alternative available treatments before asking the patient to sign the consent for surgery.
   2. The nurse may need to repeat, reinforce, or clarify information about the surgical procedure and expected outcomes of the procedure for those patients who raise questions later about these issues.

E. Arrange for any support service personnel requested or required by the patient.
   1. Priest, minister, or rabbi.
   2. Social worker, to assist with financial or family problems.
   3. Psychologist or psychiatrist, if patient is extremely anxious or depressed.

F. Instruct patient concerning self care measures that he will be expected to perform post-operatively.
   1. Deep breathing (diaphragmatic-abdominal method) as follows:
      a. Lie supine with knees flexed.
      b. Inhale slowly through the nose, distending the abdomen as the diaphragm descends.
      c. Exhale slowly through the mouth while contracting the abdominal muscles so as to force air from the lungs.
      d. Instruct patient that he will be expected

to take 10 deep breaths each hour during the 1st several hours following surgery.

2. Coughing
   a. Lie flat or sit up in bed.
   b. Take in a deep breath through the nose and exhale slowly through the mouth.
   c. Interlace the fingers of the 2 hands together and place the hands against the incisional area.
   d. Take in a short breath and cough so as to bring up secretions from deep in the lung airways.
3. Turning
   a. From a supine position, grasp the bed's left side rail with the right hand.
   b. Flex the right knee and roll it over the left knee.
   c. Pull on the bed's left side rail to roll from the back to the left side.
   d. Reverse the procedure, so as to turn from the back to the right side by pulling on the right side rail with the left hand.
4. Leg exercises
   a. Flex and extend the hip 5 times.
   b. Flex and extend the knee 5 times.
   c. Flex and extend the ankle 5 times.
   d. Circumduct each ankle in both a clockwise and a counterclockwise direction by describing a circle with the great toe.

G. Preparation of the patient on the evening before surgery.
1. Give a complete bath to reduce the number of bacteria on the patient's skin.
2. Prepare and shave the skin of the body part to be operated upon.
   a. An antiseptic soap is applied to the skin area for 5 minutes.
   b. An extensive area of skin on either side of the proposed incision line is shaved with a sterile, disposable razor.
   c. The skin area is rinsed well to remove all soap and hair.
   d. Paint prepared skin area with povidone-iodine (Betadine) or other antiseptic, if ordered.
3. Remove colored nail polish so that the nail beds can be checked for cyanosis during and following surgery.
4. If ordered, give an enema or a series of enemas to clear the intestinal tract of food residue and gas. Enemas are most apt to be used in preparation for intestinal and gynecological surgery.
5. Food and fluids are withheld for 6 to 8 hours before surgery to prevent vomiting and aspiration during anesthesia.
6. Administer ordered medication to ensure restful sleep and raise bed's side rails to prevent the patient from falling owing to medication-induced confusion.

H. Care of the patient on the morning of surgery.
1. Ensure that the patient does not receive food or fluids.
2. Measure and record the patient's temperature, pulse, respirations, and blood pressure for use as baseline values against which the anesthesiologist can compare measurements taken during surgery.
3. Provide oral hygiene and remove dentures and bridges, storing these in labeled containers and placing them for safekeeping.
4. Remove the patient's jewelry and give it to family members to take home or mark with the patient's name and store in a locked cupboard or safe.
5. If ordered, insert Levine tube or Foley catheter, or both, and attach to drainage setup.
6. Check the patient's chart to ensure that it contains the following:
   a. Laboratory reports for current blood count, urinalysis.
   b. Reports of current chest x-ray, electrocardiogram.
   c. Patient's signed consent for surgery.
7. Check to see that the patient is wearing an identification band and allergy band.
8. Remove hairpins and wigs, apply surgical cap.
9. Remove prostheses, such as eyes, limbs, and hearing aids.
10. Administer ordered pre-operative medications, which may include the following:
    a. Sedative; to decrease anxiety, thereby lessening the amount of anesthetic drug required.
    b. Tranquilizer; to decrease anxiety and promote muscular relaxation.
    c. Narcotic; to promote relaxation.
    d. Anticholinergic; to decrease tracheobronchial and gastrointestinal secretions, so as to prevent laryngospasm, vomiting, and aspiration.
11. Raise bed's side rails, darken room, and block noise, so the patient can sleep until taken to the operating room.
12. Provide patient's family or significant others a comfortable place to wait until the operation has been completed.

CARE OF THE PATIENT DURING SURGERY

A. The operating room nurse who receives the patient should check the following:
   1. Patient's identification band
   2. Patient's chart
   3. Operating schedule to ensure that the correct patient has been transported to the operating room.

B. When the patient enters the operating room to which he has been assigned, the surgeon usually greets the patient and directs the circulating nurse in positioning the patient on the operating table so as to:
   1. Protect the patient from pressure or torsion injury to tissues.
   2. Ensure adequate respiratory exchange.
   3. Prevent circulatory impairment.
   4. Prevent muscle strain.
   5. Prevent nerve pressure injury.
   6. Facilitate surgical approach to diseased or injured tissues or organs.
      a. Dorsal recumbent position
      b. Lateral position
      c. Trendelenburg position
      d. Lithotomy position

C. The surgeon and the anesthetist check the patient's chart for current vital sign measurements, blood count results, urinalysis report, and interpretation of chest x-rays and electrocardiogram.

D. If patient's x-rays were brought to the operating room, they are mounted on an x-ray viewbox, which is placed within the surgeon's line of vision during the procedure.

E. The anesthetist will insert an I.V. line for administration of fluids and medications during surgery. He may also insert an arterial line in order to obtain arterial blood samples for blood gas analysis during the procedure.

F. The anesthetist will select the type of anesthesia to be given on the basis of the patient's history and physical findings, age, general condition, and the surgical procedure to be performed.
   1. General anesthesia—a drug-induced absence of perception of all sensation. The drug can be administered by any of several routes.
      a. Inhalation—example, cyclopropane, ether, halothane.
      b. Intravenous—example, thiopental sodium.
      c. Rectal—example, thiopental sodium.
   2. Regional anesthesia—a drug-induced loss of painful sensation in one part of the body only, without loss of consciousness. Several types of regional anesthesia are possible.
      a. Topical—the anesthetizing drug is sprayed or dropped on the body part to be anesthetized.
      b. Infiltration—the anesthetizing drug is injected into the tissues surrounding the operative area.
      c. Field block—the anesthetizing drug is injected close to the nerves that surround the area to be anesthetized.
         (1.) Spinal—injection of a local anesthetic intrathecally into the subarachnoid space between L_2–L_3 or L_3–L_4.
         (2.) Epidural—injection of a local anesthetic into the epidural space.
            (a.) Caudal—an epidural anesthetic in which the local anesthetic is injected into the caudal canal through the sacral hiatus.
            (b.) The number of spinal segments that are blocked depend upon the site of injection (fewer segments are blocked with caudal than with lumbar injection), the amount of drug injected, and the patient's position (fewer segments are blocked when the patient's head is elevated than when he is supine).
      d. Intravenous—injection of a local anesthetic into a limb's vessel to which a tourniquet has been applied to obstruct circulation.
   3. Hypothermia—reduction of body temperature to 28 to 30° C (82 to 86° F) can be used as a means of inducing anesthesia and reducing the rate of tissue oxidation for certain operative procedures.
      a. Brain surgery
      b. Heart surgery
      c. Great vessel surgery
   4. Muscle relaxants can be given to block acetylcholine receptors at the myoneural junction, permitting the use of smaller doses of general anesthesia than would otherwise be needed. Commonly used muscle relaxants are as follows:
      a. Curare
      b. Pancuronium
      c. Succinylcholine

G. During the surgical procedure, the circulating

nurse and the scrub nurse should protect the patient from unnecessary injury by:

1. Ensuring complete sterility of all drapes, instruments, dressings, sponges, sutures, and prostheses that come into contact with incised and exposed tissues.
2. Keeping needed supplies and equipment available for the surgeon and anesthetist so as to prevent unnecessary delay during the surgical procedure.
3. Keeping the operating room at the desired temperature and free of drafts and electrical hazards.
4. Preventing unauthorized individuals from entering the operating room.
5. Monitoring the aseptic techniques of members of the surgical team and notifying team members of inadvertent contamination, so that contaminated gloves, gowns, drapes, sponges, or instruments can be exchanged for sterile ones.
6. Keeping accurate and up-to-date count of sponge use and retrieval.
7. Recording lot and item number of any prostheses implanted within the patient.

H. Following completion of the operation and final sponge count, the operating room nurses dress the patient in a clean gown and move him to a stretcher for transportation to the recovery room or surgical intensive care unit.

1. In moving the patient to the cart, care should be taken to prevent patient injury due to the following:
   a. Exposure; cover patient with a warm cotton flannel blanket.
   b. Tissue damage; abrupt or forceful pulling may place strain on the sutures and weaken wound closure.
   c. Sudden position change; abrupt change from supine to side-lying position or from lithotomy to supine position, or a sudden drop from the operating table to a lower level stretcher may provoke a hypotensive episode.
2. As soon as the patient has been placed on the stretcher, he should be secured with restraints over his knees and elbows, and the stretcher's side rails should be elevated to prevent falls and extremity injuries during the trip to the recovery room.

I. Post-operative patients will be transferred either to the surgical intensive care unit or to the recovery room, depending upon the type of surgery that they have undergone, their general condition, the number and type of special care procedures that will be necessary for their care (hypothermia, dialysis, respirator, blood transfusions, and so forth) and their need for constant nursing attendance.

1. Patients having undergone brain, heart, or great vessel surgery, or kidney transplant, and patients having suffered cardiac or respiratory arrest during surgery will be transferred to a surgical intensive care unit.
2. Patients having undergone thoracic, abdominal, pelvic, or extremity surgery, who are in relatively stable condition following the operation, will be transferred to the recovery room.

J. On admitting the patient to the recovery room or to the surgical intensive care unit, the nurse should question the anesthetist who accompanies the patient to determine the exact nature of the surgical procedure performed (may not be the same as that listed on the surgical schedule), the patient's overall condition, any complications that developed during surgery, and the presence of any tubes or drains.

1. The nurse assesses the patient on admission and at frequent intervals during the patient's stay in the unit and records information concerning the following:
   a. Time of admission to the unit
   b. Presence of oropharyngeal airway—patient usually pushes the airway from his mouth with returning consciousness.
   c. Presence or absence of pharyngeal reflex; if reflex is absent, patient should be positioned on his side.
   d. Level of consciousness
      (1.) Reaction of the pupil to light
      (2.) Presence of voluntary movement
      (3.) Type of response to
         (a.) Calling the patient's name.
         (b.) Touching the patient's hand or face.
         (c.) Commanding the patient to open his eyes, raise his hand.
         (d.) Compressing his fingernail with a pen.
   e. Vital signs
      (1.) Take pulse, respiration, and blood pressure every 15 minutes until stable, then every 30 minutes for 2 hours.
      (2.) Take temperature every 2 hours.
      (3.) Notify physician if heart rate is above 120 or below 60 beats per minute; systolic pressure is above 150 or below 90 mm Hg; temperature is above 101° F.
   f. Skin color, especially of the lips, circum-

oral region, and nails; cyanotic or pale. Cold, moist skin may indicate shock.

g. Wound dressing
   (1.) Note amount of bleeding or drainage.
   (2.) Note color and odor of drainage.
   (3.) Reinforce dressings as necessary.
   (4.) Summon surgeon if excessive bleeding or drainage occurs.

h. Drainage tubes and attachments to drainage collection devices; ensure that drainage tubes are unobstructed.
   (1.) Nasogastric tube
   (2.) Foley catheter (if no Foley catheter is present assess patient for bladder distention 8 hours following surgery and obtain order to catheterize if necessary).
   (3.) T-tube
   (4.) Chest tube

i. Intravenous infusions
   (1.) Check the type of fluid running.
   (2.) Check the amount of fluid remaining in the bottle or bag, the rate of fluid flow, and the condition of the skin around the intravenous infusion site.
   (3.) Check orders for fluids to be given next, fluid flow rate, and medications to be added to intravenous fluids.

j. Keep accurate intake and output record during patient's stay in the unit.

k. Assist patient to turn, cough, deep breathe, and to perform leg exercises every 2 hours.

l. Check orders for analgesic and anti-emetic medications and administer one or both to prevent pain (which can precipitate shock) and vomiting (which can cause aspiration and pneumonia).

m. Check chart for special orders that apply to specific surgical procedures or specific patient conditions.
   (1.) Check peripheral pulses and capillary refill time following vascular and orthopedic surgical procedures.
   (2.) Check intracranial pressure following cranial surgery.
   (3.) Check for needed hormone replacement in endocrine disorders.

K. When the patient's condition has stabilized sufficiently that he can be safely monitored by staff of the regular surgical unit, he will be discharged from the recovery room or the surgical intensive care unit by the anesthesiologist or surgeon and returned to a regular surgical unit for continuing post-operative care.

L. The ward nurse who admits the patient following discharge from the recovery room or surgical intensive care unit should assess the patient's condition and record information relating to the following:
   1. Respiratory status
   2. Neurological status
   3. Cardiovascular status
   4. Gastrointestinal status
   5. Wound condition
   6. Drainage tubes
   7. Intravenous fluids
   8. Genitourinary status
   9. Psychological status

M. The admitting nurse should check the patient's chart or contact the surgeon (or both) for orders concerning the following:
   1. Fluids and foods permitted.
   2. Regular and p.r.n. drugs ordered.
   3. Drainage tubes and suction needed.
   4. Wound care provided.
   5. Mobility permitted.
   6. Special treatments needed.

N. Nursing goals during the patient's early post-operative period should include the following:
   1. Ensure adequate respiratory function.
      a. Use of incentive spirometer.
      b. Regular turning and coughing to re-expand lungs.
   2. Ensure adequate cardiovascular function and tissue perfusion.
      a. Prevent vascular occlusion due to poor posture and encourage early ambulation.
      b. Leg exercises.
      c. Passive and active range of motion.
   3. Ensure adequate nutrition and hydration.
      a. Administer I.V. fluids and diet as ordered.
      b. Control environment and assist patient with feeding as needed to provide adequate food intake.
   4. Ensure adequate elimination.
      a. Keep accurate records of intake and output.
      b. Keep indwelling catheter patent by avoiding kinking and irrigating as necessary.
      c. Report failure to have bowel movement by 3rd day after last food intake so physician can order stool softener or enema.
   5. Provide adequate comfort, rest, and safety.
      a. Administer ordered analgesics p.r.n.
      b. Administer ordered anti-emetics p.r.n.

c. Change patient's position frequently, and use pillows and other comfort devices as necessary.
d. Keep bed's side rails elevated.
e. Keep patient's call bell within easy reach.
f. Keep room well lighted and floor free of obstructions for the patient with ambulatory privileges.

6. Promote wound healing.
   a. Ensure proper drainage by changing dressings as needed and by using gauze wicks as ordered.
   b. Protect wound sterility by employing aseptic technique during dressing changes and suture removal.
   c. Assess wound for symptoms of infection: redness, tenderness, heat, and drainage.
   d. Encourage proper nutrition.
   e. Protect against wound dehiscence by applying firm hand pressure over wound dressing when patient retches or coughs and by applying scultetus binder, if ordered, to support an abdominal wound in an obese patient.
7. Facilitate transition from institutional to home living through appropriate discharge planning and health teaching of patient and significant others.

CARE OF THE PATIENT WITH FLUID AND ELECTROLYTE DISORDER

A. Physiology

1. Total body mass is approximately 60% water. About 66% of total body water is intracellular, 25% is in the interstitial compartment, and 9% is intravascular.
2. Body water contains a variety of dissolved organic and inorganic substances. Electrolytes are substances that break down into positively and negatively charged particles in solution. The normal concentration of the major cations (positively charged particles) and anions (negatively charged particles) in intracellular, interstitial, and intravascular compartments is as follows:

Electrolyte	Intracellular (mEq/L)	Interstitial (mEq/L)	Intravascular (mEq/L)
Na^+	15	141	142
K^+	145	5	5
Ca^{++}	2	3	5
Mg^{++}	27	1	2
Cl^-	6	114	102
HCO_3^-	10	30	27
$HPO_4^=$	100	2	2
$SO_4^=$	20	1	1
Protein$^-$	65	1	16
Organic acids	0	4	3

3. Body fluids are in dynamic equilibrium due to continuous fluid intake and excretion and movement of electrolytes and fluid between the 3 fluid compartments. The following values are the average amounts of fluid intake and loss through various routes in the normal adult in a 24-hour period.

Intake		Output	
Route	*Volume (ml)*	*Route*	*Volume (ml)*
Imbibed water	1200	Kidneys	1200
Water in food	1000	Feces	300
Water from oxidation	300	Lungs and skin	1000
	2500		2500

4. Water moves from one compartment to another by diffusion, osmosis, and active transport.
   a. In simple diffusion electrolytes and small organic compounds are propelled by random motion from areas of high concentration to areas of low concentration.
   b. Osmolality refers to the number of particles dissolved in a kilogram (liter) of solvent. Normal serum osmolality ranges from 285 to 305 mOsm/L.
   c. Osmotic pressure in each fluid compartment is determined by the number of particles in solution rather than by particle size or activity.
   d. Active transport—ATP (adenosine triphosphate), a high energy compound in certain cell membranes, facilitates movement of solute particles *against* a concentration gradient, or from an area of low concentration to an area of high concentration. The "sodium-potassium pump" is a type of active transfer by which sodium is continuously moved out of the cell in order to maintain the difference in electrical potential inside and outside the cell, which is needed to effect nerve conduction and muscle contraction.
5. Neuroendocrine regulation of fluid and electrolyte balance.

a. When osmolality of interstitial fluid in the thirst center of the hypothalamus increases to above normal, thirst develops.
b. Antidiuretic hormone (ADH) is secreted by the posterior pituitary when serum osmolality increases above normal, causing kidney tubular cells to reabsorb greater amounts of water.
c. When sodium ion concentration of body fluids falls below normal or intravascular volume decreases, renin is produced by the kidney cortex. Renin converts angiotensinogen in circulating plasma to angiotensin I and II, which cause vasoconstriction and stimulate the adrenal cortex to secrete aldosterone. Aldosterone promotes resorption of Na^+ and Cl^- in the distal renal tubule.
d. Cortisol, another adrenal cortex hormone, also increases sodium reabsorption in the distal renal tubule.

6. Acid-base balance.
   a. The normal pH (hydrogen ion concentration) of body fluids ranges from 7.35 to 7.45.
   b. The enzymes that catalyze metabolic reactions of most cells operate only within this normal range of pH.
   c. A decrease in pH below this range represents an increase in hydrogen ion concentration or acidity; an increase in pH above this range represents a decrease in hydrogen ion concentration or alkalinity.
   d. The 3 systems that regulate the pH of body fluids are a buffer system, respiratory regulation, and renal regulation.
      (1.) A buffer system is a combination of an acid and a base, which can, under different conditions, either take up or give up hydrogen ions so as to neutralize either an acid or a base.
         (a.) Bicarbonate buffer system—metabolism of carbohydrates and fats yields CO_2 and H_2O, which then combine to yield carbonic acid, which in turn dissociates into hydrogen ions and bicarbonate ions as follows:

$$\text{Glucose} + O_2 \rightarrow \underset{\text{Lungs}}{\overset{\uparrow}{CO_2}} + H_2O \rightarrow H_2CO_3 \rightleftharpoons H^+ + \underset{\text{Urine}}{\underset{\downarrow}{HCO_3}}$$

The bicarbonate buffer system maintains the pH of body fluids within normal limits because kidneys can increase or decrease the amount of bicarbonate excreted, and changes in respiratory rate can increase or decrease the amount of CO_2 eliminated.
         (b.) Protein buffer system—some of the amino acids making up the cellular and serum proteins have free acid radicals, which can dissociate into a base plus a hydrogen ion. The high concentration of proteins in cells and serum makes the protein buffering system responsible for 3/4 of all buffering in the body.
         (c.) Phosphate buffering system—provides an effective intracellular buffer and consists of NaH_2PO_4, a weak acid, and Na_2HPO_4, a weak base. When a strong acid, like HCl, is added to a mixture of these 2 compounds, HCl is removed and additional amounts of the weak acid are formed as follows:

$$HCl + Na_2HPO_4 \rightarrow NaH_2PO_4 + NaCl$$

When a strong base, like NaOH, is added to the 2 compounds, the sodium hydroxide is eliminated and additional amounts of the weak base are formed as follows:

$$NaOH + NaH_2PO_4 \rightarrow Na_2HPO_4 + H_2O$$

Consequently, although pH is changed somewhat, the change resulting from addition of a weak acid or base is less than that resulting from addition of a strong acid or base.

      (2.) Respiratory regulation of pH—CO_2 produced by metabolism of carbohydrates diffuses from cells to interstitial fluid, to blood. Excess hydrogen ion in the blood and tissue fluid stimulates the respiratory center in the medulla, increasing respiratory rate and causing increased expiration of CO_2.

(3.) Renal regulation of pH—carbonic anhydrase, an enzyme in renal tubular cells, facilitates the combination of H_2 and CO_2 to form carbonic acid, which dissociates into H^+ and HCO_3^-. The bicarbonate ions are either resorbed from tubular filtrate or excreted in the urine, depending upon the body's need for base. Hydrogen ions are secreted by tubular cells into the urine.

Nursing Care of Patients with Common Fluid and Electrolyte Disorders

1. Water and sodium imbalance.
   a. Since sodium is the major cation in the extracellular fluid and has the ability to attract water, Na^+ is primarily responsible for regulating water volume in interstitial and intravascular spaces.
   b. In isotonic disturbances, Na^+ and H_2O increase or decrease proportionately.
      (1.) Common causes of isotonic depletion are hemorrhage, excessive diaphoresis, vomiting, and diarrhea. Prevention includes monitoring trauma victims and post-operative patients closely for signs of hemorrhage and promptly controlling hemorrhage by appropriate means; advising persons who work or exercise in extreme heat to replace fluid and sodium lost through diaphoresis; and monitoring patients for untoward gastrointestinal irritation by anti-inflammatory drugs and antibiotics.
      (2.) Common causes of isotonic excess are too rapid infusion of intravenous saline, congestive heart failure, and prolonged cortisone use. Prevention includes the following:
         (a.) Refraining from increasing the rate of intravenous infusion when fluid administration falls behind schedule.
         (b.) Reporting early signs of cardiac decompensation in susceptible persons.
   c. Hypo-osmolar disturbances due to loss of Na^+ in excess of water or gain of water in excess of Na^+. Prevention includes monitoring patients on prolonged low Na^+ diet for neuromuscular symptoms; irrigating nasogastric tubes with saline rather than with sterile water; and questioning excessive infusion of electrolyte-free fluids.
   d. Hyperosmolar disturbances due to loss of water in excess of Na^+ or intake of Na^+ in excess of water. Prevention includes recording and reporting decreased fluid intake due to coma, confusion, or dysphagia; monitoring excessive water loss due to diabetes insipidus; questioning excessive intravenous infusion of hypertonic glucose; and measuring and reporting fluid loss during ketoacidosis.
   e. Metabolic acidosis.
      (1.) Common causes.
         (a.) Excessive loss of $NaHCO_3$ during severe diarrhea.
         (b.) Decreased excretion of acid due to renal disease.
         (c.) Excessive intake of acid due to salicylism or high fat diet.
      (2.) Manifestations.
         (a.) $pH < 7.35$
         (b.) $HCO_3^- < 24$ mEq/L
         (c.) HCO_3^-/CO_2 ratio $< 20:1$
         (d.) Headache and lethargy progressing to stupor and coma
      (3.) Nursing management.
         (a.) Infuse ordered isotonic NaCl or Ringer's lactate solution together with $NaHCO_3$.
         (b.) Monitor patient for cardiac arrest due to hyperkalemia (K^+ ions leave cells and accumulate in extracellular fluid as excess H^+ ions enter cells, and K^+ ions are resorbed from renal tubular filtrate as excess H^+ ions are excreted in the urine).
   f. Metabolic alkalosis.
      (1.) Common causes.
         (a.) Excessive intravenous administration of bicarbonate or use of sodium bicarbonate as an antacid.
         (b.) Excessive H^+ ion loss by repeated emesis or continuous gastric suction.
         (c.) Hypokalemia (when serum K^+ is low, H^+ ions move into cells, allowing K^+ ions to move out of cells into the serum).
      (2.) Manifestations.
         (a.) $pH > 7.45$
         (b.) $HCO_3^- > 24$ mEq/L

(c.) HCO_3^-/CO_2 ratio > 20:1
(d.) Twitching, tremors, and hypoventilation
(3.) Nursing management.
(a.) Prevent metabolic alkalosis by advising patients against use of sodium bicarbonate to relieve dyspepsia.
(b.) Administer ordered anti-emetics to prevent excessive vomiting.
(c.) Question lack of fluid-electrolyte replacement in patients on continuous gastric suctioning.

g. Respiratory acidosis.
(1.) Common causes include decreased ventilation with excessive retention of CO_2, as in drug intoxication, emphysema, and pneumonia.
(2.) Manifestations.
(a.) pH < 7.35
(b.) pCO_2 > 40 mm Hg
(c.) HCO_3^-/CO_2 ratio < 20:1
(d.) Drowsiness, depression, and cardiac arrhythmias
(3.) Nursing management.
(a.) Improve ventilation in bedridden patients by encouraging turning, coughing, and deep breathing.
(b.) Administer prescribed treatments for underlying respiratory disease (antibiotics, bronchodilators, breathing exercises, and mechanical ventilation).
(c.) Administer low concentrations of O_2 with extreme caution to patients with chronic obstructive lung diseases.

h. Respiratory alkalosis.
(1.) Common causes include excessive loss of CO_2 due to hyperventilation related to anxiety, hysteria, or too rapid rate of mechanical ventilation, and overstimulation of respiratory center by fever, encephalitis, or meningitis.
(2.) Manifestations
(a.) pH > 7.45
(b.) pCO_2 < 40 mm Hg
(c.) HCO_3^-/CO_2 ratio > 20:1
(d.) Increased neuromuscular irritability as manifested by hyperreflexia, muscular twitching, and positive Chvostek's sign (spasm of facial muscles upon tapping facial nerve in front of the ear).
(3.) Nursing management.
(a.) Decrease respiratory rate in anxious patient by instructing patient in relaxation and meditation techniques.
(b.) Decrease respiratory rate in patient on mechanical ventilation by obtaining order to adjust ventilatory cycling rate.

i. Hypokalemia—serum K^+ < 3.5 mEq/L.
(1.) Common causes.
(a.) Inadequate intake of K^+ due to extreme dieting regimen or nausea.
(b.) Excessive K^+ loss due to thiazide diuretics, furosemide, or adrenal corticosteroid therapy.
(c.) Excessive infusion of intravenous fluids without K^+ replacement.
(d.) Excessive enemas or laxatives.
(e.) Draining of intestinal fistulas.
(2.) Manifestations.
(a.) Weakness
(b.) Lethargy
(c.) Flaccid paralysis
(d.) Paralytic ileus
(e.) Cardiac arrhythmias
(f.) Low flat T waves
(3.) Nursing management.
(a.) Prevent hypokalemia by advising patients against extreme dieting regimen and laxative abuse.
(b.) Measure and record intake and output for patients receiving thiazide diuretics and furosemide.
(c.) Estimate and record volume of wound and intestinal drainage, diarrheal stool.
(d.) Irrigate nasogastric and intestinal drainage tubes with sterile saline rather than with sterile water, to prevent washing out of K^+.
(e.) Administer ordered K^+ replacement in the form of a high K^+ diet, KCl orally with copious fluids and following meals (K^+ is irritating to gastrointestinal mucosa), or K^+ intravenously (I.V. K^+ must be well diluted and administered no more rapidly than 20 mEq/hr in order to avoid venous damage and cardiac arrest).

j. Hyperkalemia—serum K^+ > 5.5 mEq/L.
(1.) Common causes.
(a.) Excessive release of K^+ from cells damaged by burn, crush injury, or infection.
(b.) Acidosis
(c.) Rapid intravenous infusion of K^+ containing fluids.

(d.) Decreased K^+ excretion due to renal failure.
(2.) Manifestations.
(a.) Bradycardia
(b.) Tall pointed T waves
(c.) Cardiac arrest
(d.) Intestinal colic
(e.) Flaccid paralysis
(3.) Nursing management.
(a.) Provide low K^+ diet in patients with renal failure.
(b.) Administer ordered cation exchange resin, such as sodium polystyrene sulfonate (Kayexalate), orally or rectally to exchange Na^+ for K^+ and to increase K^+ excretion in feces.
(c.) Infuse ordered intravenous glucose and insulin to increase cellular storage of glycogen and K^+ in diabetic ketoacidosis.
(d.) Institute ordered peritoneal or hemodialysis when hyperkalemia is life threatening.

k. Hypocalcemia—serum $Ca^{++} < 4$ mEq/L.
(1.) Common causes.
(a.) Excessive loss of Ca^{++} due to intestinal malabsorption
(b.) Acute pancreatitis
(c.) Prolonged diarrhea
(d.) Hypoparathyroidism
(2.) Manifestations.
(a.) Increased neuromuscular irritability as revealed by tetany and laryngeal stridor
(b.) Positive Trousseau's sign (carpal spasm following tourniquet application to the arm for 1 to 5 minutes
(c.) Positive Chvostek's sign (spasm of facial muscles upon tapping facial nerve in front of the ear
(d.) Numbness and tingling of fingers and circumoral region
(e.) Arrhythmias
(3.) Nursing management.
(a.) Administration of ordered calcium lactate or calcium chloride orally or calcium gluconate intravenously (*don't add to a solution containing carbonate or phosphate, as it will form a dangerous precipitate; guard against infiltration, as it will cause tissue sloughing*).

l. Hypercalcemia—serum $Ca^{++} > 5$ mEq/L.
(1.) Common causes.
(a.) Hyperparathyroidism
(b.) Movement of Ca^{++} from bones due to patient's immobility
(c.) Increased absorption of Ca^{++} due to excessive ingestion of milk, alkali, and vitamin D
(d.) Decreased excretion of Ca^{++} in renal failure
(2.) Manifestations.
(a.) Flank pain
(b.) Kidney stones
(c.) Nausea and vomiting
(d.) Confusion
(3.) Nursing management.
(a.) Prevent hypercalcemia by advising patients against self medication with vitamin D, which increases Ca^{++} absorption from the intestine, and against excessive use of milk and antacids to relieve dyspepsia.
(b.) Encourage active range of motion for bedridden patients and early ambulation following illness, injury, and surgery to prevent mobilization of Ca^{++} from bones.
(c.) For patients with hypercalcemia, advise intake of 3000 to 4000 ml of fluid a day to prevent renal stone formation.
(d.) Infuse ordered intravenous fluid and furosemide to wash out excess Ca^{++} for rapid reduction of serum Ca^{++} levels.

m. Hypomagnesemia—serum $Mg^{++} < 1.5$ mEq/L.
(1.) Common causes.
(a.) Severe malnutrition associated with intestinal malabsorption.
(b.) Major intestinal surgery
(c.) Chronic alcoholism
(d.) Renal failure
(e.) Hypoparathyroidism
(2.) Manifestations.
(a.) Increased nervous and muscular irritability, as evidenced by hyperreflexia, twitching, positive Chvostek's sign, and convulsions.
(b.) Confusion and hallucinations
(c.) Paralytic ileus
(d.) Tachyarrhythmias
(3.) Nursing management.
(a.) Monitor patients with chronic alcoholism, chronic renal failure, intestinal surgery for symptoms of nervous and muscle hyperirritability.
(b.) Administer ordered magnesium hy-

droxide (Milk of Magnesia) orally for chronic Mg^{++} loss; $MgSO_4$ I.V. slowly when rapid replacement is needed to treat tachyarrhythmia or convulsions (have injectable calcium gluconate available to treat Mg^{++} toxicity, if it should develop).

n. Hypermagnesemia—serum $Mg^{++} > 3$ mEq/L.
  (1.) Common causes.
    (a.) Decreased excretion of Mg^{++} due to renal insufficiency.
    (b.) Overdosage with Mg^{++} during replacement therapy.
  (2.) Manifestations.
    (a.) Decreased neuromuscular irritability as revealed by lethargy and coma.
    (b.) Decreased respirations, hypotension, bradyrhythmias, and asystole.
  (3.) Nursing management.
    (a.) Question prolonged administration of intravenous Mg^{++} to a patient with poor renal function.
    (b.) Institute ordered peritoneal dialysis or hemodialysis for patient in renal failure.
    (c.) Administer ordered fluid orally or intravenously to dehydrated patients.
    (d.) Administer ordered intravenous calcium gluconate to reverse effects of Mg^{++} toxicity.

o. Internal fluid shifts.
  (1.) Edema—presence of excess fluid in interstitial spaces (edema is not visible until the interstitial fluid volume has risen to 30% above normal).
    (a.) Causes include increased capillary pressure due to venous obstruction or right heart failure; decreased plasma osmotic pressure due to decreased plasma proteins; obstruction or removal of lymphatics; and increased capillary permeability due to burns or allergy.
    (b.) Manifestations include pooling of fluid in dependent body parts (feet and ankles in ambulatory or sedentary person and sacrum of supine person); pitting of tissues for 5 to 30 seconds following finger pressure; increased girth of extremity; tawny discoloration of skin over longstanding edema.
    (c.) Nursing management.
      (1.) To mobilize edema fluid from a body part (as in a patient following a stroke in whom paralyzed arm is edematous) elevate edematous part.
      (2.) Administer ordered diuretics, and record intake and output for patients with cardiac and hepatic failure.
  (2.) Massive plasma to interstitial space fluid shift.
    (a.) Causes—in major burns or serious traumatic injuries, chemotactic substances released by injured cells cause excess fluid to move from capillaries into interstitial spaces.
    (b.) Manifestations—sudden and massive fluid movement causes increased hematocrit value, shock, and decreased consciousness.
    (c.) Nursing management.
      (1.) Use volumetric pump to infuse ordered I.V. fluid and electrolytes or plasma to replace that lost from the intravascular space.
      (2.) Monitor heart rate, respirations, central venous pressure, and pulmonary capillary wedge pressure in patients receiving fluid replacement to detect evidence of fluid overload.
  (3.) Massive interstitial to plasma fluid shift.
    (a.) Causes—3 to 5 days following a severe burn or massive traumatic injury, excess interstitial fluid is reabsorbed into capillaries.
    (b.) Manifestations—bounding pulse, hypertension, and decreased hematocrit value. If cardiac status is compromised, increased intravascular volume may precipitate congestive heart failure and pulmonary edema.
    (c.) Nursing management.
      (1.) Give ordered diuretics if cardiac function is compromised. If ordered, place rotating tourniquets on extremities to reduce intravascular volume.
      (2.) Monitor heart rate, blood pressure, central venous pressure, and pulmonary capillary wedge pressure in burn victims and massive trauma victims.
      (3.) Measure and record fluid in-

take and output in susceptible patients.

(4.) "Third spacing" of fluid—accumulation of edema fluid in the abdominal cavity, retroperitoneal space, pleural cavity, or pericardial sac.

(a.) Causes—increased venous pressure associated with right-side heart failure and decreased serum protein levels associated with liver failure.

(b.) Manifestations—increased abdominal girth and shifting, gravity dependent density in ascites; increased heart size on chest percussion and distant heart tones in pericardial effusion; and decreased resonance at the lung bases in pleural effusion.

(c.) Nursing management.

(1.) Administration of ordered treatment for cardiac failure such as bed rest, digitalis, diuretics, O_2, and so forth.

(2.) Administer ordered diuretics for ascites (furosemide or spironolactone or both).

(3.) Monitor functioning of LeVeen's shunt, if inserted in treatment for drug resistant ascites.

(4.) Assist with procedures of pericentesis, pleural tap, or pericardiocentesis when ascites, pleural effusion, or pericardial effusion threatens respiration or cardiac function or both.

CARE OF PATIENTS WITH NEUROLOGICAL DISORDERS

A. Care of Patients with Specific Neurological Disorders

1. **Epilepsy**—a disorder characterized by paroxysms of excessive neural discharge from various brain regions, with brief periods of unconsciousness, that may be associated with convulsions, unusual sensory perceptions, or aberrant behavior.

a. Causes.

(1.) Primary epilepsy results from either a genetic predisposition to seizures or an abnormal neural sensitivity to a circulatory impairment or a biochemical imbalance.

(2.) Secondary epilepsy results from the following:

(a.) Head injury, occurring either perinatally or later in life.

(b.) Infections, such as meningitis, encephalitis, and brain abscess.

(c.) Drug or alcohol intoxication.

(d.) Brain tumor

(e.) Hypoglycemia, hypocalcemia

b. Manifestations.

(1.) Grand mal (generalized convulsion)

(a.) Following a cry, there is sudden loss of consciousness, followed by rigidity of the entire body, clenched jaws, temporary cessation of respirations, cyanosis, and dilated pupils.

(b.) After a few seconds, jerky alternation of muscle contraction and relaxation (tonic-clonic) occurs, with stertorous respirations, tongue chewing, and fecal or urinary incontinence.

(c.) After a few minutes, movements cease, breathing returns to normal, and consciousness returns.

(d.) Following the seizure the patient is lethargic, with amnesia for the seizure but with memory of the warning sensations (aura) that preceded unconsciousness.

(2.) Petit mal (absence attack)—sudden brief loss of consciousness, lasting 5 to 10 seconds, during which time the individual ceases activity, stares blankly, but does not lose muscle tone, fall, or move the extremities.

(3.) Partial seizures (focal seizures) result from excessive neuronal discharge from only one region of the brain.

(a.) Partial seizures with motor manifestations (jacksonian epilepsy)—a lesion in the motor cortex provokes convulsive twitching of a single body part (often the hand), then the abnormal movements advance centrally to involve the entire limb and ipsilateral side of the body.

(b.) Partial seizures with sensory manifestations—a lesion in the parietal sensory cortex causes numbness and tingling of a hand and arm; or lesions in other sensory areas of the cortex cause unusual visual, auditory, or olfactory sensations.

(c.) Partial seizures with psychomotor manifestations (psychomotor seizures)—excessive neuronal discharges from the temporal lobe and limbic system cause an aura of anxiety and visceral symptoms, followed by involuntary and inappropriate motor activities (chewing, lip smacking, mumbling) or bizarre activity (removing clothes, aimless wandering, destructive acts). Patient has no recollection of the seizure activity following the event.

(4.) X-ray evidence of brain asymmetry, abnormal calcification, or increased intracranial pressure in patients with secondary epilepsy caused by traumatic brain injury or tumor.

(5.) Electroencephalographic evidence of abnormal electrical brain discharges, i.e., either generalized nonspecific slow wave discharges (general cerebral dysfunction) or spike and slow wave discharges from a specific focus (specific structural abnormality).

c. Nursing management.

(1.) Prevent secondary epilepsy by teaching the public the importance of wearing automobile seat belts, motorcycle helmets, football helmets, and so forth.

(2.) Inform patient that the electroencephalogram is a relatively painless hour-long procedure in which, while the patient rests in bed in a quiet darkened room, electrodes will be attached to the scalp at several positions, and the brain's electrical activity will be measured while the patient hyperventilates, then watches a moving light, and then sleeps.

(3.) Administer ordered anticonvulsant drugs, which may be given singly or in combination.

(a.) Phenytoin sodium (Dilantin) for grand mal and psychomotor epilepsy.

(b.) Paramethadione (Paradione) and trimethadione (Tridione) for petit mal epilepsy.

(c.) Primidone (Mysoline) and mephenytoin (Mesantoin) for grand mal, focal, and psychomotor epilepsy.

(4.) Provide psychological and family counseling to help patient cope with the social stigma and minimize the self consciousness and fear engendered by threat of seizure. Inform patient of services offered by the Epilepsy Foundation of America.

(5.) Protect the patient from injury during seizure; place a folded blanket or jacket under the patient's head, place a padded tongue blade between the patient's teeth (if the jaws are not yet clenched), loosen constrictive clothing, turn patient's head to the side to facilitate drainage of oral secretions, and remove nearby objects to prevent damage to flailing extremities.

(6.) Monitor for and instruct patient as to signs of drug toxicity.

2. **Common migraine**—a syndrome consisting of recurrent episodes of severe, throbbing, unilateral headache associated with visual and gastrointestinal symptoms.

a. Causes.

(1.) Predisposition to migraine may be inherited.

(2.) A drop in serum serotonin level precipitated by ingestion of certain chemicals (tyramine, glutamate, nitrate), by menstruation, or by emotional stress causes constriction, then dilation of intracranial arteries.

b. Manifestations.

(1.) Following premonitory symptoms (mood change, hunger, fluid retention, scintillating scotoma) patient develops severe pain in temporal or upper cranial region.

(2.) Pain is accompanied by photophobia, vomiting, and prostration lasting 8 to 24 hours.

c. Nursing management.

(1.) Advise patient to rest in bed in a quiet room.

(2.) Apply an ice bag to the head to cause vasoconstriction.

(3.) Administer ordered analgesics, e.g., aspirin or acetaminophen with codeine.

(4.) If analgesics are ineffective, administer ordered ergotamine tartrate, 1 mg orally or rectally to constrict dilated vessels.

(5.) Suggest that patient record a dietary history to determine foods to be avoided as possible precipitators of migraine attacks. (Various cheeses, chocolate, chicken liver, and wines contain tyramine; many processed meats contain nitrates.)

(6.) Assist patients to analyze situations surrounding migraine attacks in order to identify circumstances and events that predispose to or trigger episodes such as interpersonal conflict and imminent production deadlines.

3. **Trigeminal neuralgia** (tic douloureux)—a disorder characterized by sudden paroxysms of stabbing or burning pain in an area supplied by the maxillary or mandibular divisions of the trigeminal nerve.
   a. Cause—compression of the trigeminal nerve by an artery or vein in the posterior cranial fossa or brain stem infarct involving the 5th cranial nerve.
   b. Manifestations.
      (1.) Episodes of brief stabbing pain in the facial skin of the alae nasae, lip, or chin which are provoked by such sensory stimulation as washing the face, brushing the teeth, shaving, chewing, talking, or a cold draft. The pain lasts for a few seconds, is followed by a refractory period of a minute or so, then resumes.
      (2.) Pain clusters exacerbate in spring and fall.
   c. Nursing management.
      (1.) Assist patient to analyze circumstances of attacks, to identify trigger points, and to avoid stimulating sensitive areas.
      (2.) Administer ordered anti-epileptic drug carbamazepine (Tegretol), 100 to 200 mg B.I.D. or T.I.D. orally to relieve pain. Monitor patient for side effects, such as sedation and aplastic anemia.
      (3.) Monitor patient for nutritional inadequacy and poor oral hygiene, as patient may avoid meals and eschew toothbrushing in an effort to avoid stimulating painful attacks.
      (4.) Inform significant others that patient may decrease frequency or volume of oral communication to avoid precipitating pain but should not be socially isolated as a result of change in communication patterns.
      (5.) If drugs fail to relieve pain and the patient requires percutaneous radiofrequency rhizotomy to destroy the nerve or posterior fossa craniotomy to relieve vascular pressure on the trigeminal nerve, prepare the patient physically and psychologically for the therapy or surgery.
4. **Multiple sclerosis**—a chronic progressive upper motor neuron disease with numerous exacerbations and remissions, characterized by scattered demyelination in the brain, optic nerve, and spinal cord, followed by plaque formation on the denuded fibers (sclerosis), which impedes impulse transmission and causes widespread motor and sensory symptoms.
   a. Cause—possibly a slow acting virus or an autoimmune disorder.
   b. Manifestations.
      (1.) Evidence of 2 or more lesions of central white matter at least 1 month apart, producing such symptoms as unilateral visual loss (optic neuritis), lower extremity weakness and spasticity, incoordination (cerebellar lesion), paresthesias, loss of lower extremity position and vibratory sense, urinary frequency or incontinence, or dysarthria.
      (2.) Functional losses cause depression, but euphoria may develop in patients with substantial frontal lobe involvement.
      (3.) Marked regression of symptoms is usual during remission following initial bouts of the disease, but the amount of recovery decreases with each subsequent bout, and the disability becomes progressive.
   c. Nursing management.
      (1.) Administer ordered doses of ACTH during the acute attack to decrease edema of denuded nerve fibers.
      (2.) If ordered, give cool baths to decrease body temperature during infection, as symptoms are worsened by warm weather and fever.
      (3.) Provide bed rest during an acute attack with passive range of motion of all extremities to prevent contracture of spastic muscles.
      (4.) Administer ordered baclofen (Lioresal) or diazepam (Valium) to reduce muscle spasm.
      (5.) Encourage use of mobility devices (walkers or wheelchairs) to keep patient as active as possible for as long as possible and to prevent contractures and decubitus ulcers.
      (6.) For incomplete bladder emptying, teach patient to void at regular intervals and to use Credé's maneuver to evacuate bladder completely (hand pressure over the symphysis pubis).
      (7.) Provide self help devices (e.g., long-handled reacher, long-handled shoehorn, and long-handled bath sponge) to maximize independence in activities of daily living.
5. **Parkinson's disease**—a progressive disorder of

the basal ganglia that is characterized by abnormal involuntary movements, alteration in muscle tone, and disturbance in postural reflexes.

a. Causes.
   (1.) Loss of pigmented neurons in the substantia nigra and locus ceruleus, with resultant decrease in dopamine levels in basal ganglia.
   (2.) Tissue changes may result from viral infections, chemical or drug toxicity (manganese, CO, reserpine, phenothiazines), or arteriosclerosis.
b. Manifestations.
   (1.) Fine "pill-rolling" resting hand tremor.
   (2.) Muscle rigidity, bradykinesia.
   (3.) Mask-like facial expression, muted voice.
   (4.) Drooling, dysphagia.
   (5.) Stooped posture, shuffling gait, with gait-start hesitation.
   (6.) Unsteadiness due to loss of postural righting reflexes.
   (7.) Back pain due to bone demineralization.
c. Nursing management.
   (1.) Monitor patients on long-term reserpine or phenothiazine treatment for appearance of parkinsonian symptoms and report these to physician for possible alteration of dosage.
   (2.) For patients with severe disease, administer ordered levodopa, a precursor of dopamine that crosses the blood brain barrier and is given in combination with carbidopa (a dopa-decarboxylase inhibitor that decreases toxic effects of levodopa by slowing its metabolism in peripheral tissues). The best effects of levodopa occur during the first 2 years of use.
   (3.) For patients with less severe Parkinson's disease symptoms, administer ordered anticholinergics, such as trihexyphenidyl (Artane) or benztropin (Cogentin), ordered antihistamines, such as diphenhydramine (Benadryl), or ordered antiviral agent amantadine (Symmetrel).
   (4.) Teach patient to perform daily exercises, such as walking, swimming, or gardening, to decrease muscle rigidity and to increase muscle strength and coordination.
   (5.) Encourage patient to walk erect, consciously swinging the arms, and to raise the feet in a broad-based, heel-toe gait to improve balance.
   (6.) Teach patient to eat high residue foods, to increase fluid intake, and to establish a regular defecation time to prevent constipation.
   (7.) Provide raised toilet seat and toilet hand rails to facilitate safety and independence.

6. **Huntington's disease**—a hereditary progressive neurological disease characterized by chorea and dementia.
   a. Cause—the disease is transmitted as an autosomal dominant trait, with each offspring of a parent with Huntington's disease having a 50% chance of developing the disease. The genetic defect causes loss of neurons, gliosis (scarring), and depletion of the neurotransmitters gamma-aminobutyric acid (GABA) and acetylcholine in the basal ganglia.
   b. Manifestations.
      (1.) Chorea (writhing, twisting, involuntary movements) of entire body.
      (2.) Facial tics, grimaces, and slurred speech, which interfere with social interaction.
      (3.) Progressive neuron loss causes personality changes, such as depression, hostility, paranoia, memory loss, and intellectual deterioration.
   c. Nursing management.
      (1.) Encourage patient to ambulate as long as possible, then advise him to use the wheelchair and to remain active for as long as possible.
      (2.) Administer ordered reserpine to decrease chorea. Give prescribed phenothiazines (chlorpromazine and fluphenazine) or butyrophenones (haloperidol) to treat psychosis and tricyclic antidepressants (amitriptyline, nortriptyline, and imipramine) to relieve depression. Monitor patient for toxic effects from drugs, such as hypotension, drowsiness, and parkinsonian symptoms.
      (3.) Provide supportive counseling of patient and family to relieve guilt and despair concerning grim prognosis. Arrange for marital and genetic counseling to assist persons at risk of the disease to decide whether to have children.
      (4.) Structure patient's environment to decrease emotional stress, which tends to increase the intensity of choreiform movements.
      (5.) If choreiform movements are especially violent, pad the bed's side rails to protect the patient's limbs from injury.
7. **Myasthenia gravis**—a disorder of impulse transmission at the myoneural junction, which results in extreme weakness.

a. Cause—an autoimmune disorder, characterized by thymic enlargement and circulating antibodies that affix to acetylcholine receptors at the motor end-plate, preventing uptake of acetylcholine released by motor nerve fibers.
b. Manifestations.
    (1.) Extreme weakness of eye muscles, with eyelid ptosis and diplopia.
    (2.) Weakness of facial, tongue, pharyngeal, and laryngeal muscles, causing difficulty in speaking, chewing, and swallowing.
    (3.) Proximal limb weakness, causing difficulty in rising from a chair, climbing stairs, and lifting heavy objects.
    (4.) Prompt increase in strength of involved muscles following intravenous administration of the cholinesterase inhibitor, edrophonium (positive Tensilon test).
c. Nursing management.
    (1.) Administer ordered anticholinesterase drug (neostigmine or pyridostigmine) to permit available acetylcholine to act for as long a time as possible. Schedule drug doses before meals and before necessary physical activity to maximize strength at critical times.
    (2.) Administer ordered corticosteroids (prednisone) to suppress immune response and decrease circulating antibodies.
    (3.) If plasmapheresis is instituted to lower IgG antibodies in the serum, provide comfort measures and diversionary activities during the 2½ to 3 hours of immobility required for the treatment.
    (4.) If thymectomy is necessary to decrease the circulating antibodies to acetylcholine receptors, prepare the patient physically and psychologically for chest surgery.
    (5.) Monitor patient for symptoms of myasthenic crisis (due to worsening of muscular weakness, especially of respiratory muscles, leading to ventilatory insufficiency), and for symptoms of cholinergic crisis (due to overdose of anticholinesterase agent, causing muscular weakness and abdominal cramps). Notify physician immediately so drug dosage can be adjusted appropriately. Intravenous dose of edrophonium is given to differentiate between myasthenic crisis and cholinergic crisis, since symptoms are similar in the 2 situations.
    (6.) Provide assisted ventilation for the patient in myasthenic crisis (Ambu-bag on an emergency basis, then mechanical ventilation will be ordered).
    (7.) Teach patient to avoid persons with respiratory infections and to seek immediate treatment for any infection, since a rampant infection is a frequent precipitator of myasthenic crisis.

8. **Amyotrophic lateral sclerosis** (Lou Gehrig's disease)—an upper motor and lower motor neuron disease characterized by degeneration of motor cells and tracts in the spinal cord, brain stem, and cerebral cortex, which causes muscle weakness and atrophy, but no sensory changes.
    a. Cause.
        (1.) Unknown
        (2.) Possibly a slow acting virus or an autoimmune disorder.
    b. Manifestations.
        (1.) Symmetrical weakness and muscular atrophy beginning in the upper extremities and extending to the lower extremities.
        (2.) Muscle fasciculations and cramps.
        (3.) A mixture of spasticity and flaccidity (both upper and motor neuron lesions).
        (4.) In patients with bulbar involvement, lingual atrophy and palatal and pharyngeal paralysis, with loss of gag reflex and swallowing difficulty.
        (5.) Electromyographic evidence of muscle denervation.
    c. Nursing management.
        (1.) Inform patient that electromyography involves inserting needle electrodes into various muscles to record electrical potentials in the muscles. Slight discomfort is experienced during insertion of the electrodes; if many muscles are tested, there may be some discomfort for a few hours following the test.
        (2.) Encourage patient to perform prescribed active exercises to delay muscle atrophy and to prevent joint immobility. Explain that exercises are aimed at increasing strength in those muscle fibers that remain functional.
        (3.) Provide supportive counseling to help patient cope with frustration and depression resulting from functional losses.
        (4.) Keep orotracheal suction equipment available when feeding patient with bulbar involvement.
        (5.) Encourage use of incentive spirometer and provide assisted coughing to minimize respiratory complications in the

patient with weakness of diaphragm and intercostal muscles.

9. **Cerebrovascular accident**—abrupt onset of a neural deficit that results from an interruption of blood supply to the brain.
   a. Causes.
      (1.) Arteriosclerosis, giving rise to thrombus formation.
      (2.) Hypertension, giving rise to vascular rupture and hemorrhage.
      (3.) Embolism, from heart or carotid bifurcation.
      (4.) Severe hypotension associated with myocardial infarction, drug intoxication, or major surgery.
      (5.) High blood lipid levels, coagulation disorders, anticoagulants, and oral contraceptives increase risk of stroke in susceptible persons.
   b. Manifestations—specific pattern of motor and sensory losses depends upon the area of the brain deprived of blood. Severity and duration of symptoms depend upon the nature and extent of the lesions.
      (1.) Transient ischemic attack—temporary loss of motor, sensory, or visual function, which is caused by ischemia and which clears completely within 24 hours. Results from an obstruction to blood flow by a platelet thrombus. Should be regarded as a warning of an impending stroke.
      (2.) Middle cerebral artery disturbance—loss of movement and sensation in contralateral upper extremity and aphasia (if dominant hemisphere is involved).
      (3.) Anterior cerebral artery disturbance—loss of movement and sensation in contralateral lower extremity. Urinary incontinence, confusion, and behavioral disorders (if anterior portion of frontal lobe is involved).
      (4.) Vertebrobasilar disturbance—vertigo, nystagmus, and visual disturbances.
   c. Nursing management.
      (1.) Prevent cerebrovascular accident by persuading hypertensive individuals to do the following:
         (a.) Adhere to a prescribed drug regimen.
         (b.) Lose weight.
         (c.) Stop smoking (nicotine is a vasoconstrictor).
         (d.) Stop drinking alcohol (alcohol raises blood lipid levels).
      (2.) Refer patients with symptoms of transient ischemic attacks or slowly progressive strokes for immediate medical care, as both types of patients may be candidates for carotid endarterectomy to remove site of thromboembolus formation and to improve cerebral arterial supply.
      (3.) For patient who is comatose following a complete stroke.
         (a.) Place patient in side-lying position and provide oral suctioning as necessary to ensure an open airway.
         (b.) Provide ordered I.V. infusion of fluid, electrolytes, and nutrients while patient is comatose to promote adequate circulation and facilitate tissue healing. Record intake and output.
         (c.) Change patient's position every 2 hours to prevent decubitus ulcers, hypostatic pneumonia, and renal calculi.
         (d.) Monitor patient's vital signs, pupillary signs, and motor and sensory functions to detect worsening or improving neurological function. After neurological signs stabilize, provide passive range of motion to all joints B.I.D.
         (e.) Insert ordered indwelling catheter while patient is comatose to ensure accurate record of fluid output and to protect skin from irritation. Remove catheter when patient regains consciousness and offer bed pan or urinal every 2 hours to enourage bladder retraining. Provide scrupulous skin care to prevent irritation.
         (f.) Elevated patient's paralyzed arm on pillows to relieve edema and to prevent painful shoulder-arm syndrome.
         (g.) After patient is conscious and it has been determined that his swallowing reflex is intact, provide high bulk diet, stool softeners, and adequate fluid intake to prevent straining at stool.
         (h.) Institute ordered progressive ambulation.
            (1.) Teach patient to perform active or passive range of motion of all joints 3 times daily (patient can use functional upper extremity to move paralyzed upper extremity).
            (2.) Advance patient from long sit-

ting, to short sitting, to standing with assistance, to standing independently, while providing necessary assistance and cuing at each stage of advancement.

(3.) Assist patient to regain functional gait by assisting him to walk between parallel bars, then with a quad cane, then with a straight cane. Apply a sling to support the paralyzed upper extremity while walking (to improve balance and to prevent inadvertent injury to paralyzed extremity). Apply ankle brace or teach patient to apply brace, if ordered, to stabilize the weakened lower extremity.

(4.) Reinforce instruction given the patient by occupational therapist or physiotherapist in developing new methods and techniques (e.g., substituting single-handed for former double-handed operations) for accomplishing activities of daily living; bathing, dressing, grooming, feeding, toileting, meal preparations, and minor housekeeping tasks.

10. **Traumatic head injury**—bony or soft tissue injury, or both, resulting from falls, blows, or penetrating wounds.

a. Causes.

(1.) High speed impact during motor vehicle accident, falls from a ladder or roof, fist fighting, blows from a blunt object, or knife or gunshot wounds. Mechanical trauma to the head can cause skull fracture, hemorrhage, and bruising of brain tissue.

(2.) Expanding hematomas and edema that develop in traumatized brain tissue raise intracranial pressure and cause pressure and ischemic injury to surrounding tissue. Pressure injury to respiratory and cardiac centers causes hypoxia and hypotension, which further jeopardize brain tissue.

b. Manifestations.

(1.) Swelling, ecchymosis, or laceration at the point of traumatic impact.

(2.) Bruise behind the ear and otorrhea suggest basal skull fracture. Rhinorrhea suggests frontal skull fracture.

(3.) Decrease in level of consciousness. Patient loses orientation first to time, then to place, and last to person.

(4.) Increase in intracranial pressure as evidenced by decreasing pulse and respiratory rates and rising blood pressure and temperature.

(5.) Epidural hematoma—accumulation of blood in the epidural space following laceration of the middle meningeal artery during fracture of the temporal bone. Bleeding is arterial, so patient's condition deteriorates rapidly.

(a.) Momentary loss of consciousness at injury, followed by a lucid interval of minutes or hours, then increasing lethargy, stupor, and coma.

(b.) If expanding clot causes cerebrum to herniate through the tentorial notch, ipsilateral pupil will become dilated and fixed.

(6.) Subdural hematoma—rupture of veins in the subdural space with collection of blood that becomes encapsulated in a pseudomembrane. With time, blood cells in the clot rupture, creating a hypertonic fluid that absorbs water from surrounding tissue, creating a gradually expanding, pressure-producing mass. Because bleeding is venous, signs develop slowly.

(a.) May be a brief loss of consciousness at injury, then a long lucid interval (weeks or months).

(b.) As clot slowly grows in size, headache, confusion, personality change, and lethargy develop over weeks or months.

c. Nursing management.

(1.) For first hours and days following injury, perform neurological assessment at frequent intervals (every 2 hours) to detect evidence of increasing intracranial pressure, worsening neural status, and circulatory and respiratory embarrassment.

(a.) Glasgow coma scale—determine best response (eye opening, verbal response, and motor response) that patient can make to nurse's presence, questions, and commands; grade responses numerically. Possible scores range from 3 to 15. Score of 7 or less indicates coma.

(b.) Check size and reactivity of pupils. Unilaterally dilated and unresponding pupil suggests injury to the 3rd cranial nerve on the same side. Bilaterally fixed and dilated pupils suggest severe upper brain stem injury.

(c.) If patient is awake, check orientation to time, place, and person. Note spontaneous movement. Assess ability to respond to simple directions. Check hand grip strength and ability to perceive touch and pain sensations.

(2.) Raise head of bed 20 to 30 degrees to decrease intracranial pressure (unless patient is in shock).

(3.) For patient who is in shock, insert ordered indwelling catheter and measure urine volume hourly to determine adequacy of kidney perfusion.

(4.) Weigh patient daily, keep accurate intake and output records to detect fluid retention (from syndrome of inappropriate antidiuretic hormone secretion due to pressure injury to hypothalamus or posterior pituitary).

(5.) Examine drainage from nose or ears to detect blood or cerebrospinal fluid (a clear wet halo encircling a central pink spot). Test ear or nasal drainage with Dextrostix to determine whether glucose is present (cerebrospinal fluid contains glucose, mucus does not). Caution the conscious patient with nasal drainage of cerebrospinal fluid not to blow his nose, so as not to drive infected material into subarachnoid space.

(6.) Place patient in side-lying or semi-prone position to facilitate drainage of oral secretions.

(7.) Pad the bed's side rails to prevent self injury due to restlessness or seizure activity. Keep padded tongue blade taped to the head of the bed. Administer anticonvulsant medication (phenytoin [Dilantin] and diazepam [Valium]) as ordered.

(8.) Administer ordered O_2 to maximize oxygenation of damaged cerebral tissues.

(9.) Monitor continuous intracranial pressure measurement by subarachnoid screw or other device.

(10.) Utilize hypothermia blanket if ordered, to lower body temperature and prevent additional brain damage due to fever.

(11.) Administer ordered intravenous fluids or nasogastric tube feedings, or both, to maintain hydration and ensure positive nitrogen balance for the patient who is unable to take food and fluids orally.

(12.) Change the patient's position every 2 hours and provide passive range of motion of all joints B.I.D. to prevent decubitus ulcers, renal stones, and contracture deformities.

(13.) If hyperventilation via mechanical ventilator is used to maintain $PaCO_2$ at lower than normal levels (to decrease cerebral blood volume and intracranial pressure), monitor blood gas concentrations and ventilator settings to ensure that treatment objectives are met.

(14.) When consciousness returns, assess patient for swallowing problems, visual field cuts, motor weakness, and cognitive losses.

(15.) Provide patient and family with supportive counseling in coping with anxiety and role changes necessitated by residual physical disability.

11. **Spinal cord injury**—interruption of impulse transmission as a result of partial or complete severance of the cord. Most frequent areas of injury are the lower cervical, lower thoracic, and upper lumbar.

a. Causes.

(1.) Motor vehicle accidents
(2.) Falls
(3.) Diving into shallow water
(4.) Sport related accidents
(5.) Gunshot wounds
(6.) Improper movement of patients with spinal fractures

b. Manifestations.

(1.) Complete cord transection causes immediate loss of all movement and sensation in body parts innervated by nerves below the level of injury and temporary (weeks or months) loss of all spinal reflexes below the level of injury.

(2.) Incomplete cord transection causes varying degrees of motor and sensory losses in parts below the level of injury, with preservation of certain tracts and sparing of certain lower functions. For example, if touch and pain sensations in the perineal region are retained, there is said to be "sacral sparing."

(3.) Spinal shock—loss of all reflex activity below the level of cord injury.

(a.) Spinal shock is present from 6 weeks to 3 months after complete cord transection and may be evident for a brief time following incomplete transection.

(b.) Resolution of spinal shock is apparent when reflex activity returns below the level of injury, with conversion of previously flaccid paralysis to spastic paralysis. At the same time, autonomic functions return below the level of the injury, so bowel and bladder will begin to empty reflexively.

(4.) The level of cord injury determines the amount of motor and sensory functions retained, for example:

(a.) Lesions above C_4 cause diaphragmatic paralysis.

(b.) Lesions of the cervical spine result in quadriplegia.

(c.) With intact function at C_5, patient can contract biceps and shoulder depressors.

(d.) With intact function at C_6, patient can contract deltoid and wrist extensors.

(e.) With intact function at C_7, patient can contract triceps.

(f.) With intact function at T_1, patient can contract finger flexors.

(g.) With intact function at T_{12}, patient can contract abdominal and back muscles.

(h.) With intact function at L_5, patient can contract hip flexors.

c. Nursing management.

(1.) In giving emergency care to an accident victim, immobilize head and spine with a spine board and an extension collar before transfer to the hospital, in order to prevent flexing the spine.

(2.) Perform neurological assessment at the accident site to determine the level of cord injury. Determine patient's ability to move arms and legs, to perceive touch, pain, and position of upper and lower extremities.

(3.) When patient is admitted to the hospital, keep the spine immobilized (usually with halter traction) while spinal x-rays are taken.

(4.) Remain with patient and provide reassurance while the physician applies skeletal traction using Crutchfield's or Gardner-Wells tongs.

(5.) If patient is placed on a Stryker's frame, turn from supine to prone position every 2 hours to prevent skin irritation, pooling of respiratory secretions, and formation of renal stones.

(6.) Insert ordered nasogastric tube to prevent abdominal distention until peristalsis returns. When bowel sounds return, provide soft, then general diet, feeding patient slowly to prevent aspiration.

(7.) Administer ordered steroids parenterally to minimize cord edema and inflammation.

(8.) If decompression laminectomy is needed to relieve pressure on the cord or if spinal fusion or Harrington's rod insertion is needed to stabilize the spine, prepare the patient physically and psychologically for surgery.

(9.) If a halo brace and jacket are used to immobilize the spine following spinal fusion, get the patient up in a wheelchair as soon as possible after surgery, gradually increasing his wheelchair sitting time from 1 hour to 1½ hours to 2 hours, and so forth. Check the skin of his back and buttocks after each wheelchair interval to detect any pressure injury.

(10.) Teach patient how to lean from side to side or do push ups (depending on the level of injury) to relieve pressure over ischial tuberosities and femoral trochanters while sitting.

(11.) During spinal shock, when bladder is areflexive and lacks tone, insert ordered indwelling catheter to prevent bladder distention, which causes bladder ischemia and increases susceptibility to infection. Provide copious fluid intake (2500 to 3000 ml/day) and urine acidifiers (cranberry juice, vitamin C) to prevent urinary infection and urinary stone formation. When spinal shock resolves, and patient begins to empty his bladder reflexively, remove the indwelling catheter, start the patient on measured fluid intake (150 ml/hr from 7 A.M. to 9 P.M.) and catheterize every 4 to 6 hours to simulate normal filling and emptying pattern (prevents bladder contraction). Use a triggering mechanism, like repeated tapping over the bladder or pulling pubic hair, to provoke reflex bladder emptying in patients with cervical cord injury.

(12.) Institute a systematized bowel program, consisting of high bulk foods, stool softeners, and insertion of a bisacodyl (Dulcolax) suppository every other day, to prevent constipation. Perform daily rectal check and provide digital removal of hard stool from the lower rectum, as necessary.

(13.) Apply padded Stryker's boots while patient is in bed and sneakers while patient is in wheelchair to prevent footdrop and heel decubitus ulcers.

(14.) Apply ordered forearm splints, 2 hours on and 2 hours off, night and day, to prevent contracture deformities of hands and wrists in quadriplegic patient.

(15.) Reinforce exercise prescriptions given the patient by the physiotherapist and occupational therapist to improve muscle strength and coordination and to facilitate acquisition of skills of daily living.

(16.) Provide supportive counseling to patient and family as they cope with the numerous intrapersonal and interpersonal changes necessitated by physical disability.

(17.) Inform patient and family of the services available to them through various community agencies and groups (e.g., spinal cord clubs, wheelchair sports groups, housing for disabled, meals on wheels, and transportation for disabled).

12. **Herniated intervertebral disc**—extrusion of the soft inner nucleus pulposus through tears in the outer fibrous covering of the disc.

a. Cause.

(1.) Aging causes the nucleus to become dehydrated and lose resiliency.

(2.) Repeated trauma causes the fibrous covering to tear.

b. Manifestations.

(1.) The most common site of herniation is L_{4-5}.

(2.) A "tearing feeling" in the back is experienced by patient on lifting a heavy load, twisting, or turning.

(3.) If herniation is at L_{4-5}, low back pain radiates down the posterior thigh, with worsening on coughing, lateral bending, lifting, and defecating.

(4.) If herniation is in the cervical area, patient experiences stiff neck and shoulder pain that radiates to the arm and hand.

c. Nursing management.

(1.) Provide strict bed rest on a firm mattress, with headrest elevated 20 to 30 degrees and knees flexed.

(2.) Administer ordered acetaminophen or aspirin to relieve pain.

(3.) Administer ordered muscle relaxant, i.e., baclofen (Lioresal) or diazepam.

(4.) Administer ordered adrenal steroids for anti-inflammatory effect.

(5.) Use log rolling technique to turn patient in bed and to place patient on bedpan.

(6.) Apply abdominal corset, if ordered, to provide additional back support for patient with lumbar disc problem; apply cervical collar, if ordered, to provide additional support for patient with cervical disc problem.

(7.) Encourage obese patient with disc problems to institute a weight reduction diet.

(8.) If patient is treated with injection of the enzyme chymopapain into the disc space to dissolve the disc (an experimental treatment), administer ordered corticosteroid before the injection of chymopapain to prevent anaphylactic reaction.

(9.) If conservative treatment is ineffective and a posterior laminectomy is performed to remove the herniated disc, and a posterior spinal fusion is performed to stabilize the spine, prepare the patient physically and psychologically for the operation.

(a.) Pre-operatively

(1.) Inform patient that log rolling technique will be used to turn patient following surgery.

(2.) Determine whether patient will be placed on a Stryker's frame post-operatively. If so, describe the frame and how he will be cared for while on the frame.

(3.) Teach patient the purpose and technique of deep breathing and coughing post-operatively.

(b.) Post-operatively

(1.) Place patient on Stryker's frame (if ordered) or hard mattress with a bed board.

(2.) Maintain patient's spine in perfect alignment at all times.

(3.) Check motor and sensory functions of upper and lower extremities every 2 hours. If cervical laminectomy was performed, check patient frequently for evidence of dyspnea.

(4.) Check wound dressing for bloody or clear drainage (cerebrospinal fluid) and report either to surgeon immediately.

(5.) Turn patient every 2 hours to prevent skin, respiratory, and renal problems.

(6.) When patient is lying on his back, place pillows under full length of both legs to relieve strain on lower back muscles.

(7.) Administer ordered analgesic for pain at operative site.

(8.) Provide physical assistance and cuing as patient relearns to walk. Provide straight backed chair for sitting.

(9.) Teach good body mechanics (bending at knees and hips, holding objects close to the body, sleeping on a firm mattress with a bed board) to prevent future disc problems.

CARE OF PATIENTS WITH EYE AND EAR DISORDERS

A. Care of Patients with Selected Disorders of the Eye

1. **Cataract**—opacity of the crystalline lens or lens capsule. Cataracts tend to occur bilaterally but to progress independently.

a. Causes.

(1.) Aging—change in the metabolism of lens proteins occurs with age.

(2.) Radiation

(3.) Trauma such as a metallic foreign body striking the lens.

(4.) Recurrent uveitis

(5.) Diabetes mellitus

(6.) Congenital due to genetic defects or maternal rubella during the 1st trimester.

(7.) Toxic, untoward reaction to ergot, phenothiazine, dinitrophenol, or long-term corticosteroid therapy.

b. Cataract development proceeds through several stages.

(1.) In the immature cataract the lens is only slightly opaque, with the lens cortex mostly clear.

(2.) In the mature cataract the lens is entirely opaque, and the lens can easily be separated from its capsule.

(3.) In the hypermature cataract the degraded protein molecules have been absorbed or have escaped, leaving only a shrunken yellow lens and a wrinkled capsule.

(4.) The hypermature cataract predisposes to spontaneous dislocation of the lens and narrow angle glaucoma.

c. Manifestations.

(1.) Painless gradual blurring and loss of vision.

(2.) The normally black pupil appears to be milky white.

(3.) Patient sees halos around lights and experiences blinding glare from automobile headlights and bright sunlight.

(4.) If opacity is central, patient can see better in dim light than in bright light.

(5.) "Yellow" vision

d. Nursing management.

(1.) Prepare patient physically and emotionally for cataract removal when the vision in the other eye is better but so decreased as to interfere with activities of daily living.

(a.) Reinforce information given the patient by his physician concerning the operative procedure.

(b.) Intracapsular extraction, in which lens and capsule are removed in total through an incision at the corneoscleral junction, is usually performed under local anesthesia following strong pre-operative sedation. In the procedure of cryoextraction, a cooled cryoprobe is touched to the lens, which becomes firmly attached to the probe, permitting lens removal.

(c.) Extracapsular extraction, which is often used for congenital or traumatic cataract, consists of removal of the anterior capsule and lens, leaving the posterior lens capsule in place. In some younger patients a vibrating probe is introduced through the anterior chamber into the lens nucleus. Ultrasonic vibrations of the probe emulsify the lens nucleus, which is then aspirated.

(d.) Intra-ocular lens implantation—in some patients, a prosthetic lens is secured into the pupillary site after the cataract has been removed.

(2.) Pre-operatively, orient patient to his

room, bedside table, personal belongings, and other room occupants in order to decrease disorientation during the period when the eye is bandaged following surgery. Inform patient that post-operatively the eye will be bandaged and covered with an eyeshield, and the head of the bed will be elevated slightly. Advise patient that he should move slowly and avoid straining, bending, and stooping for 3 weeks post-operatively.

(3.) Administer ordered mydriatic (to dilate pupil) and cycloplegic (to paralyze muscles of accommodation) exactly at the ordered time pre-operatively so as to facilitate the surgical procedure. Elevate the bed's side rails, and remain with the patient following administration of pre-operative sedative and eye medications so as to minimize anxiety and prevent injury due to confusion and visual impairment.

(4.) Post-operatively, turn patient from his back to unoperated side, and avoid turning patient toward the operated side to prevent increased intra-ocular pressure in the operated eye.

(a.) Check patient's condition at regular intervals, and reorient patient frequently to surroundings, time, and prescribed care measures.

(b.) Cover operated eye with an eyeshield at night and while ambulating to prevent injury.

(c.) Report signs of increased intra-ocular pressure (pain and nausea) immediately.

(d.) Administer ordered liquid or soft diet and stool softeners to prevent straining at stool, which can increase intra-ocular pressure and strain the suture line.

(e.) Advise relative or friend to remain with the patient during hospitalization and early post-discharge period to provide needed cuing and assistance.

(f.) Provide radio and audiotapes as diversionary activities during the period of visual impoverishment following surgery.

(g.) If patient is given cataract lenses (biconvex), instruct patient that for clear vision he must turn his head so as to view objects through the center of the lens. Provide assistance while patient becomes accustomed to the cataract lenses, as objects appear larger than they are and handling objects and climbing stairs are hazardous.

2. **Glaucoma**—abnormally increased intra-ocular pressure, causing damage to the optic nerve. Responsible for 12% of all blindness in the United States.

a. Types and causes.

(1.) Chronic open angle glaucoma—most common form, often familial in occurrence; due to obstruction of the trabecular network and the canal of Schlemm, which blocks the outflow of aqueous humor from the anterior chamber. May also result from an overproduction of aqueous humor.

(2.) Narrow angle or angle closure glaucoma—due to anatomically narrow angles between the anterior iris and the posterior corneal surface, a shallow anterior chamber, or a bulging of the iris into the anterior chamber.

(3.) Secondary glaucoma develops following eye trauma, uveitis, or eye tumors.

(4.) Congenital glaucoma occurs within the 1st 6 months of life owing to congenital defects in eye structures.

b. Manifestations.

(1.) Chronic open angle glaucoma

(a.) Usually bilateral

(b.) Usually painless, but may have slight aching of eyes.

(c.) Increased fogginess of vision, not correctable with glasses.

(d.) Gradual loss of peripheral vision.

(e.) Seeing halos around lights.

(f.) Cupping and atrophy of the optic disc.

(2.) Acute closed angle glaucoma—a medical emergency.

(a.) Sudden onset

(b.) Unilateral inflammation of the eye.

(c.) Pain, feeling of pressure in the eye.

(d.) Moderate pupil dilation, which is nonreactive to light.

(e.) Blurring of vision.

(f.) Photophobia.

(g.) Seeing halos around lights.

(h.) Nausea and vomiting.

(i.) If untreated, will produce blindness in 3 to 4 days.

c. Nursing management.

(1.) Chronic open angle glaucoma

(a.) Instill ordered miotic, like pilocarpine, 1 to 4%, into the eye to constrict the pupil and contract the ciliary musculature, which opens the angle and facilitates aqueous humor outflow. A plastic reservoir of pilocarpine (Ocusert) can be placed in the upper or lower conjunctival sac to enable the drug to diffuse into the sac at a steady rate.

(b.) Administer ordered carbonic anhydrase inhibitor, like acetazolamide (Diamox) to decrease the rate of aqueous humor production.

(c.) Administer ordered β-blocker, like timolol (Timoptic), to decrease production of aqueous humor.

(d.) Teach the patient the importance of taking only those medications prescribed for him, only in ordered doses, and to instill eye medications only into the ordered eye.

(e.) Instruct patient and family concerning the correct method of instilling medications; wash hands, steady hand containing medicine dropper against the forehead or cheek, pull down lower lid, direct gaze upward, drop medication into the conjunctival sac without touching dropper to eye tissues, close lids lightly, and apply pressure over lacrimal duct opening at inner canthus (with sterile cotton ball) to prevent systemic absorption of drug.

(f.) Advise patient to wear a Medic Alert bracelet to inform caregivers of his diagnosis and treatment.

(g.) Inform patient to keep his home well lighted, as his pupils will not dilate in dim light as long as he is taking miotics.

(h.) Instruct patient to avoid using mydriatics (like atropine) and sympathomimetics (which may be found in cold and allergy medications), either of which would counteract the effects of pilocarpine.

(i.) If medical treatment is unsuccessful, and a surgical filtering procedure must be performed to create an opening for aqueous humor outflow, prepare the patient physically and emotionally for the surgical procedure.

(2.) Acute closed angle glaucoma—a medical emergency.

(a.) Instill ordered pilocarpine 4% solution into the eye to cause miosis, to pull the iris out of the chamber angle, and to open the outflow path for aqueous humor.

(b.) Administer ordered carbonic anhydrase inhibitor, i.e., acetazolamide (Diamox), to decrease aqueous humor production.

(c.) Administer ordered osmotic agent, such as mannitol or urea I.V., to decrease aqueous humor production.

(d.) After the intra-ocular pressure has been reduced and the eye is less inflamed, prepare patient physically and emotionally for a peripheral iridectomy, or removal of a small piece of the iris, so as to create a hole through which aqueous humor can drain from the anterior chamber.

(e.) Assist patient to ambulate immediately after surgery.

(f.) Administer ordered mydriatics and miotics to mobilize the pupil and prevent development of posterior synechiae.

3. **Keratitis**—inflammation of the cornea, which may be acute or chronic, and may progress to corneal ulceration.

a. Causes.

(1.) Infection by herpes simplex Type I virus, the most common cause.

(2.) Occasionally, a bacterial or fungal infection.

(3.) Exposure, due to failure or inability to close the eyelids, as occurs following stroke or brain damage.

(4.) Vitamin A deficiency

b. Manifestations.

(1.) Excessive lacrimation

(2.) Photophobia

(3.) Eye pain

(4.) Blepharospasm

(5.) Blurred vision

c. Nursing management.

(1.) Provide bed rest.

(2.) Administer ordered idoxuridine eyedrops and ointment into the eye (for treatment of herpetic keratitis).

(3.) Instill ordered atropine to dilate the pupil and to put the ciliary body and iris at rest, thus favoring healing.

(4.) If patient doesn't experience relief after 1 week of treatment, administer ordered adenine arabinoside (Vira-A) or trifluorothymidine.

(5.) Administer ordered broad-spectrum antibiotic topically or systemically to prevent secondary bacterial infection.
(6.) After infection has subsided, administer ordered corticosteroids, which are given to decrease inflammation and to prevent scarring.
(7.) For keratitis due to exposure, instill ordered moisturizing ointment, and cover eye with a plastic bubble eyeshield.
(8.) Teach patient to avoid trauma, stress, fever, and sun exposure, as these trigger flare-ups of keratitis in a susceptible patient.
(9.) For the patient with severe corneal scars in whom a corneal transplant is to be performed, prepare the patient physically and emotionally for the procedure.
(a.) Provide emotional support for the patient who is waiting for a donor cornea to become available or who is distressed at the realization that the donor cornea is obtained from a cadaver.
(b.) Pre-operatively, inform patient that his eye that will be operated upon will be covered with a patch for 24 hours following surgery. Instill ordered miotic, like pilocarpine, into the eye to constrict the pupil and to flatten the iris over the lens.
(c.) Post-operatively, allow the patient bathroom privileges and assist him to ambulate during the first few hours following the procedure. Instill ordered steroid or antibiotic eye medications or both. Instruct patient to wear dark glasses while photophobia continues and to wear eyeshield at night to prevent eye injury.

4. **Uveitis**—inflammation of the uveal tract, which consists of the iris (iritis), the ciliary body (cyclitis), and the choroid (choroiditis). Results in disturbance of the eye's vascular supply. May be granulomatous or non-granulomatous.
a. Causes.
(1.) Local infection
(2.) Improperly healed corneal abrasions
(3.) Rheumatoid arthritis
(4.) Systemic debilitating diseases such as tuberculosis, histoplasmosis, and sarcoidosis.
b. Manifestations.
(1.) Severe eye pain
(2.) Photophobia
(3.) Blurred vision
(4.) Pupil constriction (due to spasm of the iris).
(5.) Eye is red due to vasodilation.
c. Nursing management.
(1.) Provide bed rest with music or other suitable diversion to relieve boredom and frustration.
(2.) Administer ordered mydriatic, like atropine, to dilate the pupil and prevent adhesions between the anterior lens capsule and the iris.
(3.) Apply ordered warm moist compresses to the eye to decrease pain (usually for 5 minutes Q.I.D.).
(4.) Advise patient to wear dark glasses to decrease photophobia.
(5.) Instill ordered corticosteroid medication into the eye to decrease inflammation.
(6.) Follow physician's orders (e.g., administration of antituberculosis drugs) for treatment of underlying systemic debilitating diseases.
(7.) Teach patient and family the proper method for instillation of medications into the eye (see nursing management for chronic open angle glaucoma).
(8.) Teach the patient the need for long-term follow-up care because of the likelihood of recurrence and possible complications, such as glaucoma, cataract, and retinal detachment.

5. **Retinal detachment**—separation of the rod and cone layer of the retina from the pigment epithelium of the choroid, which is usually unilateral. Separation is incomplete at first, but if untreated, will become complete, with total loss of vision.
a. Causes.
(1.) Degenerative changes of aging; a hole develops as the vitreous shrinks and pulls away from the retina, allowing fluid from the vitreous and transudate from the choroid vessels to seep behind the retina, undermining it still further.
(2.) Traction injury during cataract surgery.
(3.) Traumatic injury to the globe.
(4.) Retinopathy associated with hypertension, diabetes mellitus, and glomerulonephritis.
(5.) Myopia predisposes to retinal detachment.
b. Manifestations.
(1.) Occurs suddenly.

(2.) Initially, patient may experience floating spots (due to blood cells that are freed when the retina tears) or flashes of light (due to vitreous traction on the retina).
(3.) Gradual, painless vision loss occurs as if a curtain were descending over one eye. The area of visual loss depends upon the area of detachment.
(4.) Funduscopic examination reveals folds in the retina and ballooning out of the detached area of retina.

c. Nursing management.
(1.) Position patient in bed so the area of detachment is dependent.
(2.) Caution patient against sneezing, coughing, straining, and bending over.
(3.) Administer ordered stool softeners to prevent straining at stool.
(4.) If surgery is scheduled to re-attach retina to the choroid, prepare patient physically and emotionally for the procedure. Determine which type of intervention is to be used in order to answer patient's questions.
(a.) Laser beam surgery may be used to provoke an inflammatory response in the pigment epithelium, to which the loosened retina is approximated, so that an adhesion will form to bind the 2 tissues together.
(b.) Scleral buckling—indenting the area of sclera that lies over the retinal defect, so as to bring the choroid and retina into contact again.
(1.) Following a buckling procedure, carefully check the surgeon's orders for the patient's position, and instruct patient as to which bed positions he may assume and which he should avoid. Bathroom privileges are allowed after recovery from anesthesia.
(2.) Administer ordered anti-emetics, like perchlorperazine or trimethobenzamide, to prevent vomiting.
(3.) Administer ordered softeners to prevent straining at stool.
(4.) Keep operated eye covered with an eye patch for 24 hours following surgery.
(5.) Administer ordered analgesics (often narcotics) to relieve eye pain.
(6.) Inform patient that reading will not be allowed for 2 to 3 weeks.
(7.) If ordered, administer steroid and antibiotic eye drops.
(8.) Teach patient and family the proper procedure for instillation of eye medications.

B. Care of Patients with Selected Disorders of the Ear

1. **Otitis media**—inflammation of the middle ear, which may be acute or chronic, serous or suppurative.

a. Causes.
(1.) Obstruction of the eustachian tube, which prevents normal ventilation of the middle ear, creates negative pressure in the middle ear, and leads to serous exudation into the middle ear.
(2.) Respiratory tract infection, with organisms ascending from the nasopharynx through the eustachian tube.
(3.) Allergic reactions, with exudation of serous fluid into the middle ear.

b. Manifestations.
(1.) Severe deep, throbbing pain.
(2.) Moderate to high fever (with suppurative otitis media).
(3.) Mild conductive hearing loss.
(4.) Sensation of fullness in the ear; popping or crackling on swallowing.
(5.) Dizziness, nausea, and vomiting.
(6.) Drainage from the external auditory canal, if the tympanic membrane ruptures.

c. Nursing management.
(1.) Serous otitis media
(a.) Teach patient how to inflate the eustachian tube by Valsalva's maneuver so as to facilitate drainage of fluid from the middle ear.
(b.) Administer ordered decongestant spray (usually 0.25% phenylephrine) or phenylpropanolamine orally to shrink swollen mucosa.
(c.) Administer ordered antihistamines to relieve nasal allergy.
(d.) Assist physician with needle aspiration of the eardrum to remove serous fluid from the middle ear.
(2.) Purulent otitis media
(a.) Provide bed rest.

(b.) Administer ordered antibiotics systemically to control infection.

(c.) Administer ordered aspirin or acetaminophen to decrease fever.

(d.) If myringotomy is performed, maintain flow of drainage by placing sterile gauze wick loosely into the external auditory canal.

(e.) If ordered, apply dry heat to the ear to relieve pain.

(f.) Caution patient not to blow his nose or to get his ear wet when bathing.

(g.) Instruct patient on the need to take the complete course of ordered antibiotics, even if symptoms abate before all doses have been administered.

(h.) Advise patient to perform Valsalva's maneuver several times daily to facilitate drainage from the middle ear.

(i.) Advise patient to avoid persons with upper respiratory infections and to avoid forceful nose blowing.

2. **Mastoiditis**—purulent bacterial infection of the air cells of the mastoid antrum.
   a. Cause.
      (1.) Direct extension of infection from acute suppurative otitis media, often with β-hemolytic *Streptococcus, Staphylococcus, Haemophilus influenza.*
      (2.) Immunosuppression and chronic systemic illnesses predispose to mastoiditis.
   b. Manifestations.
      (1.) Aching pain in the mastoid area.
      (2.) Low-grade fever
      (3.) Headache
      (4.) Possible drainage from the ear if the tympanic membrane is ruptured.
   c. Nursing management.
      (1.) Administer ordered parenteral antibiotics to control infection.
      (2.) Assist physician to perform myringotomy to remove pus from the middle ear.
      (3.) Monitor patient for evidence of facial nerve paralysis (facial asymmetry) or labyrinthine irritation (vertigo) and report immediately, as either may indicate the need for mastoidectomy.
      (4.) Following mastoidectomy, check wound dressing frequently for evidence of drainage and bleeding; check for evidence of facial nerve paralysis, and monitor for symptoms of meningitis (fever, stiff neck, vomiting, and disorientation).
      (5.) Assist with ambulation, as vertigo will result from trauma to inner ear tissues during surgery.
3. **Otosclerosis**—slow formation of spongy bone in the labyrinth of the inner ear, especially in the oval window, with eventual fixation of the footplate of the stapes, impairing hearing by air conduction.
   a. Cause—genetic; transmitted as an autosomal dominant trait. Pregnancy may precipitate onset of the condition.
   b. Manifestations.
      (1.) Slowly progressive unilateral hearing loss, usually first detected in patients between 20 and 40 years of age.
      (2.) Greatest difficulty is hearing softly spoken tones.
      (3.) Tinnitus
      (4.) Bone conduction is greater than air conduction on tuning fork test.
   c. Nursing management.
      (1.) In conversing with the patient with decreased hearing, provide adequate light, look directly at the patient while speaking to him, and speak slowly. Speak to the patient directly rather than through the hospital's nurse to patient intercom system. If the patient speaks too loudly, inform him of that fact and help him to modulate his tones downward.
      (2.) Following stapedectomy and replacement with a prosthesis, administer ordered antibiotics systemically to prevent infection.
      (3.) Monitor the patient post-operatively for tinnitus, vertigo, and fluctuations in hearing, and report these symptoms immediately, as they would suggest incomplete closure of the oval window, with leaking of perilymph into the middle ear.
      (4.) For 24 hours post-operatively, maintain patient in flat position with his affected ear upward to maintain the graft in proper position.
      (5.) Advise the patient to avoid loud noises and sudden pressure changes for 6 months, to avoid straining, bending, and heavy lifting for several weeks, and to avoid blowing the nose for 1 week, to prevent displacement of the prosthesis and introduction of infection into the middle ear.
4. **Ménière's disease**—a chronic disorder of the labyrinths of the inner ear, most common between 40 and 60 years of age.

a. Cause.
   (1.) Overproduction or decreased absorption of endolymph, causing endolymphatic hydrops and hypertension, with degeneration of the vestibular and cochlear hair cells.
   (2.) Autonomic nervous system dysfunction may predispose to Ménière's disease by causing temporary constriction of the blood vessels of the inner ear.

b. Manifestations.
   (1.) Rotational vertigo
   (2.) Tinnitus
   (3.) Sensorineural hearing loss
   (4.) A sense of fullness in the ear
   (5.) Nausea and vomiting
   (6.) Violent attacks of vertigo and nausea and vomiting, lasting from 10 minutes to several hours.
   (7.) Nystagmus
   (8.) Loss of balance and falling.
   (9.) While recumbent, patient lies on same side as affected ear, looking toward the affected ear.
   (10.) Attacks become less frequent as unilateral hearing loss progresses to total hearing loss.
   (11.) Diagnosed by precipitation of an attack with instillation of 0.2 ml of ice water into each ear, while the patient lies with head elevated 30 degrees.

c. Nursing management.
   (1.) Administer ordered diphenhydramine or promethazine subcutaneously to relieve vertigo.
   (2.) Keep bed's side rails up at all times during an attack to prevent falls.
   (3.) Provide low sodium diet to prevent fluid retention.
   (4.) Administer ordered diuretics, such as acetazolamide or chlorothiazide, to prevent fluid retention.
   (5.) Administer ordered niacin.
   (6.) Advise patient to stop smoking, so as to avoid provoking vasospasm.
   (7.) Teach patient to avoid sudden position changes and exposure to glaring light.
   (8.) If medical treatment is unsuccessful and surgical intervention is necessary either to shunt endolymph from the labyrinth or to section the vestibular portion of the 8th cranial nerve, prepare patient physically and emotionally for the operation.

CARE OF PATIENTS WITH ENDOCRINE DISORDERS

A. The pituitary gland or "master gland" produces hormones that control hormone secretion by other endocrine glands. In turn, hormonal secretion by the pituitary is controlled by neural signals or hormones (called releasing or inhibiting factors) from the hypothalamus.

B. The hypothalamic hormones that govern hormonal secretion by the pituitary are as follows:
   1. **Thyrotropin releasing factor**—causes anterior pituitary to release thyroid stimulating hormone.
   2. **Corticotropin releasing factor**—causes anterior pituitary to release adrenocorticotropin.
   3. **Growth hormone releasing factor**—causes anterior pituitary to release growth hormone.
   4. **Luteinizing hormone releasing factor**—causes anterior pituitary to release both luteinizing and follicle stimulating hormone.
   5. **Prolactin inhibiting factor**—inhibits anterior pituitary from releasing prolactin.

C. The hormones produced by the various endocrine glands and the effects of these hormones are indicated in the table on the following page.

Nursing Care of Patients With Selected Endocrine Disorders

1. **Hyperpituitarism**—hypersecretion of one or more pituitary hormones.
   a. Cause.
   A secreting tumor of 1 of the 3 basic cell types found in the anterior pituitary gland.
      (1.) Chromophobe adenoma—largest and most common of pituitary tumors; often secretes excess growth hormone and ACTH.
      (2.) Eosinophilic adenoma—secretes excess growth hormone and prolactin.
      (3.) Basophilic adenoma—smallest pituitary tumor; secretes excess ACTH.
   b. Manifestations.
      (1.) Chromophobe adenoma may initially produce symptoms of disturbed growth (due to excess growth hormone) or disturbed electrolyte balance (due to excess ACTH), but then the rapidly enlarging

Hormone	Physiological Effect
Anterior Pituitary Gland	
Growth hormone (somatotropin)	Stimulates growth of cartilage, bone, and muscle by increasing rate of protein synthesis.
Thyrotropin (TSH)	Stimulates thyroid gland to secrete thyroid hormones.
Adrenocorticotropin (ACTH)	Stimulates adrenal cortex to secrete cortisol and adrenal androgens; permits aldosterone secretion in response to angiotensin.
Follicle stimulating hormone (FSH)	Stimulates development of ovarian follicle and secretion of estrogen.
Luteinizing hormone (LH)	Stimulates formation of corpus luteum and secretion of progesterone.
Prolactin (lactogenic hormone)	Stimulates mammary development and milk production.
Melanocyte stimulating hormone	Stimulates cells in the dermis to form the pigment melanin.
Posterior Pituitary Gland	
Antidiuretic hormone (vasopressin)	Increases resorption of water from renal tubules into the blood.
Oxytocin	Stimulates the pregnant uterus to contract.
Thyroid Gland	
Thyroxin (T_4)	Increases the metabolic rate of most body tissue cells (onset 2 to 3 days; peak 12 days).
Triiodothyronine (T_3)	Increases the metabolic rate of most body tissue cells (onset 6 to 12 hrs; peak 3 days).
Thyrocalcitonin	Lowers blood calcium level by inhibiting bone resorption.
Parathyroid Gland	
Parathormone	Increases absorption of calcium from bowel; promotes bone resorption, elevating blood calcium level.
Adrenal Cortex Gland	
Cortisol (glucocorticoid)	Stimulates gluconeogenesis by the liver, decreases protein synthesis, stimulates protein catabolism in all body cells except liver, increases mobilization and oxidation of fatty acids from adipose tissue.
Aldosterone (mineralocorticoid)	Fosters resorption of Na^+ and elimination of K^+ by renal tubular cells.
Adrenal sex hormones (mostly androgen, some estrogen)	Stimulates genital development at puberty.
Adrenal Medulla	
Epinephrine	Excites both alpha and beta receptors. Dilates pupil, stimulates sweating, increases rate and force of cardiac contraction, constricts blood vessels, dilates bronchi, increases liver glycogenolysis, increases basal metabolic rate.
Norepinephrine	Primarily excites alpha receptors. Constricts blood vessels, raising blood pressure.
Islet Cells of Pancreas	
Insulin (secreted by beta cells of the islet)	Stimulates liver glycogenesis, decreasing blood glucose levels; inhibits gluconeogenesis; promotes glucose transport into muscle cells and fat cells.
Glucagon (secreted by alpha cells of the islet)	Stimulates liver glycogenolysis, increasing blood glucose levels.
Ovary	
Estrogens	Stimulate development of secondary sex characteristics in the female; foster proliferation of endometrial endothelium during the 1st half of the menstrual cycle.
Progesterone	Stimulates secretory development of endometrium during last half of the menstrual cycle.
Testis	
Testosterone	Stimulates development of secondary sex characteristics in the male; fosters protein anabolism.

tumor may destroy normal pituitary tissue, producing hypopituitarism.

(2.) Eosinophilic adenoma causes gigantism when it occurs in children and acromegaly when it occurs in adults (due to excess growth hormone).

(3.) Basophilic adenoma causes Cushing's disease (due to excess ACTH) with truncal obesity, flushed face, hirsutism, skin striae, hypertension, and diabetes.

(4.) Tumors of all 3 cell types may cause headache due to increase in intracranial pressure, and visual losses, due to pressure injury to the optic fibers in the optic chiasm, which is located just above the sella turcica.

c. Nursing management.

(1.) Support patient during completion of the several tests performed during the diagnostic work-up.

(a.) Radioimmunoassay of various hormones in serial blood samples.

(b.) Analysis of 24-hour urine collection for concentrations of hydroxycorticosteroids and ketosteroids.

(c.) Skull x-ray.

(d.) Tomograms of sella turcica—serial x-rays of sella turcica taken at different depths in the horizontal and vertical dimensions.

(e.) Visual field examination—while in front of the examiner, the patient covers one eye at a time and looks straight ahead. Then, while the examiner moves a small object beyond the patient's field of vision toward the center of his field of vision, the patient reports when he first sees the object.

(f.) CAT scan of skull—serial x-rays are taken while the x-ray machine is rotated through a 180 degree arc around the head. The amount of x-ray energy absorbed by various brain tissues in each exposure is fed into a computer, which combines this information to yield a photograph showing various tissue densities. If a contrast medium is to be given the patient during the procedure, hold food and fluids for 6 to 8 hours before the examination. Remove any wigs and hairpins and instruct the patient to lie completely still throughout the procedure. Following the CAT scan procedure, monitor patient for allergic reactions to the contrast medium.

(g.) Carotid angiogram—following administration of a sedative and disinfection of the skin of the neck, a radiopaque dye is injected into the common carotid artery, and serial x-rays are taken of the head to reveal obstruction or displacement of brain vessels, or both, by the tumor.

(2.) If patient is to have transphenoidal removal of the tumor, answer any questions that he may have about the surgical procedure and advise him pre-operatively that he will have nasal packing in place on returning from the operating room. Caution him against nose blowing and sneezing, post-operatively, and have him practice breathing through his mouth.

(3.) Post-operatively, monitor the patient and protect him from neurological and endocrine problems arising from the surgical procedure.

(a.) While patient recovers from anesthesia, place the patient in side-lying position to keep airway open. Following recovery from anesthesia, place patient in Fowler's position to facilitate venous return flow from the head.

(b.) Check wound dressing frequently for evidence of hemorrhage or cerebrospinal fluid leak. Check any yellow drainage for glucose content, which indicates that the drainage is cerebrospinal fluid.

(c.) Check vital signs every 30 minutes for 8 hours, then every 3 hours for 2 days to detect indications of increased intracranial pressure, which include increased temperature; decreased pulse; increased blood pressure; and rapid, shallow, and irregular respirations. Report abnormal findings to physician immediately.

(d.) If an intraventricular catheter or a subarachnoid screw has been inserted for measurement of intracranial pressure, measure cerebrospinal fluid pressure at the ordered intervals, using aseptic technique in handling measuring devices and solutions so as to prevent meningitis and encephalitis.

(e.) Check neural signs every 30 minutes for 8 hours, then every 3 hours for 2 days to detect indications of increased intracranial pressure, such as decreasing level of consciousness, pupil inequality, dilated and fixed pupil, weak hand grip, and inability to move on command or in response to painful stimulus.

(f.) Weigh patient daily and keep record of intake and output and urine specific gravity to detect signs of diabetes insipidus. Report urine output of more than 200 ml/hr with specific gravity of less than 1.005.

(g.) Administer ordered intravenous fluids at proper flow rate to prevent development of cerebral edema and increased intracranial pressure.

(h.) Administer ordered analgesic to control headache and to relieve tenderness of oral mucosa.

(i.) Provide frequent oral hygiene with hydrogen peroxide and normal saline solution to remove dried blood.

(j.) Observe patient for frequent swallowing, which may indicate saturation of nasal pack with cerebrospinal fluid.

(k.) Administer ordered hormones.

(1.) Corticosteroids to decrease cerebral edema.

(2.) Vasopressin (Pitressin) to replace antidiuretic hormone, if it is secreted in inadequate amounts owing to surgical trauma of the posterior pituitary gland.

(3.) ACTH and thyroid hormone, if the entire pituitary gland was removed.

(4.) If the patient is given radiotherapy to shrink the size of the tumor or control metastases, monitor the patient for development of sensory and motor dysfunctions caused by demyelination secondary to radiation injury of brain blood vessels.

(5.) If patient is given chemotherapy to shrink the primary tumor or prevent metastases, monitor patient for such neurotoxic effects of the drug as confusion, lethargy, and ataxia, and report these effects as indicating a need for a change in drug dosage.

(6.) Provide sexual counseling for patient in whom endocrine imbalances resulting from surgery produce decreased libido or impotence.

2. **Panhypopituitarism**

a. Cause.

Failure of both the anterior and posterior pituitary to secrete hormones as a result of glandular destruction by tumor, postpartum pituitary hemorrhage, or hypophysectomy (as palliative treatment for breast cancer).

b. Manifestations.

These depend upon the specific hormone deficiencies that exist and may include the following:

(1.) Amenorrhea

(2.) Infertility

(3.) Hypoglycemia

(4.) Myxedema

(5.) Adrenal crisis

c. Nursing management.

(1.) Administer ordered cortisone or hydrocortisone to prevent hypotension, hypoglycemia, and electrolyte imbalance.

(2.) Administer ordered conjugated estrogens (Premarin) or methyltestosterone to restore normal sexual functioning.

(3.) Administer ordered levothyroxine to maintain normal metabolic rate.

(4.) Administer ordered vasopressin (Petressin) to replace deficient ADH.

(5.) Teach patient and family the necessity for long-term medical management and hormone replacement therapy.

(6.) Teach patient and family the expected effects and toxic effects of replacement hormones administered.

3. **Diabetes insipidus**

a. Cause.

Failure of the posterior pituitary to secrete ADH.

b. Manifestations.

(1.) Excretion of large volumes (5 to 15 L/day) of very dilute urine (specific gravity 1.001 to 1.005).

(2.) Severe dehydration

(3.) Hypovolemic shock

c. Nursing management.

(1.) Administer ordered vasopressin (Pitressin) in oil I.M. or desmopressin (synthetic vasopressin) intranasally 2 to 3 times a day to replace deficient ADH.

(2.) Keep intake and output records, or instruct patient to keep intake and output records as a basis for assessing the adequacy of drug replacement therapy.

(3.) If desmopressin is administered, check patient's nasal mucosa for irritation by the drug.

4. **Graves's disease**—syndrome of hyperthyroidism, exophthalmos, and pretibial myxedema.

a. Cause.

Autoimmune reaction in which a long-acting thyroid stimulator (an autoantibody) causes thyroid enlargement and hypersecretion of T_4 and T_3, which increase the basal metabolic rate of all body tissues. The circulating antibody causes edema and cellular infiltration of extra-ocular muscles and deposition of hydrophilic mucopolysaccharide in orbital and periorbital tissues.

b. Manifestations.

(1.) Nervousness, tremor, restlessness

(2.) Polyphagia, weight loss

(3.) Heat intolerance, excess diaphoresis

(4.) Tachycardia, wide pulse pressure

(5.) Proximal muscle weakness

(6.) Neck swelling, if thyroid gland is enlarged.

(7.) Protruding eyes (exophthalmos), stare, lid lag, failure of eyes to converge.

(8.) Non-pitting edema of pretibial and ankle tissues.

(9.) Elevation of T_4 and T_3 levels of serum,

with T_3 elevated to a greater extent than T_4.

(10.) Increased uptake of ^{131}I by the thyroid gland.

c. Nursing management.

(1.) Provide mental and physical rest in a cool, quiet environment.

(2.) Facilitate relaxation by providing pastimes that relate to the patient's personal interests and involve use of large, rather than small, muscle groups.

(3.) Administer ordered propylthiouracil or methimazole (Tapazole) to inhibit T_3 and T_4 production. Monitor patient for skin rash, nausea, and petechiae.

(4.) Administer ordered propranolol (Inderal) to decrease heart rate and cardiac output. Monitor patient for insomnia, disorientation, hypotension, dyspnea, and purpura.

(5.) If hyperthyroidism is treated by administration of ^{131}I, prepare patient for administration of the drug by explaining the effect of radioiodine on the gland, by instructing the patient to imbibe liberal quantities of fluid and void frequently for the 1st 48 hours following administration of the drug.

(6.) If hyperthyroidism is treated by thyroidectomy, prepare the patient physically and mentally for surgery by providing a high calorie, high carbohydrate, high protein, high fluid diet and by screening visitors so as to protect the patient from upsetting or tiring conversations.

(7.) Post-operatively, protect patient from surgical complications and the metabolic hazards resulting from inadvertent spillage and absorption of thyroid hormone from the gland during the operation.

(a.) Monitor patient closely for wound hemorrhage and wound edema, which can cause respiratory obstruction.

(b.) Monitor patient closely for symptoms of thyroid storm, such as extreme fever, tachycardia, dyspnea, and congestive heart failure.

(c.) Administer ordered O_2 to meet increased cellular O_2 needs in the presence of hypermetabolism.

(d.) Administer ordered intravenous fluids at the proper rate to avoid precipitating congestive heart failure in the presence of increased cardiac output.

(e.) If ordered, maintain patient on hypothermia blanket to prevent hyperthermia resulting from hypermetabolism.

(f.) Maintain patient in Fowler's position to minimize edema of the operative site.

(g.) Support the back of the patient's head while moving and turning him so as to prevent strain on the suture line.

(h.) Check patient for the following evidence of hypoparathyroidism due to accidental removal of parathyroid glands during thyroidectomy; muscular hyperirritability, positive Chvostek's sign, and positive Trousseau's sign.

5. **Myxedema**—syndrome of hypothyroidism and deposition of hydrophilic mucopolysaccharide in subcutaneous tissues.

a. Causes.

Destruction or removal of thyroid tissue by the following:

(1.) Thyroiditis

(2.) Excessive dose of ^{131}I

(3.) Removal of excess thyroid tissue during subtotal thyroidectomy.

b. Manifestations.

(1.) Weakness, lethargy

(2.) Dry coarse skin, dry brittle hair

(3.) Memory loss

(4.) Cold intolerance

(5.) Non-pitting edema of extremities and periorbital tissues

(6.) Elevated serum cholesterol and triglyceride levels

(7.) Husky voice

(8.) Constipation

(9.) Menorrhagia

c. Nursing management.

(1.) Administer ordered levothyroxine orally daily.

(2.) Teach patient the importance of long-term medical follow-up, and explain the need for life-long hormone replacement.

(3.) Monitor patient for evidence of excessive dosage of levothyroxine (symptoms of hyperthyroidism).

(4.) For myxedema coma, administer ordered hydrocortisone, parenteral levothyroxine and O_2. Assist physician with tracheal intubation. Maintain patient on mechanical ventilation.

6. **Hyperparathyroidism**—excessive secretion of parathormone, which causes rapid absorption of calcium from bone and resulting hypercalcemia.

a. Causes.
   (1.) Functioning adenoma of the parathyroid gland.
   (2.) Generalized parathyroid hyperplasia and hypertrophy.
   (3.) Carcinoma of the parathyroid gland.
   (4.) Secondary hyperparathyroidism results from compensatory oversecretion of parathormone in response to the hypocalcemia associated with osteomalacia or chronic renal disease.
b. Manifestations.
   (1.) Weakness of proximal muscles and easy fatigability.
   (2.) Memory loss, emotional lability, and depression.
   (3.) Arthralgia, x-ray evidence of subperiosteal bone resorption, or nephrolithiasis.
   (4.) Pruritus
   (5.) Polyuria, nocturia, and passage of calcium oxalate or phosphate stones.
   (6.) Serum calcium level of more than 10.1 mg/dl.
   (7.) Elevated levels of serum immunoreactive parathormone.
c. Nursing management.
   (1.) Force fluids to 3000 ml/day to prevent formation of renal stones.
   (2.) Provide low calcium diet to decrease calcium absorption from the bowel.
   (3.) Strain urine to detect passage of gravel.
   (4.) Prepare patient for surgical removal of parathyroid tumor by answering the patient's questions about the operation. Surgical removal may involve removal of a single diseased gland, or if all are hyperplastic, removal of 3 parathyroid glands and half of the fourth. (The half gland that remains will maintain normal amounts of circulating parathormone.) Post-operatively, the patient should be monitored for evidence of hypocalcemia (tetany, cardiac arrhythmia, and laryngospasm) and of respiratory obstruction due to hemorrhage or edema of neck tissues.

7. **Hypoparathyroidism**—hyposecretion of parathormone, with abnormally low serum calcium levels and abnormally high serum phosphorus levels.
   a. Causes.
      (1.) Accidental removal of parathyroid glands during thyroidectomy.
      (2.) Surgical removal of malignant tumor of the parathyroid gland.
      (3.) Autoimmune destruction of the parathyroid glands.
      (4.) Prolonged hypomagnesemia (magnesium is required for parathormone release).
   b. Manifestations.
      (1.) Numbness and tingling of the hands and circumoral region.
      (2.) Positive Chvostek's sign (spasms of facial muscles upon tapping the facial nerve just anterior to the ear).
      (3.) Positive Trousseau's sign (carpal spasm following application of a blood pressure cuff to the arm).
      (4.) Tetany, convulsions
      (5.) Dry hair, brittle nails
      (6.) Cardiac arrhythmias, laryngospasm
      (7.) Cataracts
      (8.) Serum calcium level less than 8 mg/dl.
   c. Nursing management.
      (1.) Provide bed rest in quiet, nonstressful environment to prevent anxiety-induced hyperventilation, which produces hypocapnea and alkalosis, which increase hypocalcemia.
      (2.) Administer ordered vitamin D_2 or D_3 (calcitriol).
      (3.) Administer ordered calcium gluconate, calcium chloride, or calcium carbonate orally.
      (4.) Provide high calcium, low phosphorus diet.
      (5.) If ordered, administer aluminum hydroxide gel to bind dietary phosphate in the intestine and prevent its absorption.
      (6.) Keep endotracheal tube and tracheostomy tray at bedside for emergency use in the event of laryngospasm.

8. **Cushing's disease**—a metabolic disorder that results from excess secretion of glucocorticoids.
   a. Causes.
      (1.) Secreting adrenocortical tumor (Cushing's syndrome).
      (2.) Pituitary adenoma that secretes excess ACTH (Cushing's disease).
   b. Manifestations.
      (1.) Central obesity, buffalo hump.
      (2.) Round face, ruddy complexion.
      (3.) Acne, hirsutism, purple abdominal striae.
      (4.) Increased serum sodium concentration, decreased serum potassium concentration.
      (5.) Hypertension
      (6.) Increased serum glucose concentration.
      (7.) Decreased resistance to infection, delayed wound healing.
      (8.) Plasma cortisol concentration of more than 15 μg/dl both morning and evening

(normally 8 to 25 μg/dl in the morning and less than 8 μg/dl in the evening).

(9.) Urinary 17-hydroxyketosteroid level more than 10 mg/gm of creatinine (normally 3 to 7 mg/gm of urinary creatinine).

(10.) Failure of a dose of dexamethasone to depress plasma cortisol level.

c. Nursing management.

(1.) If patient is to be treated by surgical removal of a functional adrenal tumor:

(a.) Promote physical and mental rest pre-operatively.

(b.) Provide low calorie, low carbohydrate, low sodium, high protein, adequate potassium diet to promote weight loss and tissue repair.

(c.) Monitor patient closely for hypertension, infection, glycosuria, and edema.

(d.) Raise the bed's side rails to protect confused patient from falls, as osteoporosis predisposes to fractures, and hormone imbalance predisposes to delayed healing.

(e.) Administer ordered glucocorticoid parenterally on the morning of surgery to protect the patient from adrenocortical insufficiency during adrenalectomy.

(f.) Post-operatively, monitor patient closely for evidence of shock (due to adrenocortical insufficiency) and infection (due to long-standing metabolic imbalance). Administer ordered corticosteroids. Instruct patient about need for long-term hormone replacement therapy.

(2.) If pituitary irradiation is used to treat a pituitary tumor, inform patient that full therapeutic effect of irradiation is not apparent for several months. Monitor patient for toxic effects of radiation.

(3.) If metyrapone (Metopirone) is administered to block cortisol production by the adrenal cortex, monitor patient for nausea and vertigo (toxic effects of the drug).

(4.) Provide psychological support for the patient in dealing with loss of self esteem resulting from the disfiguring characteristics of the disorder.

9. **Addison's disease**—chronic adrenal cortical insufficiency, with deficient secretion of glucocorticoids and mineralocorticoids.

a. Cause.

(1.) Destruction of adrenal cortex by tuberculosis, amyloidosis, or tumor.

(2.) Autoimmune reaction resulting in atrophy of the adrenal cortex.

b. Manifestations.

(1.) Weakness, fatigue, emaciation

(2.) Nausea, vomiting, diarrhea

(3.) Weak pulse, hypotension

(4.) Hypoglycemic episodes, such as headache, nervousness, trembling, diaphoresis.

(5.) Low serum sodium level, high serum potassium level.

(6.) Bronze skin discoloration.

(7.) Failure of plasma cortisol and urinary 17-hydroxycorticosteroid levels to rise following I.V. administration of 25 U of ACTH.

c. Nursing management.

(1.) Administer ordered cortisol orally after meals and with milk to decrease the risk of peptic ulcer.

(2.) Administer ordered aldosterone daily to raise serum sodium level.

(3.) Provide liberal intake of salt to prevent extracellular fluid depletion.

(4.) Teach patient the need for the following:

(a.) Life-long hormone replacement therapy.

(b.) A Medic Alert bracelet indicating diagnosis and maintenance therapy.

(c.) Increased doses of adrenocortical hormones in times of stress (illness, surgery).

10. **Diabetes mellitus**—chronic multisystem disorder that is characterized by disturbances in carbohydrate and fat metabolism and results from insufficient production of insulin by beta cells of the pancreatic islet.

a. Causes.

(1.) Predisposition to diabetes is transmitted as a mendelian recessive trait.

(2.) In Type I diabetes (insulin dependent), the beta cells are impaired by a virus or an autoimmune reaction and fail to produce insulin.

(3.) In Type II diabetes (noninsulin dependent), an age-related impairment of beta cell function is present, with deficient release of insulin from the pancreas or blockage of insulin effect in the peripheral tissues.

b. Manifestations.

(1.) Polyphagia with weight loss and weakness.

(2.) Polydipsia and polyuria

(3.) Glycosuria and acetonuria
(4.) Positive glucose tolerance test results; excessively rapid and sustained rise in serum glucose level following ingestion of a glucose-containing beverage.
(5.) Blurred vision, cataracts, and retinopathy (microaneurisms, exudates, and neovascularization).
(6.) Peripheral neuritis—decreased vibratory and fine touch sensations in symmetrical, stocking-like distribution.
(7.) Arteriosclerosis of coronary, cerebral, and peripheral arteries, increasing the patient's susceptibility to myocardial infarction, stroke, and gangrene.

c. Nursing management.
(1.) Provide ordered 1200 calorie diet to facilitate weight loss in the obese patient. Generally, carbohydrates constitute 50% of the allowed calories, fats 30%, and proteins 20%, with most of the carbohydrates in the form of polysaccharides, lactose, and fructose.
(2.) For the Type II diabetic whose symptoms cannot be controlled on diet alone, administer ordered oral hypoglycemic agent, such as tolbutamide (Orinase) or chlorpropamide (Diabinese), which stimulates beta cells to release insulin.
(3.) For the Type I diabetic, administer ordered insulin subcutaneously; often a combination of a rapid acting (Regular or Semilente), intermediate acting (Globin Zinc, NPH or Lente), and long acting (Protamine zinc or Ultralente) in order to maintain fairly constant levels of blood glucose.
(4.) Teach insulin-dependent patient to test urine daily for glucose and acetone.
(5.) Teach patient and primary caregiver the following:
(a.) Symptoms, causes, and consequences of hyperglycemia and hypoglycemia.
(b.) Symptoms and causes of ketoacidosis.
(c.) Proper treatment for hypoglycemia.
(d.) Procedures for insulin administration.
(e.) Testing of urine and blood ("fingerstick" sample) for glucose.
(f.) Principles of proper skin and foot care.
(g.) Complications of diabetes.
(h.) Need for life-long medical follow-up and supervision.

CARE OF PATIENTS WITH RESPIRATORY DISORDERS

1. **Lower respiratory disorders**—classified as either obstructive (blocking of airways) or restrictive (limited lung elasticity).
2. **Acute tracheobronchitis**—acute bacterial infection and inflammation of the mucosal lining of the trachea and bronchial tree.

a. Cause.

Usually an extension of an acute upper respiratory infection to the lower respiratory tree. Lowering of resistance and impairment of tracheobronchial ciliary movement (from smoking) predispose to bacterial invasion of tracheobronchial mucosa.

b. Manifestations.
(1.) Dry, irritating cough develops following an upper respiratory infection.
(2.) Cough with mucopurulent sputum, lasting 10 to 14 days.
(3.) No x-ray film evidence of pulmonary consolidation.
(4.) Streptococci or pneumococci obtained on sputum culture.
(5.) Fever (101° to 102° F orally), fatigue, and malaise lasting 3 to 5 days.
(6.) Tracheobronchitis is especially hazardous in elderly patients, immunocompromised patients, and patients with compromised respiratory function.

c. Nursing management.
(1.) Provide bed rest in a room with humidified air.
(2.) Push fluid intake of 3000 to 4000 ml/day.
(3.) Provide high protein, high carbohydrate diet to facilitate tissue healing.
(4.) Administer ordered expectorant medications, such as Glyceryl Guaiacolate or potassium iodide with copious amounts of fluid.
(5.) Administer ordered acetylsalicylic acid or acetaminophen orally to reduce fever.
(6.) Administer ordered bronchodilator, such as ephedrine, aminophylline, or isoproterenol if inflammatory bronchospasm causes dyspnea.
(7.) Administer ordered antibiotics to prevent secondary infection, such as pneumonia, in elderly or immunocompromised patients.
(8.) Protect debilitated patients from overexertion and from exposure to visitors and staff members with upper respiratory infections.

3. **Pneumonia**—acute inflammation of lung tissue, produced by an infectious agent and causing obliteration of alveolar spaces by inflammatory exudate.
   a. Causes.
      (1.) Inhalation of such infective agents as bacteria (pneumococci, Friedlander's bacillus, staphylococci, and streptococci), viruses, and fungi (*Histoplasma, Coccidioides*, and *Blastomyces*).
      (2.) Inhalation of noxious gases causes chemical pneumonitis, upon which bacterial pneumonia can easily be superimposed.
      (3.) Predisposing factors include debilitating conditions like cancer, malnutrition, upper respiratory infection, chronic obstructive lung disease, immobility, and aspiration.
   b. Manifestations.
      (1.) Precipitous onset with fever (101° to 105° F orally), shaking chills, diaphoresis, and chest pain that is increased by coughing.
      (2.) Tachypnea (30 to 40/min), dyspnea, grunting respirations, and flaring of the alae nasae.
      (3.) In lobar pneumonia (consolidation of all alveoli of a single lobe of the lung), the patient lies on his affected side to splint the chest wall.
      (4.) In lobar pneumonia, breath sounds are absent over the consolidated lobe. In bronchial pneumonia (diffuse patches of inflamed and consolidated alveoli adjacent to bronchial tubes), areas of diminished breath sounds are scattered throughout both lungs.
      (5.) Pleurisy (inflammation of visceral pleura resulting from extension of infection to the lung surface) causes stabbing chest pain on deep inspiration and pleural friction rub.
      (6.) Flushed cheeks, cyanotic lips and nail beds.
      (7.) In both lobar and bronchial pneumonia, when alveoli are filled with solid inflammatory coagulum, cough is dry and nonproductive. After neutrophils have phagocytized the bacteria and the coagulum has liquefied, sputum may be rusty looking due to red blood cells, which enter into alveolar exudate from damaged pulmonary capillaries. In late stages of pneumonia, sputum becomes copious and purulent due to increased numbers of white blood cells and dead tissue cells in the coagulum.
      (8.) Rapid pulse, with wide pulse pressure.
      (9.) Increased white blood cell count, with increased proportion of polymorphonuclear leukocytes.
      (10.) Abdominal distention due to paralytic ileus.
   c. Nursing management.
      (1.) Provide absolute bed rest.
      (2.) Administer ordered O_2.
         (a.) Since normal PaO_2 is 80 to 100 mm Hg and tissue damage occurs when PaO_2 falls below 55 mm Hg, the goal of O_2 therapy should be to keep PaO_2 above 55 mm Hg.
         (b.) Normally, $PaCO_2$ above 40 to 45 mm Hg stimulates respiratory centers to increase respiratory effort. In patients with chronic obstructive lung disease, who have a chronic elevation of $PaCO_2$ above 45 mm Hg, it is a low PaO_2 that stimulates respiratory centers to increase the rate and depth of respiration. Therefore, high concentrations of O_2 should not be given to a patient with chronic obstructive lung disease, because a marked rise in PaO_2 could obliterate accustomed respiratory drive. Since chronic obstructive lung disease predisposes to pneumonia, many patients with pneumonia may face this hazard.
         (c.) When hypoxemia is diagnosed following blood gas analysis, O_2 should be administered continuously until PaO_2 again reaches safe levels.
         (d.) A variety of O_2 delivery systems are available to meet the needs of diverse types of patients. In some delivery systems the O_2 concentration is measured in liters delivered per minute. In some systems, O_2 concentration is measured in percent of O_2 in inspired air.
            (1.) A low flow system delivers O_2 in amounts that vary with changes in the patient's breathing. Nasal cannula; flow rate is from 2 to 6 L/min. At a flow rate of 4 L/min, the patient receives from 21 to 40% of O_2, depending upon respiratory rate and depth. Nasal catheter; flow rate is from 2 to 6 L/min. O_2 concentration at a given flow rate varies with the patient's respiratory rate and pattern.

Gas flow can cause drying of the respiratory mucosa or distention of the stomach. The catheter should be changed from one nostril to the other every 8 hours. Standard mask; small holes in the side permit elimination of exhaled air and facilitate inhalation of room air to mix with O_2. The flow rate is from 6 to 12 L/min, which supplies an O_2 concentration of 40 to 65%, depending upon respiratory rate.

(2.) High flow system; delivers a fixed amount of O_2, as long as flow exceeds the patient's peak inspiratory demand. Venturi mask; O_2 enters the mask in such a manner as to draw in large amounts of room air. Delivers a fixed O_2 concentration. Air entrance ports must be unencumbered by bed linens for the mask to function properly. The flow rate is from 4 to 10 L/min and provides from 24 to 100% of O_2. Provides a specific O_2 concentration to a patient with an irregular ventilation pattern.

(3.) Administer ordered codeine to relieve pleuritic pain and to allow full respiratory excursions. Strong acting narcotics are not used, as they would depress the respiratory centers.

(4.) Push fluids to 3000 ml/day, orally or intravenously, to loosen pulmonary secretions and to replace fluids lost because of diaphoresis and fever.

(5.) Administer ordered 7- to 10-day regimen of antibiotics. The specific drug used is selected on the basis of organisms grown on sputum culture. Penicillin or erythromycin for pneumococcal or streptococcal pneumonia. Chloramphenicol or cephalothin for *Klebsiella pneumoniae*. Nafcillin or cephalothin for staphylococcal pneumonia.

(6.) Provide high protein, high carbohydrate, high caloric liquid diet for febrile, dyspneic patient.

(7.) If paralytic ileus develops, administer nothing by mouth, insert ordered nasogastric tube to drain gastric secretions, and infuse ordered intravenous fluids to replace 3rd space losses.

(8.) Monitor patient for complications. Atelectasis; diminished or absent breath sounds in lung tissue distal to inflamed bronchus. Shock; vascular collapse due to circulating bacterial toxins (most common in gram-negative infections). Pleural effusion; transudation of a large amount of fluid into the pleural sac in response to irritation of the visceral pleura. Large effusions impede lung expansion, causing dyspnea and dullness to percussion over areas where resonance is normally heard. Lung abscess; localized, circumscribed collection of pus within lung tissue that develops when infected secretions stagnate in a cavity formed by alveolar or bronchiolar necrosis. If the abscess erodes into a bronchus, copious purulent sputum results. Empyema; a collection of infected exudate in the pleural space, due to direct extension of microorganisms to the pleural space from an underlying pulmonary infection.

(9.) As inflammatory coagulum liquefies, teach the patient techniques for productive coughing, and provide frequent oral hygiene to improve comfort and appetite.

4. **Bronchiectasis**—a chronic disease characterized by patchy and irreversible dilation of medium sized bronchi, with destruction of elastic and muscle fibers in the bronchial walls, recurrent infection, and hypersecretion of mucus.

a. Causes.

(1.) Congenital immobility of cilia, leading to bronchial obstruction and subsequent infection of retained secretions.

(2.) Early childhood respiratory infections and IgA deficiency (hypogammaglobulinemia) predispose to bronchiectasis.

b. Manifestations.

(1.) Chronic cough with copious purulent sputum, which is worst on arising and retiring.

(2.) Hemoptysis

(3.) Fetid breath

(4.) Sputum sample separates into 3 layers on standing.

(5.) Anorexia, weight loss, fatigue, exertional dyspnea.

(6.) Bronchial obstruction and pooled secretions seen on bronchoscopy.

(7.) Sacculated or fusiform bronchial dilations with fluid levels seen in middle and lower lung lobes on chest x-ray films following instillation of radiopaque material into the tracheobronchial tree.

(8.) Repeated pulmonary infections.

(9.) Finger clubbing develops if hypoxemia is present for a long time.

c. Nursing management.

(1.) Push high fluid intake (3000 ml/day), and administer aerosol nebulizer treatment to liquefy lung secretions.

(2.) Provide chest physiotherapy (vibration, percussion, and cupping), ordered bronchodilators, and postural drainage B.I.D. to remove stagnant bronchial secretions.

(3.) Prepare patient for bronchoscopy, if ordered, to remove tenacious sputum that cannot be removed by postural drainage.

(a.) Inform patient that he will lie on his back with a small pillow under his shoulders during the procedure; that his throat will be anesthetized before the procedure; and that during the procedure he should lie quietly, practice relaxation exercises, and breathe through his nose.

(b.) Give no food or fluids for 6 to 8 hours before bronchoscopy.

(c.) Remove any dentures, and store for safekeeping.

(d.) Check to see that a signed consent form is on the patient's chart.

(e.) Administer ordered sedative or tranquilizer.

(4.) Administer ordered antibiotics (ampicillin, tetracycline, or cephalothin) for treatment of acute respiratory infections.

(5.) Provide high protein, high carbohydrate diet to support tissue repair and meet energy needs during hypermetabolic state.

(6.) Administer ordered humidified O_2 if blood gas analysis reveals hypoxemia.

(7.) Teach patient the importance of high fluid intake, avoidance of persons with respiratory infections, and hazards of smoking (irritates mucosa, increases tracheobronchial secretions, and paralyzes cilia).

(8.) If disease is confined to one or two lobes and symptoms do not respond to medical management, patient may undergo lobectomy or pneumonectomy to preserve normal remaining lung tissue and prevent recurring pneumonia. If chest surgery is required, prepare patient physically and psychologically, and monitor closed chest drainage apparatus post-operatively to facilitate expansion of remaining lung tissue.

(a.) Pre-operatively, urge patient to stop smoking to decrease bronchial irritation; provide postural drainage and chest physiotherapy to remove airway secretions; provide incentive spirometry to maximize lung inflation; administer aerosolized bronchodilator and antibiotics to remove secretions and control infection; and teach proper coughing techniques.

(b.) Post-operatively, maintain patient in low Fowler's position; support the incision and encourage patient to breathe deeply and cough every hour; administer ordered narcotic to facilitate deep breathing; and monitor closed chest drainage apparatus.

(1.) Normally, lung adheres to the chest wall, despite normal elastic recoil of lung tissue, due to subatmospheric pressure in the pleural space. During lung surgery, air enters the pleural space and the lung collapses. Following thoracotomy, chest tubes are inserted and attached to closed chest drainage to remove air and secretions from the pleural space during inspiration and prevent reflux of the same air and secretions during expiration.

(2.) The typical closed chest drainage setup consists of a 1-, 2-, or 3-bottle (compartment) system that provides a collection device for secretions removed, prevents ingress of atmospheric air to the pleural space (by a water seal), and applies suction to the pleural catheter. In a 1-bottle system, the drainage tube is attached to a glass tube that protrudes from the drainage bottle cap, the other end of which is 1 inch below the water level in the bottom of the bottle. Air, blood, and secretions flow through the drainage tube by gravity; secretions mix with water in the bottle; and air exits the bottle through a short glass tube that protrudes through the bottle cap. In a 2-bottle system secretions are collected in the 1st bottle, and the water seal is provided in the 2nd bottle. In a 3-bottle system, the 1st bottle collects secretions, the 2nd provides the water seal, and the 3rd controls the amount of suction applied. To ensure the continuity and effectiveness of the closed drainage system, all tubing connections and bottle stoppers should be taped; drainage bottles should be kept below the patient's chest level; tubing should be fastened to the bed linens to prevent pulling, kinking, and compression; the patient should turn, cough, and deep breathe at frequent intervals; the tubing should be "milked" in the direction of the drainage bottle to remove clots; and forceps should be attached to the bed's head to clamp the chest tube if the water seal is accidentally broken. If, despite precautions, air leaks into the drainage tube and enters the pleural space, it will increase pressure in the pleural space, collapse the lung, and push the heart toward the unaffected side of the chest (tension pneumothorax). An intact water seal system must be reestablished immediately to prevent serious respiratory and cardiac complications.

5. **Chronic obstructive lung disease**—a group of respiratory disorders characterized by chronic, persistent obstruction to bronchial air flow, including bronchial asthma, chronic bronchitis, and emphysema.
   a. Bronchial asthma—a disorder characterized by episodic paroxysms of wheezing dyspnea, which are due to widespread narrowing of airways.
      (1.) Causes.
         (a.) Extrinsic asthma—an inherited immune disorder with increased levels of IgE and reversible hypersensitivity of tracheobronchial muscles to specific allergens.
         (b.) Intrinsic asthma—an abnormality of the parasympathetic nervous system that results in hyperresponsiveness of tracheobronchial smooth muscle to a variety of nonantigenic stimuli, with resulting bronchospasm, mucosal edema, and production of thick, tenacious sputum.
      (2.) Manifestations.
         (a.) Episodes of non-productive cough and wheezing, with dyspnea and feeling of tightness in the chest.
         (b.) Bronchospasm causes prolongation of expiration and distal air trapping, with resulting increase in the anteroposterior chest diameter.
         (c.) With severe dyspnea, use of accessory muscles of respiration and retraction of intercostal, supraclavicular, and suprasternal spaces.
         (d.) Attacks often occur at night or following severe emotional stress. Attacks may last several hours and may resolve spontaneously, changing to productive cough and expectoration of plugs of thick and tenacious mucus.
         (e.) Blood gas analysis during an attack reveals hypoxemia, acidosis, and hypocapnea (due to increased ventilation).
         (f.) Pulmonary function test results reveal increased residual volume, decreased compliance, decreased forced expiratory volume, and decreased peak expiratory flow rate.
         (g.) Status asthmaticus—severe and continuing asthmatic attacks, with dyspnea, requiring intubation and

mechanical ventilation. PCO_2 is more than 65 mm Hg; PO_2 is less than 45 mm Hg; and pH is less than 7.35.

(3.) Nursing management.

(a.) Acute asthmatic attack.

(1.) Administer ordered epinephrine, 0.2 to 0.5 ml of 1 to 1000 solution S.C.; isoproterenol or metaproterenol by aerosol inhalation; or theophylline ethylenediamine (aminophylline) 0.5 mg/kg/hr, I.V., to relieve bronchospasm.

(2.) Administer low concentrations of O_2 as ordered by mask in the hypoxemic patient with PCO_2 elevation.

(b.) Maintenance therapy.

(1.) Perform ordered skin sensitivity tests to identify allergens that trigger attacks.

(2.) Encourage patient to keep a daily diary to identify allergic and nonallergic stimuli responsible for provoking asthmatic attacks.

(3.) Advise patient to avoid or remove allergens (pollen, dust, dander, feathers, pets, and molds) from living and working environments.

(4.) Advise patient to apply filters to home and business air conditioning systems.

(5.) Reinforce instructions given by physician for treatment of chronic sinusitis; increase fluid intake, increase humidification, apply local heat, and use vasoconstrictive drugs.

(6.) Advise patient to have yearly influenza vaccination.

(7.) Persuade patient to stop smoking and to avoid noxious fumes and known allergens. Advise desensitization to known allergens that can't be avoided.

(8.) Instruct patient to prevent asthmatic attacks by inhalation of ordered cromolyn sodium (Intal), 20 mg, by inhaler Q.I.D., which blocks release of histamine and serotonin from mast cells. Advise patient that cromolyn should be taken following administration of a bronchodilator.

(9.) Teach the patient the action, indication, and toxic effects of ordered bronchodilators, adrenergics, and antihistamines.

b. Chronic bronchitis—chronic inflammation of tracheobronchial tree by chronic exposure to mucosal irritants without airway hyperreactivity.

(1.) Causes.

(a.) Repeated or continuous low-grade exposure of bronchial mucosa to chemical or infectious irritants, such as cigarette smoke, industrial fumes, environmental dust, chronic sinusitis, or chronic pulmonary infections.

(b.) Continuous airway irritation leads to mucosal edema, increased mucus secretion, decreased ciliary action, and decreased resistance to infection.

(2.) Manifestations.

(a.) Habitual cough, productive of odorless mucoid or purulent sputum, which is worst upon arising.

(b.) Repeated lower respiratory tract infections, with worsening cough and sputum production following each infection.

(c.) Sputum cultures reveal pneumococci, staphylococci, streptococci, *Haemophilus influenzae*, or Friedlander's bacilli.

(d.) Severe episodes of coughing may induce bronchospasm and wheezing.

(e.) As the disease progresses, sputum becomes purulent, and bronchial scarring leads to retention of secretions, emphysema, and cor pulmonale.

(f.) When bronchitis becomes severe, symptoms of respiratory obstruction appear; prolonged expiration, intercostal and supraclavicular retractions, pursed lip breathing, wheezing, hypoxia, hypercapnea, and cyanosis.

(3.) Nursing management.

(a.) Emphasize to patient the importance of eliminating his exposure to bronchial irritants, such as smoking, industrial fumes, and dust.

(b.) Administer ordered antibiotic to

treat bronchial infection (ampicillin or tetracycline).

(c.) Push high fluid intake (3000 ml/day) to liquefy bronchial secretions.

(d.) Administer ordered bronchodilator (epinephrine, isoproterenol, or aminophylline) by inhaler, B.I.D., followed by deep breathing and deliberate coughing to remove retained secretions.

(e.) Administer ordered low flow O_2 by mask if patient is hypoxemic.

(f.) Advise obtaining influenza vaccination every year and pneumonia vaccination every third year.

6. **Pulmonary emphysema**—chronic lung disease that is characterized by destruction of alveolar walls, leading to a decreased number of enlarged air spaces (blebs) and destruction of pulmonary capillary network.

a. Causes.

(1.) Congenital plasma protein abnormality (deficiency of alpha$_1$-antitrypsin) predisposes to the disease.

(2.) Cigarette smoking causes emphysema through inflammation of lung mucosa, paralysis of ciliary action, and release of leukocytic proteases.

(3.) Chronic bronchitis

b. Manifestations.

(1.) Insidious onset of fatigue and dyspnea that occurs at first on exertion, then at rest, and is due to airway collapse during expiration.

(2.) Pursed lip breathing.

(3.) Inefficient cough, producing small amounts of tenacious sputum.

(4.) If chronic bronchitis is also present, expiratory rales and wheezing occur.

(5.) Chest is rigid and fixed in inspiratory position.

(6.) Accessory muscles of respiration (sternocleidomastoid, scalenes, and pectorals) are used to elevate the chest during inspiration.

(7.) Distant breath sounds

(8.) Ruddy complexion

(9.) Finger clubbing occurs if hypoxemia is chronic.

(10.) X-ray film evidence of overaeration of the lungs; flattened diaphragm, widened rib spaces.

(11.) Pulmonary function test results show decreased vital capacity, decreased forced expiratory volume, and increased residual volume.

(12.) Blood gas analysis shows decreased PaO_2, increased $PaCO_2$.

(13.) Blood count reveals increased red blood cell count, increased hematocrit value (as compensation for chronic hypoxemia).

(14.) Severe, prolonged emphysema predisposes to repeated lung infections, right ventricular failure, and respiratory failure.

c. Nursing management.

(1.) Describe the effect of smoking on ciliary action and respiratory secretions and advise patient to stop smoking.

(2.) Push high fluid intake (3000 ml/day) to liquefy bronchial secretions.

(3.) Administer aerosolized bronchodilators (epinephrine, isoproterenol, or metaproterenol), if ordered, to relieve bronchospasm.

(4.) Administer ordered ultrasonic nebulizer to liquefy tenacious secretions.

(5.) Institute postural drainage and assisted coughing to remove secretions.

(6.) Teach patient diaphragmatic breathing exercises to decrease rate and increase depth of respirations.

(7.) Teach patient to use pursed lip breathing to prevent airway collapse during exhalation.

(8.) Encourage physical conditioning exercises to increase motor endurance.

(9.) Administer ordered antibiotics to treat underlying bronchial infection.

(10.) Administer ordered low flow O_2 (no more than 2 L/min) by portable cylinder to correct hypoxemia.

(11.) Teach patient the importance of high protein, high carbohydrate, high fluid diet; of the need to avoid persons with respiratory infections; and the reasons for avoiding extremes of hot and cold.

(12.) Assist patient to plan work and recreational activities to fit diminished physical capacity.

7. **Respiratory failure**—progressive obstruction of respiratory passages leads first to respiratory insufficiency, or inability to meet the body's O_2 needs during exertion, and finally to respiratory failure, or inability to meet the body's O_2 needs at rest. Respiratory failure is also defined as a PaO_2 of less than 50 mm Hg, with or without elevation of $PaCO_2$.

a. Causes.

Any combination of obstructive and restrictive lung disorders can cause acute or chronic respiratory failure.

(1.) Acute respiratory failure develops over a short period of time and is life threatening.

(2.) Chronic respiratory failure develops over a long period of time and is characterized by Pa_{O_2} of less than 50 mm Hg and Pa_{CO_2} of more than 45 mm Hg, while the patient is partially functional.

b. Manifestations.

(1.) Symptoms of acute hypoxia.

(a.) Decreased judgment

(b.) Motor instability

(c.) Tachycardia giving way to bradycardia.

(d.) Cyanosis of lips and nail beds; when the concentration of reduced hemoglobin in the capillaries is greater than 5 gm/100 ml.

(e.) Drowsiness, apathy, and fatigue.

(f.) Increased reaction time

(g.) Plethora

(2.) Symptoms of hypercapnea

(a.) Apprehension

(b.) Confusion

(c.) Drowsiness

(d.) Tachycardia

(e.) Sweating

(f.) Headache

(g.) Muscular twitching

c. Nursing management.

(1.) Determine that airway is open, or establish open airway. Clear secretions from mouth and throat, tilt head backward, and pull jaw forward. If respirations don't resume, give mouth-to-mouth resuscitation.

(2.) Institute O_2 therapy if ordered to ensure oxygenation of vital tissues. Provide humidification to prevent drying of tracheobronchial mucosa and to liquefy secretions.

(3.) If patient does not resume spontaneous respirations, assist physician with intubation and institution of mechanical ventilation. Ventilators are of different types as follows:

(a.) Pressure ventilator—a prescribed airway pressure is achieved by the machine with each respiratory cycle.

(b.) Volume ventilator—a prescribed tidal volume is delivered with each respiratory cycle.

(c.) Both pressure and volume respirators can be set either to cycle automatically or to assist the patient's own respiratory effort once inhalation is initiated.

(4.) Auscultate lungs and aspirate airway as needed to remove retained secretions.

8. **Pulmonary embolism**—obstruction of a pulmonary artery by a thrombus that is dislodged from its origin in the peripheral venous circulation or the right side of the heart. If the embolus is large, interruption of blood supply to a large area of lung tissue causes infarction of the ischemic area. Multiple pulmonary emboli are usually present and are most apt to be located in the right lower lobe of the lung.

a. Causes.

(1.) Usually, a clot is mobilized from a lower extremity vein in which blood stasis, venous trauma, or blood hypercoagulability causes clot formation; limb movement causes the tail of the clot to break loose and move with venous return flow toward the heart.

(2.) Thrombi from pelvic veins or the right side of the heart (due to atrial fibrillation or myocardial infarction) may develop into emboli and enter into the pulmonary circulation.

(3.) Varicosities, prolonged bed rest, pregnancy, and oral contraceptives predispose to lower extremity venous thrombi and emboli.

b. Manifestations.

(1.) Massive pulmonary embolism.

(a.) Sudden central chest pain

(b.) Cough, with blood tinged sputum.

(c.) Dyspnea

(d.) Low-grade fever

(e.) Symptoms of right ventricular overload (distended neck veins, hepatojugular reflux, loud pulmonic second heart sound), and circulatory collapse (hypotension, syncope).

(f.) Decreased lung perfusion causes decreased Pa_{O_2}.

(g.) Wedge shaped lung opacity on chest x-ray.

(h.) Elevation of serum lactic dehydrogenase (LDH) level.

(i.) Evidence of obstruction in pulmonary blood flow on radioactive (^{99m}Tc) lung scan.

(2.) Moderate size pulmonary embolism.

(a.) Sudden pleuritic pain

(b.) Cough, with blood tinged sputum.
(c.) Pleural friction rub or pleural effusion.
(d.) Dullness to percussion over infarcted lung tissue.
(e.) Recurrent medium sized pulmonary emboli may cause right ventricular failure.

c. Nursing management.
(1.) Monitor elderly bedridden patients closely for signs of thrombophlebitis (pain, heat, swelling of the lower extremity) and report promptly.
(2.) Administer ordered heparin I.V. for 10 days, monitoring daily clotting time and partial thromboplastin time.
(3.) Keep patient at complete bed rest to decrease cellular O_2 need.
(4.) Administer ordered O_2 by nasal cannula or face mask.
(5.) When patient has been regulated on heparin dose so that clotting time is 2 to 2½ times normal (raised from 7 to 14 minutes), administer ordered daily oral dose of warfarin (beginning 5 days before discontinuation of heparin I.V.). Goal is to keep prothrombin time 1.5 to 2 times normal (from 13 seconds to 20 to 26 seconds).
(6.) In massive pulmonary embolism, administer ordered thrombolytic agents, like streptokinase or urokinase I.V., to convert plasminogen to plasmin, which lyses the clot. During administration of thrombolytic agents, patient must be monitored closely for bleeding.
(7.) If there is repeated embolization from the lower extremity or pelvic veins and the inferior vena cava is clipped or an umbrella-like device is inserted to block the movement of clots to the lung, prepare the patient physically and psychologically for surgery.
(8.) Teach the patient on long-term Coumadin (Warfarin) therapy that the following potentiate Coumadin's action: alcohol, broad-spectrum antibiotics, aspirin, and steroids.

9. **Pulmonary tuberculosis**—a chronic communicable infection of lung tissue.
a. Cause.
(1.) Inhalation of *Mycobacterium tuberculosis*; antigens in the causative organism stimulate the production of specific leukocytes that either surround the mycobacterium to form a cell mass called a tubercle or engulf the mycobacterium and carry it to the hilar lymph nodes, which then become infected.
(2.) Poor nutrition, malignancy, alcoholism, and immunosuppression predispose to tuberculosis by lowering resistance.

b. Manifestations.
(1.) Primary or first infection
(a.) Tuberculous pneumonia develops in the lower portion of the upper lobe, and the hilar lymph nodes become infected.
(b.) If the area of pneumonia is small, the patient may be asymptomatic.
(c.) The primary infection sensitizes body tissues; within 4 to 8 weeks following the initial lesion a positive skin reaction occurs to intracutaneous injection of 0.1 ml of purified protein derivative of the *Mycobacterium*. A positive reaction consists of a visible and palpable induration of at least 10 mm diameter within 48 to 72 hours.
(2.) Secondary infection
(a.) If the patient is reinfected by inhaling additional mycobacteria, or the wall of lymphocytes that surrounded the primary infection breaks down, mycobacteria are distributed throughout the now sensitized lung tissue and initiate an active infection.
(b.) If the tubercle becomes necrotic and cells liquefy into a cheesy material, freed microorganisms are carried by lymph channels to multiple sites in the body, where new tubercles develop.
(c.) Secondary infections cause anorexia, weight loss, weakness, pallor, fatigability, especially in the afternoon, fever in the afternoon, night sweats, persistent cough, mucoid or purulent sputum, hemoptysis, asymmetrical chest expansion, and dullness to percussion over the lung lesion. Acid-fast aerobic rods are found in the sputum and chest x-ray film shows patchy infiltrate in the lung apex or cavitation elsewhere in the lung.

c. Nursing management.
(1.) Report each case of tuberculosis to the staff of the local health department, who will follow up persons in close contact

with the tuberculous patient for case finding and treatment referral.

(2.) Administer ordered antituberculosis drugs, and teach patient the importance of continuing drug therapy for the prescribed interval. Two of the following drugs are given for a full year and are chosen on the basis of drug sensitivity test results:

(a.) Isoniazid, orally, 100 mg T.I.D.; given with 25 mg of vitamin B_6 to prevent peripheral neuritis, which is a toxic effect of the drug.

(b.) Rifampin, orally 600 mg/day; rifampin is excreted by the liver, so it can't be used in patients with liver disease.

(c.) Ethambutol, orally, 15 mg/kg/day; ethambutol may cause optic neuritis.

(d.) *Para*-aminosalicylic acid, 4 gm orally, T.I.D. with meals.

(3.) Provide high protein, high carbohydrate, high calorie diet to facilitate tissue healing. Teach patient the number of servings from each of the major food groups that he will need to ingest daily to maintain adequate nutrition.

(4.) Assist patient to plan daily schedule to provide balanced periods of rest and exercise to decrease tissue O_2 needs.

(5.) Teach patient to cough into tissues and then to burn tissues to avoid contaminating friends and family members.

(6.) Inform patient that his contact will be treated prophylactically for 1 year with isoniazide.

CARE OF PATIENTS WITH CARDIOVASCULAR DISORDERS

1. **Myocardial infarction**—a localized area of myocardial necrosis, with actual or potential jeopardy of cardiac pumping effectiveness.

a. Causes.

Sudden occlusion of a coronary artery caused by either thrombus formation in a vessel narrowed and roughened by subintimal arteriosclerotic plaques or by embolization of a clot from the left side of the heart into the coronary circulation.

b. Manifestations.

(1.) Often, a history of angina; paroxysms of anterior chest pain provoked by physical exertion, exposure to cold, eating a heavy meal, or experiencing strong emotion.

(2.) Severe, crushing substernal pain that is unrelieved by rest and nitroglycerine, which radiates into the left arm, left subscapular region, or neck.

(3.) Shock—systolic blood pressure of less than 80 mm Hg, tachycardia, gray pallor, cold skin, and urine output of less than 30 ml/hr.

(4.) Extreme apprehension and restlessness.

(5.) Pulmonary edema—dyspnea, orthopnea, rales, and cough with production of thin, watery, blood tinged sputum.

(6.) Elevation of serum enzyme levels (creatine phosphokinase-MB_1 (CPK-MB_1), serum glutamate oxaloacetate transaminase (SGOT), and lactate dehydrogenase (LDH_1).

(7.) Audible fourth heart sound.

(8.) Pericardial friction rub.

c. Nursing management.

Patient will be cared for in coronary care unit.

(1.) Provide complete bed rest in semi-Fowler's position without flexion of the knees for 24 to 48 hours to decrease cardiac work, lower diaphragm, increase lung expansion, and decrease venous return without compressing popliteal veins.

(2.) Start ordered intravenous infusion of 5% dextrose in water at 5 to 10 ml/hr to ensure that an intravenous line is available for administration of emergency drugs if patient's condition requires it.

(3.) Administer ordered morphine sulfate, 1 to 4 mg I.V., to relieve pain and apprehension.

(4.) Administer ordered O_2 (with humidity) at 3L/min by nasal cannula to relieve dyspnea and maximize coronary oxygenation.

(5.) If ordered, administer furosemide (Lasix) or ethacrynic acid (Edecrin), I.V., for rapid diuresis in a patient with pulmonary edema.

(6.) If ordered, administer digoxin or deslanoside (Cedilanid), I.V., to digitalize patient rapidly, decrease tachycardia, and increase myocardial force.

(7.) Assist patient to bedside commode for bowel movement.

(8.) Administer, orally, ordered stool softener daily to prevent straining at stool.
(9.) Monitor patient closely (take vital signs every 1 to 2 hours) to detect following signs of worsening condition; arrhythmia, shock, myocardial rupture, congestive heart failure, morphine toxicity, and respiratory failure.
(10.) Omit bathing patient during acute stage, but feed, wash his face and hands, and shave patient to conserve his energy.
(11.) Administer ordered, low sodium liquid diet (without caffeine-containing beverages) in frequent small feedings to avoid overdistending the stomach and to diminish fluid retention. Restrict fluid intake as ordered (often 1500 to 2000 ml/day) to prevent circulatory overload.
(12.) Insert ordered Foley catheter and measure urine output and specific gravity every 1 to 2 hours to determine adequacy of renal perfusion. Report output of less than 30 ml/hr and specific gravity of more than 1.020.
(13) Change patient's position every 2 hours to prevent pressure injury to edematous sacral tissues.
(14.) If ventricular fibrillation or asystole occurs, administer cardiopulmonary resuscitation and (if ordered) precordial shock.
(15.) When symptoms abate, and ambulation is ordered, assist patient to resume activities of daily living gradually, so as to avoid undue cardiac stress. Monitor patient's vital signs to determine his response to increasing activity.
(16.) Teach patient and family the purpose and toxic effects of all prescribed medications, and stress the need for ongoing health supervision following hospital discharge.
(17.) Provide supportive counseling of patient and family as they cope with the need to alter long-standing habit patterns in decreasing cardiac risk factors. Provide information and encouragement with regard to the following:
(a.) Stopping smoking.
(b.) Decreasing intake of high carbohydrate, high fat, high cholesterol, high sodium foods.
(c.) Resuming sexual activities. Many experts advise that when patient can ascend 2 flights of stairs without difficulty, sexual intercourse with the partner can be resumed.
(d.) Return to employment, former family roles, and community responsibilities.

2. **Congestive heart failure**—inability of the heart to pump enough blood to meet tissue needs for O_2 and nutrients. Symptoms of heart failure may develop suddenly (acute failure), as following myocardial infarction, or slowly (chronic failure), as following long-standing hypertension or generalized, diffuse coronary arteriosclerosis.

a. Types.
(1.) Left-sided heart failure—inability of the left ventricle to pump blood from the pulmonary circulation into the systemic circulation.
(2.) Right-sided heart failure—inability of the right ventricle to pump blood from the systemic venous circulation through the pulmonary circuit.
(3.) High output failure—inability of the heart to meet excessive tissue demands for O_2 and nutrients, despite normal or higher than normal minute volume, as in hyperthyroidism or severe anemia.
(4.) Low output failure—inability of the heart to pump out enough blood under sufficient pressure to perfuse peripheral tissues.

b. Causes.
(1.) Arteriosclerotic narrowing and thrombotic occlusion of coronary arteries, with reduced O_2 supply to heart muscle.
(2.) Acute rheumatic fever—an immune disorder that causes connective tissue inflammation which can cause lesions in all 3 layers of the heart.
(a.) Rheumatic pericarditis may cause pericardial effusion or adhesions, either of which would interfere with normal cardiac contractions.
(b.) Rheumatic myocarditis is characterized by perivascular inflammation and causes tachycardia and arrhythmia.
(c.) Rheumatic endocarditis is characterized by inflamed valve leaflets that contract on healing so the valve doesn't open or close completely.
(1.) With mitral stenosis, the left atrium is unable to empty completely, and increased left atrial pressure is referred backward to the pulmonary circulation, causing pulmonary edema.
(2.) With mitral insufficiency, the blood regurgitates from the left ventricle to the left atrium dur-

ing ventricular systole, resulting in inadequate cardiac output to meet tissue needs.

c. Pathophysiology of congestive heart failure.
   (1.) Disproportion between hemodynamic load and myocardial ability to cope with it.
      (a.) Preload, or degree of myocardial stretching at the end of diastole (the blood volume that must be moved by contraction), that is increased in excessive intravenous infusion of fluids and decreased in massive hemorrhage.
      (b.) Afterload, or force the ventricle must develop to eject the stroke volume, that is increased in aortic valve stenosis and systemic hypertension.
      (c.) Decreased myocardial contractility that occurs following necrosis of large areas of myocardium in coronary occlusion.
      (d.) Incoordination of myocardial contraction or failure of upper and lower cardiac chambers to synchronize contractions so as to move blood effectively into and out of the heart, which occurs in most cardiac arrhythmias.
   (2.) When the heart is stressed by internal and external factors, certain compensatory mechanisms develop to maintain needed cardiac output.
      (a.) Tachycardia—due to reflex stimulation of the heart by distention of superior and inferior vena cava.
      (b.) Cardiac hypertrophy—increased thickness of the myocardium due to increased size of myocardial fibers. At first muscle mass and capillaries increase proportionately. Later, muscle mass outgrows its blood supply.
      (c.) Cardiac dilation—as end-diastolic volume and pressure increase, cardiac chambers dilate, stretching the muscle fibers and (initially) increasing their force of contraction.
      (d.) When compensatory measures can no longer be maintained, cardiac output drops, and metabolism of vital tissues can no longer be maintained (forward failure); the volume of blood remaining in the ventricle following contraction gradually increases, blocking venous return to the heart and causing venous engorgement (backward failure).

d. Manifestations of congestive heart failure.
   (1.) Left-sided heart failure—congestion of pulmonary circulation.
      (a.) Dyspnea—due to increased muscle work required to move stiff lungs.
      (b.) Tachypnea—reflex response to tissue anoxia.
      (c.) Orthopnea—dyspnea while lying flat that is relieved by sitting up (due to increased venous return in supine position).
      (d.) Cough and expectoration of thin, watery sputum; increased pressure in pulmonary capillaries causes transudation of fluid into alveoli.
      (e.) Paroxysmal nocturnal dyspnea—urgent respiratory distress that wakes patient (due to increased venous return in supine position).
      (f.) Pulmonary edema—increased pulmonary capillary pressure pushes fluid from the capillaries through interstitial spaces into alveoli, causing rales, dyspnea, and frothy blood tinged sputum.
      (g.) Cheyne-Stokes respirations—alternating cycles of apnea and hyperventilation due to failure of respiratory control by poorly perfused respiratory centers.
      (h.) Cardiac enlargement due to hypertrophy of myocardial fibers in response to increased preload or afterload.
      (i.) Abnormal rhythm (gallop)—appearance of a third or fourth heart sound during diastole due to vibrations of the ventricular walls when rapidly inflowing blood is stopped by atrioventricular valve closure.
   (2.) Right-sided heart failure—symptoms of systemic venous congestion.
      (a.) Distended neck veins in the upright position due to inability of the failing right ventricle to handle venous return flow.
      (b.) Dependent edema (pedal edema if standing, sacral edema if recumbent) due to transudation of fluid from capillaries distended by increased systemic venous pressure.

(c.) Ascites due to transudation of fluid from peritoneal capillaries.
(d.) Distended liver, tender to pressure, due to increased systemic venous pressure.
(e.) Anasarca—accumulation of fluid in all body tissues in severe and prolonged right-sided heart failure.

e. Nursing care of the patient in congestive heart failure.

(1.) Provide complete mental and physical rest in a cool, quiet room to decrease cardiac work load. Reassure patient and restrict visitors to decrease anxiety and sympathetic nervous system stimulation.

(2.) Maintain patient in Fowler's position with his arms elevated on pillows at his sides to relieve dyspnea and decrease the work of respiratory muscles.

(3.) Administer ordered sedative or tranquilizer to encourage relaxation.

(4.) Assist patient to bedside commode, rather than providing a bed pan, to decrease cardiac strain.

(5.) Administer ordered O_2 by nasal catheter, at 5 L/min.

(6.) Administer ordered digoxin to decrease heart rate, increase myocardial contractile force, slow heart rate, and increase cardiac output. Digitalizing dosage is 0.5 mg, × 6 in 24 hours. Maintenance dosage is 0.5 mg/day. Take apical pulse rate before administration; if rate is less than 60/min, hold digoxin administration and consult physician.

(7.) Monitor patient for signs of digitalis toxicity, such as anorexia, nausea, diarrhea, visual disturbances, and arrhythmia. Since digitalis is eliminated by the kidney, renal disease leads to toxicity.

(8.) Check laboratory reports to determine serum potassium concentration. Hypokalemia sensitizes the myocardium to digitalis and enhances the drug's effects.

(9.) Administer ordered diuretic.
(a.) Hydrochlorothiazide inhibits resorption of sodium and potassium in distal tubules; 500 mg, orally, each day.
(b.) Furosemide (Lasix) inhibits resorption of sodium in proximal and distal tubules; 20 to 40 mg, orally, each day.
(c.) Spironolactone (Aldactone) is an aldosterone antagonist, thereby increasing excretion of sodium and chloride; 25 mg, orally, Q.I.D.

(10.) Keep accurate records of the intake and output, and weigh patient daily to assess the efficacy of diuretic therapy.

(11.) Provide ordered diet, which is apt to be a low calorie (if patient is obese), low residue, low sodium diet (if patient is retaining sodium). Sodium may be restricted to 500 to 1000 mg/day. If ordered, restrict fluid intake to less than 1000 ml/day (for patients refractive to treatment).

(12.) Change patient's position every 2 hours, and keep back and buttocks clean and dry to prevent hypostatic pneumonia and decubitus ulcers (edematous tissues are unusually prone to pressure injury).

(13.) Provide passive range of motion to all joints T.I.D. to prevent venous stasis and thrombosis.

(14.) Apply anti-embolism stockings to prevent lower extremity phlebothrombosis.

(15.) If patient develops acute pulmonary edema:
(a.) Administer ordered morphine sulfate to decrease the anxiety and the volume of venous return to the heart.
(b.) Administer ordered O_2, 40 to 50%, by face mask to decrease dyspnea and hypoxia.
(c.) Administer ordered digoxin or deslanoside (Cedilanid) I.V. for rapid digitalization.
(d.) Administer ordered furosemide (Lasix) or ethacrynic acid (Edecrine) I.V. to reduce circulating blood volume rapidly by immediate diuresis.
(e.) Administer ordered theophylline ethylenediamine (aminophylline), 250 mg, I.V. slowly to decrease bronchospasm and dilate coronary arteries.
(f.) Administer ordered venous vasodilators, nitroglycerine, or isosorbide dinitrate (Isordil) to dilate venous capacitance vessels and decrease venous return to the heart.
(g.) If ordered, apply rotating tourniquets to extremities, 3 limbs at a time, rotating to a different 3-limb combination at 15-minute intervals. By obstructing venous return from 3 extremities at a time, the volume of circulating blood can sometimes

be decreased to a point that the failing heart can function with improved efficiency.

(16.) After patient recovers from congestive heart failure:

(a.) Advise him to resume activities of daily living very gradually.

(b.) Teach him the action, dose, and toxic effects of all maintenance drugs, e.g., digitalis, diuretics, potassium, and tranquilizers.

(c.) Help patient to plan modifications of daily routines, so as to provide balanced periods of rest and exercise.

(d.) Instruct patient and family regarding the signs and symptoms of heart failure.

(e.) Explain the purpose and particulars of sodium restriction and diet modification.

(f.) Advise patient to avoid the following high sodium foods and fluids; smoked meat and fish, canned soup and vegetables, potato chips, olives, pickles, and commercial baked goods.

(g.) Advise patient to season foods with pepper, paprika, onion, garlic, lemon, vinegar, and chili powder, rather than salt.

3. **Arrhythmias** due to myocardial inflammation (rheumatic carditis) or myocardial ischemia (coronary disease) impair the heart's pumping efficiency by reducing diastolic filling time, decreasing stroke volume, or increasing myocardial O_2 need. Common arrhythmias include the following:

a. Sinus tachycardia—100 to 180/min with a P wave before each QRS complex due to fever, congestive heart failure, hypertension, hyperthyroidism, and volume depletion.

b. Atrial flutter—regular atrial rate of 220 to 360/min, with ventricular rate 1/3 to 1/2 of atrial rate (due to atrioventricular block); electrocardiogram reveals sawtoothed P waves with regularly occurring QRS due to rheumatic heart disease, coronary heart disease, or cor pulmonale.

c. Atrial fibrillation—atrial rate of more than 350/min with irregularly irregular ventricular rhythm of 100 to 150/min. Electrocardiogram reveals no discrete P waves; occurs in rheumatic carditis, coronary artery disease, and thyrotoxicosis.

d. Ventricular tachycardia—3 or more ectopic ventricular beats in succession (bizarre QRS complexes of more than 0.14 sec) with regular ventricular rate of 120 to 200/min; occurs in acute myocardial infarction and chronic arteriosclerotic heart disease. Markedly decreases cardiac output and often leads to ventricular fibrillation.

e. Ventricular fibrillation—completely chaotic myocardial electrical activity leading to ineffectual or absent ventricular contractions and death unless a more effective rhythm can be restored through cardioversion.

f. Sinus bradycardia—sinus rate of less than 60/min, with normal P waves; may result from diaphragmatic infarction, myxedema, or increased intracranial pressure; may produce severe hypotension.

g. Atrioventricular block

(1.) Primary—all atrial impulses are transmitted to ventricular muscle but are delayed (PR interval more than 0.2 sec).

(2.) Secondary—every 3rd or 4th atrial impulse is not transmitted to the ventricle.

(3.) Tertiary—complete block, with no atrial impulses transmitted to the ventricles. In secondary or tertiary block, when the ventricular rate and force produce insufficient cardiac output to meet tissue needs, a temporary or permanent pacemaker may be inserted.

4. **Hypertension**—prolonged, pathological elevation of arterial blood pressure (systolic of more than 150 mm Hg; diastolic of more than 90 mm Hg).

a. Causes.

(1.) Obesity

(2.) Excessive sodium intake in sodium sensitive individuals.

(3.) Arteriosclerosis

(4.) Cushing's syndrome

b. Manifestations; none or as follows:

(1.) Headache and dizziness in the morning.

(2.) Increasing fatigability.

(3.) Long-standing untreated hypertension may be associated with nocturia, visual blurring, enlarged left ventricle, and funduscopic changes (narrowed arterioles, hemorrhages, and exudates).

c. Nursing management.

(1.) Persuade obese individuals to adhere to weight reduction diet.

(2.) Advise patient to stop smoking (nicotine is a vasoconstrictor).

(3.) Teach patient which foods are to be avoided when adhering to a low sodium diet, if patient is sodium sensitive.

(4.) Administer ordered antihypertensive drugs. Treatment is started with a small dose of a diuretic, adding more drugs in a stepwise fashion if needed to maintain diastolic pressure at 85 mm Hg.
(a.) Step I—chlorothiazide (increases urinary excretion of sodium).
(b.) Step II—reserpine (impairs cellular storage of norepinephrine), methyldopa (decreases tissue concentrations of norepinephrine), or propranolol (blocks sympathetic stimulation).
(c.) Step III—hydralazine (relaxes vascular smooth muscle), guanethidine (prevents release of norepinephrine), or minoxidil (dilates peripheral vessels).
(5.) Assist patient to identify situations and events that cause him emotional stress and help him to minimize or eliminate these from his life (financial risk, marital discord, and business competition).
(6.) Help patient to plan daily schedule so he will obtain 8 hours of sleep each night and will have 2 to 3 periods of rest and relaxation throughout the day.

Care of Patients with Vascular Disturbances

1. **Shock**—widespread and severe reduction in tissue perfusion, with consequent impairment of cellular function.
a. Causes (and types).
(1.) Hypovolemic shock is due to marked decrease in intravascular fluid following massive hemorrhage, loss of plasma in major burns, or loss of body fluid in prolonged vomiting.
(2.) Cardiogenic shock is due to decrease in cardiac output following myocardial infarction or serious arrhythmia.
(3.) Vasogenic shock is due to widespread vasodilation, such as that caused by endotoxins released by gram-negative organisms (septic shock).
(4.) Neurogenic shock is due to general loss of vasomotor tone, such as during spinal anesthesia, and barbituric intoxication.
b. Manifestations.
(1.) Cool moist skin (except in septic shock in which skin is warm).
(2.) Pallor (except in cardiogenic shock in which skin is cyanotic).
(3.) Decreased temperature due to disturbance of hypothalamic thermoregulatory center and lowered tissue metabolism.
(4.) Increased pulse rate and respiratory rate.
(5.) Decreased systolic and diastolic blood pressure (a systolic pressure of 70 mm Hg is necessary to maintain adequate coronary circulation).
(6.) Slow capillary refill following compression of fingernail.
(7.) Oliguria (less than 20 ml/hr) or anuria due to reduced glomerular perfusion.
(8.) Weakness due to poor perfusion of peripheral tissues.
(9.) Metabolic acidosis—pH less than 7.35, P_{CO_2} more than 45 mm Hg, and HCO_3^- less than 24 mEq/L.
(10.) Restlessness and anxiety due to increased sympathetic activity.
(11.) Confusion, lethargy, and coma due to cerebral anoxia.
c. Nursing management.
Goal is to improve tissue perfusion, especially to vital tissues of brain, myocardium, and kidney.
(1.) Reassure patient that he will receive prompt and vigorous treatment in order to allay his anxiety and decrease sympathetic nervous system hyperactivity.
(2.) Assist physician to insert central venous pressure line to determine right atrial pressure and guide fluid replacement therapy. Monitor central venous pressure every hour during treatment. Normal central venous pressure in the superior vena cava is 5 to 8 mm Hg, but treatment may be directed toward maintaining pressure slightly above this level.
(3.) Assist physician to attach patient to cardiac monitor to permit continuous monitoring for premature ventricular contractions or other arrhythmias caused by myocardial ischemia.
(4.) If patient is being cared for in an intensive care unit, a Swan-Ganz catheter may be inserted to measure pulmonary capillary wedge pressure, in order to monitor left ventricular end-diastolic pressure and guide fluid replacement therapy. Measure capillary wedge pressure every hour during treatment (normal is 12 mm Hg).
(5.) If an arterial line has been inserted, draw arterial blood samples as ordered for determination of arterial blood gas

analysis, pH, and degree of hypoxia and acidosis, and to monitor patient's response to treatment. If arterial blood pH is less than 7.3, prepare $NaHCO_3$, 44.6 mEq, for intravenous infusion to correct acidosis.

(6.) Maintain patient at bed rest with legs elevated, trunk horizontal, and head flat to mobilize the blood pooled in the lower extremities.

(7.) Keep patient warm by applying extra bed covers and by increasing room temperature. Do not apply external heat to body because poorly perfused tissues are susceptible to burn injury.

(8.) Infuse ordered blood, plasma, albumin, Ringer's lactate solution, or sodium chloride solution, I.V., at prescribed rate to restore circulating blood volume.

(9.) If ordered, insert nasogastric tube to remove gastrointestinal secretions, since with decreased splanchnic circulation there is delay in gastric emptying and danger of vomiting and aspiration.

(10.) Instill ordered antacids through the nasogastric tube to prevent development of stress ulcer.

(11.) Insert ordered indwelling catheter and measure urine output and specific gravity every hour; report output of less than 30 ml/hr.

(12.) Administer ordered O_2 by face mask (often 50% concentration) to achieve PaO_2 at 70 mm Hg.

(13.) Infuse ordered vasoactive drugs (vasoconstrictors or vasodilators, singly or in combination, depending upon the primary mechanism of shock causation) and cardiotonic drugs.

(a.) Sympathomimetic amines increase cardiac output by increasing strength of cardiac contraction. Different drugs in the group have different effects on peripheral circulation.

(1.) Norepinephrine (Levophed) increases myocardial contractility; dilates coronary vessels; and constricts vessels in skin, muscle, and abdominal organs.

(2.) Epinephrine increases myocardial contractility, dilates coronary vessels, and constricts vessels of kidney and abdominal organs.

(3.) Isoproterenol (Isuprel) increases myocardial contractility; dilates vessels in skeletal muscle (not useful in cardiogenic or septic shock).

(b.) Vasodilators used after sufficient volume replacement to dilate peripheral vessels, to reduce preload by inducing blood pooling in peripheral veins, and to reduce afterload by decreasing peripheral resistance against which the left ventricle must eject blood. Goal is to adjust dose of vasodilator to maintain a mean arterial pressure of 70 mm Hg.

(1.) Sodium nitroprusside relaxes vascular smooth muscle; dilates veins to reduce preload and dilates arterioles to reduce afterload.

(2.) Dopamine in moderate doses dilates vessels in kidney and mesentery, slightly dilates vessels in brain and myocardium. (In larger doses, constricts vessels in most vascular beds.)

(14.) Administer ordered adrenocorticoids to stabilize cellular membranes, making them more resistant to injury from biochemical changes occurring in shock. Adrenocorticoids also cause sodium ion retention and increased blood volume.

(15.) If tissue anoxia causes metabolic acidosis, physician may insert an endotracheal tube and order mechanical ventilation to remove CO_2 and thereby increase blood pH.

(16.) If patient in cardiogenic shock doesn't respond to drug therapy, physician may insert an intra-aortic balloon pump to improve peripheral circulation. A balloon-tipped catheter is inserted through the femoral artery, threaded backward to the descending thoracic aorta, and connected to a gas-driven pump. The balloon at the catheter tip is inflated during ventricular diastole, deflated before systole. This counterpulsation displaces blood back into the aorta during ventricular diastole to improve coronary perfusion. Because it increases mean arterial pressure, it also increases perfusion of liver, kidney, and brain.

(17.) Alternatively, the physician may order an external counterpulsation device. Tubular pants are applied to the legs; the pants are filled with air and attached to a pump. The pants are inflated during ventricular diastole, and deflated during systole to augment venous return flow to the heart and increase cardiac output.

(18.) Throughout treatment, provide emotional support to the patient by informing him of the purpose and nature of each treatment and by providing needed comfort measures. Provide family members with emotional support and information about the patient's condition and treatment.

2. **Thrombophlebitis**—inflammation of a vein wall with formation of a clot. (If a clot forms in a vein without antecedent inflammation of the vein wall, the condition is phlebothrombosis.) Venous clots consist mostly of red blood cells and adhere to the vein wall but have a free-floating tail, which extends proximally and can break free to form an embolus. Thrombophlebitis is most common in veins of the lower extremity.

a. Causes.

(1.) Venous stasis, as in pregnancy; long period of bed rest; congestive heart failure; long bus or plane trips.

(2.) Change in clotting factors as in ulcerative colitis, in which increases in Factor V, Factor VIII, and fibrinogen occur.

(3.) Local trauma to vein wall caused by constrictive garters or pelvic surgery.

(4.) Increased platelet stickiness as occurs in malignancy.

b. Manifestations.

(1.) Calf pain, which is worse on climbing stairs.

(2.) Rapidly developing swelling, tenderness, and warmth of involved lower extremity.

(3.) Positive Homans's sign—increased resistance to ankle flexion and occurrence of calf pain on forcible flexion of the ankle.

(4.) When tail of the thrombus breaks loose, it is carried through the heart and lodges in a branch of the pulmonary artery, causing pulmonary infarction, with sudden chest pain, hemoptysis, dyspnea, and respiratory failure.

(5.) Use of an ultrasonic Doppler flow detector over the femoral, popliteal, and posterior tibial veins will reveal continuous blood flow with no changes during the respiratory cycle. (Normally, blood flow velocity decreases during inspiration and increases during expiration.)

(6.) Phlebography—x-ray of the limb, following injection of a radiopaque dye into a vein of the foot, that will reveal the clot as a radiolucent area in an opaque vein.

c. Nursing management.

(1.) Provide complete bed rest for 4 to 7 days to permit the thrombus to become adherent to the vessel wall, preventing embolization.

(2.) Elevate foot of bed on blocks, without bending the knees, to facilitate venous return, decrease edema, and prevent extension of the thrombus.

(3.) Apply ordered warm moist packs to the leg to decrease vasospasm and pain.

(4.) Administer ordered anticoagulant drugs for 4 weeks following thrombophlebitis and 6 months following pulmonary embolism.

(a.) Heparin, 5000 Units I.V. bolus, then continuous I.V. infusion to prolong clotting time to 20 minutes (prevents conversion of fibrinogen to fibrin). Heparin prevents extension of existing thrombus but does not cause dissolution of existing thrombus.

(b.) On 5th day of heparin therapy, administer ordered warfarin (Coumadin) 10 to 15 mg/day, orally, to keep prothrombin time 1½ to 2 times normal (prevents formation of prothrombin). Heparin is discontinued when desired prothrombin time has been achieved.

(c.) During heparin and Coumadin therapy, no aspirin is to be administered, as the patient is at risk of bleeding.

(d.) Check daily hematocrit value, urinalysis, and stool guaiac test results for evidence of bleeding. If bleeding develops during heparin administration, notify physician and ready protamine sulfate to be given as heparin antidote. If bleeding develops during warfarin administration, notify physician and ready vitamin K to be given as an antidote.

(e.) Occasionally, a fibrinolytic drug (streptokinase or urokinase) is given intravenously to break down fibrin strands and dissolve a venous clot. When streptokinase is used, monitor patient carefully for evidence of allergic response to the drug, such as itching, urticaria, periorbital edema, bronchospasm, and dyspnea. When either fibrinolytic drug is used, monitor patient for evidence of bleeding and perform venipuncture as infrequently as possible.

(5.) If repeated pulmonary emboli occur and venous ligation or inferior vena cava plication is necessary (insertion of a grid or umbrella-like structure in the vena cava to filter out emboli), prepare patient physically and psychologically for surgery.

(6.) Prevent thrombophlebitis in susceptible patients.
  (a.) Ensuring adequate fluid intake to prevent dehydration and hypercoagulability of blood.
  (b.) Providing passive range of motion or bed exercises to improve venous return.
  (c.) Applying elastic stockings to prevent venous pooling.
  (d.) Avoiding knee flexion to prevent venous compression.
  (e.) Changing intravenous catheters every 48 hours to prevent vein infection.

(7.) Teach patients at risk for thrombophlebitis the following:
  (a.) Not to sit in one position for more than 2 hours.
  (b.) To get up and walk around every hour or so during long bus or plane rides.
  (c.) To avoid wearing tight girdles and garters.
  (d.) To wear support hose.
  (e.) To avoid crossing the legs.
  (f.) To ensure adequate fluid intake.

3. **Varicose veins**—dilated, tortuous veins, with incompetent valves, which are most common in the saphenous vein of the lower extremities and veins of the perineal region.

a. Causes.
  (1.) Congenitally defective valves (familial tendency).
  (2.) Pregnancy, obesity, ascites, and abdominal tumor, which obstruct venous return flow.
  (3.) Extreme height that increases venous pressure by lengthening the venous column for return flow to the heart.
  (4.) Occupations requiring prolonged standing, e.g., barber, beautician, nurse, and salesperson.

b. Manifestations.
  (1.) Dark, enlarged, tortuous veins engorged with blood.
  (2.) Easy fatigability of limb and edema following weight bearing.
  (3.) Cramping leg pain.
  (4.) Subcutaneous edema overlying the vein.
  (5.) Tawny skin discoloration due to extravasation of blood into subcutaneous tissues and itchy, eczematoid rash; may develop indolent, painless ulcer above the medial malleolus.
  (6.) Retrograde blood flow occurs past incompetent valves in the Trendelenburg's test.
    (a.) Elevate the leg to drain the veins.
    (b.) Apply a tourniquet to occlude the superficial veins.
    (c.) Have patient stand, and release the tourniquet.
    (d.) The veins distend immediately, indicating back flow due to incompetent valves.

c. Nursing management.
  (1.) Prevent varicose veins by instructing clients not to wear constrictive garters and girdles, not to sit with legs crossed, and not to stand or sit for long periods of time.
  (2.) Instruct patient with varicose veins to wear elastic stockings at all times and never to wear a girdle.
  (3.) Advise obese patients to adhere to a weight reduction diet.
  (4.) Advise patients to elevate the legs for 15 to 20 minutes every 2 to 3 hours throughout the day.
  (5.) If sclerosing solution (3% sodium tetradecyl sulfate) is injected to obliterate the vein in a patient with a chronically swollen extremity, maintain pressure bandages on the leg from toe to thigh, and assist the patient to ambulate frequently following the injection.
  (6.) Saphenous vein ligation and stripping are performed only when absolutely necessary, because the vein may be needed as an autograft in coronary or peripheral vascular surgery.
  (7.) Cleanse venous ulcer daily with sodium chloride and hydrogen peroxide, and cover with sterile gauze. If ordered, pour Debrisan, a dextranomer in bead

form, into the ulcer to absorb microorganisms and wound secretions between dressing changes.

(8.) If skin grafting is necessary to cover a varicose ulcer that doesn't respond to topical treatment, cleanse graft donor site with germicidal soap on the morning of surgery and, following surgery, protect the grafted site from pressure and friction. Use aseptic technique in dressing changes, and report accumulations of blood or serum under the graft.

(9.) Instruct patient in the types of foods to be included in a high protein, high vitamin C diet to facilitate healing of the ulcer or graft.

(10.) Teach patient to lubricate the healed graft site with skin lotion daily and to wear elastic stockings on both lower extremities.

4. **Aortic aneurysm**—dilation or sacculation of the aorta due to localized weakening of the wall; occurs in the ascending aorta, arch, descending thoracic aorta, or (most commonly) abdominal aorta.

a. Causes.

(1.) Arteriosclerosis, which destroys elastic fibers in the aortic wall.

(2.) Syphilis, which destroys elastic and muscle fibers in the aortic wall.

b. Manifestations.

(1.) Pulsating abdominal mass, with a systolic bruit over the mass.

(2.) In a thin individual, increased width of the abdominal aorta may be palpable on physical examination.

(3.) If the aortic wall is arteriosclerotic, calcifications in the wall may be visible on x-ray and will reveal focal widening of the vessel.

(4.) Blood pressure in the thigh is lower than in the arm (normally, blood pressure is 15 mm Hg higher in the thigh).

(5.) In a dissecting aortic aneurysm (a cavity formed by blood that forces its way between the layers of the aortic wall), there is sudden, severe, tearing pain with shock and collapse.

(6.) Evidence of local dilation of the aorta on ultrasonogram and on aortogram, following injection of radiopaque dye.

c. Nursing management.

(1.) Early diagnosis of abdominal aortic aneurysm is facilitated by auscultating the central upper abdomen on physical assessment to detect a systolic bruit over a widened, calcified aorta.

(2.) Prepare patient for diagnostic tests.

(a.) Ultrasonogram. Inform the patient that a conducting gel will be applied to the abdominal skin and a transducer will be moved back and forth over the abdomen to pass sound waves into the abdomen and detect sound reflected back from various internal organs. The reflections will be displayed on an oscilloscope, enabling the physician to visualize abdominal structures.

(b.) Aortogram. Inform the patient that a catheter will be inserted into the femoral artery and a radiopaque dye injected, at which time the patient will experience a burning sensation, following which a series of x-rays will be taken to determine the exact location and size of the aneurysm.

(3.) Administer ordered propranolol (Inderal) or methyldopa (Aldomet) to decrease systolic blood pressure to 120 mm Hg and to decrease the possibility of aneurysmal rupture.

(4.) If symptoms and x-ray reveal dissection and it becomes necessary to resect the aneurysm and insert a vascular graft, provide post-operative care to prevent complications.

(a.) Maintain patient flat in bed without flexing knees.

(b.) Monitor vital signs every 15 minutes until stable.

(c.) Measure central venous pressure hourly to assess fluid status and to detect early indications of shock.

(d.) Check femoral, popliteal, posterior tibial, and dorsalis pedis pulses hourly.

(e.) Check skin color and temperature, movement, and sensation in both lower extremities hourly.

(f.) Check urine output hourly to detect renal damage due to aortic clamping during surgery.

(g.) Encourage patient to dorsiflex and plantar flex the feet at intervals, and keep anti-embolism stockings smoothly and evenly applied to the legs.

(h.) Report complaints of back pain immediately, as possible indication of retroperitoneal hemorrhage or occlusion of the aortic graft.

(i.) Encourage patient to cough and deep breathe every hour while the nurse applies hand pressure over the abdominal wound for support.

5. **Arteriosclerotic obliterative disease of the lower extremities**—subintimal deposition of lipid and cholesterol in large and medium sized arteries and intimal roughening over plaques, with vascular narrowing and formation of fibrin clots; intravascular clots and vessel narrowing obstruct blood flow.
   a. Causes.
      (1.) High fat diet, causing elevation of blood lipids.
      (2.) Hypertension
      (3.) Cigarette smoking
      (4.) Diabetes mellitus
      (5.) Lack of physical exercise
      (6.) Familial tendency to hyperlipidemia, arteriosclerosis.
   b. Manifestations.
      (1.) Intermittent claudication—cramping leg pain and leg muscle fatigue on exercise, which is relieved with rest.
      (2.) Diminished or absent pulses in lower extremities (dorsalis pedis, posterior tibialis, popliteal, and femoral).
      (3.) Coldness, numbness, paresthesias of involved extremity.
      (4.) Position-related color changes—pallor of soles on elevating the legs 45 degrees for 3 to 4 minutes and flushing of soles only 20 to 30 seconds after the legs are placed in the dependent position (due to anoxic injury to capillaries and venules).
      (5.) Dry, thin, shiny skin of the feet and legs, with absence of hair growth (atrophic changes).
      (6.) Hard, thick, deformed nails.
      (7.) Decreased pedal arterial pressure, as revealed by Doppler velocitometer (pressure should be equal to or higher than brachial artery pressure).
      (8.) Decreased pulse volume below the level of obstruction, as revealed by oscillometry.
      (9.) Visualization of arterial block on x-ray film following injection of radiopaque dye.
      (10.) Ischemic rest pain at night, which is relieved slightly by leg dependency.
      (11.) Painful ulcerations of toes following minor trauma to foot or leg.
   c. Nursing management.
      (1.) Prepare patient for *arteriography*.
         (a.) Inform patient that following injection of a radiopaque dye into the femoral artery (patient will experience a burning sensation), serial x-rays will be taken of the leg to determine the location of arterial block and degree of vascular patency beyond the block.
         (b.) Following the procedure, monitor the patient for symptoms of allergic reaction to the dye, e.g., dyspnea, nausea, diaphoresis, and tachycardia. Check the dye injection site for evidence of hemorrhage or thrombosis.
      (2.) If there is no ulcer or gangrene, help the patient to begin a program of graduated walking to increase collateral circulation in the extremities. Teach the patient to exercise to the point of pain, then rest until the pain disappears.
      (3.) Persuade the patient to regulate his diet to reduce weight, and if the patient is diabetic provide instruction and support needed to bring diabetes under good control.
      (4.) Urge patient to stop smoking, explaining that nicotine is a vasoconstrictor.
      (5.) Provide scrupulous daily foot care. Teach patient to wash feet daily in warm water and mild soap, rinse completely, and pat dry. Suggest that emollients be applied to lubricate the skin of the feet and prevent fissuring. Advise the patient to wear white cotton or wool hose. Teach the patient the importance of wearing hard soled, well fitted shoes and slippers. Advise patient never to go barefoot, even in the house. Teach patient to wear bed socks for cold feet, but never to apply hot water bottles or heating pads to the feet or legs.
      (6.) In a patient with a small arterial obstruction of short duration, angioplasty may be used to recanalize the obstructed vessel. An inflatable balloon catheter is inserted into the vessel, the balloon is inflated, compressing the soft plaque against the vessel wall, widening the vessel lumen. Following the procedure, monitor the patient carefully for evidence of circulatory impairment distal to the site of catheter insertion.
      (7.) If obstructive symptoms worsen despite conservative treatment and an aorto-iliac or femoro-popliteal bypass graft becomes necessary, maintain graft patency post-operatively.

(a.) Check vital signs frequently post-operatively, and notify surgeon immediately of a fall in blood pressure, as an adequate systolic blood pressure is necessary to maintain circulation through the graft and prevent thrombus formation.

(b.) Encourage patient to cough and deep breathe to foster circulation and maximize oxygenation of the blood.

(c.) Keep leg fully extended to prevent compression and obstruction of the graft.

(d.) Check lower extremity pulses, capillary refill time, skin color and temperature, and motor and sensory function at frequent intervals to detect early signs of circulatory impairment.

(e.) When ambulation is ordered, caution patient against sharp flexion of the operated extremity and advise against crossing the legs or sitting for long periods.

(8.) If the graft fails, gangrene develops, and amputation becomes necessary, prepare the patient emotionally and physically for the amputation.

(a.) Pre-operatively, teach the patient to do push ups and weight lifting to strengthen arm muscles in preparation for crutch walking.

(b.) Post-operatively, elevate the stump on a small pillow to decrease edema (no longer than 24 hours so as to prevent hip contracture deformity).

(c.) During the early post-operative period, keep a tourniquet attached to the head of the bed to be applied to the stump if hemorrhaging occurs.

(d.) Dress the stump with several layers of sterile gauze, and wrap with elastic bandage to prevent edema. If immediate prosthetic fitting was done at surgery (wound covered with sterile gauze and a plaster cast applied to the stump to prevent bleeding and edema and to shape the stump for later prosthetic use), check the cast for evidence of bleeding or drainage and assure that the cast is securely applied to the limb and attached to the waist belt. If cast is accidentally dislodged place patient flat, and summon physician immediately to replace cast to prevent stump edema.

(e.) When progressive ambulation is ordered, help patient to sit on edge of bed, then stand at the bedside, and then walk to the chair with crutches (or pylon and cane). After temporary prosthesis is applied, help patient to walk between parallel bars, then with walker, and then with cane.

(f.) Teach patient and family members the reasons and procedures for stump dressing and wrapping, proper care of the prosthesis, and proper care of the remaining foot.

CARE OF PATIENTS WITH DIGESTIVE DISORDERS

1. *Oral cancer*—malignant tumor of the lip, tongue, floor of the mouth, or salivary glands.

a. Causes.

Continuous irritation from tobacco, hot pipe stem, alcohol, jagged teeth, ill fitting dentures, or poor oral hygiene.

b. Manifestations.

(1.) Leukoplakia (pearly crinkled patches) may cover the surface of the tumor.

(2.) A painless lump or ulcer develops at the point of chronic irritation.

(3.) With time, enlargement of the tumor causes pain, increased salivation, hemorrhage, and difficulty in chewing and swallowing.

(4.) Enlarged submandibular or cervical lymph nodes, or both, indicate metastatic spread of the tumor.

(5.) Numerous dividing cells are seen on cytological study of tissue scraped from the tumor or ulcer.

c. Nursing management.

(1.) Prevent oral cancer by advising clients to stop smoking (explaining that tobacco tars are irritating to oral as well as lung tissue); by advocating regular dental examinations and prompt attention to carious or broken teeth.

(2.) Facilitate early diagnosis of oral cancer by palpating as well as observing oral structures during physical assessment of patients.

(3.) Provide information and emotional support to the patient who is undergoing diagnostic work-up of a suspected oral lesion.

(4.) If radiation is used to shrink the tumor, relieve complaints of dry mouth by urging increased fluid intake, by lubricating oral tissues with glycerine or mineral oil, and by stimulating saliva flow with sugar free lozenges or gum.

(5.) Provide a bland, soft diet with increased liquid intake to minimize irritation of oral tissues.

(6.) If tumor irritation causes increased salivation, encourage the patient to swallow more frequently or remove excessive secretions by mechanical suctioning.

(7.) If tumor has metastasized to cervical nodes, wide excision of tumor and nodes with radical neck resection may be done. If skin flaps are used to cover denuded areas, check drainage tubes for evidence of hemorrhage.

(8.) Post-operatively, irrigate nasogastric tube to keep it patent and to prevent regurgitation and aspiration of stomach contents; aspirate tracheostomy, using care to avoid injury to operative suture line.

(9.) Elevate head of bed during ordered gastrostomy feedings to prevent regurgitation and aspiration of stomach contents.

(10.) Encourage patient to turn, deep breathe, and cough every hour or two to prevent hypostatic pneumonia.

(11.) Irrigate mouth with ordered solution (usually half strength H_2O_2) to prevent infection of the suture line and to decrease unpleasant mouth odor.

(12.) Check patient frequently for evidence of hemorrhage from irritated or traumatized neck vessels. If hemorrhage occurs apply direct pressure to control bleeding, and summon the surgeon.

(13.) If patient is unable to swallow saliva, place a gauze wick in the mouth and apply suction to mouth frequently to prevent aspiration of secretions and contamination of the neck wound.

(14.) Encourage patient to ventilate fear and anger (in writing if unable to vocalize) concerning facial disfigurement and threats of debility, pain, and death.

(15.) After gastrostomy tube is removed, administer frequent small servings of high calorie, high protein, high vitamin, but mechanically and chemically bland diet. Keep suction machine at the bedside, ready for use if necessary.

2. **Mandibular fracture**—break in the continuity of the mandible with or without displacement of bone fragments.

a. Cause.

Impact injury to the lower face due to blow from a fist, a vehicular accident, or a fall.

b. Manifestations.

(1.) Displacement of the jaw to one side.

(2.) Malocclusion of the teeth.

(3.) Preauricular pain on closing the jaws.

c. Nursing management.

(1.) If a simple fracture of the jaw is immobilized by wiring or banding the lower and upper teeth together, protect the airway post-operatively.

(a.) Maintain the patient in side-lying position to drain oral secretions.

(b.) If nasogastric tube is in place irrigate the tube as needed, and administer ordered anti-emetic agent to prevent vomiting and aspiration.

(c.) Remove excessive oral secretions by mechanical suctioning.

(d.) Keep metal clippers or scissors at the bedside in plain view to cut wire or rubber bands if patient should vomit.

(2.) If a compound fracture is immobilized with arch bars, wires, or pins affixed to bone fragments (may be stabilized with a plaster helmet), protect the airway, and prevent dislocation of fragments.

(a.) Caution patient to position himself, so as not to apply pressure to the extra-oral stabilizing equipment.

(b.) Aspirate secretions from the mouth by mechanical suction.

(c.) Provide frequent oral hygiene with a soft brush, H_2O_2, or $NaHCO_3$ mouth wash.

(d.) Administer a high calorie, high protein liquid diet through a straw.

3. **Esophageal stricture**—muscular or fibrotic narrowing of the esophagus, which interferes with swallowing.

a. Cause.

Inflammatory scarring following ingestion of a strong acid or base, radiation, or mechanical trauma.

b. Manifestations.

(1.) Dysphagia

(2.) Regurgitation of recently chewed food.

c. Nursing management.

(1.) Prepare patient for esophagoscopy.

(a.) Hold food and fluids for 6 to 8 hours before the examination to prevent regurgitation and aspiration of gastric contents.

(b.) Remove patient's eyeglasses and dentures, and have patient void before the procedure.

(c.) Administer ordered sedative-hypnotics (usually meperidine and phenobarbital) 30 to 60 minutes before the procedure to enable patient to relax and cooperate with the examiner.

(d.) Inform patient that his posterior pharynx will be sprayed with a topical anesthetic (cocaine or tetracaine) to inactivate the gag reflex; that he will be placed in a recumbent position, with head and shoulders extending over the edge of the table; and that he should lie completely still while the esophagoscope is inserted and manipulated.

(e.) Following the examination, instruct the patient to take nothing by mouth until the gag reflex has returned (test by tickling the back of the throat with a cotton tipped applicator).

(f.) If narrowed portion of esophagus is dilated by peroral or oral-gastrostomy passage of bougies of increasing size, inform patient to take nothing but clear liquids for 12 to 24 hours before bouginage, and inform him that he will be asked to gargle with a topical anesthetic lidocaine (viscous Xylocaine) before passage of the bougies.

(g.) After completion of the prescribed series of dilations when patient is allowed to return to a normal diet, teach the patient to chew his food well and to take plenty of liquids with meals.

(h.) If the stricture is surgically excised, with end-to-end anastomosis of remaining esophageal segments, provide post-operative care to protect the suture lines and to ensure adequate nutrition.

(1.) Maintain closed chest drainage apparatus until lung reexpansion is complete; tape tubing and bottle connections, keep collection bottle below level of the patient's chest, encourage coughing and deep breathing, record amount and type of drainage from the chest tube, and clamp chest tube immediately in the event that the water seal is accidentally broken.

(2.) Irrigate the nasogastric tube, and maintain gastric suctioning until the surgical anastomoses have healed.

(3.) Administer ordered intravenous or nasogastric tube feedings, or both, to divert food and fluids from the operative site.

(4.) When oral feedings are resumed, keep a suction machine at hand to prevent aspiration if the patient has difficulty swallowing.

4. **Hiatus hernia**—protrusion of the upper part of the stomach through the esophageal opening of the diaphragm with regurgitation of acid gastric juices into the esophagus, causing ulceration and bleeding.

a. Cause.

Congenital weakness or traumatic injury to the diaphragm, often associated with increased intra-abdominal pressure, as from obesity or ascites.

b. Manifestations.

(1.) Heartburn

(2.) Substernal pain

(3.) Dysphagia

(4.) Sensation of fullness shortly after initiating feeding.

(5.) Hematemesis

c. Nursing management.

(1.) Provide frequent small, bland meals.

(2.) Urge obese individual to adhere to a low calorie diet for weight loss.

(3.) Teach patient to avoid coughing, heavy lifting, bending forward, wearing tight girdles, and eating bedtime snacks.

(4.) Advise patient to elevate the head of the bed 6 inches to prevent esophageal reflux of gastric contents during sleep.

5.) Administer ordered antacids for heartburn.

(6.) Teach patient to eat slowly and to avoid highly seasoned foods and alcoholic beverages.

(7.) If surgery is required to place the herniated tissue into the abdomen, to narrow the esophageal hiatus, and to increase the esophagogastric angle to stop reflux of gastric juice, prepare patient physically and emotionally for surgery.

(8.) Post-operatively, monitor the chest tubes and water seal suction used to reexpand the lung (if the thoracic approach has been used). Limit oral intake to fluids during the first 24 hours, then add foods in gradually increased amounts in order to prevent gastric overloading.

5. **Peptic ulcer**—erosion of mucosa and submucosa (a chronic ulcer may also penetrate the muscularis and may perforate the serosa) in those areas of the gastric tube that are exposed to acid and pepsin in gastric juice (lower esophagus, stomach, and duodenum).

a. Cause.

Imbalance between acid and pepsin and mucosal resistance.

(1.) Excessive production of HCl by the gastric glands and/or deficient production of protective mucus by glands of the esophagus, stomach, or duodenum, leading to chronic mucosal inflammation and erosion.

(2.) Smoking promotes peptic ulceration by inhibiting pancreatic bicarbonate production.

(3.) Aspirin promotes peptic ulceration by breaking the mucosal barrier to hydrogen ions.

(4.) Caffeine promotes peptic ulceration by stimulating increased HCl secretion by parietal cells of the gastric glands.

b. Manifestations.

(1.) Burning or gnawing epigastric pain 2 to 3 hours after meals and during the night, which is relieved by ingestion of food or antacids, or both. Pain episodes occur in clusters of days or weeks most often during spring or fall.

(2.) Excessive salivation and nausea occur in some patients.

(3.) If ulcer penetrates to erode a large vessel, hematemesis occurs.

(4.) If repeated ulcerations extend to the muscularis and scarring occurs in the pyloric region or duodenum, obstruction to gastric emptying causes epigastric distention and vomiting of undigested food.

(5.) If ulcer penetrates through all 4 layers of the gastrointestinal wall and gastric or intestinal contents leak into the peritoneal cavity, sudden intense abdominal pain, abdominal muscle rigidity, absent bowel sounds, and shock develop.

(6.) Radiographic evidence of an ulcer crater in the esophageal, gastric, or duodenal wall following barium ingestion.

(7.) Visualization of ulcer crater, hyperemia, and tissue friability on gastroscopic examination.

c. Nursing management.

(1.) Administer ordered histamine H_2 receptor antagonist to inhibit gastric acid secretion; cimetidine (Tagamet), 300 mg orally, Q.I.D. with meals and at bedtime (h.s.); ranitidine (Zantac), 150 mg, orally, B.I.D. with breakfast and dinner.

(2.) Administer ordered antacids orally to buffer excess HCl, e.g., magnesium hydroxide, aluminum hydroxide, calcium carbonate, or mixtures of 2 or 3 of these in a dose of 30 ml 1 hour after meals (p.c.) and h.s.

(3.) If ordered, administer sucralfate, a complex of a sulfated disaccharide and aluminum hydroxide, which coats and protects the ulcer crater from injury by acid and pepsin.

(4.) If diet modification is ordered (controversial), advise patient to eliminate alcohol, caffeine, meat extracts, pepper, mustard, roughage, gas forming foods, and bedtime snacks.

(5.) Emphasize the importance of obtaining adequate rest and sleep and reducing psychological stress.

(6.) Urge patient to stop smoking, if this will not be accompanied by increased anxiety.

(7.) Assist patient to plan for needed adjustments in lifestyle. Provide information about groups offering support to stop smoking and to stop drinking alcohol. Teach patient relaxation techniques for relieving stress.

(8.) For patient who suffers repeated relapses, fails to respond to medical management, or develops life threatening complications from the ulcer (penetration, perforation, obstruction, or intractable pain), prepare for a surgical procedure designed to decrease acidity, decrease motility, relieve obstruction, or close perforation. Provide information about the procedure to be performed.

(a.) Vagotomy and pyloroplasty—vagus nerve trunks are cut to decrease acid secretion, and pylorus is widened to prevent gastric stasis. (Vagotomy decreases antral peristalsis, one stimulus for pyloric opening.)

(b.) Partial gastrectomy—removal of distal 75% of the stomach (to remove the ulcer and decrease gastrin and acid production) and anastomosis of the gastric remnant to the duodenal stump (Billroth I procedure) or to the jejunum (Billroth II procedure).

(9.) Prepare patient for ordered diagnostic tests.

(a.) Gastric analysis.

Inform patient that food and fluids will be held for 6 to 8 hours before the test, that a nasogastric tube will be inserted, and that the patient will be placed in a semirecumbent position and gastric contents removed by syringe suction. Following I.M. injection of a secretagogue (histamine or pentagastrin), additional samples of gastric contents will be obtained. Samples of gastric secretions will be analyzed for acidity and enzyme content.

(b.) Upper gastrointestinal x-ray series.

Inform patient that food and fluids will be held for 8 to 10 hours before the test and that a laxative will be given to empty the gastrointestinal tract. Instruct the patient to refrain from smoking on the morning of the examination, since smoking stimulates gastric motility. Inform patient that he will be given a radiopaque liquid to drink (barium) and that passage of the liquid from the mouth through the pharynx and esophagus into the stomach will be viewed on fluoroscopy while serial x-rays are taken of the various organs outlined by the barium.

(c.) Gastroscopy.

Inform patient that food and fluids will be held for 6 to 8 hours before the test and that a sedative-hypnotic (usually meperidine) and atropine will be given 30 minutes before the procedure to increase relaxation and decrease secretions. Inform the patient that he will gargle with a local anesthetic to eliminate the gag reflex and will be placed in a recumbent position with neck hyperextended (if a rigid gastroscope is used) or will sit facing the physician (if a flexible gastroscope is used); he will be asked to remain immobile while the instrument is advanced slowly and the physician scrutinizes the interior of the esophagus and stomach through the lighted tube.

(10.) Infuse ordered dextrose in saline I.V. to replace fluids lost by vomiting or third space displacement, if perforation and peritonitis have developed.

(11.) Administer blood transfusions, if ordered, to restore blood volume, blood pressure, and tissue oxygenation following gastric or duodenal hemorrhage.

(12.) Pre-operatively, irrigate nasogastric tube and maintain suction to remove acid and blood from the stomach.

(13.) If ordered, irrigate stomach with iced, normal saline solution to control bleeding by cold constriction of vessels in the ulcer base.

(14.) Maintain accurate record of intake and output to obtain information upon which to plan fluid replacement therapy.

(15.) Provide scrupulous oral hygiene in the patient with a nasogastric tube in place to prevent oral infections and to increase comfort.

(16.) Post-operatively, check drainage from nasogastric tube to detect post-operative hemorrhage.

(17.) Irrigate nasogastric tube only on a specific order from the physician, to protect operative suture lines from injury.

(18.) Encourage patient to move, cough, and deep breathe, as high abdominal incision may cause patient to limit respiratory excursions.

(19.) When oral fluids are given for the first time following surgery, aspirate gastric residual 60 minutes after fluid is given to determine whether tissue edema has subsided enough that the stomach can empty properly. When nasogastric tube is removed, advance the patient slowly from clear liquids to soft foods to general diet given in small feedings several times a day.

(20.) Following either vagotomy or gastric resection, monitor patient for symptoms of "dumping syndrome" (due to entry of hypertonic chyme into the jeunum and withdrawal of fluid from the blood into the jejunum). Patient complains of nausea, weakness, faintness, palpitation 5 to 30 minutes following a meal. Advise patient to avoid or minimize symptoms by eating frequent dry, small meals, avoiding drinking fluid for 2 to 3 hours after meals; avoiding highly concentrated carbohydrate foods; and by lying down for several minutes following meals.

6. **Viral hepatitis**—infectious communicable disease that is characterized in the acute phase by inflammation and necrosis of hepatocytes and bile duct obstruction, which lead either to acute liver failure or to regeneration of normal liver structure.
   a. Causes.
      Several different viruses may cause hepatitis.
      (1.) Hepatitis A virus causes short incubation hepatitis or infectious hepatitis and is transmitted by fecal-oral route.
      (2.) Hepatitis B virus causes long incubation hepatitis or serum hepatitis and is transmitted primarily by the parenteral route (transfusion, needle puncture).
      (3.) Non-A, non-B hepatitis viruses are transmitted primarily by blood transfusion.
   b. Manifestations.
      (1.) Malaise, fatigue, and mild fever.
      (2.) Anorexia and nausea, aversion to cigarettes and coffee.
      (3.) Arthralgia
      (4.) Right upper quadrant tenderness and liver enlargement.
      (5.) Clay colored stool due to lack of bilirubin in the bowel.
      (6.) Dark urine due to presence of bilirubin.
      (7.) Jaundice, lasting several days or weeks.
      (8.) Pruritus due to irritation of dermal tissues by bile salts.
      (9.) Elevation of serum enzyme levels; SGOT, SGPT, and LDH may reach 500 to 1000 IU in late prodromal or early icteric phase of the disease.
      (10.) Elevation of serum bilirubin level often to 15 mg/dl (normal is 0.3 to 1.1 mg/dl).
      (11.) Presence of HB_sAg in serum (hepatitis B antigen).
   c. Nursing management.
      (1.) Prevent transmission of hepatitis A virus by taking the following steps:
         (a.) Enforcing proper hand washing technique by patients, caregivers, and food handlers.
         (b.) Advising the public not to eat shellfish from polluted waters.
         (c.) Instructing and supervising health workers in proper sterilization and handling of instruments and supplies used in vascular puncture and enforcing proper disposal of single-use needles, syringes, and tubing.
         (d.) Advising administration of immune serum globulin to passively immunize travelers to areas with high risk for hepatitis A virus infection.
      (2.) For the patient with hepatitis, provide bed rest with bathroom privileges during the acute phase of the disease.
      (3.) Administer ordered anti-emetics, like hydroxyzine, for severe nausea and vomiting.
      (4.) Provide a low fat, high carbohydrate diet in frequent feedings if patient is anorexic.
      (5.) Administer ordered vitamin K I.M., if prothrombin time is elevated.
      (6.) Instruct patient to avoid alcohol.
      (7.) Advise patient to regulate his activity and rest so as to avoid fatigue.
      (8.) If severe nausea and vomiting occur, infuse ordered I.V. fluids or parenteral hyperalimentation. Keep accurate intake and output records to guide fluid replacement therapy.
      (9.) Institute isolation techniques to prevent spread of hepatitis to others through contamination by patient's body fluids.
      (10.) Advise patient to resume physical activity slowly to avoid a relapse of hepatitis.

7. **Cirrhosis**—irreversible alteration of liver structure, characterized by fibrotic distortion of lobular architecture and areas of hepatocyte regeneration.
   a. Causes.
      (1.) Excessive alcohol (ethanol) consumption (>80 gm/day), which injures hepatocytes by destroying mitochondria, impairing protein synthesis, producing cellular hypoxia, and causing intracellular deposition of fat globules.
      (2.) Malnutrition from a poorly balanced diet or impaired intestinal absorption predisposes to hepatocyte injury by alcohol (ethanol).
      (3.) Chronic active hepatitis and chronic bil-

iary tract obstruction may lead to destruction of liver cells and their replacement by fibrous tissue.

b. Manifestations.
   (1.) Hepatomegaly due to fatty infiltration (early stage); small, hard, nodular liver due to fibrotic scarring (late stage).
   (2.) Splenomegaly due to increased portal system pressure.
   (3.) Ascites due to fluid transudation from intestinal capillaries in response to increased portal system pressure.
   (4.) Dilated periumbilical veins and hemorrhoidal veins due to increased portal system pressure.
   (5.) Mild jaundice and slightly increased serum bilirubin level (normal is 0.3 to 1.1 mg/dl) due to inability of damaged hepatocytes to remove unconjugated bilirubin from the serum.
   (6.) Decreased serum albumin concentration and reversal of normal 2:1 albumin to globulin ratio due to inability of damaged hepatocytes to produce normal amounts of albumin.
   (7.) Elevation of serum enzyme levels of SGOT, SGPT, and LDH due to release of these enzymes from damaged hepatocytes.
   (8.) Elevated prothrombin time due to failure of damaged hepatocytes to produce normal amounts of prothrombin.
   (9.) Hypoglycemia due to faulty glycogenolysis and gluconeogenesis.
   (10.) Hematemesis, if rupture of esophageal varices (dilated veins at the gastric cardia, resulting from increased portal system pressure) occurs.
   (11.) Anemia due to marrow depression by alcohol (ethanol) and blood loss from rectal or esophageal varices.

c. Nursing management.
   (1.) Persuade patient that abstinence from alcohol is necessary to preserve life. Provide information about support groups (e.g., Alcoholics Anonymous) for those who experience difficulty in alcohol withdrawal.
   (2.) Provide a high calorie, high carbohydrate, high vitamin diet with 75 to 100 gm of protein a day; restrict sodium to less than 1000 mg/day if ascites or dependent edema is a problem.
   (3.) Administer ordered oral ferrous sulfate for iron deficiency anemia (given with food to prevent gastrointestinal irritation) or oral folic acid for folic acid deficiency anemia.
   (4.) Administer ordered vitamins A, D, E, and K parenterally for patients with fat malabsorption (steatorrhea), resulting from inadequate bile in the intestine.
   (5.) Monitor for evidence of respiratory difficulty (may occur as a result of interference with respiratory excursions in the patient with massive ascites).
   (6.) If ordered, restrict sodium intake to 500 mg/day, and restrict fluid intake to 1500 ml/day to minimize ascites formation.
   (7.) For the ascitic patient with hypoalbuminemia, administer ordered chlorothiazide or spironolactone for diuretic effect. Keep accurate intake and output record and weigh daily to determine the amount of fluid retention.
   (8.) Monitor patient for evidence of gastrointestinal bleeding (apprehension, tachycardia, hematemesis, and pallor of shock).
      (a.) For patient who develops bleeding from esophageal varices, infuse ordered I.V. vasopressin (Pitressin) to constrict splanchnic vessels, and assist with insertion of a Sengstaken's tube (has an esophageal balloon to exert pressure against the bleeding varix, and a gastric balloon to hold the tube and esophageal balloon in proper position).
         (1.) While Sengstaken's tube is in place, apply suction to oral secretions to avoid aspiration, as esophageal balloon prevents swallowing of secretions.
         (2.) Deflate esophageal balloon at ordered intervals to prevent decubitus ulcer of esophagus.
   (9.) If a surgical procedure is required to prevent future variceal bleeding, prepare the patient physically and psychologically for the operation.
      (a.) Ligation of varices.
      (b.) Portacaval anastomosis shunts blood from the portal system to the inferior vena cava (around the liver) in order to decrease pressure in the portal system.
   (10.) If ascites increases despite alcohol abstinence, sodium restriction, and diuretics, prepare patient for either of the following procedures to remove ascites:
      (a.) Paracentesis—used in an emer-

gency to rapidly remove fluid from the peritoneal cavity to relieve respiratory embarrassment.

(b.) LeVeen's peritoneojugular shunt—surgical implantation of a tube with a one-way valve to drain ascitic fluid from the peritoneal cavity and carry it up through the abdominal and thoracic walls to empty into the jugular vein.

(11.) If acute alcoholic hepatitis develops in a patient with cirrhotic liver damage, provide complete bed rest, infuse ordered 5% dextrose I.V., and institute "reverse isolation" to protect the patient against infection and vasomotor collapse.

(12.) Monitor the cirrhotic patient for evidence of hepatic encephalopathy (cerebral toxicity resulting from increased blood concentrations of ammonia, amines, and mercaptans due to shunting of blood from portal to systemic circulation). Symptoms of hepatic encephalopathy include flapping tremor, muscle clonus, positive Babinski's reflex, and confusion.

(13.) Change patient's position frequently, and caution patient against scratching pruritic areas, to prevent breakdown of malnourished skin.

(14.) Teach patient the reasons for alcohol abstinence, high carbohydrate intake, and sodium restriction. Teach family members the symptoms and significance of hypoglycemia and hepatic coma.

8. **Pancreatitis**–inflammation of the pancreas that usually involves disturbances in pancreatic exocrine or endocrine function. Acute pancreatitis is characterized by digestion of pancreatic tissue by trypsin, a proteolytic enzyme produced by pancreatic acinar cells. Chronic pancreatitis is characterized by persistent pain and deficient production of pancreatic enzymes or hormones or both.

a. Cause.

Activation of proteolytic and lipolytic pancreatic enzymes in the pancreas rather than in the small intestine.

(1.) Chronic alcoholism causes edema of duodenal wall and spasm of the sphincter of Oddi, which blocks flow of pancreatic juices into the duodenum.

(2.) Gallstones may block the ampulla of Vater, causing bile to regurgitate into the duct of Wirsung, where it activates enzyme precursors in the pancreatic juice (trypsinogen).

(3.) Some drugs, like chlorothiazide and glucocorticoids, may provoke pancreatitis.

b. Manifestations.

(1.) Steady, severe epigastric or left upper quadrant pain, which radiates to the back and often develops following excessive alcoholic intake.

(2.) Vomiting, which does not relieve epigastric pain.

(3.) Fever, tachycardia, hypotension.

(4.) Upper abdominal tenderness and some rigidity of abdominal muscles.

(5.) Elevated serum and urinary amylase levels; serum amylase level rises to 300 to 500 Somogyi units within a few hours after onset of pain and remains elevated for about 3 days. Urinary amylase level remains elevated longer.

(6.) Shock due to release of a myocardial depressant factor by damaged pancreatic tissue and loss of intravascular fluid into peritoneal and retroperitoneal spaces.

(7.) Decreased bowel sounds due to decreased intestinal motility caused by peritoneal inflammation.

(8.) Hyperglycemia, if destruction of islet cells reduces insulin production.

(9.) Steatorrhea, if destruction of acinar cells reduces lipase production.

c. Nursing management.

(1.) Infuse ordered electrolyte and colloid solutions to replace intravascular fluid lost into the retroperitoneal space. Maintain accurate record of intake and output to guide fluid replacement therapy.

(2.) Measure vital signs frequently, and report immediately any fall in blood pressure.

(3.) Measure central venous pressure and urine volume every hour to monitor cardiac function and tissue perfusion.

(4.) Give nothing by mouth, and maintain nasogastric suction (irrigate nasogastric tube as needed to ensure patency) to keep stomach empty (removes HCl that stimulates secretin production which, in turn, stimulates pancreatic secretion).

(5.) Administer ordered antacids through the nasogastric tube to neutralize HCl and prevent secretin production.

(6.) Administer ordered meperidine (Demerol) 50 mg subcutaneously for pain (morphine causes spasm of the sphincter of Oddi).

(7.) Administer ordered anticholinergics, like atropine, to inhibit spasm of the sphincter of Oddi.

(8.) Test urine for glucose and acetone to detect diabetes resulting from islet cell destruction.

(9.) Monitor patient for respiratory difficulty due to increased alveolar capillary permeability.

(10.) Monitor patient for symptoms of tetany (muscular twitching and spasm) caused by hypocalcemia resulting from formation of calcium soaps in fat necrosis.

(11.) If pancreatic pseudocyst is suspected (accumulation of fluid resulting from inflammation, hemorrhage, and necrosis of pancreatic tissue), prepare patient for ultrasonography. If diagnosis is confirmed, prepare patient for surgical procedure to drain or resect the pseudocyst.

(a.) Ultrasonography; inform patient that after a lubricant is applied to the skin of the abdomen, a transducer will be moved back and forth over the abdomen to send sound waves into the body and to detect sound waves deflected back to the surface. The pattern of these deflections reveals the location and size of normal and abnormal abdominal structures.

(b.) Computerized body tomography (CAT scan); inform patient that images derived from channeling multiple x-rays through the body at different depths and at different angles are fed into a computer, which then analyzes the characteristics of the structure being studied and renders both a print-out of information and a photograph of the part.

(c.) Post-operatively, maintain gastric suctioning; infuse ordered intravenous fluids; encourage turning, coughing, and deep breathing; and, when the nasogastric tube is withdrawn and oral feeding is resumed, advance the patient slowly from a clear liquid diet to a soft diet and, finally, a low fat diet given in frequent small feedings.

(12.) Persuade the patient to eliminate coffee, which stimulates pancreatic secretion, and alcohol, which causes edema of the duodenal mucosa and spasm of the sphincter of Oddi.

(13.) If chronic pancreatitis causes deficient enzyme production, administer ordered supplemental trypsin, lipase, and amylase (Viokase). If islets are destroyed and diabetes develops, administer ordered insulin.

9. **Ulcerative colitis**—chronic disease of the large bowel that is characterized by congestion, edema, ulceration, and abscess formation in the mucosa and submucosa.

a. Cause.

Unknown; but probably multiple, such as viral infection, autoimmune disorder, together with a familial predisposition.

b. Manifestations.

The disease is characterized by numerous exacerbations and remissions.

(1.) Cramping lower abdominal pain and diarrheal stools, containing mucus, pus, and blood.

(2.) Severe tenesmus, with scanty hard stools.

(3.) Anal fissures and abscesses.

(4.) Weight loss, anorexia, anemia.

(5.) Visualization of inflamed, hyperemic, granular mucosa of the rectum and sigmoid colon on proctosigmoidoscopy.

(6.) X-ray evidence of superficial mucosal erosions and loss of hautral markings in rectosigmoid area following barium enema.

c. Nursing management.

(1.) Administer low fiber, bland diet, with frequent small feedings so as not to stimulate gastrocolic reflex.

(2.) Provide ordered liquid nutritional supplements to facilitate weight gain.

(3.) Instruct patient to eliminate milk products (if lactose deficient on the basis of diet history or serum test results). Advise patient to also eliminate spices, caffeine, alcohol, and excessively fatty foods.

(4.) If patient is acutely ill with malnourishment and dehydration, provide complete bed rest; infuse ordered intravenous fluids; or administer ordered parenteral hyperalimentation to put bowel at rest and restore fluid balance.

(5.) Administer prescribed ferrous sulfate intramuscularly for iron deficiency anemia (oral iron salts are not well tolerated because they are irritating to gastrointestinal mucosa).

(6.) Administer ordered diphenoxylate or atropine to decrease bowel motility in severe diarrhea; monitor patient for abdominal distention and prostration, as these drugs may cause toxic megacolon (dilation of the colon and thinning of the intestinal wall).

(7.) Administer ordered sulfasalazine (Azulfidine), 1 gm, orally, Q.I.D. to arrest bowel inflammation.

(8.) Administer ordered prednisone, 10 mg, orally, for anti-inflammatory effect during severe exacerbations of diarrhea.

(9.) Empty bed pan or commode promptly, provide adequate ventilation of the patient's room, and provide room deodorizer to remove odors resulting from frequent bowel movements.

(10.) Bathe the perineal area with mild soap and warm water and dry gently following each diarrheal stool to prevent perineal excoriation.

(11.) Advise patient on bed rest to turn frequently to avoid pressure areas, as skin is friable due to malnourished state.

(12.) Teach patient the need for continuous medical supervision and regular colonoscopy and mucosal biopsy (ulcerative colitis predisposes to cancer of the colon).

(13.) If medical treatment is unsuccessful and hemorrhage or toxic megacolon occur, prepare patient for total colectomy and ileostomy.

(14.) Post-operatively, teach the patient to care for the ileostomy. Since small bowel contents are liquid, the patient must wear a collection pouch over the stoma at all times (unless a continent ileostomy or ileal pouch has been created). Secure the faceplate of the collection pouch to the abdominal skin with stoma adhesive and Karaya gel to prevent leakage of intestinal contents (which contain digestive enzymes).

(15.) Encourage patient to first observe, then assist, and then execute changing of the collection pouch so that he becomes proficient in self care procedures and techniques before discharge from the hospital.

(16.) Introduce the patient to representatives from self help groups, such as Ileoptimists and National Ostomy Association, to provide him with peer support from experienced ileostomy patients.

10. **Cancer of the colon**—malignant tumor of the large bowel, 50% of which occur in the distal 10 inches of the large bowel and 33% of which are within length of the examining finger on digital rectal examination.

a. Cause.

(1.) Diet high in fat and animal protein (especially beef) and low in roughage predisposes to colon cancer, possibly because carcinogens in the fecal mass are in longer contact with the bowel wall when transit time is prolonged.

(2.) Familial polyposis and ulcerative colitis predispose to colon cancer.

b. Manifestations.

(1.) Change in bowel habit, either constipation or constipation alternating with diarrhea.

(2.) Cancer of the right colon is more apt to cause pain, nausea, and vomiting.

(3.) Cancer of the left colon is more apt to cause rectal bleeding and constipation.

(4.) X-ray evidence of stricture or ulceration following barium enema.

(5.) Finding of occult blood on testing of stool.

(6.) Finding numerous dividing cells in a biopsy specimen or cytology smear obtained during colonoscopy.

c. Nursing management.

(1.) Provide information and emotional support for the patient while diagnostic tests are being performed.

(a.) Colonoscopy; inform the patient that a clear liquid diet should be followed for 3 days before the test and that all food and fluids will be held for 8 hours before the test; that he will be given a laxative the night before the test and enemas until return solution is clear on the morning of the test. Explain that he will be given a sedative-hypnotic before the test (meperidine or diazepam) and that he will be placed in the left side-lying position while the fiberoptic colonscope is introduced, then turned from side to side as the tube is advanced throughout the full length of the colon.

(b.) Colon roentgenography; inform the

patient that he will be given no food or fluids for 8 to 10 hours before the examination; that he will be given a laxative on the night before and enemas until return solution is clear on the morning of the examination; that he will be placed in left side-lying position while a radiopaque liquid (barium) is instilled rectally; that he will be asked to retain the barium while several x-rays are taken of the bowel; and that following the examination he will be given a laxative or an enema to remove the barium and prevent impaction.

(c.) Removal of rectosigmoid polyps through a sigmoidoscope for histological examination; administer cleansing enemas before the polypectomy, and monitor patient for hemorrhage following the procedure.

(2.) If it is necessary to resect the tumor and anastamose remaining bowel segments (for malignancy in the ascending and transverse colon) or to perform an abdominoperineal resection of the tumor and creation of a permanent colostomy (for malignancy of the sigmoid, rectum, or anus), prepare the patient physically and emotionally for the operation.

(a.) Provide a high calorie, high protein, low residue diet for several days before surgery to empty the bowel and facilitate healing.

(b.) Administer ordered intestinal antiseptic; such as phthalylsulfathiazole or neomycin, orally for several days pre-operatively to decrease bacteria in the colon (to minimize or prevent peritoneal contamination during surgery).

(c.) Administer ordered intravenous fluids or blood transfusions pre-operatively to correct dehydration and anemia.

(d.) Administer serial enemas on the evening before surgery to empty the bowel and decrease intra-operative peritoneal contamination.

(e.) If ordered, insert nasogastric tube and indwelling catheter pre-operatively to prevent intra-operative and post-operative distention of the bowel and bladder.

(f.) If the patient is to have a colostomy and his surgeon approves, arrange for a representative of a local ostomy group to visit the patient pre-operatively to answer any questions that he may have about living with a colostomy.

(g.) For temporary colostomy, after the bowel loop is opened by the surgeon on the 3rd post-operative day, encourage the patient to observe, then to assist with colostomy irrigations (if these are ordered to train the bowel to empty at regular times) and colostomy pouch changes.

(h.) Have patient sit on toilet or on a chair in front of the toilet for colostomy irrigation and colostomy pouch change. Using an enema bag and catheter or a bulb syringe, irrigate the colostomy with 500 to 700 ml of warm saline to distend the bowel and stimulate peristalsis, evacuating stool and gas.

(i.) If rectoperineal resection has been done, remove the rubber drains slowly from the perineal wound according to the surgeon's order, irrigate the wound with H_2O_2 and normal saline, and pack the wound with sterile gauze to remove inflammatory debris and facilitate healing.

(j.) Inform the patient of sources from which colostomy supplies (irrigating bags, catheters, bulb syringes, colostomy pouches, belts, gauze dressings, deodorizing solutions, Karaya gel, stoma adhesive, and so forth) can be obtained.

(k.) Arrange for the patient to meet and talk with a completely rehabilitated colostomy patient who can provide practical advice concerning the patient's problems and concerns.

(3.) If a chemotherapeutic agent, such as 5-fluorouracil, is given to inhibit tumor growth in a patient with metastases from colon cancer, monitor for symptoms of drug toxicity, such as nausea, diarrhea, alopecia, weakness, and hemorrhage.

(4.) If radiation is used to reduce tumor size and inactivate metastatic cells, either pre-operatively or in a patient whose condition makes surgery impossible, examine the skin of the irradiated area daily for evidence of irritation. Bathe the part with water only (no soap), pat dry, and do not apply powders or lotions unless prescribed by the radiotherapist. Do not wash off skin markings placed on the radiation site by the radiotherapist. Instruct patient to avoid constrictive clothing and exposure to sunshine for the irradiated skin area.

(5.) Provide supportive counseling for the patient and the family as they cope with shock, denial, anger and depression associated with the diagnosis of cancer and the prescribed treatment.

11. **Hemorrhoids**—varicose veins of the anal canal; those that are covered by mucosae are internal hemorrhoids; those that are covered by skin are external hemorrhoids.

a. Causes.

(1.) Hereditary weakness of the veins, absence of venous valves.

(2.) Obstruction of venous return, as in portal hypertension.

(3.) Precipitating causes are pregnancy, straining at stool, pelvic tumor, and prolonged standing.

b. Manifestations.

(1.) Bright red rectal bleeding associated with defecation.

(2.) A feeling of moisture in the anal region associated with prolapse of an internal hemorrhoid.

(3.) Pain is most common with thrombosis of a prolapsed internal hemorrhoid.

(4.) Pallor, dyspnea, weakness, if iron deficiency anemia results from repeated hemorrhoidal bleeding.

c. Nursing management.

(1.) For bleeding internal hemorrhoids, administer ordered stool softeners, bulk laxatives, lubrication with an emollient ointment, and sitz baths several times a day.

(2.) If conservative treatment is ineffective and a constricting rubber band is placed around the bleeding internal hemorrhoid to cause it to slough and fall off, monitor the patient following the procedure for rectal hemorrhage.

(3.) If a prolapsed, thrombosed, painful hemorrhoid is ligated and excised, monitor the patient post-operatively for hemorrhage and urinary retention.

(a.) Administer ordered sitz baths to decrease discomfort and facilitate healing.

(b.) Administer ordered stool softeners and laxatives, and encourage patient to defecate when he feels the urge to do so in order to prevent constipation and fecal impaction.

(c.) Encourage patient to eat a high bulk diet and to drink increased liquids to prevent contipation, which would traumatize the surgical site.

(4.) Teach the patient the need for regular proctoscopic examination after the age of 40 years, since there are causes for rectal bleeding other than hemorrhoids.

CARE OF PATIENTS WITH GENITOURINARY DISORDERS

1. **Diagnostic work-up**—prepare patients for and support them during performance of tests.

a. Urine culture and sensitivity tests; obtain an early morning catheterized urine specimen and send it to the laboratory, where plates of culture media are inoculated with the urine and incubated for 72 hours. Microorganisms obtained from resulting cultures are identified by staining and microscopic examination. Discs impregnated with various antibiotics are applied to cultured organisms to determine which antibiotic will inhibit growth of offending organisms.

b. Kidney-ureter-bladder x-ray; a plain film of the abdomen is taken to reveal the size and position of the kidney, as well as the presence of stones.

c. Intravenous pyelogram; administer ordered laxative on the evening before the test to remove feces and gas from the intestinal tract. If ordered, withhold fluids for 8 hours before the test to facilitate concentration of the dye in the urine (would not be done in older patients with inadequate renal function). An iodine containing radiopaque dye is injected intravenously and serial x-rays are taken. The dye is excreted to assess renal function and to detect dilation of the renal pelvis, ureter, or bladder, and to detect stones or diverticula. During and following the test the patient should be observed for evidence of allergic reaction to the dye, such as chills, fever, hives, tachycardia, or shock.

d. Cystogram; administer ordered laxative on the evening before the test to remove feces and gas from the colon. A catheter is inserted into the bladder, a radiopaque dye is instilled, and x-rays are taken to determine whether stones or diverticula are present and to determine whether vesicoureteral reflux occurs (backflow of urine from bladder into ureter) with increase in bladder pressure. Vesicoureteral reflux would contraindicate use of suprapubic pressure to empty a flaccid bladder.

e. Cystometrogram; a retention catheter is inserted and measured amounts of saline are instilled into the bladder at a constant rate while intravesicular pressures are recorded. The patient indicates when he feels the desire to void and when he feels that the bladder is completely full. The catheter is withdrawn and the patient is directed to cough to test for stress incontinence. The changes in bladder pressure during fluid instillation and micturition permit diagnosis of constricted bladder, spastic bladder, dilated autonomous bladder, motor paralytic bladder, and bladder-sphincter dyssynergia (failure of coordination of detrusor contraction and sphincter relaxation).

f. Cystoscopy; administer ordered sedative or tranquilizer before procedure. A telescope with a light source and a series of reflecting mirrors is inserted through the urethra and into the bladder. Sterile saline is instilled to distend the bladder and permit visualization of the bladder, ureteral orifices, and urethra. Observe the patient following the procedure for hematuria and urinary retention. If ordered, administer smooth muscle relaxants and warm sitz baths to decrease discomfort due to procedure.

g. Ultrasonography; high frequency sound waves are projected into the abdomen, projected back by tissues of varying densities, and converted to electrical energy that is displayed graphically on an oscilloscope. Ultrasonography can be used to differentiate between solid tissue masses (tumor) and fluid filled masses (hydronephrosis). No specific preparation is needed for the test other than an explanation of the purpose and procedure.

2. **Health history**—while taking patient's health history, question patient concerning the following functional urinary disorders:
   a. Frequency—need to urinate at short intervals due to bladder infection or neurogenic bladder disorder.
   b. Urgency—strong desire to urinate that is difficult to resist due to cystitis, prostatitis, or urethritis.
   c. Dysuria—painful or difficult voiding.
   d. Nocturia—frequent voiding during the night due to renal diseases that cause loss of concentrating power, and due to diabetes mellitus and diabetes insipidus.
   e. Hesitancy—difficulty in initiating or maintaining the urinary stream due to urethral obstruction.
   f. Oliguria—urine volume of 400 ml/day or less, due to shock, acute renal failure, or incompatible blood transfusion.
   g. Hematuria—blood in the urine, gross or microscopic, due to bladder or kidney carcinoma or acute glomerulonephritis.
   h. Pain.
      (1.) Dull pain in costovertebral angle because of distention of the renal capsule due to tumor, or hydronephrosis.
      (2.) Colicky pain radiating from costovertebral angle to the retropubic area caused by ureteral obstruction by a stone or a stricture.
      (3.) Burning pain during and after voiding due to bladder inflammation.

3. **Urinary retention**—inability to release urine, which has accumulated in the bladder, despite a desire to do so.
   a. Causes.
      (1.) Obstruction at or below the bladder outlet.
         (a.) Prostatic hypertrophy
         (b.) Urethral stricture
      (2.) Spasm of urinary sphincters following pelvic surgery.
      (3.) Neurogenic bladder dysfunction, as follows spinal cord injury.
   b. Manifestations.
      (1.) Bladder distention—dullness to percussion and a palpable swelling in the suprapubic area.
      (2.) Passing small amount (25 to 50 ml) of urine at frequent intervals.
      (3.) Lower abdominal pain and fullness.
      (4.) If retention is not relieved, detrusor muscle hypertrophies, bladder trabeculae and diverticula develop, and retained urine becomes infected.
   c. Nursing management.
      (1.) Assist female patient to the bathroom or commode, and allow male patient to stand at the urinal to provide a position and an environment that facilitate voiding.
      (2.) Pour warm water over perineum, or

have patient sit in a warm tub to relieve sphincter spasm.

(3.) Administer ordered analgesics liberally post-operatively, since abdominal pain may inhibit voiding.

(4.) If patient cannot void despite facilitative measures, obtain an order to catheterize the patient. No more than 1000 ml of urine should be removed from the bladder at one time, to avoid provoking bladder spasm.

(a.) If urethra is blocked by stricture or prostatic hypertrophy, assist physician with suprapubic catheterization. With the bladder distended and the patient in prone position, paint the suprapubic skin with ordered antiseptic. Support patient while physician injects skin with a local anesthetic, makes a puncture wound through the anterior abdominal wall into the bladder with a trocar (cannula), threads a catheter through the cannula, and secures the catheter to the skin with sutures. Attach the catheter to a closed drainage system.

(b.) Perform ordered urethral catheterization by cleansing the external urinary meatus with ordered antiseptic and inserting either a straight or a retention catheter through the urethra and into the bladder. If an indwelling catheter is used, inflate the balloon with sterile saline and attach the catheter to a closed drainage system. Leg bag or bedside drainage bag must be kept below the bladder level to facilitate proper drainage and prevent reflux of urine into the bladder.

4. **Urinary incontinence**—inability to voluntarily control discharge of urine from the bladder.

a. Causes.

(1.) Psychological factors that upset conditioned reflexes associated with micturition, such as excessive dependence or regression associated with illness.

(2.) Damage to internal or external urinary sphincter, as may occur following obstetrical trauma.

(3.) Instability of detrusor muscle, as that due to bladder infection, spinal cord injury, and multiple sclerosis.

b. Manifestations.

(1.) Enuresis—urinary incontinence during the night because of a sleep-arousal disorder or a behavioral problem.

(2.) Stress incontinence—urinary dribbling associated with coughing, sneezing, laughing, and lifting due to incompetence of urinary sphincter.

(3.) Urgency incontinence—inability to hold urine once the desire to void is experienced caused by interruption of cerebral cortical control over the micturition reflex.

(4.) Continuous incontinence—the bladder empties whenever the micturition reflex is stimulated because of lack of voluntary control of urinary sphincter.

c. Nursing management.

(1.) Administer ordered antiseptic or antibiotic to patient with bladder infection.

(2.) Teach patient to perform Kegel exercises; voluntary contraction of perineal muscles 10 times Q.I.D. to strengthen urinary sphincter muscles and pelvic floor muscles and thereby prevent stress incontinence.

(3.) Encourage patient to drink 2000 to 2500 ml/day of fluid, spaced at regular intervals from 8:00 A.M. to 8:00 P.M., and institute a voiding schedule of every 2 hours to retrain the bladder for voluntary control.

(4.) If ordered, attach an external urine collection device. A condom attached to a drainage tube is effective in keeping the incontinent male patient dry and in preventing skin maceration. Each day at bedtime, remove the condom; wash, rinse, and dry the penis; and expose the skin of the genitals to air for an hour before reapplying the external collecting device. Attach the condom collection device with elastic tape to prevent circulatory constriction during erections.

5. **Neurogenic bladder**—malfunction of the bladder that results from a disorder of the central or peripheral nervous system.

a. Types, causes, and manifestations.

(1.) Uninhibited bladder—inability to resist the urge to void, with expulsion of urine as soon as the need to void is experienced; due to injury of the upper motor neuron, as in cerebrovascular accident and multiple sclerosis.

(2.) Reflex bladder—no sensation of bladder fullness and bladder empties reflexively whenever a certain volume of urine has accumulated. Micturition reflex is triggered by stimulating the skin of the thigh or penis; due to spinal cord transection above the sacral segments.

(3.) Sensory paralytic bladder—although motor control of the bladder is possible, patient cannot perceive bladder fullness and does not initiate voiding reflex. Urine retention and overflow occur; due to diabetic polyneuropathy.

(4.) Motor paralytic bladder—sensation of bladder fullness occurs, but patient cannot initiate voiding response; due to interruption of motor outflow from sacral cord segments 2, 3, and 4, as in poliomyelitis.

(5.) Autonomous bladder—patient unable either to perceive bladder fullness or to initiate bladder emptying owing to interruption of micturition reflex through sacral cord segments 2, 3, and 4. Bladder can be emptied only through external compression or catheterization; due to transection of the sacral cord.

(6.) Bladder disorder during spinal shock (1st 3 months following spinal cord injury). During the period of spinal shock, all reflexes at and below the level of spinal cord injury are blocked. While micturition reflex (sacral S_2, S_3, S_4 level) is absent, bladder is atonic, and micturition does not occur either voluntarily or reflexively, so patient must have an indwelling catheter inserted or be catheterized intermittently. When spinal shock resolves, spinal reflexes below (but not at) the level of injury return. If cord damage is above sacral S_2, S_3, S_4 level, the micturition reflex returns. The indwelling catheter can be removed, and reflex bladder emptying can be triggered by stroking the thigh, pulling pubic hair, or tapping over the bladder area.

6. **Urinary tract infection**—because of anatomical differences, females are more prone to urinary infections that males.

a. Causes.

(1.) Usually gram-negative microorganisms, e.g., *Escherichia coli*, *Proteus vulgaris*, *Pseudomonas aeruginosa*, and *Aerobacter aerogenes*.

(2.) Normal urinary tract tissues are resistant to infection, but irritation of urinary mucosa is caused by catheter, cystoscope, or stone; ischemia of the bladder wall caused by distention, stagnation of urine, alkaline urine, and glycosuria all predispose to infection.

b. Manifestations.

(1.) Burning on urination

(2.) Frequency and urgency to void.

(3.) Pain in suprapubic, perineal, low back, or flank regions.

(4.) Fever, chills, malaise

(5.) Bacteria, protein, pus cells in urine.

(6.) More than 100,000 colonies of bacteria/ml on urine culture.

c. Nursing management.

(1.) Force fluids to 2500 to 3000 ml/day to dilute microorganisms and flush live organisms and tissue debris from the urinary tract.

(2.) Administer ordered course (10 to 14 days) of antiseptic or antibiotic drug, usually sulfisoxazole, nitrofurantoin, methenamine mandelate, ampicillin, gentamycin, cephalosporin, or tetracycline.

(3.) Administer ordered ascorbic acid or cranberry juice to acidify the urine. Bacterial multiplication is slowed in acid urine, and certain urinary antiseptics are more effective in an acid medium.

(4.) Administer ordered sitz baths, and advise patient to avoid sexual intercourse to decrease inflammation in urethritis.

(5.) Teach outpatient the importance of taking the full course of prescribed medication even though symptoms of urinary tract infection may disappear after only a few days of treatment. A full course of treatment is needed to prevent development of drug resistant organisms.

(6.) Instruct female patient in proper method of perineal cleansing (from front to back) following a bowel movement to prevent contamination of urethral opening with coliform organisms.

(7.) Establish a voiding schedule of every 2 hours for patient with urinary retention so as to prevent bladder distention and bladder wall ischemia.

7. **Urinary calculosis**—development of stones in either the kidney or bladder.

a. Causes.

Any factor that predisposes to precipitation and accretion of mineral salts in the urinary tract.

(1.) Infection

(2.) Obstruction of urine outflow

(3.) Presence of a foreign body, such as a catheter.

(4.) Urine retention and stagnation

(5.) Abnormalities of calcium metabolism due to immobility, hyperparathyroidism.

(6.) Metabolic disorders, such as cystinuria or gout.

b. Manifestations.

(1.) Colicky pain in the mid-back, which radiates to the genitals (if stone blocks urine flow).

(2.) Passage of small stones (gravel); must strain urine through several layers of gauze to retrieve smallest stones.

(3.) Laboratory analysis may reveal stone composition as follows:

(a.) Calcium phosphate or carbonate or magnesium phosphate or carbonate, usually resulting from infection.

(b.) Uric acid, xanthine, cystine, or oxalate due to metabolic imbalances, some of which result from genetic predisposition.

(4.) Nursing management.

(a.) Prevent stone formation in susceptible persons by teaching them to drink large quantities of fluid (3000 to 4000 ml/day) and to void frequently to prevent urine concentration and stagnation.

(b.) Move bed bound patients frequently, and teach them to perform bed exercises, since immobility provokes movement of calcium salts from bones.

(c.) Restrict intake of calcium-rich foods and liquids in immobilized individuals.

(d.) Check patient's laboratory reports to detect elevation of serum calcium, phosphate, or uric acid levels, and call physician's attention to excessive concentrations of any of these compounds, so that appropriate diet modifications or medications can be ordered.

(e.) For immobilized patients, spinal cord–injured patients, and patients with indwelling catheters, send urine samples for culture and sensitivity testing to identify any urinary tract infections that would predispose to stone formation.

(f.) If x-ray reveals a kidney or bladder stone too large to be passed naturally, prepare patient for surgical procedure to crush or remove the stone. Post-operatively, monitor patient closely for bleeding, urinary obstruction, urinary retention, urinary tract infection, and recurrent stone formation.

(g.) Teach patient with tendency for stone formation of continuing need for high fluid intake, urine acidification with cranberry juice or ascorbic acid, prescribed dietary modifications (low calcium, low purine, or low oxalate), and continuous medical follow-up to identify long range complications.

8. **Bladder cancer**—most frequent neoplasm of the urinary tract. Most bladder cancers originate as papillomatous growths on the posterior bladder wall in the region of the trigone and invade the bladder wall and obstruct urine flow from the bladder.

a. Causes.

Exposure to various carcinogens.

(1.) Aniline dyes used in textile and printing industries.

(2.) Asbestos

(3.) Smoking

(4.) Cyclamate

(5.) Cyclophosphamide (Cytoxan)

(6.) Chronic irritation by infection or stone.

b. Manifestations.

(1.) Intermittent, gross, painless hematuria.

(2.) Frequency, urgency, dysuria.

(3.) Pelvic and back pain, if tumor metastasizes.

(4.) Palpation of tumor on digital rectal examination.

(5.) Visualization of tumor mass on cystoscopy and histological diagnosis of tumor on biopsy.

c. Nursing management.

(1.) Prepare patient for diagnostic cystoscopic examination or excision of tumor through the cystoscope.

(a.) Administer enemas to empty the bowel on the evening before the procedure. If patient is to have general anesthesia, hold food and fluids for 8 hours before cystoscopy. Administer ordered sedative-hypnotic, and instruct patient to lie completely still during the procedure.

(2.) If patient receives radiation therapy,

monitor for radiation skin injury, wash skin with water and without soap, and do not apply skin lotions or powders.

(3.) If cystectomy is required for removal of invasive tumors, prepare patient physically and psychologically for body image–changing surgery. In conjunction with cystectomy, pelvic lymph nodes are dissected to block metastases and an ileal conduit urinary diversion procedure is performed.

(a.) A portion of the terminal ileum is isolated, ureters are transplanted into the isolated segment, and the distal end of the isolated ileal segment is sutured to the anterior abdominal wall to form a stoma to which a collection appliance is attached. Urine flows into the ileal conduit and is continually pushed from the conduit to the abdominal surface by peristalisis (electrolytes like Cl^- are not resorbed).

(1.) Following surgery, check stoma for patency, and check peristomal skin for irritation and hemorrhage.

(2.) Empty collection device every 3 to 4 hours.

(3.) Weigh patient daily and measure intake and output to detect fluid retention as evidence of renal dysfunction.

(4.) Counsel and support patient and family to enable them to cope with changed body image resulting from urinary diversion procedure.

(5.) Teach patient procedures for peristomal skin care and changing urine collection device. Use Karaya powder and Karaya seal wafers to relieve skin irritation around stoma. Irrigate collection device with dilute white vinegar and insert deodorant tablets or solution in the pouch to reduce noxious odors.

(6.) Provide sexual counseling for patient and partner to facilitate sexual adjustment following urinary diversion procedure.

9. **Glomerulonephritis**—inflammation of the glomeruli.

a. Causes.

Immunological response of glomerular tissue to circulating antibodies (usually antibodies to group A streptococcal antigens), which results in decreased patency of glomeruli; obstruction of tubules; and red blood cells, white blood cells, and proteinaceous casts in urine.

b. Manifestations.

(1.) Acute glomerulonephritis.

(a.) Acute onset of malaise, fever, and chills 10 to 21 days following streptococcal pharyngitis.

(b.) Edema of hands and feet.

(c.) Dyspnea resulting from pulmonary congestion due to sodium and water retention.

(d.) Bloody urine

(e.) Moderate hypertension

(f.) Elevated antistreptolysin O titer in serum.

(g.) Increased blood urea nitrogen and creatinine.

(2.) Chronic glomerulonephritis—granular, contracted kidney due to fibrous tissue scarring.

(a.) Malaise, headache, dizziness.

(b.) Edema, polyuria, nocturia.

(c.) Hypertension

(d.) Low, fixed urine specific gravity.

(e.) Elevated blood urea nitrogen, creatinine.

(f.) Anemia

(g.) Nephrotic syndrome, with ascites, hydrothorax, anasarca, and increased intracranial pressure.

c. Nursing management.

(1.) Acute glomerulonephritis.

(a.) Admister ordered penicillin to treat streptococcal infection.

(b.) Administer ordered antihypertensive medicines.

(c.) Administer ordered diuretics to relieve edema.

(d.) Implement ordered fluid restriction if edema is present.

(e.) Provide bed rest, with frequent position changes to prevent pneumonia.

(f.) Administer ordered corticosteroids to block immune response to streptococcal antigens.

(g.) Weigh patient daily, and keep intake and output records to monitor fluid retention.

(2.) Chronic glomerulonephritis.

(a.) Administer ordered antihypertensive medications.

(b.) Provide ordered low sodium, low potassium diet.
(c.) Restrict fluid intake to 1500 ml/day.
(d.) If blood urea nitrogen and creatinine levels are elevated, provide ordered low protein diet. If blood urea nitrogen and creatinine levels are normal, provide ordered high protein diet.
(e.) Administer ordered blood transfusion to treat severe anemia.

10. **Renal failure**—cessation of renal function, with accumulation in the blood of excess nitrogenous wastes, electrolytes, and water; may occur suddenly or gradually.
   a. Causes of acute renal failure.
      (1.) Prerenal: decreased renal blood flow, as occurs in hemorrhage, shock, sepsis, burns, and congestive heart failure.
      (2.) Intrinsic: post-streptococcal glomerulonephritis, acute pyelonephritis, subacute lupus erythematosus, and sickle cell disease.
      (3.) Postrenal: bilateral obstruction to urine outflow, such as kidney stones, blood clots, bladder tumor, benign prostatic hypertrophy, and urethral stricture.
   b. Causes of chronic renal failure.
      (1.) Chronic glomerulonephritis
      (2.) Chronic pyelonephritis
      (3.) Polycystic kidney
      (4.) Renal nephrosclerosis
      (5.) Hypertension
      (6.) Diabetes mellitus
   c. Manifestations of acute renal failure.
      (1.) Initial oliguria or anuria, with later diuresis.
      (2.) Elevated blood urea nitrogen and creatinine levels.
      (3.) Electrolyte imbalance, elevated serum potassium level.
      (4.) Metabolic acidosis
      (5.) Anorexia, nausea, vomiting.
      (6.) Headache, drowsiness, irritability.
      (7.) Hypertension
   d. Manifestations of chronic renal failure.
      No symptoms develop until 75% of glomerular filtration power is lost.
      (1.) Initial salt wasting, with decreased serum sodium level, hypotension, and dry skin.
      (2.) Later sodium retention and hypertension, potassium retention and muscular irritability.
      (3.) Pulmonary edema, congestive heart failure (due to sodium and fluid retention).
      (4.) Stomatitis, gastrointestinal ulceration, and bleeding.
      (5.) Drowsiness, confusion, irritability due to cerebral edema.
      (6.) Anemia, thrombocytopenia due to marrow depression.
      (7.) Calcium and phosphorus imbalance, leading to hypersecretion of parathormone, which causes bone demineralization and pathological fractures.
      (8.) Elevated blood urea nitrogen and creatinine levels: decreased serum pH, decreased serum bicarbonate level.
      (9.) Urine specific gravity of less than 1.010, proteinuria, urinary casts.
      (10.) Decreased libido, infertility.
   e. Nursing management of patient in renal failure.
      (1.) Implement ordered fluid restriction (usually 400 ml plus volume of previous day's fluid output). If patient is edematous, measure daily output.
      (2.) Provide gentle mouth care to increase appetite for patient with stomatitis and gingivitis.
      (3.) If patient has uremia and develops gastrointestinal symptoms, provide low protein diet (20 to 40 gm/day) with enough carbohydrate and fat to provide needed calories.
      (4.) If serum sodium or potassium level is above normal, restrict sodium or potassium intake (in early stage of renal failure, kidneys may waste sodium).
      (5.) If serum potassium level is more than 7 mEq/L, administer ordered, orally or rectally, cation exchange resin (e.g., polystyrene sulfonate) to remove potassium from the bowel. Administer ordered sorbitol to prevent constipation and sodium retention.
      (6.) Administer ordered phosphate-binding antacids, such as aluminum hydroxide gel, to reduce phosphate levels.
      (7.) Administer ordered ferrous sulfate or folic acid, or both, to treat anemia.
      (8.) Administer ordered peritoneal dialysis in which the peritoneum is used as a semipermeable membrane across which ions and molecules diffuse from the blood to a dialysate solution, which is then removed from the body.
         (a.) Assist physician with insertion of intraperitoneal catheter. While patient is under local anesthesia, a catheter is inserted through the an-

terior abdominal wall, 1 to 2 inches below the umbilicus, into the peritoneal cavity, and is sutured in place.

(b.) Introduce 1 to 2 L of warm dialysis fluid into the peritoneal cavity by gravity in 10 minutes, allow the fluid to remain in the abdomen for 30 minutes, then drain it out for 20 minutes. Repeat cycle continuously for 24 to 48 hours to treat acute renal failure in a hospitalized patient. When peritoneal dialysis is used to treat chronic renal failure in an outpatient, the dialysate is instilled 4 times daily, left in the peritoneal cavity for 4 hours, then removed.

(c.) Monitor patient for catheter displacement or obstruction.

(d.) Check character of returned dialysate fluid; fecal material would indicate bowel perforation and cloudy fluid would indicate peritonitis.

(e.) Monitor patient for respiratory distress due to pressure of dialysate solution on the diaphragm.

(f.) Monitor patient's vital signs at intervals during dialysis to detect cardiorespiratory stress caused by too rapid shifts of fluid and electrolytes.

(g.) Weigh patient before and after procedure to detect weight loss.

(h.) Measure amount of fluid instilled and drained during each cycle. It is expected that outflow would be 100 to 200 ml more than inflow. If less fluid drains out than was instilled, have patient change position to bring abdominal fluid level in contact with catheter opening.

(9.) Administer ordered hemodialysis, in which a synthetic semipermeable membrane in a machine is used to effect diffusion of ions, molecules, and water from the blood to a dialysate bath: can be used to remove toxic substances, such as barbiturates, or excess nitrogenous wastes of chronic renal failure.

(a.) Prepare patient for a surgical procedure in which an arteriovenous fistula is created in the forearm or an external shunt is attached to an artery and vein in the forearm. Following either procedure, the arm vein dilates.

(b.) When patient is to be dialyzed, prime the hemodialyzer with dialyzing fluid, insert a large bore needle into the arterial limb of the fistula (or attach a tube to the arterial limb of the external shunt), add heparin to the patient's blood as it enters the machine, and allow the blood to flow into the membrane compartment of the dialyzer.

(c.) Check the setup to ensure that the dialysate contains major electrolytes in desired (ordered) extracellular concentrations and that the membrane in the dialyzer is intact, so that excess water and electrolytes in the patient's blood will diffuse across the membrane into the dialysate and be discarded.

(d.) Check the setup to ensure that purified blood is returned from the hemodialyzer, treated with protamine sulfate to neutralize the heparin added to the afferent tubing, and then delivered into the venous limb of the fistula or shunt.

(e.) During dialysis monitor patient to detect untoward effects of the procedure.

(1.) Check blood test reports to detect anemia (failed kidney no longer produces hemopoietin)

(2.) Monitor patient for cerebral edema and seizures, which are symptoms of electrolyte disequilibrium. Rapid decrease in plasma concentration of urea causes fluid to shift from blood to brain tissue by osmotic pressure gradient.

(3.) Observe patient for evidence of anxiety, depression, and risk of suicide.

(4.) Monitor patient for bone pain and pathological fractures. Calcium malabsorption and faulty conversion of vitamin D to its active metabolites by the damaged kidney causes osteomalacia and reactive hyperparathyroidism.

(5.) Observe patient for motor and speech dysfunctions (cerebrovascular accident) and tachycardia, dyspnea, and edema (congestive heart failure).

(6.) Check results of serological tests for hepatitis B antigen.
(7.) Question patient concerning decreased libido and impotence resulting from metabolic imbalance and psychological stress.

11. **Renal transplantation**—the kidney may be obtained from a living donor (a biological relative is preferred because of greater probability of tissue-type compatability) or from a cadaver donor (following sudden terminal illness in an otherwise healthy individual).
    a. Assist physician in preparing living kidney donor and kidney recipient psychologically and physically for procedure to ensure that donor's decision was not made under pressure and that both are in optimum condition for surgery.
    b. Immediately following surgery, administer ordered hemodialysis until the new kidney is fully functional.
    c. Following transplantation, administer ordered immunosuppressive drug to decrease chances of organ rejection.
        (1.) Corticosteroids
        (2.) Chemotherapy agent, such as cyclophosphamide (Cytoxan).
    d. Post-operatively, hold oral food and fluids and keep nasogastric tube in place until bowel sounds indicate that peristalsis has returned.
    e. Monitor patient closely for the following signs of transplant rejection:
        (1.) Fever
        (2.) Leukocytosis
        (3.) Hypertension
    f. If ordered, maintain reverse isolation to protect patient against gram-negative and viral infections from patients, hospital staff, and visitors.
    g. Encourage patient to cough and deep breathe every 2 hours to prevent respiratory infections.
    h. Help patient and family to plan for close medical follow-up for the rest of the patient's life.

CARE OF PATIENTS WITH MUSCULOSKELETAL DISORDERS

1. **Dislocation (subluxation)**—displacement of a bone from its normal position in a joint, so that the articulating surfaces of opposing bones are no longer in contact.
    a. Cause.
        (1.) Genetic defect of socket—congenital dislocation of the hip, for example.
        (2.) Trauma to the joint, as occurs in falls or sport-related injuries.
    b. Manifestations.
        (1.) Deformity of the joint.
        (2.) Shortening or lengthening of the extremity.
        (3.) Pain
        (4.) Loss of joint movement or restriction of movement.
    c. Nursing management.
        (1.) Prevent subluxation in susceptible individuals (e.g., shoulder subluxation in the hemiplegic patient) by protecting the weakened joint from injury. In assisting the hemiplegic patient to move from supine to sitting position, the nurse should slide her hand behind his upper back and pull the patient forward rather than pull on his paralyzed arm.
        (2.) If physician manipulates dislocation by closed reduction, administer ordered analgesic following reduction and monitor extremity for evidence of circulatory impairment or nerve damage (which may occur owing to soft tissue injury during the initial trauma or during the manipulation required for reduction).
        (3.) Inform patient that the affected part will be immobilized for 3 to 6 weeks in a splint or cast to permit healing of soft tissues.
        (4.) When the affected joint is removed from the cast or splint, advise active motion to prevent muscle atrophy and contraction of fibrous tissue elements of the joint capsule.
2. **Fracture**—a break in the continuity of a bone, which is usually accompanied by associated soft tissue injury.
    a. Causes.
        (1.) Direct force against the bone.
        (2.) Forceful twisting of the bone.
        (3.) Violent muscle contractions.
        (4.) Disease processes that weaken the bone structure so that the forces of normal use cause the bony structure to collapse as in osteoporosis and Cushing's syndrome.
    b. Types of fracture.
        (1.) Open (compound)—fracture is accompanied by a break in the skin over the

fracture site through which bony fragments may protrude.
(2.) Closed (simple)—skin over the fracture site is intact.
(3.) Comminuted—contains several fracture lines, with the result that the bone is broken into several pieces.
(4.) Impacted—one fragment is telescoped or driven forcibly into the adjacent fragment.

c. Manifestations.
(1.) Pain and muscle spasm
(2.) Swelling
(3.) Deformity (change in contour, angulation, length).
(4.) Abnormal movement
(5.) Ecchymoses due to bleeding from torn vessels
(6.) Impaired sensation caused by tearing or compression of nerves.
(7.) Crepitus on movement.
(8.) Shock is especially apt to occur in association with fractures of large bones, such as the femur or humerus, when there is excessive bleeding into surrounding soft tissue.
(9.) Visualization of fracture line and dislocation of fragments on x-ray film.

d. Nursing management.
(1.) Before moving patient from the site where the injury took place, immobilize the joint above and the joint below the fracture, using sticks or rolled newspapers; the patient's uninjured leg may be positioned to stabilize the injured one.
(2.) Cover any surface wound with a clean (sterile, if possible) dressing.
(3.) Control bleeding from any surface wound by direct pressure.
(4.) Maintain an open airway, if necessary to wait for further medical attention.
(5.) Apply cold to relieve pain and swelling.
(6.) Keep patient lying flat, and cover with blankets to prevent shock.
(7.) Assess for head and spinal injuries before moving patient. Apply spine board before moving patient if any symptoms of head or spinal injury are observed.
(8.) Transport patient to hospital for treatment.
(9.) Assist physician with closed reduction and immobilization of the fracture with cast or traction.
(10.) If closed reduction is ineffective or impossible, prepare patient physically and psychologically for open reduction procedure.

(a.) Cast application and maintenance.
(1.) Before cast is applied, explain to the patient that the chemical reaction that occurs when plaster of Paris is mixed with water generates heat, so the newly applied cast will feel warm.
(2.) Encase the limb or body part to which the cast will be applied in Stockinette, and pad the bony prominences with cotton wadding or felt, as directed by the physician.
(3.) Assist cast application by submerging the plaster bandage roll in water until bubbling ceases; then hand the wet plaster bandage to the physician, who will apply the plaster and mold it to the injured part while an assistant holds the part in proper alignment. When the case is finished, pull the stockinette over the edge of the plaster and fasten it to the outer cast surface with adhesive tape or a circle of wet plaster.
(4.) While the cast is drying (12 to 48 hours), place the patient on a firm mattress and support the cast on plastic or rubber covered pillows; leave the cast uncovered to air dry. Cover the patient's exposed skin to prevent chilling, and turn the patient every 2 to 3 hours to permit even drying of the cast. When turning the patient, handle the cast with the palms to avoid indenting the cast's surface with the fingers.
(5.) Monitor the patient for any untoward effects of the cast. For a leg or arm cast, compress the nail briefly, release, and note the speed with which color returns to the nail in order to test for circulatory obstruction. Compare the skin color of fingers or toes on the extremity with the cast with the skin color of the same parts on the extremity without the cast, as a test for circulatory embarrassment. Ask patient to wiggle his fingers or toes and to detect

tactile stimulation of the digits with his eyes closed in order to test for motor and sensory ischemic nerve damage. Check the hand or foot of the extremity with the cast for edema, which can be minimized by elevating the extremity with the cast on a pillow. Observe the surface of the cast for evidence of bleeding. Check vital signs every 2 hours to detect shock due to blood loss. Note odor of patient's skin under the cast, as foul odor could signify infection or gangrene.

(6.) Notify physician immediately concerning symptoms of bleeding, swelling, circulatory impairment, and motor or sensory loss; prepare equipment for immediate cast removal.

(7.) In turning the patient in a hip spica cast, move the patient to the side of the bed and turn the patient toward the uninvolved leg, without grasping the crossbar of the cast to move the patient.

(8.) Instruct the patient to drink liberal quantities of fluid in order to prevent formation of urinary calculi, which may develop owing to movement of calcium from the bones during periods of immobility.

(9.) Encourage coughing and deep breathing to prevent hypostatic pneumonia.

(b.) Application and maintenance of traction involves pulling on a body part in 2 directions (the direction of force and the direction of counter force) to relieve muscle spasm, alleviate pain, correct overriding of bone fragments, and maintain proper alignment of bone.

(1.) Types of traction; skin traction in which tape or sponge rubber is attached to the skin and ropes and weights are attached to the tape or sponge rubber to exert pull on the musculoskeletal tissues. Skeletal traction in which securing of pins, wires, or tongs into bone and attachment of ropes and weights to the pins, wires, or tongs to exert pull on musculoskeletal tissues.

(2.) Traction is of 2 varieties with reference to line of pull. Running traction (straight traction) in which traction force pulls in 1 direction against the long axis of the body, e.g., Buck's traction and Bryant's traction. Balanced traction (suspension traction) in which traction force exerts a pull on the affected part while, at the same time, the part is suspended in a sling or splint to which weights are applied, so as to exert a counter force. With balanced traction, the amount of pull on the part remains the same even when the patient moves about in bed.

(3.) To ensure that the ordered amount of traction is continuously applied, maintain traction setup. Ensure that patient remains in proper body alignment at all times and that tape does not slip or release from the site of skin attachment. Check skin of the application site for irritation or breakdown. Report any complaints by patient of "burning" under the tape. Keep traction ropes taut, unencumbered by the patient's body, bed, bed linen, ropes, or other equipment. Ensure that the rope rides easily over the pulleys. When checking the position of ropes, monitor for fraying and breakage. Ensure that weights are securely fastened and hang free of the bed, bed linen, nearby furniture, and the floor. When checking the position of weights, see that knots are securely tied, with rope ends taped to prevent fraying and loosening. Check that height of bed elevation blocks or bars is that ordered by the physician. The amount of bed elevation determines the amount of counter force provided by the patient's body weight.

(4.) While the patient is in traction, provide care to prevent complications of immobility. Prevent skin irritation and breakdown by keeping bed linen smooth and free of crumbs and by checking the skin of the back for discoloration and excoriation. Teach patient the importance of twice daily active range of motion of parts other than those immobilized by traction. Instruct patient in muscle setting exercises, e.g., quadriceps setting and abdominal setting, if ordered. Encourage patient to cough and deep breathe every hour to prevent pooling of respiratory secretions. Push liberal fluid intake (2500 to 3000 ml) to prevent formation of urinary stones resulting from mobilization of calcium from bones unstressed by use. Instruct patient to use uninvolved extremity and overhead trapeze to lift himself without disrupting traction pull for bed pan placement, bed making, and pressure relief. For skeletal traction, check that pins or wires are immobile and skin exit wound is dry. If ordered, cleanse pin site with antiseptic and apply bacteriostatic ointment. Cover sharp edges of pin with cork or adhesive tape. Regularly check peripheral pulses, speed of capillary refill, and color and temperature of extremity to which traction is applied to detect evidence of circulatory impairment. Ask patient to flex and extend digits of extremity to which traction is applied to detect evidence of neural damage due to pressure. Check for calf tenderness or Homans's sign in extremities, so as to detect evidence of deep vein thrombosis.

(5.) Provide diversionary activities in order to decrease patient's frustration and depression associated with immobility and confinement.

(6.) When traction is removed, gradually and progressively restore patient to upright position and to full range of motion of the immobilized part, taking into consideration the orthostatic hypotension, muscle atrophy, and weakness to which immobility has subjected him.

Care of the Patient with Selected Musculoskeletal Disease

1. **Gout**—metabolic disorder that is characterized by inflammation of selected joints following deposition of urate crystals in joint tissues.
   a. Cause.
      Genetic defect in purine metabolism (either overproduction of uric acid or retention of uric acid), with deposition of urate crystals in joints, skin, and other tissues.
   b. Manifestations.
      (1.) Involved joint (often the first metatarsophalangeal) is hot, swollen, red, and painful.
      (2.) Elevation of serum uric acid level.
      (3.) Formation of tophi, or nodular deposits of urate crystals in joints (visible on x-ray), and subcutaneous tissues (e.g., ear lobes).
      (4.) Elevation of white blood cell count and red blood cell sedimentation rate.
   c. Nursing management.
      (1.) Provide bed rest, with elevation of inflamed joint during acute attack.
      (2.) Advise low purine diet; avoiding such foods as liver, kidney, sweetbreads, and anchovies.
      (3.) Push liberal fluid intake to foster urinary excretion of urate.
      (4.) Administer ordered colchicine on hourly basis for 8 hours or until toxic symptoms develop (nausea, vomiting, and diarrhea) to treat acute attack.
      (5.) Administer ordered allopurinol to suppress uric acid formation in patients being treated with chemotherapeutics for malignancy, and monitor patient for

skin rash and gastrointestinal disturbance.

(6.) Administer ordered uricosuric medicine, such as probenecid or sulfinpyrazone, to promote uric acid excretion. Teach patient to maintain 3000 ml/day fluid intake while receiving probenecid.

(7.) Assist patient to institute dietary and habit changes so as to avoid foods and beverages that provoke gouty attacks.

2. **Rheumatoid arthritis**—chronic systemic inflammatory disease of connective tissue.

a. Cause.

Unknown, but possibly a virus or bacterium or an autoimmune disorder.

b. Manifestations.

(1.) Fatigue, malaise, low-grade fever, anorexia, weight loss, and lymphadenopathy.

(2.) Pain, swelling, subluxation, contracture deformity of small and medium sized joints in bilateral, symmetrical distribution. Common deformities are fusiform, shortened fingers, ulnar deviation of fingers, swan neck or boutonniere deformity of fingers, and flexion contractures of wrist, elbow, shoulder, hip, and knee.

(3.) Subcutaneous nodules on elbows and extensor surface of extremities.

(4.) Muscular pain and stiffness

(5.) Elevated red blood cell sedimentation rate, leukocytosis, and anemia.

(6.) Presence of rheumatoid factor and C-reactive protein in serum.

c. Nursing management.

(1.) Administer ordered acetylsalicylic acid (aspirin) to relieve joint inflammation, 1 to 1½ gm Q.I.D. to maintain blood levels at 23 to 30 mg/dl. Arrange for patient to take the medicine after meals or with antacids to decrease gastrointestinal irritation.

(2.) If aspirin is ineffective, administer ordered nonsteroid anti-inflammatory drug, such as indomethacin, phenylbutazone, or ibuprofen. Monitor patient for signs of gastrointestinal irritation.

(3.) Monitor patient for and teach patient about the toxic effects of ordered drugs.

(a.) All anti-inflammatory drugs may cause gastrointestinal irritation, peptic ulcer, and gastrointestinal bleeding.

(b.) Indomethacin also may cause depression, confusion.

(c.) Phenylbutazone also may cause leukopenia, thrombocytopenia.

(d.) Ibuprofen also may lower prothrombin time and cause bleeding tendencies.

(4.) If aspirin and nonsteroid anti-inflammatory drugs are unsuccessful in controlling symptoms, administer ordered corticosteroids (only given for a short term). Monitor patient for gastrointestinal bleeding, fluid retention, and psychosis.

(5.) If ordered, administer gold salts, e.g., aurothioglucose, intramuscularly, weekly, to relieve synovitis in patients who don't respond to less severe treatment. Monitor patient for dermatitis, stomatitis, and proteinuria.

(6.) If immunosuppressive agents, such as cyclophosphamide and azathioprine, are given to block autoimmune response, monitor the patient for evidence of anemia and infection.

(7.) Administer ordered dry or moist heat to decrease muscle spasm and reduce edema of involved joints. If ordered, submerge the part in a warm paraffin bath to provide penetrating heat to inflamed joints. Use caution to prevent skin burns.

(8.) Provide frequent rest periods throughout the day to prevent fatigue.

(9.) Maintain patient in optimum body alignment to prevent contracture deformities. Allow no pillows under the knees and only a small flat pillow under the head.

(10.) Institute passive or active range of motion of all joints to but not beyond the point of pain, Q.I.D. If the joint is excessively painful, use isometric exercises to strengthen muscles without moving the joint.

(11.) Provide supportive splinting of inflamed joints to relieve pain.

(12.) Teach patient the importance of avoiding soft, low chairs and soft soled shoes in preventing deformities of involved joints.

(13.) Teach patient and family methods of adapting clothing, utensils, furniture, and home arrangements so as to facili-

tate greatest possible independence in activities of daily living and conservation of energy.
(a.) Elevated toilet seat
(b.) Front zipper or Velcro closures for dresses, shirts, coats, jackets, and slacks.
(c.) Long-handled zipper pull, shoe horn, and reacher.

3. **Osteoarthritis**—chronic, progressive, noninflammatory degeneration and atrophy of articular cartilage, with eventual damage to underlying bone.
a. Cause.
(1.) Trauma of use, accentuated by obesity, poor posture, and occupationally related excessive joint stress.
(2.) Biochemical abnormality of cartilage metabolism.
b. Manifestations.
(1.) Joint pain, worst following prolonged exercise or weight bearing.
(2.) Morning stiffness, which is relieved by motion and heat.
(3.) Aching joint pain, associated with weather changes.
(4.) Feeling of grating on joint motion.
(5.) Enlargement of distal interphalangeal joint (Heberden's nodes).
(6.) X-ray evidence of narrowed joint spaces, erosion of articulating bony surfaces, increased density of subchondral bone, and formation of bony spurs at joint margins.
(7.) Limitation of joint motion.
c. Nursing management.
(1.) Prevent osteoarthritis in susceptible individuals by advising weight loss in those who are obese to diminish joint stress.
(2.) Administer ordered acetylsalicylic acid (aspirin) to relieve pain. Give the drug with food or milk to prevent gastrointestinal irritation.
(3.) Administer ordered nonsteroid anti-inflammatory drugs, such as indomethacine and phenylbutazone (Butazolidine), to relieve joint pain when aspirin is ineffective.
(4.) Administer ordered diazepam or other antispasmodic drug to relieve muscle spasm.
(5.) Advocate use of orthopedically fitted shoes.
(6.) Teach patient how to maintain good body alignment while reclining, sitting, walking, and lifting so as to prevent additional joint stress.
(7.) Advise patient to schedule several rest periods throughout the day.
(8.) Teach patient to use moist heat and mild exercise to relieve pain and stiffness.
(9.) If ordered, apply cervical collar or traction to relieve nerve pressure secondary to cervical osteoarthritis.
(10.) If prosthetic replacement of severely damaged weight bearing joints becomes necessary, prepare patient physically and psychologically for surgery.
(a.) Teach patient isometric exercises to strengthen muscles post-operatively without moving surgically traumatized tissues.
(b.) Teach patient how to use a trapeze to move himself about in bed and relieve pressure on skin of the back.
(c.) Give patient a thorough bath with hexachlorophene emulsion (pHisoHex) on the evening before surgery to decrease the number of skin bacteria and reduce possibility of surgical wound infection.
(11.) Following total hip replacement (insertion of prostheses for femoral head and acetabular cup).
(a.) Maintain operated hip in abduction and straight alignment while patient is supine and while patient is being turned from back, to unoperated side, to prone to prevent skin pressure damage.
(b.) Apply support hose to prevent venous congestion and deep vein thrombosis, to which the patient is susceptible by immobility and by vascular damage during surgery.
(c.) Encourage patient to cough and deep breathe hourly to prevent hypostatic pneumonia.
(d.) Direct patient to flex ankle and knee of uninvolved extremity and to flex ankle of involved extremity. Five days post-operatively, if ordered, instruct patient in quadriceps setting and gluteal setting exercises to strengthen muscles around the prosthetic hip and prevent dislocation.
(e.) Provide overhead trapeze so patient can lift himself at intervals to re-

lieve pressure and facilitate bed linen changes, toileting, and back care.

(f.) When ordered, assist patient to standing position at bedside. Allow weight bearing as ordered to walk from bed to chair or toilet. Provide cane or walker for greater safety in walking.

(g.) Before hospital discharge, teach patient to avoid sitting in low soft chairs, crossing the legs, bending the hip more than 90 degrees, taking long auto rides, and instruct him to place a pillow between his knees and sleep on his back to prevent hip dislocation.

4. **Osteoporosis**—metabolic disorder in which bone degenerates because of imbalance between bone formation and bone absorption.
   a. Causes.
      (1.) Hyperparathyroidism
      (2.) Cushing's syndrome
      (3.) Reduction of estrogen levels in post-menopausal females.
      (4.) Prolonged negative calcium balance due to inadequate dietary intake of calcium.
   b. Manifestations.
      (1.) Low back pain, which radiates around the trunk and is precipitated by heavy lifting.
      (2.) Gradually increasing kyphosis, decreasing height, and musculoskeletal aching.
      (3.) X-ray evidence of vertebral compression (especially in lower thoracic and lumbar regions).
      (4.) X-ray evidence of decreased bone density.
   c. Nursing management.
      (1.) Prevent osteoporosis by encouraging post-menopausal females to remain physically active and to ingest foods and beverages containing calcium.
      (2.) If estrogen is given to post-menopausal female to decrease the rate of bone resorption, teach her the importance of regular breast self examination and annual vaginal examination and Papanicolaou's stain of cervical smear.
      (3.) If corset or brace is ordered to maintain proper trunk alignment, teach patient to perform regular skin examinations to identify pressure and irritation from the support device.
      (4.) Warn patient that periods of inactivity foster calcium resorption and bony weakness, and instruct patient in suitable exercise techniques to prevent calcium mobilization from bones.

CARE OF PATIENTS WITH IMMUNOLOGICAL DISORDERS

A. Care of Patients with Specific Immune System Disorders

1. Hypersensitivity (allergy)—increased immune reaction to an allergen, causing tissue injury.
   a. Type I hypersensitivity reaction (immediate); anaphylaxis.
      (1.) Causes.
         (a.) Offending allergen may be horse serum, insect venom, foods, antibiotics, local anesthetics, or iodinated radiopaque dye.
         (b.) Antigen reacts with an IgE antibody attached to tissue mast cells or basophilic white blood cells, releasing lysozymes, histamine, and chemotactic factors.
      (2.) Manifestations.
         (a.) Skin rash
         (b.) Urticaria
         (c.) Angioedema
         (d.) Wheezing and dyspnea
         (e.) Decreased blood pressure to shock levels.
      (3.) Nursing management.
         (a.) Monitor patients receiving iodinated radiopaque dye or experiencing insect sting for symptoms of allergic response. Administer ordered antihistamine, such as chlorpheniramine (Chlor-trimeton), parenterally, and ordered sympathomimetics, such as epinephrine, parenterally.
         (b.) Question patient for history of allergic drug reactions before administering antibiotics or local anesthetics.
         (c.) Instruct patient with known allergy to wear Medic Alert bracelet.
         (d.) If offending allergen was injected into an arm or leg, apply a tourniquet to the extremity to halt absorption of the offending substance.

(e.) Administer ordered epinephrine, 0.2 to 0.5 ml of 1:1000 solution, subcutaneously.
(f.) Assist physician with endotracheal intubation if laryngeal edema causes respiratory obstruction.
(g.) Administer ordered sympathomimetic drugs, such as metaproterenol (Alupent) or theophylline (Aminophylline) I.V. to relieve bronchospasm.
(h.) Administer ordered norepinephrine (Levophed) to raise blood pressure in patients with severe shock.

b. Type II hypersensitivity reaction—cytotoxic and cytolytic reactions, e.g., incompatible blood reaction.
(1.) Cause.
An antibody (IgG or IgM) reacts with an antigen on a target cell, activating complement, which then destroys the target cell.
(2.) Manifestations.
(a.) Chills
(b.) Fever
(c.) Muscle aching
(d.) Oliguria or anuria if acute renal failure develops.
(3.) Nursing management.
(a.) Discontinue blood transfusion; send blood sample to laboratory for typing check.
(b.) Administer fluid intravenously to keep patient well hydrated.
(c.) Administer ordered diuretics if oliguria develops.
(d.) Administer ordered ion exchange resins or institute ordered hemodialysis or peritoneal dialysis if serum potassium level becomes dangerously high.

c. Type III hypersensitivity reaction—immune complex reaction, e.g., systemic lupus erythematosus.
(1.) Cause.
Antigen-antibody complexes in the circulation activate complement, initiating an inflammatory reaction. Activated enzymes destroy the target cells. Chemotactic substances released by mast cells and basophils attract polymorphonuclear leukocytes to the inflammation site.
(2.) Manifestations (systemic lupus erythematosus).
(a.) Butterfly shaped rash across the nose and malar eminences.
(b.) Fever
(c.) Weight loss
(d.) Arthralgia
(e.) Proteinuria and hematuria
(f.) Pleural friction rub
(g.) Antinuclear antibodies (IgG or IgM) in the serum.
(h.) Lupus erythematosus cells in the serum.
(3.) Nursing management.
(a.) Teach patient to avoid sunlight, ultraviolet radiation, and penicillin, which accentuate skin lesions.
(b.) Provide bed rest to patient in acute stage to relieve fatigue.
(c.) Administer ordered corticosteroids for pleurisy, pericarditis, or glomerulonephritis. Monitor patient for edema, emotional changes, and gastrointestinal bleeding.
(d.) Administer ordered imunosuppressive drugs to patients who are unresponsive to other treatments.
(e.) Reassure patient and family that with proper management many complications of the disease can be avoided.

d. Type IV hypersensitivity reactions—delayed cellular hypersensitivity, e.g., tuberculin skin reaction, contact dermatitis, and transplant rejection.
(1.) Cause.
Sensitized T cells react with antigen, without involving humoral antibody or complement. Lymphokines released by the T cells destroy the antigen.
(2.) Manifestations.
(a.) After intracutaneous injection of tuberculin, a 10-mm wheal of erythema and induration develops in 48 hours if the individual has previously experienced a tuberculous infection.
(b.) Following initial healing of skin allograft or homograft, the graft becomes infiltrated with lymphocytes, macrophages, and plasma cells, which damage blood vessels, causing graft necrosis.
(3.) Nursing management.
(a.) For contact allergy, teach patient which allergens his sensitivity test results indicate hypersensitivity to,

how to avoid those substances, and advise application of ordered 1% hydrocortisone cream.

(b.) For transplant rejection.

(1.) Administer ordered corticosteroids to suppress inflammation at transplant site.

(2.) Administer ordered cytotoxic drug, such as azathioprine (Imuran) or methotrexate (Amethopterin), to depress lymphoid tissue response.

(3.) Administer ordered antilymphocyte serum (prepared in horses by immunizing them with human T cells) to deplete patient's sensitized T cells.

B. General Approach to Prevention and Management of Hypersensitivity Reactions

1. Interview patient to identify previous medical history of hypersensitivity to one or more of the following:
   a. Foods, such as eggs, milk, strawberries, wheat, and shellfish.
   b. Soaps, lotions, or cosmetics.
   c. Cat or dog hair; other animal dander.
   d. Plants; often roses, poison ivy, and sumac.
   e. Pollen; often of trees, grasses, and weeds.
   f. Molds
   g. Fabrics, such as wool.
2. Instruct and prepare patient for the following laboratory tests ordered during diagnostic work-up:
   a. Differential white blood cell count; eosinophilia is common in allergies.
   b. Determination of serum level of IgE, which is elevated in many allergic conditions; normal level is 0 to 150 IU.
3. Assist in performance of skin tests to identify agents responsible for Type I, II, and III hypersensitivity reactions (antibody mediated).
   a. Advise patient to avoid taking antihistamines or subcutaneous epinephrine before skin tests are done, as these drugs would inhibit skin reactions.
   b. Either inject dilute preparations of common offenders (pollens, fungi, dust, and foods) intradermally or apply substances in liquid or paste form over a skin scratch.
   c. Read test results in 15 to 30 minutes. Redness and induration indicate a positive reaction to the test substance.
4. Administer ordered twice weekly subcutaneous injections of solutions of the offending allergens in progressively increasing strength to desensitize the patient to identified allergens.
5. Inform patient of food and contactants to which he evidenced a positive reaction in skin sensitivity tests. Advise patient to avoid eating identified food allergens; to avoid contact with identified fabrics, animals, plants, and cosmetics; and to install humidifiers and air filters at home and at work.
6. Instruct patient to sleep with the windows closed and to avoid trips to rural areas during pollen season.
7. If the patient suffers an allergic attack, administer ordered drugs to yield symptomatic relief.
   a. Antihistamines, such as chlorpheniramine (Chlor-Trimeton), diphenhydramine (Benadryl), or tripelennamine (Pyribenzamine), for hay fever and urticaria. Advise patient not to drive or operate heavy machinery while taking antihistamines, as drowsiness is a possible side effect.
   b. Corticosteroids for anti-inflammatory effect in severe allergic reactions (used only on a short term basis); monitor patient for toxic symptoms; hypertension, weight gain, mood change, and gastrointestinal bleeding.

C. Care of Patients with Inadequate Immune Response

1. Malignant tumor—a new growth of cells that reproduces in a disorganized manner, invades surrounding tissue, and spreads to distant parts of the body, endangering life and health.
   a. Cause.

      Malignant transformation of cells due to interaction of multiple factors.

      (1.) Viruses, e.g., Epstein-Barr virus.
      (2.) Physical irritants, e.g., sunlight.
      (3.) Chemical irritants, e.g., tar, plastics, asbestos.
      (4.) Dietary characteristics, e.g., high protein, high fat, low fiber.
      (5.) Hormones, e.g., estrogen, androgen.
      (6.) Immunological incompetence—malignant cells are continuously being developed in the body and are normally destroyed by T-lymphocytes. In immunosuppressed individuals, malignant cells escape destruction and multiply.
   b. Characteristics of malignant tumors.

      (1.) Larger than normal cells.
      (2.) Larger than normal nuclei.

(3.) Cells vary considerably in size and shape.
(4.) Cells bear little resemblance to normal cells of the tissue.
(5.) Greater than normal percentage of cells in the tissue undergo mitosis at any one time.
(6.) Unregulated cellular growth; cells are uninhibited by contact with normal cells in surrounding tissue.
(7.) Tumor cells are not contained or confined within a capsule.
(8.) Tendency to invade surrounding tissue.
(9.) Less cohesiveness with adjacent cells; cells break loose and are carried to distant sites by lymph and blood and seed new tumors (metastases) of the original cell type in distant tissues.

c. Types of malignant tumors.

Tumors are classified with reference to the type of tissue from which they arise.

(1.) Epithelial tissue
(a.) Squamous cell carcinoma—skin.
(b.) Basal cell carcinoma—glandular tissue.
(2.) Connective tissue
(a.) Fibrosarcoma—fibrous tissue.
(b.) Chondrosarcoma—cartilage.
(c.) Osteogenic sarcoma—bone.
(3.) Endothelial tissue
(a.) Hemangiosarcoma—blood vessel.
(b.) Multiple myeloma—bone marrow.
(c.) Lymphosarcoma—lymphoid tissue.
(4.) Muscle
(a.) Leiomyosarcoma—smooth muscle.
(b.) Rhabdomyosarcoma—striated muscle.
(5.) Nervous tissue
(a.) Glioblastoma—glial cells.
(b.) Malignant meningioma—meninges.

d. Manifestations of malignant tumors.

(1.) General
(a.) Malaise
(b.) Weight loss
(c.) Anorexia
(d.) Weakness, fatigue
(e.) Cachexia
(2.) Specific

Depend upon the normal functions of the tissues involved.

(a.) Creates symptoms by pressure, displacement of surrounding tissues, obstruction of blood supply and lumens of tubes.
(b.) Pressure on sensitive tissue, such as bone; involvement of nervous tissue may cause pain.
(c.) Tumors involving serous membranes (pleurae) may cause serous effusions.
(d.) Surface ulcerations of tumors may become infected (e.g., breast).

e. Prepare patient for procedures used in diagnosis of malignant tumors.

(1.) Cytological examination—Papanicolaou's smear of malignant cells from cervical scraping; aspiration of digestive or respiratory secretions. Smeared cells are chemically fixed with a mixture of ether and ethyl alcohol and examined microscopically to look for anaplastic changes.
(a.) For cervical scraping, instruct patient to empty her bladder before procedure. Provide drapes and screens to prevent exposure. Teach patient how to use deep breathing and meditation to promote muscle relaxation.
(2.) Biopsy—surgical or needle excision of tumor tissue that is then fixed either by rapid freezing (for immediate microscopic examination) or by embedding in paraffin (following which thin tissue sections are mounted, stained, and examined microscopically to search for changes in cell architecture and arrangement).
(a.) Prepare patient by cleansing the skin of the biopsy site with ordered antiseptic, administering ordered pre-operative sedative. If a colon biopsy specimen is to be obtained, prepare patient by administering ordered laxatives and enemas to cleanse the bowel before colonoscopy.
(3.) X-ray films
(a.) X-ray of the chest or abdomen may indicate blocking of tubular structures by tissue masses, e.g., of bronchus or bowel.
(b.) X-ray of bone may reveal focal changes in radiolucency or pathological fractures resulting from bony tumor.
(c.) Mammography employing ordinary x-ray film or a photographic process (xeroradiography) is used to diagnose breast cancer.
(4.) High frequency ultrasonography—since substances of different densities reflect

sound waves to different degrees, the pattern of sound wave reflections can be used to identify the presence and location of abnormal masses of tissue in chest and abdomen.

(a.) Patient preparation consists of little more than an explanation of the purpose and procedure for the test.

(5.) Radioisotope technique—the movement and concentration of a radioisotope within the body can be tracked by scanning machines. Since tumors distort normal blood vessel patterns and since abnormal tumor tissue metabolizes chemical elements and their isotopes in a different fashion than does normal tissue, radioisotopes can be used to identify malignant tumors.

(a.) Thyroid tumors take up and concentrate ^{131}I.

(1.) Following ingestion of a test dose of radioiodine, the patient should be advised to drink fluids and void at frequent intervals for 24 hours to prevent bladder irritation by ^{131}I, which is eliminated in urine.

(2.) Liver tumors take up and concentrate ^{198}Au.

(6.) Serum analysis for carcinoembryonic antigen, an antigen that is produced by carcinomas of colon and pancreas.

f. Nursing care of patients receiving various types of treatment for malignant disease.

(1.) Surgical removal of tumor tissue.

(a.) Provide emotional support and information about the prescribed treatment.

(1.) Radical excision—removal of entire tumor, together with lymph nodes that drain the area. Used in treating early stages of skin, breast, gastric, cervical, and rectal malignancies. Post-operatively, provide the patient the opportunity to ventilate feelings about radically changed body image, in addition to administering care directed toward protecting patient against the specific complications of the surgical procedure.

(2.) Palliative surgery—removal of as much tumor tissue as possible so as to relieve obstruction or pressure and to reduce the body's tumor burden in preparation for radiotherapy or chemotherapy. Used to treat late stages of gastrointestinal and ovarian carcinoma. Post-operatively, maintain ordered gastrointestinal intubation, intravenous fluid therapy, parenteral nutrition, analgesic pain control, and support patient and family as they work through the stages of grief associated with chronic illness and dying.

(3.) Radiotherapy — administration of high dose, focussed radiation to destroy rapidly dividing tumor cells. Used pre-operatively to shrink tumor tissue or postoperatively to prevent metastases by destroying cells that have broken loose from the tumor during surgical manipulation. External radiation employing x-ray machines is used to treat deep internal malignancies, such as brain, esophageal, and bladder malignancies. Interstitial radiation, using radioisotope filled needles or beads which are embedded in the tumor tissue, is effective in treating malignancies of the tongue and cervix. During a course of radiotherapy, bathe the patient's skin with water only, pat dry, and avoid all powders and lotions. The patient should be cautioned to refrain from washing off the skin markings used to locate radiation dose and to avoid direct sunlight, as irradiated skin is especially liable to heat injury. Advise patient to avoid clothing or jewelry that constrict or chafe the skin. Provide small frequent feedings for the patient who suffers anorexia, nausea, and vomiting as a result of radiation enteritis. Administer ordered antiemetic, such as promethazine

(Phenergan) before meals. Provide ordered vitamin supplements for patients whose oral intake is restricted severely or for long periods of time. Administer soft or puréed nonfiber foods to the patient with radiation pharyngitis and enteritis. Provide dilute NaCl or $NaHCO_3$ solution irrigations for the patient with radiation stomatitis or pharyngitis.

(4.) Chemotherapy—systemic or regional administration of drugs that destroy cells of the primary tumor and the metastases. Drugs that destroy malignant cells are of several types. Alkylating agents interfere with the structure of DNA, e.g., cyclophosphamide (Cytoxan) and nitrogen mustard (Mustargen). Antimetabolites inhibit the synthesis of nucleic acids, e.g., methotrexate (amethopterin) and 5-fluorouracil.

(c.) Anticancer antibiotics bind with or alter the structure of DNA, e.g., doxorubicin (Adriamycin), and bleomycin (Blenoxane). Plant alkyloids disrupt the mitotic spindle, interrupting cell division, e.g., vinblastine (Velban), and vincristine (Oncovin). Steroid hormones alter hormone balance in the body, suppressing tumor growth in hormone sensitive tissue. Examples include estrogen and androgen. Chemotherapeutic drugs are given orally, intramuscularly, or intravenously when malignant disease is widely disseminated and by local intra-arterial infusion when malignancy is localized to a particular organ. When the drug is locally infused into the tumor, a substance, such as leucovorin calcium or folinic acid is injected intramuscularly to block the effect of the antimetabolite on normal body tissue. Observe and question patient about toxic effects of chemotherapeutic drugs, e.g., nausea, vomiting, diarrhea, stomatitis, leukopenia, thrombocytopenia, and anemia. Push fluid intake to 2000 to 3000 ml/day, and hold food and fluid before administration of the chemotherapeutic drug to decrease gastrointestinal symptoms. Teach patient to report symptoms of infection immediately, as leukopenia resulting from bone marrow depression would lower resistance to infection. Advise patient to wear wigs and scarves to cover the head during periods of temporary hair loss.

(5.) Immunotherapy — procedures that are employed to strengthen the patient's immune reaction to malignant cells. In active immunotherapy, the patient is injected with an antigen that stimulates B-lymphocytes to form antibodies. Active specific immunization; patient is injected with a vaccine that is prepared from his own tumor tissue. Active nonspecific immunity; patient is injected with bacille Calmette-Guérin (BCG) vaccine, which stimulates his reticuloendothelial system to activate macrophages and attract lymphocytes to the tumor. Monitor patient for allergic reaction to the vaccine (fever, chills, malaise). Administer ordered aspirin to relieve symptoms. Check injection site; report irritation and ulceration. In passive immunotherapy, the patient is injected with antitumor antibodies or immunologically active lymphocytes that have been obtained from a patient who has been cured of a malignancy. Passive immunity lasts only weeks or months. In adaptive immunity, the patient is first passively immunized with antitumor antibodies or immunologically competent lymphocytes from a person who has been cured of malignancy; then patient is actively immunized by incubating the patient's lymphocytes with tumor cells in the laboratory, then reinjecting the sensitized lymphocytes into his body. Protect patient from untoward effects of his illness and treatment. Protect patient who is receiving radiation or chemotherapy from infection by screening visitors and by separating him from other patients with infections. Monitor patient for symptoms of malignancy of other organs and tissues.

Medical Surgical Nursing Bibliography

Barrows, J. (1984). Turning the tide against acute pulmonary edema. *Nursing 84, 14*:58–63.

Baum, P. (1983). Carotid endarterectomy: One strike against stroke. *Nursing 83, 13*:50–58.

Beland, I. & Passos, J. (1981). *Clinical Nursing: Pathophysiological and Psychosocial Approaches*, 4th ed. New York: MacMillan Company.

Billings, D. & Stokes, L. (1982). *Medical Surgical Nursing*. St. Louis: C. V. Mosby Co.

Binkley, L. (1984). Keeping up with peritoneal dialysis. *American Journal of Nursing, 84*:729–733.

Boss, B. (1983). The dementias. *Journal of Neurosurgical Nursing, 15*:87–97.

Brunner, L. & Suddarth, D. (1984). *Textbook of Medical Surgical Nursing*, 5th ed. Philadelphia: J. B. Lippincott.

Camunas, C. (1980). Transphenoidal hypophysectomy. *American Journal of Nursing, 80*:1820–1823.

Cohen, S. (1980). Pulmonary function tests in patient care. *American Journal of Nursing, 80*:1135–1161.

Cohen, S. (1981). New concepts in understanding congestive heart failure, part 2: How the therapeutic approaches work. *American Journal of Nursing, 81*:357–380.

Covington, R. & Walker, J. (1984). *Current Geriatric Therapy*. Philadelphia: W. B. Saunders.

Dossey, B. & Passons, J. (1981). Pulmonary embolism: Preventing it, treating it. *Nursing 81, 11*:26–33.

Doyle, J. (1983). All leg ulcers are not alike: Managing and preventing arterial and venous ulcers. *Nursing 83, 13*:58–63.

Dudas, S. (1984). Rehabilitation concepts of nursing. *Journal of Enterostomal Therapy, 11*:6–15.

Eisenberg, M., Sutkin, S. & Jansen, M. (eds.) (1984). *Chronic Illness and Disability through the Life Span*. New York: Springer Publishing Company.

Erickson, R. (1981). Solving chest tube problems. *Nursing 81, 11*:62–67.

Fahey, V. (1984). An in-depth look at deep vein thrombosis. *Nursing 84, 14*:34–41.

Felver, L. (1980). Understanding the electrolyte maze. *American Journal of Nursing, 80*:1591–1595.

Fuchs, P. (1980). Oxygen delivery systems. *Nursing 80, 10*:34–43.

Fuchs, P. (1983). Providing tracheostomy care. *Nursing 83, 13*:139–142.

Gandy, F. & Veigh, G. (1984). Helping the amputee stand on his own again. *Nursing 84, 14*:46–49.

Gurevich, I. (1983). Viral hepatitis precautions. *American Journal of Nursing, 83*:572–586.

Guyton, A. (1981). *Textbook of Medical Physiology*, 6th ed. Philadelphia: W. B. Saunders.

Guyton, A. (1982). *Human Physiology and Mechanisms of Disease*, 3rd ed. Philadelphia: W. B. Saunders Company.

Hassey, K., Bloom, L. & Burgess, S. (1983). Radiation: Alternative to mastectomy. *American Journal of Nursing, 83*:1567–1570.

Hickey, J. (1981). *The clinical practice of neurological and neurosurgical nursing*. Philadelphia: J. B. Lippincott.

Hincker, E. & Malasonos, L. (eds.) (1983). *The Little, Brown Manual of Medical Surgical Nursing*. Boston: Little, Brown and Company.

Holloway, N. (1979). *Nursing the Critically Ill Adult*. Reading, Massachusetts: Addison Wesley Publishing Company.

Honigman, R. (1982). Thyroid function tests. Nursing 82, *12*:68–71.

Johnston, S. & Patt, Y. (1981). Caring for the patient on intra-arterial chemotherapy. *Nursing 81, 11*:108–112.

Lamanske, J. (1977). Helping the ileostomy patient to help himself. *Nursing 77*, 7:34–39.

Knobf, M. (1984). Breast cancer: The treatment revolution. *American Journal of Nursing, 84*:1110–1128.

Krause, M. & Mahan, L. (1984). *Food Nutrition and Diet Therapy*, 7th ed. Philadelphia: W. B. Saunders.

Lamphier, R. & Lamphier, R. (1981). Upper GI hemorrhage: Emergency evaluation and management. *American Journal of Nursing, 81*:1814–1817.

Larson, C. (1984). The critical path of adrenocortical insufficiency. *Nursing 84, 14*:66–69.

Leibrandt, R., Cohen, L. & DiCarlantonio, M. (eds.) (1981). *Diseases*. Horsham, Pennsylvania: Intermed Communications, Inc.

Levenson, L. & Levenson, J. (1977). Corneal transplantation. *American Journal of Nursing*, 77:1160–1162.

Levitt, D. (1981). Multiple myeloma. *American Journal of Nursing, 81*:1345–1347.

Lighty, M. (1984). Solving the puzzles of patients' fluid imbalances. *Nursing 84, 14*:34–41.

Luckman, J. & Sorensen, K. (1980). *Medical Surgical Nursing, A Psychophysiologic Approach*, 2nd ed. Philadelphia: W. B. Saunders.

Luke, B. (1979). Nutrition in renal disease: The adult on dialysis. *American Journal of Nursing*, 79:2155–2157.

Peterson, F. (1983). Assessing peripheral vascular disease at the bedside. *American Journal of Nursing*, 83:1549–1551.

Petton, S. (1984). Easing the complications of chemotherapy. *Nursing 84, 14*:58–63.

Phipps, W., Long, B. & Woods, N. (eds.) (1979). *Medical Surgical Nursing: Concepts and Clinical Practice*. St. Louis: C. V. Mosby Co.

Rakel, R. (ed.) (1984). *Conn's Current Therapy*. Philadelphia: W. B. Saunders.

Reed, W. (1982). Givng more than dialysis. *Nursing 82, 12*:58–63.

Resler, M. & Tumulty, G. (1983). Glaucoma update. *American Journal of Nursing, 83*:752–756.

Rifas, E. (1983). Teaching patients to manage acute asthma. *Nursing 83, 13*:77–82.

Saunders, W., Havener, W., Keith, C. & Havener, G. (1979). *Nursing Care in Eye, Ear, Nose, and Throat Disorders*, 4th ed. St. Louis: C. V. Mosby Co.

Schwartz, S., Shires, G., Spencer, F. & Storer, E. (eds.) (1979). *Principles of Surgery*, 3rd ed. New York: McGraw-Hill Book Co.

Sheridan, E., Patterson, H. & Gustafson, E. (1982). *Falconer's The Drug, The Nurse, The Patient*, 7th ed. Philadelphia: W. B. Saunders.

Spivak, J. & Barnes, H. (1978). *Manual of Clinical Problems in Internal Medicine*, 2nd ed. Boston: Little, Brown and Company.

Stark, J. (1982). How to succeed against acute renal failure. *Nursing 82, 12*:26–33.

Stark, J. & Hunt, V. (1983). Helping your patient with chronic renal failure. *Nursing 83, 13*:56–63.

Taylor, J. & Ballenger, S. (1980). Neurological dysfunctions and nursing intervention. New York: McGraw-Hill Book Co.

Thompson, M. (1981). Managing the patient with liver function. *Nursing 81, 11*:101–107.

Tobiason, S. (1979). Benign prostatic hypertrophy. *American Journal of Nursing, 79*:286–290.

Varricchio, C. (1981). The patient on radiation therapy. *American Journal of Nursing, 81*:334–337.

Vogt, G., Miller, M. & Esluer, M. (1985). *Mosby's Manual of Neurological Care*. St. Louis: C. V. Mosby Co.

Walters, J. (1981). Coping with a leg amputation. *American Journal of Nursing, 81*:1349–1352.

Yanko, J. (1984). Head injuries. *Journal of Neurosurgical Nursing, 16*:173–180.

Section
MEDICAL SURGICAL NURSING PRACTICE QUESTIONS

1 • Eight weeks after suffering a closed head injury in a motor vehicle accident, 38-year-old Harvey Conklin was admitted to the emergency room of his neighborhood hospital with severe headache and right leg weakness. He was drowsy, irritable, disoriented as to place and time; he had an oral temperature of 99°F, a pulse rate of 68/min, respirations of 16/min, and blood pressure of 160/100 mm Hg. A brain CAT scan revealed a left subdural hematoma, so burr holes were drilled, and a liquefied clot was evacuated. When interviewing Mr. Conklin's wife concerning the history of his present illness, the nurse would be apt to learn that, in addition to his present symptoms, he had experienced which of the following?

1. Slight intellectual impairment
2. Momentary loss of vision
3. Rhythmic lateral oscillation of the eyes
4. Drainage of clear fluid from the nose

2 • Which of the following directions by the nurse would be best suited to assessing Mr. Conklin's response to command?

1. "Pour a glassful of water from this pitcher."
2. "Tell me who you are and who brought you here."
3. "Touch your nose with your finger."
4. "Close your eyes, raise your right arm, and touch your left ear."

3 • During the first few hours following Mr. Conklin's operation, the recovery room nurse should monitor his respiratory rate, depth, and character because:

1. Clot pressure on the motor cortex would have impaired diaphragmatic efficiency.
2. Increasing respiratory rate is a symptom of increasing intracranial pressure.
3. Elevation of $PaCO_2$ dilates cranial vessels and increases intracranial pressure.
4. Coughing provokes the Valsalva's maneuver and increases cardiac output and intracerebral pressure.

4 • During the period of observation that preceded Mr. Conklin's surgery, which of the following should the nurse consider to be the best index of his neurological status?

1. Vital signs
2. Eye movements
3. Motor activity
4. State of consciousness

5 • If either pre-operatively or post-operatively, the nurse discovers that Mr. Conklin's corneal reflex is absent, she should institute which of the following protective measures?

1. Cleanse the lid margins with saline, and apply warm compresses to the eye.
2. Keep the head flat, and manually raise and lower the eyelid on an hourly basis.
3. Tape the eyelid closed with vertically applied strips of adhesive tape.
4. Place methyl cellulose drops into the eye, close the lid, and apply an eyeshield.

6 • The physician ordered that a sputum specimen be obtained from Ben Kaufman, 40 years of age, a patient with right and left lower lobe bronchiectasis who was hospitalized for treatment of a superimposed acute respiratory infection. At which time of day should the nurse expect that the patient's cough would be most troublesome, and his sputum most copious?

1. On arising
2. At mid-day
3. At mealtime
4. On retiring

7 • The nurse should supervise Mr. Kaufman closely during periods of increased respiratory difficulty, as paroxysms of coughing would predispose to:

1. Laryngospasm.
2. Pneumothorax.
3. Syncope.
4. Convulsions.

8 • In which of the following positions would Mr. Kaufman probably be most comfortable?

1. Lying flat on his back with a small pillow under his shoulders.
2. Reclining on his left side with his right arm and leg supported on pillows.
3. Resting in a semi-Fowler's position with his arm supported at his sides on pillows.
4. Sitting upright at 90 degrees with his arms resting on an over-the-bed table.

9 • Because Mr. Kaufman was anorexic and malnourished, the physician ordered a high protein, high vitamin diet, with 5 small meals a day. Which of the following nursing measures should be employed to improve Mr. Kaufman's nutritional status?

1. Encourage liberal fluid intake between meals.
2. Provide frequent and thorough oral hygiene.
3. Institute postural drainage immediately before meals.
4. Encourage vigorous bed exercises immediately before meals.

10 • Postural drainage was instituted twice daily to foster removal of Mr. Kaufman's excessive tracheobronchial secretions. The respiratory specialist ordered that Mr. Kaufman be placed for 5 minutes in each of the following positions; head dependent, prone, left lateral, supine, and right lateral. Which of the following interventions should the nurse undertake during the procedure to increase the effectiveness of postural drainage?

1. Direct the patient to breathe in and out of a paper bag 4 to 5 times with each change of position.
2. Encourage the patient to drink a full glass of water before the procedure to liquefy secretions.
3. Use a bulb syringe to aspirate secretions from the mouth just before each change of position.
4. Strike the chest wall with cupped hands over the uppermost portions of the chest.

11 • Walt Proxmire, 35 years old, developed chronic renal failure secondary to chronic glomerulonephritis. When dietary management, diuretics, and antihypertensive medications failed to control his symptoms, he was admitted to the hospital. An arteriovenous fistula was established in his left arm, and hemodialysis was instituted for 3 hours, 3 times each week. In arranging for Mr. Proxmire's care during hospitalization, the nurse should record which of the following precautions in the nursing care plan?

1. Encourage fluid intake to 2500 ml/day to prevent renal calculus formation.
2. Avoid skin lotions and oils that interfere with excretion of fluids and salts through perspiration.
3. Encourage vigorous daily exercise to minimize muscle wasting, bone absorption, and renal calculi.
4. Perform venipunctures and blood pressure measurements only on the right arm.

12 • When informing Walt Proxmire and his wife about his expected response to hemodialysis, the nurse should explain that:

1. Since Walt will be unable to eat or drink during hemodialysis, it is advisable that he consume a full meal immediately before the procedure.
2. Because he must remain awake and alert during hemodialysis to report sensory perceptions, dialysis will be performed in the morning when he is well rested.
3. He will experience greater subjective benefit on the day after rather than immediately following hemodialysis.
4. Since movement causes blood pressure changes that alter blood and dialysate flow, Walt will be sedated to minimize position changes during the procedure.

13 • In planning Mr. Proxmire's instruction for self care at home, the nurse should be aware that he will probably be discharged from the hospital with instructions for which type of diet?

1. Low protein, high carbohydrate, high fat diet.
2. Adequate protein, high calorie, low fluid diet.
3. Low carbohydrate, low calorie, high potassium diet.
4. Low calorie, low fat, low bulk diet.

14 • In counseling and supporting Mrs. Proxmire following Mr. Proxmire's discharge from the hospital, the nurse should be aware that for many hemodialysis patients and their wives, the greatest source of psychological stress is:

1. Financial problems arising from the cost of the patient's hemodialysis.
2. Decrease in shared family activities due to diminution of the patient's strength.
3. Increased friction between husband and wife due to the husband's continuous presence in the home.
4. Alteration in sexual relations between husband and wife due to the patient's diminished desire and potency.

15 • Following each hemodialysis treatment, the nurse should observe Walt closely for evidence of which of the following complications?

1. Bleeding tendencies
2. Pulmonary edema
3. Carpopedal spasm
4. Leg cramps

16 • Nettie White, widowed and 60 years old, grew progressively more weak and confused until her landlady brought her to the health maintenance organization of which Mrs. White was a member. A physician's examination revealed lemon yellow pallor, inability to walk, loss of position and vibratory sense in the lower extremity, pulse of 96/min, and respirations of 26/min at rest. When blood studies, bone marrow biopsy specimen, and gastric analysis confirmed a diagnosis of pernicious anemia, Mrs. White was hospitalized for a transfusion of packed red blood cells and was started on regular intramuscular injections of vitamin B_{12}. By carefully questioning Mrs. White's landlady, the admitting nurse would be apt to learn that Mrs. White had recently complained of:

1. Excess salivation.
2. Chest pain.
3. Abdominal distention.
4. Leg cramps.

17 • Which of the following devices should the nurse employ to protect Mrs. White from possible complications of her disease?

1. Bed board
2. Trapeze
3. Inflatable rubber ring
4. Padded boots

18 • In planning for Mrs. White's care the nurse should include which of the following advice in the nursing care plan and in the predischarge instructions?

1. No passive or active exercise of extremities, which could initiate bleeding into the joints.
2. Remain out of bed during waking hours so as to prevent decubitus ulcers, hypostatic pneumonia, and renal calculi.
3. Use blankets and wear socks to bed, rather than applying hot water bottle or heating pad to relieve problem of cold feet.
4. Brush the teeth thoroughly and rinse the mouth with antiseptic after each meal to prevent oral infections.

19 • In preparing Mrs. White for self care following hospital discharge, the nurse should inform her that:

1. Since the cause of pernicious anemia cannot be eliminated, Mrs. White will require regular injections of vitamin B_{12} for the rest of her life.
2. Because Mrs. White's anemia was so severe before treatment was begun, she will require additional transfusions at a later date.
3. After several months of vitamin B_{12} therapy, Mrs. White can expect relief of all of her circulatory and neurological symptoms.
4. After a year or two of follow-up therapy, Mrs. White's condition will be improved enough that the vitamin B_{12} injections can be discontinued.

20 • Until Mrs. White's symptoms begin to subside, the nurse should expect that she will be given a diet of which type?

1. High protein, high vitamin liquids.
2. Bland, soft, unseasoned foods.
3. High carbohydrate, high fat, low protein foods.
4. High bulk, high residue, high fluids.

21 • Nell Tripp, 50 years of age, consulted her physician with complaints of nervousness and eye irritation. Physical examination revealed an enlarged thyroid gland and exophthalmos. Findings of increased serum levels of T_4, T_3, and thyroid stimulating hormone (TSH) and increased uptake of ^{131}I on thyroid scan confirmed a diagnosis of hyperthyroidism. Treatment was an oral dose of 7 millicuries (mc) of ^{131}I. In taking Mrs. Tripp's health history, the physician's office nurse would be apt to learn that, in addition to nervousness and eye problems, Mrs. Tripp had experienced which of the following symptoms?

1. Weakness of the proximal muscles of the arms and legs.
2. Dry, flaking skin.
3. Decreased tolerance to cold.
4. Coarse intention tremor.

22 • In the interval between diagnosis and administration of ^{131}I treatment, the nurse should expect that which of the following drugs will be prescribed for Mrs. Tripp?

1. Potassium iodide
2. Propylthiouracil
3. Physostigmine
4. Propranolol

23 • Since Mrs. Tripp was not hospitalized following radioactive iodine therapy, what should she be taught concerning self care following the treatment?

1. Increase oral fluids and empty the bladder often during the first 24 hours following ^{131}I administration.
2. Avoid ingestion of food or fluids for 8 hours following administration of radioactive iodine.
3. Take an antacid or a drink of milk to relieve dyspepsia resulting from gastric irritation by ^{131}I.
4. Avoid bulky and high fiber foods for 3 days to prevent irritation of irradiated gastrointestinal mucosa.

24 • During the 3 weeks between ^{131}I administration and her return to euthyroid level, Mrs. Tripp will probably be given which of the following types of drug?

1. Antihypertensive
2. Tranquilizer
3. Cardiotonic
4. Anticonvulsant

25 • Which of the following interventions should the nurse suggest to relieve Mrs. Tripp's complaints of itching and redness of her eyes?

1. Wear sunglasses to decrease light stimulation and protect the eyes from injury by foreign bodies.
2. Irrigate the eyes with boric acid solution several times each day.
3. Instill methylcellulose drops into the eyes 4 times a day, and wear eyeshields at night.
4. Take aspirin 2 to 3 times each day to relieve conjunctival inflammation and irritation.

26 • Seventy-year-old Zella Merkel was hospitalized for removal of a cataract from her right eye and insertion of an intra-ocular lens implant. As part of her pre-operative instructions the nurse should inform Mrs. Merkel that which of the following devices will be used during the early post-operative period to protect her from post-operative complications?

1. Posey's belt will be applied to keep her from falling out of bed.
2. Cloth mittens will be tied on her hands to keep her from rubbing her eyes.
3. An eye patch and metal shield will be placed over the operated eye to prevent accidental trauma.
4. An ice bag or cold pack will be applied to the eye to decrease conjunctival inflammation and lid edema.

27 • Mrs. Merkel's pre-operative preparation will probably include which of the following?

1. Trimming the lashes in the eye to be operated upon to 3 mm in length.
2. Shaving the brows and facial hair from the right side of the face.
3. Scrubbing the face with hexachlorophene, and painting the periorbital skin with povidone-iodine (Betadine).
4. Washing the face with soap and water and painting it with alcohol.

28 • In which position should Mrs. Merkel be placed when she is returned to her room following surgery?

1. Supine, with head slightly elevated.
2. Head elevated at a 30 degree angle.
3. Foot of the bed elevated 4 to 5 inches.
4. Right side-lying position.

29 • Post-operatively, the nurse should instruct Mrs. Merkel to avoid eye injury by:

1. Remaining in bed until her new contact lens has been fitted.
2. Cupping her hand over the operated eye when turning in bed or ambulating.
3. Moving slowly and avoiding either bending at the waist or lifting.
4. Squeezing her eyelids shut tightly on retiring to ensure total lid closure.

30 • If, during the first few hours following surgery, Mrs. Merkel should become nauseated and vomit her food or medications, the nurse should interpret these symptoms as possible indicators of:

1. Untoward reaction to the anesthetic agent
2. Anxiety related to the operation and its outcome.
3. A rise in intra-ocular pressure.
4. Cerebrovascular spasm caused by reflex response to pain.

31 • Mrs. Merkel's preparation by the nurse for discharge should include teaching her to:

1. Irrigate the eye with an eyecup.
2. Instill eye drops and eye ointments.
3. Apply warm, moist eye compress.
4. Prepare and apply an iced towel eye compress.

32 • Dom Iago, 65 years of age, was diagnosed as having chronic open angle glaucoma during the course of a regular eye examination. When his intra-ocular pressure continued to rise despite treatment with timolol, pilocarpine, and acetazolamide, he was hospitalized. An iridectomy and a trabeculectomy (surgical filtering operation) were performed. In evaluating Mr. Iago's health history at the time of hospitalization, the nurse should be aware that which of the following is a possible untoward effect of acetazolamide?

1. Headache
2. Palpitations
3. Diarrhea
4. Paresthesias

33 • In planning Mr. Iago's care during hospitalization, the nurse should take into consideration the fact that his glaucoma is apt to have caused which of the following visual difficulties?

1. Loss of color vision
2. Inability to read small print
3. Loss of peripheral vision
4. Inability to rotate and laterally abduct the eye

34 • In preparing Mr. Iago for surgery, the nurse should be prepared to reinforce the following information about expected surgical outcome (which also would have been explained by his surgeon):

1. The operation will not restore sight already lost but will prevent further loss.
2. There will be a slow return of peripheral vision during the 6 to 12 months following surgery.
3. The surgery will result in marked improvement in peripheral vision, with slight loss of acuity in central vision.
4. Following the operation, there will be no further need for systemic or topical medications to treat glaucoma.

35 • Mr. Iago should be maintained in which of the following positions for the first 24 hours postoperatively?

1. Supine, with head immobilized by pillows.
2. Trendelenburg, with hands restrained.
3. Turned toward the side of the operated eye.
4. Low Fowler's position, with a small pillow under the neck.

36 • In preparing Mr. Iago for self care following discharge, the nurse should emphasize the importance of:

1. Restricting intake of oral fluids to 1500

ml/day to decrease production of aqueous humor.
2. Limiting physical activity to that required for daily living and job requirements.
3. Utilizing a high bulk diet and stool softeners to prevent constipation.
4. Avoiding reading and television watching so as to prevent eyestrain.

37 • Tim Casey, a recent nursing graduate, was found to have a fluid-filled cavity in his right upper lung lobe on routine chest x-ray. Because Tim's current Mantoux test result was positive, whereas a test result 2 years before had been negative, and because his sputum cultures revealed acid-fast bacilli, a diagnosis of pulmonary tuberculosis was made. He was hospitalized briefly for institution of treatment with isoniazid and ethambutal, to which the causative organism had responded on sensitivity testing. In preparing a room for Tim's admission to the hospital, the nurse should institute which of the following precautions against infection transmission?

1. Post signs on the patient's door directing visitors and staff persons to don gown, cap, and mask before entering the room.
2. Place a container of disposable masks on the bedside table for Tim to wear while there are visitors or staff members in his room.
3. Assign Tim to a private room with hand washing facilities; soap dispenser, towel holder, and covered, foot-controlled waste container.
4. Install an ultraviolet light on the head of the bed or the bedside stand to destroy airborne tubercle bacilli.

38 • In obtaining Tim's health history at the time of hospital admission, the nurse might expect to learn that Tim had experienced which of the following symptoms as a result of his active tuberculosis?

1. Weight loss despite polyphagia.
2. Expiratory prolongation and wheezing.
3. Afternoon temperature elevation.
4. Orthopnea and paroxysmal nocturnal dyspnea.

39 • On the day following hospital admission, Tim coughed up 5 ml of bright red blood. Which nursing action would be appropriate?

1. Inform Tim that bronchial irritation and bleeding are an expected effect following initiation of drug treatment.
2. Encourage him to remain immobile in supine position to decrease heart rate and blood pressure.
3. Assist him to sit upright with arms resting on the over-the-bed table.
4. Turn him to his right side, and summon the physician immediately.

40 • In order to achieve the most therapeutic effect, Tim's isoniazid and ethambutol should be administered:

1. Each in divided doses at regular intervals throughout the day.
2. One drug before breakfast and the other before retiring.
3. One drug with breakfast and the other drug with lunch.
4. Both at the same time shortly after arising.

41 • Thirty-five-year old Edna Cavers consulted a physician with complaints of weight loss, weakness, and diarrheal stools containing mucus and blood. Proctosigmoidoscopy revealed diffusely ulcerated, inflamed, and friable colonic mucosa with scarring and narrowing of the intestinal lumen. A diagnosis of ulcerative colitis was made, and Edna was treated with sulfasalazine and low residue diet for 1 year. When drug therapy failed to control her symptoms, she was hospitalized and a colectomy and pouch ileostomy were performed. In preparing Mrs. Cavers for self care following the diagnosis of her disease, the nurse should advise her that which of the following foods must be eliminated on a low residue diet?

1. Milk
2. Farina
3. Baked potato
4. Roasted chicken

42 • In preparing Mrs. Cavers to care for herself at home following diagnosis and institution of medical therapy, the nurse should inform her to report which of the following symptoms to her physician as a possible toxic effect of sulfasalizine?

1. Deafness and tinnitus
2. Repeated sore throat and infections
3. Jaundice and urticaria
4. Periorbital and pedal edema

43 • In anticipating Mrs. Cavers' pre-operative care, the nurse should assume that treatment will be needed to resolve which fluid and electrolyte imbalance?

1. Hypernatremia
2. Hypokalemia
3. Hypercalcemia
4. Hypophosphatemia

44 • Mrs. Cavers' preparation for colectomy and ileostomy will include which of the following interventions?

1. Serial tap water enemas until returns are clear the night before surgery.
2. Administration of a stool softener and a laxative on the day before surgery.
3. Administration of a liquid diet and neomycin or phthalylsulfathiazole (Sulfathalidine) orally for 3 to 4 days before surgery.
4. Withholding all solid food for a week before surgery.

45 • During Mrs. Cavers' pre-operative instruction, the nurse should clarify which of the following points with regard to expected effects of a pouch ileostomy?

1. Since small intestine contents are liquid, it will be necessary for Mrs. Cavers to wear a collection device continuously for life.
2. Until ileostomy function can be regulated by diet management, Mrs. Cavers will need to wear an ileostomy bag.
3. For several months after surgery, her ileostomy will drain continuously, but eventually the pouch contents can be drained several times a day with a catheter.
4. Mrs. Cavers will wear an ileostomy bag to collect fecal drainage until the ileum is later anastomosed to the rectum.

46 • Which of the following should be applied to the abdominal skin surrounding the ileostomy valve to prevent skin irritation?

1. Talcum powder
2. Zinc oxide paste
3. Tincture of benzoin
4. Karaya gum

47 • Bob Pine, 60 years of age, consulted a urologist because of complaints of urinary frequency, urgency, and hematuria. Excretory urograms and cystoscopy revealed narrowing of the bladder neck and trabeculations of the bladder wall. A biopsy specimen of tissue from the bladder neck revealed transitional cell carcinoma. Mr. Pine was hospitalized and a radical cystectomy was performed and an ileal conduit was created. Mr. Pine's pre-operative excretory urogram was done on an out-patient basis. The doctor's office nurse should direct him to prepare for the procedure in which fashion?

1. "Take this dose of castor oil on the evening before the test, and hold all food and fluids after midnight of the night before."
2. "Avoid solid food for 2 days before the test, and take serial enemas until return solutions are clear on the morning of the test."
3. "Hold all solid food during the 12 hours preceding the test and insert a rectal suppository 2 hours before the test."
4. "Drink fluids to 3000 ml/day during the 48 hours preceding the test, and hold all food after supper on the previous evening."

48 • Mr. Pine was returned to the recovery room following surgery with ureteral catheters in place and a temporary collection pouch over the stoma. During the first 24 hours following surgery, Mr. Pine's care should include:

1. Attaching the ureteral catheters to low suction apparatus.
2. Irrigating the ureteral catheters with normal saline.
3. Measuring the volume of urinary drainage every hour.
4. Limiting fluid intake to 1000 ml.

49 • During Mr. Pine's early post-operative period, which of the following observations should be reported immediately to the surgeon as a possible indication of serious complication?

1. Dusky color of stomal tissue.
2. Edema of stomal tissue.
3. Reddening of peristomal skin.
4. Ammoniacal odor of urinary drainage.

50 • During the discharge instruction, the nurse should teach Mr. Pine how to decrease the risk of urinary tract infection by:

1. Irrigating the urinary drainage pouch with white vinegar solution.
2. Avoiding ingestion of gas-forming foods and liquids.
3. Emptying the pouch as infrequently as possible to decrease contamination.
4. Ingesting 2000 ml of fluids each day, including cranberry juice.

51 • Ina Wallace, 45 years of age, came to the Walk-In Clinic of the City Hospital for treatment of a draining 2-cm ulcer over the medial malleolus of the left leg. Physical examination revealed obesity and severe varicosities of both legs. Medical history revealed that a previous leg ulcer had been treated by a private physician with Unna's paste boot. Phlebography revealed intact deep venous circulation and incompetent superficial veins in both legs. Following a Trendelenburg test, Mrs. Wallace was scheduled for a vein stripping. Mrs. Wallace's medical history revealed that she had recently experienced leg cramps on walking long distances. The nurse should interpret this symptom as evidence that:

1. Mrs. Wallace has significant arteriosclerosis of leg arteries as well as varicose veins.
2. In addition to venous dilation, Mrs. Wallace is suffering from hypocalcemia.
3. Blood stasis has caused inflammation or infection of dilated leg veins.
4. Chronic venous congestion has caused sluggish capillary blood flow and muscle ischemia.

52 • At the time that Mrs. Wallace's leg ulcer was being treated with Unna's paste boot, she would have been instructed to minimize venous congestion by:

1. Wearing thigh-high elastic stockings for 24 hours every day.
2. Sleeping with the foot of the bed elevated 6 inches.
3. Sitting in a soft easy chair rather than in a straight wooden chair.
4. Avoiding walking rapidly, walking long distances, and climbing stairs.

53 • The purpose of the Trendelenburg test is to determine:

1. Adequacy of arterial flow to the leg.
2. Thrombus formation in veins of the lower extremity.
3. Competence of valves in the communicating veins of the leg.
4. Retrograde congestion of capillaries in the extremity.

54 • The purpose of the Unna's paste boot that was used to treat an earlier ulcer was to:

1. Decrease tissue O_2 need by decreasing movement of the extremity.
2. Relieve itching of inflamed skin and subcutaneous tissue surrounding the ulcer.
3. Destroy bacteria and absorb inflammatory exudate from the ulcer base.
4. Stimulate healing of ulcerated tissue while preventing edema of surrounding healthy tissue.

55 • Which of the following measures will be ordered following Mrs. Wallace's vein stripping operation to prevent possible complications from the procedure?

1. Application of cold compresses over the path of the ligated vein.
2. Encasing the leg in pressure bandage from the toes to the groin.
3. Application of warm moist compresses over the ankle incision.
4. Immobilizing the legs with sandbags placed along the inner and outer aspects of the limb.

56 • Ella Schaff, an 18-year-old black woman with systemic lupus erythematosus, had been satisfactorily managed on a maintenance dose of prednisone when she suddenly developed fever, chest pain, and arthralgia. Medical workup revealed an oral temperature of 102°F, pulse of 100/min, respirations 24/min, cervical and axillary lymphadenopathy, hematocrit value 37 ml/100 ml, and red blood cells and proteinaceous casts in the urine. Ella's problems were diagnosed as an acute exacerbation of systemic lupus erythematosus, and she was hospitalized for treatment. In taking Ella's medical history at the time of hospitalization, the nurse should be alert for mention of which of the following as a possible cause for her exacerbation of illness?

1. Exposure to sunlight
2. Insect bites
3. Inhalation of paint fumes
4. Excessive alcohol consumption

57 • In planning for Ella's care during hospitalization, the nurse should assume that she will receive drugs of which type in treating this exacerbation of lupus?

1. Vitamins
2. Antibiotics
3. Anticoagulants
4. Immunosuppressives

58 • Which of the following nursing interventions would probably be most effective in increasing Ella's sense of well-being during hospitalization?

1. Scheduling frequent rest periods and 10 hours of sleep each night.
2. Encouraging frequent and vigorous oral hygiene with a stiff toothbrush.
3. Providing a hot shower soon after arising to increase joint mobility.
4. Applying talcum powder between skin folds to absorb perspiration.

59 • During their interactions, the nurse noted Ella's habit of referring to herself in negative, self deprecating terms. Which feature of her disease would probably contribute most to her negative self concept?

1. The speed and unpredictability with which her symptoms have exacerbated.
2. The facial disfigurement caused by the butterfly rash over the nose.
3. The waning of energy and strength with multiple system involvement.
4. The decrease in weight and loss of feminine body contours.

60 • Which type of diet would be most appropriate in combating Ella's weight loss and malnutrition?

1. High bulk, high vitamin, high liquid diet.
2. High carbohydrate, low protein, low fat diet.
3. High protein, high calorie, soft diet.
4. High calcium, low potassium, soft diet.

61 • Leo Helm, 18 years old, suffered a complete T_6 spinal cord injury when he was shot during a robbery attempt. A spinal fusion was performed to stabilize the spinal fracture and Taylor's back brace was used for support when Leo was allowed to sit in a wheelchair. For the first few weeks following his injury, the neurological examination of his lower extremities would reveal:

1. Absent deep tendon reflexes.
2. Hyperactive deep tendon reflexes.
3. Increasingly higher levels of sensory paralysis.
4. Decreasing levels of motor paralysis.

62 • During the 2 days that elapsed between Leo's hospital admission and the spinal fusion procedure, he could best be cared for if positioned on a:

1. Tilt table.
2. Circolectric bed.
3. Stryker's frame.
4. Recovery bed.

63 • Immediately following his injury, Leo was unable to urinate and his bladder was distended when he was brought to the hospital emergency room. He was catheterized on admission, with removal of 450 ml of yellow urine. The most likely cause for Leo's urinary problem is:

1. Renal ischemia.
2. Bladder laceration.
3. Spinal shock.
4. Autonomic hyperreflexia.

64 • In teaching Leo and his parents about needed bowel and bladder care, the nurse should inform them that, in time, Leo should regain some control over both functions because:

1. His initial bowel and bladder incontinence is due to anxiety as much as to nervous tissue injury.
2. Some of the severed spinal cord fibers will heal, reestablishing some control over bowel and bladder sphincters.
3. Return of parasympathetic nervous system activity will permit reflex emptying of bowel and bladder.
4. With training, collateral nerve fibers will develop and impulses will circumvent severed nerve pathways.

65 • The nurse should explain to Leo that, on recovery from spinal shock, he can expect to experience:

1. Return of sensation in the lower extremities.
2. Uncontrollable reflex movements of the legs.
3. Voluntary control of bowel emptying.
4. Reduction of post-void residual urine volume to less than 30 ml.

66 • Ken Beadle, a 22-year-old college student, sought medical attention for fever, malaise, nausea, and vomiting. Physical examination revealed scleral icterus, hepatomegaly and dehydration. Laboratory tests revealed prolonged prothrombin time, elevation of serum glutamic oxaloacetic transaminase (SGOT) and serum glutamic pyruvic transaminase (SGPT). Since hepatitis B surface antigen (HB_sAg) was not found in the serum, diagnosis of hepatitis A was made. Ken's health history on admission may reveal which of the following symptoms of hepatitis in addition to his complaints of fever, malaise, and vomiting?

1. Periorbital edema
2. Subcutaneous nodules
3. Dark urine
4. Tarry stools

67 • The nurse should base Ken's nursing care plan on the knowledge that which of the following will be needed to minimize liver cell damage during the acute phase of his illness?

1. Blood transfusion
2. Bed rest
3. High flow O_2 therapy
4. Induced hypothermia

68 • In teaching Ken how to prevent spread of viral hepatitis to his friends and relatives, the nurse should inform him that hepatitis A virus is most often spread by which route?

1. Fecal-oral contamination
2. Parenteral injection
3. Genital contact
4. Direct skin contact

69 • Which type of diet would be best suited for Ken during the acute phase of his illness?

1. Low sodium, high potassium, restricted fluids.
2. Low protein, low carbohydrate fluids.
3. Low calorie, high iron, high vitamin diet.
4. High protein, high carbohydrate, low fat.

70 • If Ken's symptoms are not relieved by rest, and persistent anorexia leads to malnutrition, which of the following drugs is apt to be ordered?

1. Thiamine
2. Cimetidine
3. Prednisone
4. Penicillin

71 • Belle Trask, 35 years old, had been treated for psoriasis for several years with coal-tar ointment, when she consulted her physician because of a severe exacerbation of skin lesions. He discontinued the coal-tar ointment and ordered a corticosteroid cream to be applied to Mrs. Trask's skin lesions. In addition to application of coal-tar ointment, Mrs. Trask's previous treatment would probably have included:

1. A cold shower T.I.D. to constrict skin vessels and decrease inflammation.
2. Daily removal of softened skin scales in an oatmeal bath.
3. Liberal application of talcum powder to absorb excess skin moisture.
4. Use of infrared light to apply heat to subcutaneous fat and connective tissue.

72 • The prescribed corticosteroid cream should be applied in which fashion?

1. Apply a thin film of cream, rub it into the skin, apply an occlusive dressing, and leave overnight.
2. Apply a thick layer of cream over the most severe lesions, and leave the area open to air.
3. Remove scales with brisk scrubbing in a warm bath, then apply cream to hemorrhagic areas.
4. Apply cream only to areas of intact skin between psoriatic plaques and scales.

73 • After 2 weeks of treatment with corticosteroid cream, Mrs. Trask's lesions were less severe, and the physician initiated PUVA therapy, i.e., a combination of orally administered methoxsalen (psoralen) and ultraviolet light, wavelength A. The nurse should inform Mrs. Trask that the function of psoralen is to:

1. Increase the production of vitamin D by epithelial cells.
2. Constrict blood vessels in the skin and subcutaneous tissue.
3. Block histamine release from mast cells.
4. Absorb ultraviolet energy and affix it to epithelial cell nuclei.

74 • While receiving PUVA therapy, Mrs. Trask can minimize its complications by:

1. Avoiding sun exposure on the 2 days a week that she receives therapy.
2. Taking the methoxsalen on an empty stomach between meals.
3. Refraining from bathing on the day of treatment.
4. Avoiding the use of oily lotions and bath preparations.

75 • In preparing Mrs. Trask for self care at home, the nurse should warn her against:

1. Oily skin lubricants and lotions.
2. Transmission of infection to others.
3. Removing skin scales and crusts.
4. Bogus cures for psoriasis.

76 • When coal-tar ointment, corticosteroid cream, and PUVA therapy are not effective in treating psoriasis, which of the following drugs is sometimes used to relieve symptoms?

1. Hydroxychloroquine
2. Penicillamine
3. Aurothioglucose
4. Methotrexate

77 • Ed Wiggins, 45 years of age, sought medical attention for recurring episodes of vertigo. Results of audiometry, a caloric test, and electronystagmography led the physician to diagnose Ménière's disease. The physician prescribed bed rest, diphenhydramine (Benadryl) and diazepam (Valium). In addition to vertigo, Mr. Wiggins' health history is apt to reveal that he has also experienced which of the following symptoms?

1. Decreased hearing acuity
2. Fine muscle tremor
3. Momentary visual loss
4. Unilateral numbness and tingling

78 • During an acute attack of Ménière's disease, Mr. Wiggins will be most comfortable in which position?

1. Sitting upright with the neck hyperextended.
2. Sitting with head resting on crossed arms on an over-the-bed table.
3. Low Fowler's position with eyes closed.
4. Lying on the side of the unaffected ear.

79 • Until symptoms of the acute attack abate, which of the following devices should the nurse provide to protect Mr. Wiggins from injury?

1. Bed side rails
2. Cloth hand restraints
3. Sandbags alongside the head
4. Padded tongue blade

80 • Following institution of bed rest and administration of parenteral diphenhydramine and diazepam, Mr. Wiggins' vertigo slowly diminished in intensity over a period of 4 days. To minimize his vertigo during this time, the nurse should advise him to avoid:

1. Eating solid food.
2. Sitting upright.
3. Exposure to glaring light.
4. Turning the eyes to the side.

81 • Bertha Schultz, 60 years of age, consulted her physician with complaints of burning pain and a vesicular eruption over the left side of her back and the lower anterior area of her chest. The character and distribution of the pain and skin lesions led to a diagnosis of herpes zoster. The physician prescribed bed rest, calamine lotion, and propoxyphene, and scheduled the patient for a follow-up visit in 3 weeks. During this follow-up visit, the physician performed a complete physical examination, Papanicolaou's cervical smear, proctoscopic examination, chest x-ray, complete blood count, and urinalysis to detect evidence of:

1. Allergy.
2. Vitamin deficiency.
3. Neuromuscular disease.
4. Malignancy.

82 • On Mrs. Schultz's following visit to the physician, the doctor's office nurse should question Mrs. Schultz specifically regarding:

1. Presence and severity of neuritic pain.
2. Amount and character of urinary output.
3. Her appetite for protein and fatty foods.
4. Known contacts with children with infectious diseases.

83 • In preparing Mrs. Schultz to care for herself at home, the nurse should instruct her to notify her physician in the event that:

1. The skin vesicles rupture or crusting develops.
2. The pain becomes stabbing in nature.
3. Vesicles develop in the peri-ocular region.
4. Scars remain after resolution of the skin vesicles.

84 • In addition to calamine lotion and propoxiphene, which of the following types of drugs are frequently ordered for the patient with herpes zoster?

1. Antihistamines
2. Antibiotics
3. Anticonvulsants
4. Antipyretics

85 • In preparing Mrs. Schultz to provide self care, the nurse should teach her to apply calamine lotion in which fashion?

1. Spray the calamine lotion on the vesicles, let dry, and immediately remove the residue with a hot shower.
2. Apply the calamine lotion sparingly on only the opened vesicles and cover with a pressure dressing.
3. Paint the vesicles with calamine lotion and cover the area with a piece of plastic to prevent drying of the lesions.
4. Apply calamine lotion liberally to the rash, let dry, and cover with cotton batting to prevent trauma to vesicles.

86 • Leon Ward, 45 years old and obese, complained to his physician of heartburn after meals and during the night. A chest x-ray and upper gastrointestinal barium x-rays revealed a hiatus hernia. The physician ordered a 1200-calorie reducing diet and antacids and advised Mr. Ward to stop smoking. In addition to losing weight and giving up smoking, the nurse should advise Mr. Ward to avoid which of the following in order to prevent heartburn?

1. Protein foods
2. Physical exercise
3. Heavy lifting
4. Carbonated beverages

87 • On examining the patient, the physician noted that Mr. Ward was recovering from a recent cold and bronchitis. This observation would probably lead the physician to order which of the following as part of Mr. Ward's current therapy?

1. Antibiotic
2. Antihistamine
3. Expectorant
4. Cough suppressant

88 • What of the following tests should be used in order to identify possible complications of Mr. Ward's disorder?

1. Gastric washings
2. Schilling's test
3. Bronchoscopy
4. Stool guaiac test

89 • In preparing Mr. Ward for self care, the nurse should advise him to do which of the following to prevent episodes of heartburn?

1. Eliminate bulk and fiber from the diet.
2. Sleep with the head of the bed elevated 6 inches.
3. Drink a cup of warm milk at bedtime.
4. Lie down for a brief nap after each meal.

90 • Mr. Ward should be advised that which of the following types of diet will decrease the frequency and severity of heartburn?

1. Hourly intake of a mixture of milk and cream.
2. Frequent small bland meals.
3. High protein, high fat, low carbohydrate.
4. High fiber, high vitamin, high liquid.

91 • Joe Holt, 25 years of age, sought medical attention for weakness and markedly enlarged cervical lymph nodes. When a lymph node biopsy specimen revealed Hodgkin's disease, Joe was treated with 4500 rads of total lymphoid radiotherapy over a 4-week period. In taking Joe's medical history at the time of his initial visit to the physician, the office nurse would be likely to learn that in addition to cervical adenitis, he had experienced which other symptom?

1. Pruritus
2. Shaking chills
3. Eructation
4. Vertigo

92 • In preparing Joe's parents to care for their son during his 4 weeks of radiation therapy, the nurse should inform them that all but which of the following are common untoward effects of total lymphatic irradiation?

1. Dry mouth
2. Dysphagia
3. Dyspnea
4. Skin rash

93 • Joe and his parents should be given the following advice concerning the care of the skin in the area of irradiation:

1. Protect irradiated skin areas from exposure to wind and direct sunlight.
2. Apply zinc oxide ointment to the skin of the treated area to prevent fissuring.
3. Shave the treatment area daily to remove hair and standardize radiation exposure.
4. Wash the irradiated area thoroughly after each treatment with warm water and soap.

94 • After 3 weeks of radiation therapy, Joe developed an area of itching, redness, burning, and oozing on the skin of the left supraclavicular region. The radiologist ordered that vitamin A and D ointment be applied to the area. The preferred method for application would be to spread the ointment:

1. Liberally over the irritated area, cover with a gauze square, and seal the edge with adhesive tape.
2. Thinly over the reddened area, cover with a plastic square, and seal the edges with water resistant type.
3. On a gauze square, apply the dressing to the irritated skin, and secure with a halter made of tubular elastic dressing.
4. On a piece of sterile gauze and fasten the gauze to the inside of the patient's clothing over the area of irritation.

95 • In order to answer questions from Joe and his parents about long-term treatment of his disease, the nurse should expect that, if his disease continues to progress to a more advanced stage, Joe will probably be treated with which of the following drug combinations?

1. Hydroxychloroquine, penicillamine, and gold salts.
2. ACTH, prednisone, and desoxycorticosterone acetate.
3. Ampicillin, gentamycin, and chloramphenicol.
4. Nitrogen mustard, vincristine, and prednisone.

96 • Olive Sipe, 43 years of age, had suffered with hemorrhoids for many years. When she was no longer able to relieve hemorrhoidal pain and itching with applications of commercial lubricants and anesthetics, she consulted a proctologist, who diagnosed both internal and external hemorrhoids and scheduled Mrs. Sipe for a hemorrhoidectomy. In taking Mrs. Sipe's health history, the nurse should be aware that all *but which one* of the following may predispose to development of hemorrhoids?

1. Chronic constipation
2. Multiple pregnancies
3. Arteriosclerosis
4. Hereditary predisposition

97 • Mrs. Sipe's pre-operative preparation will probably include:

1. Holding all food for 24 hours and holding all liquid for 12 hours before surgery.
2. Administering serial enemas until return solutions are clear on the evening before surgery.
3. Administering a tap water enema 2 or 3 hours before surgery.
4. Inserting a bisacodyl (Dulcolax) suppository 2 hours before surgery.

98 • When Mrs. Sipe is returned to her room following surgery, the nurse may expect to find which of the following in place?

1. Nasogastric tube
2. Intravenous fluid line
3. Indwelling catheter
4. Rectal tube

99 • Which of the following types of drugs will be given Mrs. Sipe to prevent post-surgical complications?

1. Anticoagulant
2. Antibiotic
3. Stool softener
4. Cholinergic

100 • Which of the following treatments will be ordered on the first post-operative day to relieve post-operative discomfort?

1. Small, low tap water enema
2. Warm sitz baths
3. Ice pack to the perineum
4. Glycerine suppository

Answer Sheet for Medical Surgical Nursing Practice Questions

Question	1	2	3	4
1.	‖	‖	‖	‖
2.	‖	‖	‖	‖
3.	‖	‖	‖	‖
4.	‖	‖	‖	‖
5.	‖	‖	‖	‖
6.	‖	‖	‖	‖
7.	‖	‖	‖	‖
8.	‖	‖	‖	‖
9.	‖	‖	‖	‖
10.	‖	‖	‖	‖
11.	‖	‖	‖	‖
12.	‖	‖	‖	‖
13.	‖	‖	‖	‖
14.	‖	‖	‖	‖
15.	‖	‖	‖	‖
16.	‖	‖	‖	‖
17.	‖	‖	‖	‖
18.	‖	‖	‖	‖
19.	‖	‖	‖	‖
20.	‖	‖	‖	‖
21.	‖	‖	‖	‖
22.	‖	‖	‖	‖
23.	‖	‖	‖	‖
24.	‖	‖	‖	‖
25.	‖	‖	‖	‖
26.	‖	‖	‖	‖
27.	‖	‖	‖	‖
28.	‖	‖	‖	‖
29.	‖	‖	‖	‖
30.	‖	‖	‖	‖
31.	‖	‖	‖	‖
32.	‖	‖	‖	‖
33.	‖	‖	‖	‖
34.	‖	‖	‖	‖
35.	‖	‖	‖	‖
36.	‖	‖	‖	‖
37.	‖	‖	‖	‖
38.	‖	‖	‖	‖
39.	‖	‖	‖	‖
40.	‖	‖	‖	‖
41.	‖	‖	‖	‖
42.	‖	‖	‖	‖
43.	‖	‖	‖	‖
44.	‖	‖	‖	‖
45.	‖	‖	‖	‖
46.	‖	‖	‖	‖
47.	‖	‖	‖	‖
48.	‖	‖	‖	‖
49.	‖	‖	‖	‖
50.	‖	‖	‖	‖
51.	‖	‖	‖	‖
52.	‖	‖	‖	‖
53.	‖	‖	‖	‖
54.	‖	‖	‖	‖
55.	‖	‖	‖	‖
56.	‖	‖	‖	‖
57.	‖	‖	‖	‖
58.	‖	‖	‖	‖
59.	‖	‖	‖	‖
60.	‖	‖	‖	‖
61.	‖	‖	‖	‖
62.	‖	‖	‖	‖
63.	‖	‖	‖	‖
64.	‖	‖	‖	‖
65.	‖	‖	‖	‖
66.	‖	‖	‖	‖
67.	‖	‖	‖	‖
68.	‖	‖	‖	‖
69.	‖	‖	‖	‖
70.	‖	‖	‖	‖
71.	‖	‖	‖	‖
72.	‖	‖	‖	‖
73.	‖	‖	‖	‖
74.	‖	‖	‖	‖
75.	‖	‖	‖	‖
76.	‖	‖	‖	‖
77.	‖	‖	‖	‖
78.	‖	‖	‖	‖
79.	‖	‖	‖	‖
80.	‖	‖	‖	‖
81.	‖	‖	‖	‖
82.	‖	‖	‖	‖
83.	‖	‖	‖	‖
84.	‖	‖	‖	‖
85.	‖	‖	‖	‖
86.	‖	‖	‖	‖
87.	‖	‖	‖	‖
88.	‖	‖	‖	‖
89.	‖	‖	‖	‖
90.	‖	‖	‖	‖
91.	‖	‖	‖	‖
92.	‖	‖	‖	‖
93.	‖	‖	‖	‖
94.	‖	‖	‖	‖
95.	‖	‖	‖	‖
96.	‖	‖	‖	‖
97.	‖	‖	‖	‖
98.	‖	‖	‖	‖
99.	‖	‖	‖	‖
100.	‖	‖	‖	‖

Section

ANSWERS AND RATIONALES FOR MEDICAL SURGICAL NURSING PRACTICE QUESTIONS

1. (1) In chronic subdural hematoma, the symptoms are similar to those of a brain tumor and include variable degrees of intellectual impairment, fluctuating levels of consciousness, hemiparesis, and, occasionally, convulsive seizures. Momentary visual losses from which the patient recovers completely, within an hour or two, are characteristic of transient ischemic attacks resulting from platelet emboli that are released from the carotid bifurcation into the ophthalmic artery. Nystagmus is characteristic of labyrinthitis. Drainage of cerebrospinal fluid from the external ear canal is seen in basal skull fracture.

2. (3) In testing a patient's ability to follow simple commands, the test imposed by the nurse should not also require the patient to exercise motor dexterity, memory, or abstract reasoning; these are different central nervous system functions and should be tested separately.

3. (3) Impaired ventilation causes CO_2 retention. When the concentration of CO_2 and hydrogen ions increases in the brain's arterial blood supply, there is reflex dilation of cranial vessels, with increased intracranial pressure, which may cause further decline in the patient's level of consciousness.

4. (4) Since consciousness is the highest function of the brain and since consciousness tends to recede and return in a predictable continuum, level of consciousness is the most reliable index of neurological status. Abnormal eye movements or motor activity, or both, could signify peripheral nerve damage as well as central nervous system damage, so they are less valuable indices of overall neurological status than is a change in the level of consciousness.

5. (4) If the blink reflex is absent, the eye should be protected against injury from a foreign body by instillation of sterile mineral oil or artificial tears, closing the lid (and securing with nonallergic tape if necessary), and covering the eye with a shield. Regular adhesive tape would irritate the sensitive periorbital tissues. Cleansing the lid margin would remove crusts but would not protect against corneal drying. Manual movement of the lids is not sufficient to lubricate the conjunctiva and cornea with tears.

6. (1) Change from supine to upright position causes the secretions that have pooled in dilated bronchial segments during sleep to shift to adjacent undilated segments, stimulating the cough reflex and resulting in expectoration of a large volume of secretions.

7. (3) The Valsalva's maneuver, or forceful expiration against a closed glottis, commonly occurs during coughing. It causes increased intrathoracic pressure, which results in decreased venous return to the right atrium and decreased left ventricular output, with consequent cerebral ischemia. Therefore, paroxysms of coughing in a person with decreased cardiac reserve or impaired cerebral circulation could cause transient syncope.

8. (3) A semi-Fowler's (semi-sitting) position with the arms at the sides supported on pillows permits maximum chest wall expansion with least muscular effort. The semi-Fowler's position also fosters gravity drainage of respiratory secretions to the lung bases, leaving the upper and middle lobes clear for gaseous exchange.

9. (2) Expectoration of copious purulent sputum produces fetid breath and a bad taste in the mouth. Scrupulous oral hygiene before meals would eliminate the purulent debris and unpleasant breath odor that depresses appetite in the bronchiectatic patient. Vigorous exercise immediately before meals would tire the patient, depleting the energy available for the muscular work of eating. Postural drainage immediately before meals would stimulate paroxysms of coughing and diminish appetite. Although patients with bronchiectasis should have liberal fluid intake to liquefy secretions, administration of large volumes of fluid immediately before meals would distend the stomach and decrease appetite.

10. (4) Percussion and vibration of the chest wall will dislodge mucus that is adherent to the walls of bronchi and bronchioles so it can be removed by gravity and explosive coughing. Breathing into and out of a paper bag would increase the patient's $PaCO_2$, which is probably abnormally high. Although this patient should have liberal fluid intake, he should not drink water immediately before postural drainage treatments as the head lowered position would favor regurgitation of liquid from a full stomach. If the patient is unable to expectorate mobilized tracheobronchial secretions from the upper airway, the secretions should be aspirated using a sterile catheter and suction machine rather than a bulb syringe, the lumen of which would be easily obstructed by thickened mucus.

11. (4) In chronic renal failure, the patient is oliguric or anuric, therefore fluid intake is limited, often to 1200 or 1500 ml/day to prevent fluid overload; allowable liquid is distributed evenly throughout the day to prevent nocturnal dehydration. Forcing fluid would predispose to fluid retention, pulmonary edema, and general anasarca. Lotions should be applied to prevent the patient from scratching and infecting his extremely dry skin. Although a certain amount of activity is desirable to prevent skin pressure injury and hypostatic pneumonia, vigrous exercise should be avoided, as it would increase catabolism and cause negative nitrogen balance. Decreasing the flow of blood through the fistula even for short periods can cause clotting and obstruction. Therefore, the arm with the fistula must be protected from tight bandages, restrictive clothing, constrictive blood pressure cuffs, and infective venipuncture sites. Only Mr. Proximire's right arm should be used for venipunctures and blood pressure measurements.

12. (3) Many dialysis patients experience disequilibrium phenomena toward the end or after dialysis as a result of rapid removal of nitrogenous wastes, which creates an osmotic gradient between the blood and the tissues, causing cerebral edema. Generally, fluid-electrolyte balance is reestablished by the day following dialysis. The patient's position should be changed at intervals during the procedure to prevent skin pressure damage. Although some patients avoid eating during dialysis because the smell of food causes nausea, others become quite hungry owing to the loss of glucose and amino acids in the dialysate and ask to be fed during the procedure. Since the nurse or technician who attends the patient during dialysis will assess the effects of the procedure by monitoring vital signs, dialysate composition, and blood flow, the patient may sleep, read, listen to the radio, or enjoy other quiet pursuits during the dialysis.

13. (2) The patient on long-term hemodialysis need not limit protein intake. The protein eaten should contain complete amino acids (meat, fish, and milk) to replace the amino acids lost during dialysis and to maintain positive nitrogen balance. A high calorie intake is necessary to replace glucose lost

during dialysis, to prevent ketoacidosis, and to prevent utilization of protein as an energy source. Potassium should be restricted because the damaged kidney can no longer excrete potassium.

14. (4) Although all of the factors mentioned would contribute to marital stress between the hemodialysis patient and his wife, for most couples the patient's loss of potency constitutes the greatest source of psychological stress. Dialysis costs usually are paid by Medicare for eligible individuals. Personal contact between husband and wife may not be increased if the wife must take a job outside the home to support the family. Depending upon the activity patterns of patients before illness and treatment and the type of group activities in which family members like to engage, some husband and father hemodialysis patients actually may spend more time with their family after institution of hemodialysis than they did before illness and treatment.

15. (1) Since fluid is removed from the blood during hemodialysis, the procedure would diminish rather than increase the risk of pulmonary edema. Since the composition of dialysate is prescribed to prevent removal of calcium ions from the serum, carpopedal spasm due to hypocalcemia would not be an expected consequence of hemodialysis. Since the dialysate composition is prescribed to result in removal of potassium ions from the serum, hyperkalemic leg cramps would not be an expected outcome of treatment. To prevent clotting, heparin is added to the patient's blood as it enters the dialyzer. To counter later untoward effects, protamine sulfate is added to the blood returning from the dialyzer to neutralize the effects of heparin. In some patients a heparin rebound occurs within a few hours after dialysis because metabolic reactions break the heparin-protamine bond, and clotting time increases, so the patient may bleed from any of several sites.

16. (2) Pernicious anemia is an autoimmune disorder that is characterized by absence of the intrinsic factor, which is normally produced by parietal cells of the gastric mucosa and which is necessary for the body to absorb vitamin B_{12}. Lack of vitamin B_{12} causes glossitis, mental disturbances, symmetrical paresthesias, and loss of position and vibratory senses in fingers and feet, as well as megaloblastic anemia in which red blood cells are destroyed more rapidly than normal. The result is a marked decrease in red blood cell count (1 million to 1.5 million/mm^3) and a severe decrease in hemoglobin concentrations (5 gm/dl in some instances). The patient with pernicious anemia suffers from indigestion due to gastric achlorhydria, but abdominal distention is not an expected finding. Pernicious anemia gives rise to numbness and tingling in the lower extremities rather than to leg cramps. Severe decrease in hemoglobin concentration results in anoxia of vital tissues, such as the myocardium, with the result that anginal pain is a frequent problem.

17. (4) In addition to defective DNA synthesis, vitamin B_{12} deficiency blocks the synthesis of myelin, with resulting neuropathy, involving both peripheral nerves and the posterior and lateral columns of the spinal cord. These nervous tissue changes cause loss of position sense and muscle weakness. Padded plastic boots should be worn to maintain the feet at right angles to the lower leg and to prevent decubitus ulcers of ischemic heel tissues. There is no underlying joint or connective tissue pathology that would make a bed board necessary. Although weakness and immobility do predispose to pressure injury of the skin of the back and buttocks, the best way to protect Mrs. White from decubitus ulcers would be for the nurse to change Mrs. White's bed position every 2 hours since the patient will probably be too weak to use a trapeze for position changes. An inflatable rubber ring causes skin pressure damage to certain areas while relieving it in others.

18. (3) Pernicious anemia is not characterized by bleeding tendencies, and a certain amount of exercise will be needed to maintain muscle strength and joint motion. Until Mrs. White's severe anemia is relieved by treatment, she will be weak and easily fatigued, so her daily activities should be alternated with frequent rest periods to conserve energy and prevent injury due to falls. Since a sore mouth and tongue would make toothbrushing painful, cotton swabs and a mild alkaline mouthwash should be

used to clean the teeth, gums, and tongue. Since demyelination of peripheral nerves and sensory tracts of the spinal cord will have diminished Mrs. White's temperature perception and her anoxic tissues would be slow to heal following injury, she should be protected against burn injury by avoiding hot water bottles and heating pads.

19. (1) Lack of production of intrinsic factor, the underlying cause of pernicious anemia, is a permanent defect; Mrs. White must receive vitamin B_{12} injections for the rest of her life to remain symptom free. If she continues to receive vitamin B_{12} at regular intervals, her red blood cell count and hemoglobin concentration will gradually improve, and she will not require additional blood transfusions. Even if she continues to receive vitamin B_{12} on a regular basis, some of her neurological changes will be irreversible, though they will not increase in severity.

20. (2) Until Mrs. White's stomatitis and glossitis have subsided, it will be painful for her to eat coarse or highly seasoned foods. However, her food intake should not be limited to liquids, as that would encourage constipation in an immobilized elderly individual. Her protein intake should be adequate to facilitate red blood cell formation and tissue repair and should consist of complete proteins, i.e., those containing all of the essential amino acids.

21. (1) Excessive thyroid hormones increase the metabolic activity of most body cells, and thereby increase the amount of glucose oxidized to CO_2 and water. The excess body water of metabolism is excreted as perspiration, and the skin is warm and moist, not dry and flaky. The increased basal metabolic rate results in heat intolerance rather than cold intolerance. Greater central nervous system excitability results in a fine, rather than a coarse tremor of the hands, and this tremor is present at rest as well as with voluntary movement. Catabolism of muscle protein, infiltration of muscles with lymphocytes, and depletion of muscle glycogen stores lead to pronounced weakness of skeletal muscles, which is especially noticeable in the proximal muscles of the extremities.

22. (4) Potassium iodide is given to decrease the vascularity of the thyroid gland when surgical removal is planned. Propylthiouracil or methimazol is given when it is decided to use long-term medical therapy to block the formation of thyroid hormones. When hyperthyroidism is to be treated with radioactive iodine, propranolol (Inderal), a β-blocker, is given to decrease tachycardia, palpitations, diaphoresis, nervousness, and tremor until enough of the thyroid cells have been destroyed by ^{131}I (after about 3 weeks) to eliminate the symptoms of hyperthyroidism.

23. (1) Since the radioactive iodine that is not taken up by the thyroid gland is excreted in the urine, the patient should imbibe liberal quantities of fluids and empty the bladder at short intervals during the 24 hours following iodine administration so as to prevent irradiation of renal and bladder tissue. The ^{131}I is absorbed so rapidly from the stomach that contact between the drug and gastric mucosa is too brief to cause mucosal irritation, so dyspepsia and diarrhea do not occur.

24. (2) Until hyperthyroidism is relieved, Mrs. Tripp's sympathetic nervous system hyperactivity will make it difficult for her to obtain needed rest. Consequently, a tranquilizer, such as diazepam, may be ordered to relieve tension and promote mental and physical relaxation. An antihypertensive medication will not be necessary since slowing of the heart rate by propranolol will cause the blood pressure to decrease. A cardiotonic, such as digitalis, will not be necessary unless congestive heart failure develops. There is no reason to expect convulsions in the patient with hyperthyroidism.

25. (3) When exophthalmos is severe, the eyelids may not close completely during sleep, therefore the cornea becomes dry and irritated. Also, lymphatic infiltration and edema of the periorbital tissues cause decreased blink, so tears are not spread over the anterior surface of the eye as frequently as in normal individuals. Instillation of methylcellulose drops Q.I.D. will lubricate the anterior surface of the globe and prevent corneal and conjunctival irritation. Frequent irrigations with boric acid solution would tend to dry the conjunctiva and increase irritation. Glasses of any type would shield the eye from dirt and other particulate matter, but would not prevent corneal drying. Aspirin would relieve some of the discomfort associated with the eye changes but would not address the underlying cause of symptoms.

26. (3) If the bed's side rails are kept elevated and the nurse or a family member orients her to her surroundings at regular intervals, Mrs. Merkel should not need to be restrained with Posey's belt or cotton mittens. Neither an ice bag nor a cold pack would be applied to the eye, as the weight of either might cause rupture of the incision and loss of aqueous humor. The operated eye will be covered with a patch for 24 hours following surgery and with a patch and a metal shield at night to prevent accidental injury from the hands or the bed linen.

27. (1) The eyelashes are cut short before cataract surgery to prevent contamination of the operative field. The patient should be instructed to keep her eyes closed during the clipping, and petroleum jelly (Vaseline) should be applied to the blades of the scissors to keep the cut hairs from dropping into the patient's eye. The face should be washed well before surgery with hexachlorophene, but povidone-iodine and alcohol would cause skin irritation in many individuals, so they should be avoided.

28. (2) Since a head dependent position would increase intra-ocular pressure and increased intra-ocular pressure could cause hemorrhage within the eye, the patient should lie on the back with the head elevated 30 degrees to decrease intra-ocular pressure and prevent injury to the incision. Later, when the patient is allowed to lie on her side, she should turn only toward the side of the unaffected eye.

29. (3) In order to avoid the hazards of immobility, the patient will usually not be confined to bed throughout her entire hospitalization but may be allowed to ambulate to the bathroom with assistance soon after recovery from anesthesia. She should wear an eye patch and glasses during the day and an eye patch and shield at night to protect the eye but should not cover the eye with her hand for fear of accidentally dislodging glasses or shield and damaging the eye. She should be instructed not to squeeze her eyes shut, as this will increase intraocular pressure and may weaken the suture line.

30. (3) A sudden rise in intra-ocular pressure is usually accompanied by eye pain, nausea, and vomiting. Since, as a consequence of lens extraction, the outflow tract for aqueous humor may be obstructed, intraocular pressure may increase, causing intra-ocular hemorrhage. Because of the serious consequences of this complication, the physician should be notified immediately if the patient vomits following surgery. Since a local anesthetic is used for most cataract surgery, it would be unlikely that vomiting would result from an untoward effect from an anesthetic agent. Unless there is a rise in intra-ocular pressure, there should be no post-operative pain following cataract extraction. Post-operative anxiety might cause restlessness or behavioral changes but would not be expected to cause nausea and vomiting.

31. (2) Since Mrs. Merkel may be expected to self administer mydriatic drops or antibiotic ointment into the eye following hospital discharge, she should be taught how to apply such medications into the conjunctival sac without contaminating the eye and without injuring the eye. Use of an eyecup would be contraindicated because of the danger of mechanical injury to tissues newly operated upon. Neither warm moist compresses nor cold compresses would be applied to the eye unless inflammation or infection occurs.

32. (4) Acetazolamide is both a diuretic and a depressant of aqueous humor production. It acts by inhibiting the action of the enzyme carbonic anhydrase (which converts CO_2 and water to carbonic acid), thereby decreasing resorption of sodium, chloride, and potassium ions from renal tubules. Consequently, in some patients, the drug causes such symptoms of electrolyte imbalance as paresthesias, confusion, and anorexia.

33. (3) Elevated intra-ocular pressure gradually destroys bundles of optic nerve fibers at the nerve head. Since the fibers from the central fixation area are usually spared until late in the disease, the central visual acuity used in reading may be normal despite severe loss of peripheral vision. The ability to rotate and laterally abduct the eyes is

dependent upon action of extra-ocular muscles, which are not affected in glaucoma. Since the rods, which are responsible for color vision, are most numerous in the central, rather than in the peripheral retina, color vision is not lost early in glaucoma.

34. (1) Since injury to optic nerve fibers from increased intra-ocular pressure is irreversible, the peripheral vision that has already been lost will not be restored by iridectomy and trabeculectomy. If the procedure is successful in restoring aqueous drainage from the eye, there should be no further visual loss, either peripheral or central. Since it is possible for the surgically created pathway for aqueous drainage to become obstructed, the patient will require lifelong medical follow-up of the eye condition. If problems develop, miotics, β-blockers, or diuretics may again be prescribed to lower intra-ocular pressure.

35. (1) The patient should be kept flat and relatively immobile for 24 hours after trabeculectomy to prevent prolapse of the iris through the incision. Fowler's and side-lying positions would favor iris prolapse. Straining, coughing, squeezing the eyes shut, and the Trendelenburg position should all be avoided since they increase intra-ocular pressure.

36. (3) Following trabeculectomy and iridectomy, fluid intake need not be curtailed, mild exercise is permitted, and there is usually no restriction on use of the eyes. However, any activity that raises intra-ocular pressure, such as straining at stool, should be avoided; a high bulk diet and adequate fluid intake are therefore recommended, with stool softeners as needed to avoid constipation.

37. (3) Until drug therapy renders Tim's sputum noninfectious, he should be placed in a private room with noncirculating air flow and the discharge of room air to the outside. If the patient can comply with the instruction to cover his mouth and nose during coughing, to expectorate into paper wipes, and to dispose of sputum tissues in a closed container, staff and visitors need not wear cap, gown, and mask in the patient's room. Both patient and staff should wash hands frequently to eliminate organisms picked up from patient's tissues, linen, and skin. Ultraviolet light should be used to destroy tubercle bacilli in the patient's room, but the lamp should be positioned well above the direct line of vision of the patient or staff so as to prevent eye damage.

38. (3) The patient with active tuberculosis may have no symptoms or only mild constitutional symptoms until there has been extensive destruction of lung tissue. Weight loss is common but occurs in conjunction with anorexia rather than with polyphagia. Absorption of bacterial antigens from the pulmonary infection causes temperature elevation, which is most common in late afternoon and at night—giving rise to night sweats in some patients. Expiratory prolongation and wheezing would be suggestive of bronchospasm, which is not characteristic of pulmonary tuberculosis. Orthopnea and paroxysmal nocturnal dyspnea are characteristic of pulmonary edema, not an expected consequence of pulmonary tuberculosis.

39. (4) The expectoration of 5 ml of bright red blood would suggest that the tuberculous cavity has eroded into a bronchial artery. Placing Tim on his right side would splint the chest and minimize bleeding, while facilitating drainage of blood from the lung. Bronchial irritation is not an expected effect of the drug therapy.

40. (4) Antituberculous drugs have proved most effective when the full daily doses of both are administered at the same time on an empty stomach to achieve a peak concentration of both drugs simultaneously. Administering either drug in divided doses or administering the two separately would prevent a daily peak concentration of both and would diminish their antibacterial effect.

41. (1) The following high and medium residue foods are usually eliminated from the diet in ulcerative colitis in order to decrease colonic spasms: milk, raw fruits and vegetables, dried fruits, fried foods, whole grain cereals, nuts, and relishes. Refined cereals, baked and mashed potatoes, and roasted or broiled meats are permitted.

42. (2) Since sulfasalizine causes agranulocytosis in some patients, sudden sore throats and repeated infections should be reported so that blood studies can be performed. Those sulfonamides that are freely absorbed from the gastrointestinal tract (sulfasalizine is absorbed to a lesser extent) are more apt to cause nervous tissue injury, liver damage, or renal damage; therefore, deafness, jaundice, and edema would be unlikely occurrences during sulfasalizine therapy.

43. (2) Both sodium and potassium are lost in large quantities in diarrheal stools. Since aldosterone conserves sodium at the expense of potassium, serum potassium levels are apt to decline more than serum sodium levels. Thus, serum sodium levels may decrease somewhat but would not be elevated. Neither hypercalcemia nor hypophosphatemia, which are characteristic of hyperparathyroidism, would be expected in ulcerative colitis. Rather, diarrheal stools would lead to increased intestinal loss of calcium, with hypocalcemia.

44. (3) To empty the bowel and prevent peritoneal contamination during the operation, the patient is given a clear liquid diet for several days to reduce food residue in the colon and is given an anti-infective that is poorly absorbed from the intestinal flora. Neither laxatives nor cathartics are used to empty the bowel because thinning and increased friability of the bowel wall would predispose to perforation. Repeated enemas tend to weaken the debilitated patient, so enemas may be limited to 2 or 3 rather than continuing the irrigations until the enema returns are clear.

45. (3) It is necessary for the patient to wear an ileostomy collection device continuously when the ileum is sutured directly to the anterior abdominal wall. In a pouch ileostomy, an intra-abdominal reservoir is formed from a small loop of terminal ileum in which a nipple valve is constructed to promote continence. Although a collection device must be worn over the pouch opening immediately after surgery, the pouch slowly increases in size for the 1st 6 months post-operatively, so that eventually the pouch will hold 500 ml of liquid stool, which can be drained with a catheter several times a day. Since the small bowel contents are liquid, the time of ileostomy emptying cannot be controlled by dietary regulation. When a pouch colostomy is created, the rectum is not left in place for later anastomosis to the terminal ileum.

46. (4) When the ileostomy collection bag is changed, the skin surrounding the stoma should be washed with soap and water and covered with a protective coating of a gelatinous protective substance, which will coat and protect the skin from digestion by intestinal enzymes. Karaya is a dried gummy plant substance that will protect the skin from excoriation by irritating substances while permitting healing of underlying tissues. Because it is sticky, it will facilitate adherence to the ileostomy bag faceplate to the abdominal skin. Because it becomes gelatinous in coming into contact with a liquid, it will form a water tight seal between drainage bag and skin, and prevent leakage of fecal material. Both tincture of benzoin and zinc oxide ointment will soothe irritated skin and promote healing, but neither will protect skin from digestion by intestinal enzymes. Talcum powder would be useless in protecting the skin around the ileostomy.

47. (1) Fluids are withheld for 8 to 12 hours before the test so that fluid depletion will facilitate concentration of the radiopaque dye, providing clearer definition of the walls of the renal pelvis, ureter, and bladder. Since the kidneys are retroperitoneally placed, feces and gas must be removed from overlying bowel in order to facilitate x-ray visualization of urinary tract structures. A cathartic, such as castor oil, given on the night before the test will usually empty the bowel before the x-ray must be taken. If not, an enema or a suppository can be used on the morning of the test to ensure bowel evacuation. However, since some patients do not respond to suppositories for a half hour or more, the suppository should be inserted more than 2 hours before the urogram.

48. (3) For the first 24 hours following creation of an ileal conduit, the patient's urinary output should be measured every hour to determine whether ureteral-ileal conduit suture lines remain intact. Suction is not needed to ensure urinary drainage, as urine is moved through ureters and conduit by peristalsis. The ureteral catheters are inserted to splint the ureters during healing and not to permit irrigation of the renal pelvis. Fluid intake should not be restricted, as concentrated urine is apt to become infected and would be irritating to peristomal skin.

49. (1) Dusky color of stomal tissue may indicate embarrassed blood supply and potential necrosis of the ileal conduit and should be reported immediately. It is expected that the stomal tissue will be edematous for some time following surgery, taking 4 to 6 weeks to shrink to normal size. Normally, urine has an ammonia-like odor. If the collection pouch faceplate does not fit closely enough around the stoma, urine will irritate the peristomal skin and cause reddening.

50. (4) Cranberry juice ensures an acid urine, which discourages bacterial growth; liberal fluid intake dilutes any microorganisms that may be present in the urine. The ileal conduit is not connected in any way to the intestine, so ingestion of gas-forming foods and liquids would have no effect on ureteral function. During the day, the pouch should be emptied at 2-hour intervals to prevent stagnation of urine, which would encourage bacterial growth. During sleep the pouch should be connected to a bedside drainage bag. The pouch is irrigated with a white vinegar solution to control odors rather than to prevent urinary infection.

51. (4) Because the blood vascular system is circuitous in design, a chronic pressure increase in any part of the system is referred backward through the circuit. Therefore, venous obstruction causes capillary congestion, which in turns slows arterial blood flow. Exercise cramps in the legs indicate muscle anoxia, which can result from slowing of arterial flow and capillary congestion as well as from arterial occlusion by atheromatous plaques. Calf pain on foot dorsiflexion and tenderness over the involved vein are more characteristic of phlebitis than are exercise cramps. Carpopedal spasms are characteristic of hypocalcemia.

52. (2) Eight hours of sleep in a 24-hour period with the foot of the bed elevated 6 inches plus frequent elevation of the legs throughout the day is advised to minimize venous congestion in patients with varicose veins. Elastic stockings that extend above the knee tend to bind the popliteal space while sitting, so knee-length elastic stockings are preferred for the patient with varicose veins. The patient tends to sink so far back in a soft, deep upholstered chair that pressure is applied to the popliteal area; therefore, a high hard chair with a narrow seat is less apt to obstruct venous flow. Regular walking is advised since muscular contraction forces blood through the veins and prevents pooling. Prolonged standing and sitting are discouraged.

53. (3) In the Trendelenburg test the limb is elevated so the superficial veins will empty by gravity. A tourniquet is applied and the patient is brought to a standing position. If superficial veins remain empty, the valves in the communicating veins between the deep and superficial veins are competent. If superficial veins fill within 30 seconds, valves in the communicating veins are incompetent. To assess competence of the deep veins, a tourniquet is placed at the thigh when the patient is standing in order to fill the superficial veins; then the patient lies down with the legs elevated. If blood empties promptly from the superficial veins, the deep venous system is patent, and it will be possible to remove superficial varicose veins by surgical stripping.

54. (4) Unna's paste boot is a roller gauze dressing that is impregnated with a mixture of zinc oxide, glycerine, and gelatin, and is applied cast fashion to the ulcerated leg and covered with an elastic bandage. The dressing controls tissue edema by compression, protects the ulcer against trauma from furniture and shoes, and the zinc oxide stimulates granulation at the wound margins. Zinc oxide, glycerine, and gelatin do not have an antiseptic effect. If leg immobilization is needed to control edema, the patient should be on complete bed rest. If the patient experiences itching sensations as the ulcer begins to heal, Unna's paste boot will keep him from scratching the wound and contaminating it.

55. (2) Since bleeding may occur from torn branches of the saphenous vein, the entire limb is wrapped with a pressure bandage, and the foot of the bed is elevated from 6 to 9 inches when the patient is supine. Ambulation is begun 24 to 48 hours after surgery to prevent venous stasis and thrombosis of deep leg veins. Neither heat nor cold should be applied to the limb, as direct heat could burn edematous and poorly nourished tissues, and cold would constrict superficial vessels and delay heal-

ing of tissues traumatized by passage of the stripping wire.

56. (1) Systemic lupus erythematosus is an autoimmune disorder involving inflammation of vascular and connective tissue in multiple body organs. When the disorder is quiescent, exacerbations can be provoked by emotional stress, trauma, and ultraviolet radiation, such as exposure to sunlight. Insect bites, paint fumes, and alcohol have no known effect on the disease.

57. (4) Since the symptoms of systemic lupus erythematosus result from the deposition of antigen-antibody complexes on target tissues, immunosuppressive drugs, such as azathioprine, nitrogen mustard, and cyclophosphamide, may be given to block the autoimmune reaction. Although adenopathy is seen in systemic lupus erythematosus, the disease is not infectious. Intradermal bleeding (purpura) rather than intravascular clotting is another characteristic.

58. (1) Because systemic lupus erythematosus is characterized by generalized weakness and severe fatigue, the patient will need from 10 to 12 hours of sleep each night and should have several rest periods scattered throughout the day. Systemic lupus erythematosus is characterized by a variety of skin problems, among which are dry scaling, erythema, maculopapular rash, angioedema, urticaria, and ulceration. The skin should be kept clean and free of powders, which increase skin inflammation. Cool baths will decrease itching and scaling in some patients. Moisturizing lotions will relieve itching and cracking of dry, flaking skin. Painless ulcers of the oral mucosa are common, so cotton-tipped applicators and mild mouthwashes should be used for oral hygiene.

59. (2) In a young woman, facial disfigurement is especially threatening to the body image and self esteem. Since the butterfly rash over the nose and malar eminences of the patient with lupus frequently doesn't disappear when the disease is in remission, the patient may suffer this stigma of the disease for months or years. While loss of strength, changes in body contour, and uncertainty as to prognosis are all stressful to the patient with lupus, these problems offer less threat to her self concept and self esteem than does facial disfigurement.

60. (3) Ella's weight loss is due, in part, to anorexia, which may result from dysphagia secondary to esophageal inflammation. Therefore, a high calorie and high protein diet that is soft in consistency will facilitate ingestion of sufficient protein to replace tissue loss and sufficient carbohydrate to prevent catabolism of protein as an energy source. The patient will undoubtedly need vitamin and iron supplements to reverse the normocytic normochromic anemia that is common in systemic lupus erythematosus.

61. (1) During the period of spinal shock, which may last from 6 to 10 weeks following traumatic injury to the cord, superficial and deep reflexes are absent below the level of injury because impulses are not being transmitted through the inflamed or edematous (or both) cord segment. Following resolution of spinal shock, superficial and deep tendon reflexes will return below the level of the lesion. From the time of injury, which resulted in complete cord transection, Leo will be without movement or sensation below the level of the lesion, and the level of his motor and sensory paralysis will not change.

62. (3) Prior to fixation of Leo's thoracic vertebrae by the fusion procedure, his spine must be aligned and immobilized to prevent additional injury to the spinal cord and spinal nerves from ragged bone fragments. Placement on the Stryker's frame will maintain the spine in proper alignment while permitting turns from supine to prone position to relieve skin pressure. While the patient in a Circolectric bed can also be turned from supine to prone position, the weight that is placed on the fractured vertebrae as the patient's body rotates from supine to vertical to prone position may cause bony displacement and cord or nerve injury. The recovery bed will be too soft to immobilize the spine in anatomical position. A tilt table would not permit position change without pressure on the fractured vertebrae.

63. (3) Complete and sudden transection of the cord results in spinal shock or sudden loss of continuity between that portion of the cord below the injury and higher nerve centers. During spinal shock, which lasts from 2 to 6 weeks following injury, all motor activity, sensation, and reflexes are absent below the level of the injury. Loss

of the bladder emptying reflex (S_2, S_3, S_4 cord levels) leads to bladder distention. If hypovolemic shock had resulted from Leo's gunshot wound and he had suffered renal ischemia as a result, his kidney would not be producing urine. If the bladder had been lacerated by passage of the bullet, there would be blood in his urine. Autonomic hyperreflexia, which occurs in patients with spinal cord injuries above T_6 and is characterized by episodic hypertension, upper body flushing and sweating, and lower body pallor and chilling, may be caused by bladder distention but is not a cause of bladder distention.

64. (3) Following resolution of spinal shock, cord reflexes below the level of cord injury will return, and certain triggering stimuli can be used to provoke the bladder emptying reflex or bowel emptying reflex at desired habit times. Nerve fibers within the central nervous system cannot regenerate following injury, and collateral fibers do not develop to reroute impulses around interrupted tracts. Leo's incontinence results from bowel and bladder paralysis due to interruption of micturition and defecation reflexes mediated through S_2, S_3, S_4 segments of the cord.

65. (2) The patient should be forewarned that, on resolution of spinal shock, the return of spinal cord reflexes below the level of injury will give rise to uncontrolled leg movements in order that he will not misinterpret these reflex movements as indication of cord healing and reversal of paralysis. Since his cord transection is complete, sensation will not return below the level of injury and he will never regain voluntary control of bowel emptying. The amount of urine left in the bladder following bladder contraction is determined by the strength of the detrusor muscle and the integration of bladder contraction and sphincter relaxation.

66. (3) Viral hepatitis causes diffuse inflammation and necrosis of liver cells. Because damaged liver cells can no longer remove bilirubin from the serum and excrete it in the bile, stools become clay colored and bilirubin in the blood is excreted by the kidneys, causing the urine to be mahogany colored. Tarry stools indicate bleeding high in the gastrointestinal tract, which is not a consequence of hepatitis. Subcutaneous nodules are an index of connective tissue disorder rather than of hepatitis. Although the damaged liver cell is unable to produce serum albumin in normal amounts, periorbital edema is not an expected finding in viral hepatitis.

67. (2) In order to reduce the metabolic work of the liver cells and to maximize hepatic blood flow, the patient should remain at complete bed rest during the phase of acute liver cell inflammation and necrosis. The fever of acute hepatitis will respond to liberal fluid intake so neither ice packs nor hypothermia blankets will be necessary treatment. Inflammatory swelling rather than anoxia or anemia is the cause of liver cell death, so neither O_2 therapy nor transfusion will be required.

68. (1) Hepatitis A virus is most often transmitted by ingestion of foods and fluids that have been contaminated by the feces of an infected individual. Consequently, the patient with hepatitis A should be placed in a private room, and caregivers should wear gown and gloves when handling the patient's body fluids, feces, bed linen, and skin areas that could have been contaminated by his saliva and feces. Hepatitis A virus can be transmitted by parenteral injection but is less frequently spread in this manner than is hepatitis B virus. Hepatitis B virus is found in semen and vaginal secretions, but hepatitis A virus is not. Either hepatitis A or B can be spread by direct contact with areas of the patient's skin that have been contaminated by body fluids and excretions, but this is the less common route of transmission for hepatitis A virus than is the fecal-oral route.

69. (4) To maintain adequate nutrition in the presence of severe anorexia and vomiting, a high calorie, high carbohydrate, high protein diet should be given in frequent small feedings. Fat should be limited during the icteric phase because bile is not being secreted into the bowel. Protein is needed to permit liver cell regeneration and shouldn't be limited unless symptoms of impending hepatic coma are seen. There is no need to limit sodium, and liberal rather than restricted fluids will be needed to combat infection and inflammation.

70. (3) The anti-inflammatory effect of prednisone can relieve swelling of liver cells and obstruction of bile channels. Corticosteroids also increase the patient's sense of well-being and improve appetite. Ken's anorexia is due to nausea resulting from disturbed digestion, so it is unlikely to respond to vitamin B_1. Hepatitis virus is not killed by penicillin. Cimetidine, a histamine H_2-receptor antagonist, reduces acid production in peptic ulcer. Ken's problem is anorexia, not dyspepsia.

71. (2) The purpose of coal-tar ointment is to slow down the accelerated proliferation of epidermal cells. After the ointment has softened the scales, they should be removed by gentle friction in an oatmeal bath. Warmth, rather than cold, has a beneficial effect on psoriatic lesions. Ultraviolet light, rather than infrared light, is helpful in treating psoriasis.

72. (1) Steroid creams are used for their anti-inflammatory effect in the basal skin layer, so the cream should be rubbed into the skin and covered with an occlusive dressing to enhance tissue penetration. If left open to air, the cream would not penetrate but would dry and fall off.

73. (4) Psoralen is a photosensitizing substance that increases the absorption of ultraviolet light, which in turn blocks DNA replication in epithelial cells, thereby slowing cell proliferation.

74. (1) Since methoxsalen increases sensitivity to ultraviolet rays and it takes from 6 to 8 hours for the drug to be eliminated from the body, sun exposure should be avoided on the day of PUVA therapy in order to prevent excessive ultraviolet radiation exposure and sunburn. Methoxsalen causes nausea in some patients, which can be minimized by taking the drug with food. Bath oils are used to help moisten and remove scales during the daily bath.

75. (4) Because psoriasis is resistant to treatment and the lesions of psoriasis are disfiguring, victims of the disease waste a great deal of money on patent remedies promising quick and permanent cures of the disease. Patients should be informed that though psoriasis is characterized by remissions and exacerbations, there is no cure for the disease and it should be treated only by a reputable dermatologist. Deliberate removal of crusts is part of the prescribed treatment for psoriasis, which is neither infectious nor contagious. Skin lubricants and bath oils should be used to prevent skin drying, cracking, and itching.

76. (4) Since psoriasis is characterized by too rapid proliferation of epithelial cells, when less severe therapies fail, methotrexate, a folic acid antagonist, is given to slow cell replication by inhibiting cellular RNA and enzyme synthesis. Hydroxychloroquine, penicillamine, and aurothioglucose are used in treatment of rheumatoid arthritis.

77. (1) Ménière's disease, a disorder of the labyrinth of the inner ear, is characterized by sudden attacks of severe and disabling vertigo. Preceding these attacks, the patient often experiences tinnitus and deafness, and in connection with these attacks, the patient experiences an increased hearing loss with each one. A fine tremor is characteristic of hyperthyroidism. Momentary visual loss may result from discharge of platelet emboli from the carotid bifurcation into the ophthalmic artery. Unilateral numbness and tingling would suggest a cerebrovascular accident.

78. (4) The rotational vertigo experienced during a Ménière's attack is so severe that the individual cannot walk without falling, and nausea and vomiting occur. To relieve these symptoms the patient may instinctively assume a characteristic posture of lying on the unaffected ear and looking toward the affected ear.

79. (1) Since the vertigo of Ménière's disease causes loss of balance and a tendency to fall in the direction of the affected ear, the bed's side rails should be elevated at all times to keep the patient from falling out of bed. There is no need to immobilize his head with sandbags, as he will probably instinctively turn to his side. Cloth hand restraints would be undesirable since the patient should move about slowly in bed to prevent skin pressure injury. A padded tongue blade is unnecessary, as convulsions are not a manifestation of Ménière's disease.

80. (3) Glaring light and sudden or jarring movement will increase vertigo. However, the patient should be encouraged to move about in bed slowly to prevent skin pressure and to minimize frustration and depression. Because vertigo and nausea discourage the patient from eating the

nurse should encourage intake of any food or fluids that the patient will accept. The patient may sit upright to eat and bathe. He will experience less discomfort if the nurse stands directly in front of him during conversation, as sudden turning of the head or eyes may increase vertigo. However, when recumbent, the patient may instinctively turn his eyes toward the involved ear to relieve dizziness.

81. (4) Herpes zoster results from inflammation of nerve fibers by the varicella virus. It is believed that after a case of chickenpox has run its course, the causative virus lies dormant in nerve cells and may be reactivated and multiply to cause a rash of vesicles along the course of ganglia of posterior nerve roots. This reactivation tends to occur in patients with depressed immunocompetence due to malignancy or irradiation.

82. (1) In a few patients, severe prolonged postherpetic neuralgia causes depression and, occasionally, habituation to analgesic drugs. Dependence to propoxyphene can develop with prolonged use. Herpes zoster does not affect appetite or renal function. It is believed that herpes zoster results from reactivation of a latent varicella infection rather than from exogenous infection.

83. (3) The varicella virus may attack any of the sensory nerves. Involvement of the ophthalmic branch of the trigeminal nerve could cause keratitis, uveitis, and corneal ulceration; therefore, if vesicles develop in or around the eye, the patient should be referred to an ophthalmologist.

84. (1) Since the vesicular rash of herpes zoster is characterized by intense itching as well as by sharp pain, an antihistamine is usually prescribed to decrease discomfort and ensure restful sleep. Neither antibiotics nor topical antiseptics would be necessary unless the vesicles become secondarily infected by scratching. Fever is not present in all patients with herpes zoster and when present is usually mild or moderate in degree. The varicella virus attacks peripheral nerve ganglia rather than the motor cortex, so does not cause convulsions.

85. (4) Calamine lotion is applied to the lesions for its cooling, drying, and antipruritic effects; therefore, it should be applied liberally to cover the entire rash, allowed to dry, covered with cotton to protect the vesicles from rupture, and left in place until time for reapplication. A hot bath or shower would increase itching. A plastic wrap would prevent drying and crusting of vesicles.

86. (3) Heartburn occurs with hiatus hernia because the upper portion of the stomach slides through the diaphragmatic hiatus into the thorax, and acid gastric juice is retained in the herniated segment of stomach, causing ulceration and bleeding. Since increased intra-abdominal pressure favors gastric herniation through the hiatus, the patient should be cautioned against coughing, heavy lifting, and straining at stool. The patient should engage in regular exercise that does not require sudden changes in position or bending at the waist. Although protein does stimulate secretion of gastric juice, it is the gastric herniation and retention of acid in the herniated segment of stomach that causes pyrosis not protein intake per se.

87. (4) Coughing increases intra-abdominal pressure. An increase in intra-abdominal pressure precipitates gastric herniation through the diaphragmatic hiatus, and prolonged coughing often occurs during resolution of bronchitis; therefore, a cough suppressant would be used to eliminate a common cause for gastric herniation. If Mr. Ward is recovering from a cold and bronchitis, he will not need antibiotics or antihistamines. An expectorant would stimulate rather than decrease coughing.

88. (4) Since retention of acid gastric contents in the herniated portion of the stomach may cause ulceration and bleeding, a stool guaiac test should be done to detect bleeding from the upper portion of the gastrointestinal tract. Gastric washings are used to aspirate swallowed sputum to examine for *Mycobacterium tuberculosis*. A Schilling's test is used to detect a lack of gastric intrinsic factor in pernicious anemia.

89. (2) Since a head dependent position would encourage the gastric cardia to slide through the diaphragmatic hiatus into the thorax, the patient should remain erect after meals and should elevate the head of the bed when sleeping. Since the presence of food in the stomach stimulates secretion of acid gastric juice, the patient should avoid bedtime snacks.

90. (2) Frequent small servings of chemically bland foods will decrease gastric secretions and minimize gastric irritation. A high fat intake, such as a milk and cream diet, will delay gastric emptying and encourage retention of acid gastric juice in the herniated segment of stomach. A high fiber, high liquid diet would minimize constipation and eliminate straining at stool, but the high fiber would be mechanically irritating to inflamed gastric mucosa.

91. (1) A severe and generalized pruritus, the cause of which is unknown, may occur even before enlargement of superficial lymph nodes in Hodgkin's disease and is a prominent and distressing symptom in the late stage of the disease. Patients may complain of dyspnea or dysphagia due to pressure of cervical or mediastinal nodes on the trachea or esophagus, but eructations and vertigo are not characteristic of the disease. Although the patient with Hodgkin's disease frequently has evening fever and night sweats, chills are not a feature.

92. (3) The rapidly dividing cells of the skin and gastrointestinal mucosa are especially susceptible to radiation injury, so skin rash, dry mouth, and dysphagia result from a radiation injury. Dyspnea, if it occurs, is more apt to result from tracheal obstruction by enlarged cervical or mediastinal nodes than from radiation mucositis.

93. (1) Medicated ointments and powders should be avoided in patients receiving radiation therapy, as heavy metals, e.g., zinc, which are included in such preparations would increase the radiation dose. Since the irradiated skin is exceedingly sensitive to mechanical, chemical, and physical trauma, it should be washed with water only, should be protected from exposure to sun and wind, and should be unshaved.

94. (4) Because skin that is traumatized by radiation injury is also easily traumatized by friction, the patient should not wear constrictive clothing or dressings over areas of skin irritation and breakdown.

95. (4) In stage III Hodgkin's disease the patient is given chemotherapy in conjunction with radiation therapy. The drugs most often used in chemotherapy of Hodgkin's disease are a combination of 3 or 4 drugs: nitrogen mustard, vincristin (Oncovin), procarbazine (Matulane), and prednisone.

96. (3) Hemorrhoids are dilated sacculated veins of the anal canal, which result from increased pressure in the hemorrhoidal plexus, and are caused by hereditary weakness of venous walls, occupations requiring prolonged sitting or standing, increased abdominal pressure, straining at stool, repeated pregnancies, heart failure, and cirrhosis. Arteriosclerosis is an arterial rather than a venous disorder.

97. (3) Since it is necessary to empty the lower colon but not the entire bowel before hemorrhoidectomy, either a laxative given the evening before surgery or an enema given to 2 to 3 hours before surgery will clear the operative field. Holding all food for 24 hours would weaken the patient unnecessarily. Serial enemas or a rectal suppository could irritate the hemorrhoids and cause bleeding.

98. (4) Because there may be considerable post-operative bleeding from the surgical site if a ligature slips, a rectal tube may be well lubricated and left in place to facilitate removal of blood and flatus from the lower bowel. Neither post-operative ileus nor post-operative urinary retention would be a likely consequence of rectal surgery. The operative blood loss is not sufficient to require intravenous fluid therapy.

99. (3) Since passage of constipated stool would traumatize the operated area and the patient may avoid defecating following hemorrhoidectomy to avoid pain, a stool softener should be given. Because hemorrhage is a possible post-operative complication, an anticoagulant would be contraindicated. A cholinergic would be ill advised because it would stimulate peristalsis. An antibiotic would be unnecessary unless a post-operative infection should develop.

100. (2) Warm sitz baths will clean the operative suture line, relieve rectal pain, and increase circulation to the rectal area. Either a rectal suppository or an enema could traumatize the operative area.

UNIT IV

Psychiatric Nursing

Section

PSYCHIATRIC NURSING CONTENT OUTLINE

Psychiatric nursing interventions are applicable not only to the psychiatric nursing area but to virtually every clinical nursing area in which the professional might be practicing. Abnormal behavior can be viewed from two perspectives, and the nursing profession utilizes both when applicable. Abnormal behavior can be thought of as behavior that deviates from a given culture's norms, or it can be thought of as behavior that interferes with the well-being of the individual or the groups of which he is a member. One must ask, "Does this behavior foster the well-being of the individual or the group, or both, and does it promote self actualization?" The 1978 Institute of Mental Health report listed the following estimated incidences of major maladaptive behavior patterns in the United States:

1. One million individuals are actively schizophrenic.
2. Over 53 million people suffer mild to moderate depression.
3. 20 million people suffer from neurotic disturbances.
4. 10 million people report problems related to alcohol.
5. Approximately 26,000 people commit suicide each year.

Nursing embraces the physical and emotional assessment, care, and evaluation of these individuals in all professional practice areas.

THEORETICAL FRAMEWORKS FOR UNDERSTANDING HUMAN BEHAVIOR

Medical-Biological Model

Psychosocial Model

Psychoanalytical
Behaviorist

Humanistic
Interpersonal
Sociocultural
Interdisciplinary

I. Medical-Biological Model

A. Genetic Factors
1. Can provide a foundation for predisposition.
a. Down's syndrome
b. Affective disorders
c. Alcoholism

B. Biochemical Factors
1. Neurotransmitters
a. Catecholamines; deficiency in norepinephrine possible causal factor in depression; surplus of norepinephrine possible causal factor in mania.
b. Dopamine—decreased uptake may contribute to schizophrenia.
c. Serotonin—deficiency found in both depressed and manic persons.
2. Hormones

Stress may cause imbalance and changes in the endocrine system that in turn may trigger abnormal behavior.
3. Blood components
a. Vitamin deficiencies may cause schizophrenia.
b. Taraxein, an abnormal blood protein, may cause schizophrenia.

C. Biological Deficiencies
1. Severe malnutrition prenatally.
2. Severe malnutrition during 1st 6 months of life.
3. Altered metabolism of glucose in the brain of schizophrenics.

D. Sleep Deprivation
1. After 40 sleepless hours, psychotic-like symptoms can appear.

II. Psychosocial Model

A. Psychoanalytic

Developed by Sigmund Freud; all behavior and symptoms are caused by internal factors and significant events and are meaningful to either the conscious or unconscious mind. The beginning of neurosis has its roots in the phallic stage of development (ages 3 to 6 years)
1. Psychic structures
a. Id—consisting of instincts, biological drives, and survival impulses.
b. Ego—operates on the reality principle and controls impulses from the id and demands of the superego. Helps person engage in acceptable behavior.
c. Superego—the conscience and the ego ideal that the person strives to achieve.
2. Ego defense mechanisms; utilized if anxiety cannot be managed by the person's usual coping mechanisms. They are learned behaviors and are relatively automatic and habitual.
a. Repression—the most important *unconscious* defense mechanism in that it keeps anxiety producing situations out of conscious awareness.
b. Denial—refusal to acknowledge a painful or unacceptable thought, feeling, behavior, or event.
c. Introjection—taking on the beliefs, attitudes, and behaviors of an idealized other.
d. Projection—placing one's unacceptable feelings, thoughts, or impulses onto another person.
e. Displacement—placing unacceptable feelings, such as anger, onto a safe person or object.
f. Isolation—repression of affect (feelings) surrounding an event, though all details can be recalled and talked about.
g. Rationalization—logical, socially acceptable reason to justify maladaptive behavior.
h. Reaction formation—unacceptable feelings and thoughts are repressed, and socially correct behavior is substituted in their place.
i. Undoing—a method of atonement for unacceptable behaviors, thoughts, or feelings, such as offering apologies, doing penance, or undergoing punishment.
j. Identification—enhances feelings of worth as an individual; uses someone as a model and mimics their behavior.
k. Regression—a return to behavior that was used at an earlier developmental stage.

B. Behaviorist

This model began with the early work of Pavlov. Modern day theorist B. F. Skinner is the present day contributor to this discipline.
1. Basic principle is that all behavior is learned; research has focussed on environmental stimuli and their effects on acquisition, modification, and eradication of human responses.
a. Respondent conditioning—a response elicited by a stimulus.
b. Operant conditioning—individual makes a response in order to achieve a desired goal.
c. Reinforcement may be positive or nega-

tive; used to encourage and strengthen the desired response.

C. Humanistic

Abraham Maslow, Carl Rogers, and Fritz Perls shaped this approach.

1. Basic principle is the belief in the human being's ability to understand conscious and unconscious thoughts, to be aware of past events, and to utilize this information for self-direction and self-actualization.
   a. Focus is on values and personal growth.
   b. Holds a positive view of human nature and man's potential.
   c. Individual's sense of identity and relation to the world is important.

D. Interpersonal

Harry Stack Sullivan developed this framework. Theory focuses on positive or negative relationships between people. Social experiences are important.

1. Three modes of experience
   a. Prototaxic mode occurs during infancy. Child experiences self and environment as one undifferentiated entity.
   b. Parataxic mode may be experienced by children and adults and involves utilization of fantasy, magical thinking, and cause and effect thinking.
   c. Syntaxic mode is characterized by consensual validation. Communication utilizes mutually understood symbols and language between preadolescence, adolescence, and adulthood.
2. Anxiety occurs due to poor interpersonal relationships, disrupts interpersonal relationships, and can be relieved by participating in more secure interpersonal relationships.

E. Sociocultural

Maladaptive behavior may be caused by abnormal conditions in the surrounding environment and not by faulty internal processes.

1. If individuals become so mentally disordered that they cannot control their behavior or survive without the help of others, their behavior is considered abnormal in *any* society.
2. Cultural factors influence which form the disorder takes and its course.
3. How the individual is received and treated, and what the culture's expectations are for that individual will influence the outcome.
4. Culture influences the way psychological disorders are expressed by the individual.

F. Interdisciplinary

Though each of the theoretical frameworks discussed has merit, it is clear that no one theory can explain mental disorders. Usually, factors impact on the individual from several of these frameworks. The nurse should utilize the interdisciplinary approach that assesses the medical-biological, the psychosocial, and the sociocultural factors that are of concern to the individual. The nurse practices within an interdisciplinary team comprised of physicians, psychologists, social workers, occupational and recreational therapists, and fellow nurses.

PSYCHOSEXUAL, PSYCHOSOCIAL, AND INTERPERSONAL DEVELOPMENTAL MODELS

A. Freudian theory

Development occurs in 5 stages. Failure to achieve completion in 1 developmental area precludes the individual from progressing to the next stage.

1. Oral stage—birth to 18 months; gratification and security are primary goals. Defense mechanisms of denial, introjection, and projection develop now and are used to reduce tension.
   a. Nursing assessment would elicit information regarding feeding difficulties, sleeping patterns, and growth record.
2. Anal stage—ages 2 through 3 years; control is the mastery issue at this level, and the issue revolves around toilet training. Reaction formation and undoing are defense mechanisms used during this stage.
   a. Nursing assessment would elicit information regarding toilet training, early personality traits, developmental milestones achieved, and personal spontaneity.
3. Phallic stage—ages 3 to 6 years. Oedipal complex is resolved as male child deals with issues regarding castration anxiety. Female child resolves the Electra complex as she deals with hostility toward mother and penis envy. Child eventually identifies with parent of same sex. Repression, displacement, conversion reactions, and phobias or fetishes develop during this period.
   a. Nursing assessment would explore relationships with family members, fears, dreams, regressions, and anxiety levels.
4. Latency stage—school age. Child begins to

develop mastery in social skills; begins to identify with children of the same sex, joins clubs with children of same sex, and begins separation from home and family. Defense mechanisms of reaction formation, isolation, repression, and displacement may develop during this phase and are characterized as neurotic.

a. Nursing assessment would elicit the child's interest in the community and school programs, activity level, and performance in school.

5. Genital stage—adolescence. Sexual energy becomes focussed on a member of the opposite sex. Individual struggles with dependence versus independence. Coping mechanisms developed during this phase are sublimation, rationalization, suppression, and identification, which are mature defenses.

   a. Nursing assessment would include school performance, interest in the opposite sex and dating, attitudes toward sex, and peer group involvement.

B. Eriksonian theory

Does not stop at adolescence as Freud's theory does. Addresses psychosocial development throughout the life cycle. Developmental tasks need to be accomplished during each stage, but the most important factor is that the person's conscious experience of the world is *most* important in shaping that person's self perception. Along with Freud, Erikson believes that each stage must follow the other in an orderly sequence, because each developmental process builds upon its predecessor.

1. Trust versus mistrust—birth to 18 months. Need security and consistent caretaking. Loss of the primary caretaker would be a real developmental threat.
   a. Nursing assessment—evaluate maternal-infant bonding and any early losses or separations.
2. Autonomy versus shame and doubt—ages 2 to 3 years. Muscle control is heightened, and the child begins to move about and impact on his surroundings. As in Freud's theory, anal retention or expulsion is a focus for the child's and parent's attentions.
   a. Nursing assessment would elicit information on developmental milestones, such as walking and talking, and types of reactions to separation from the mother or the primary caretaker.
3. Initiative versus guilt—ages 3 to 6 years; successful completion of the autonomy phase prepares the child for taking on new tasks, which build self esteem. As in Freud's theory, there is rivalry for mother, but in successful completion of this phase, there is eventual identification with the same sex parent that results in reduction of guilt.
   a. Nursing assessment determines activity level of the child, the early personality traits of the child, and family relationships.
4. Industry versus inferiority—ages 6 to 11 years; child is heavily engaged in social mastery skills outside the home and is working on independence from parents versus dependence upon parents. Family support of his individual successes is important at this stage.
   a. Nursing assessment—any behavior problems, the quality and quantity of child's friendships, hobbies, academic achievement, and childhood illnesses or diseases.
5. Identity versus role diffusion—12 to 18 years; as the individual develops sexually, there will be sexual and societal experimentation. During the child's struggle into adulthood any previously unresolved developmental tasks will emerge. Authoritative parents who provide control and support are important for the child at this stage.
   a. Nursing assessment—ascertain academic performance, community involvement, and friendships.
6. Intimacy versus isolation—adolescence to young adulthood; a personal identity involving commitment to work and acknowledgement of the social and interpersonal needs of the individual emerge. One can achieve intimacy with another without giving up the self. The ability to love another provides for further development in the individual.
   a. Nursing assessment—determine the work status, social involvement, and whether there is a significant other. Is there any sexual activity?
7. Generativity versus self absorption—the developmental task of middle age. Births of children and contributions to work and to society play a key role.
   a. Nursing assessment—evaluate significant relationships, work history, and hobbies.
8. Integrity versus despair—a need to develop personal self acceptance is crucial here. Self realization of accomplishments and past successes leads to contentment and feeling of not being threatened by the following generation.

a. Nursing assessment—evaluate the individual's physical health, available support systems, and social involvement.

C. Sullivanian theory

Proposes 7 developmental stages that occur as the individual matures in relation to the interpersonal interactions in the environment. Two major goals are the satisfaction of biological needs and of the need for security and relating at an interpersonal level.

1. Infancy—birth to 18 months; prototaxic mode of experiencing. As in the Freudian and Eriksonian models, the primary task is to feel secure and develop trust. Oral gratification is important, and the infant moves into interpersonal intimacy with the mother if biological needs are met.
   a. Nursing assessment—what is or was the anxiety level between mother and child during interpersonal interactions, such as feeding, bathing, changing diapers, and putting to bed?
2. Childhood—1½ to 6 years; development of language moves the child through the prototaxic and parataxic modes of interacting to the syntaxic behavioral mode.
   a. Nursing assessment—determine what the reactions to others in the child's environment are, how separations from significant others are handled, and what the ability to accommodate behavior to social expectations is.
3. Juvenile era—grade school years; increased socialization with peers; learns to get along with authority figures other than parents. Child becomes competent in performance and expression as skill of distinguishing between fantasy and reality is developed.
   a. Nursing assessment—identify developed personality traits, performance anxiety (if present), and social experiences.
4. Preadolescent era—ages 9 through 12 years. Development of same sex friends (interpersonal relationships) with whom to share thoughts and feelings. An ability to love someone else occurs during this phase. Sexual intimacy is not a component of this stage.
   a. Nursing assessment—determine the quality and quantity of friendships.
5. Early adolescent era—interpersonal development now centers on relationships with members of the opposite sex. The ultimate goal is an integration of a need for security, a need to be free from anxiety, and a need for intimacy. This goal can be achieved only if the self is stable.
   a. Nursing assessment—elicit information regarding relationships with the opposite sex, level of self esteem, evidence of antisocial behavior, and social successes.
6. Late adolescence—the self system should stabilize during this phase. The individual works on establishing a place for himself within society. Developmentally, it is important to have a consistent and loving relationship with another individual.
   a. Nursing assessment—evaluate for job and social success.
7. Adulthood—adult role is assumed. Genital consistency is achieved; therefore, anxiety is decreased, and the adult is able to consistently invest in other interpersonal relationships.

THERAPEUTIC INTERVENTIONS IN PSYCHIATRIC DISORDERS

Psychiatric nursing embraces the notion of the therapeutic use of self in establishing a relationship with a patient and in implementing therapeutic interventions. Nursing interventions are based on theoretical frameworks that embrace the biological, sociological, and psychological disciplines. Pertinent concepts from any or all of these therapeutic interventions may be utilized in order to provide holistic care for the patient. Psychiatric nursing is the diagnosis and treatment of human responses to actual or potential health problems in order to promote, maintain, and restore the individual to the optimal level of functioning. The nursing process (assessment, analysis, planning, intervention, and evaluation) and a clinical practice based on a biopsychosocial theoretical framework provide the individual with holistic care. Nursing roles include that of the interviewer, the supporter, the teacher, the counselor, and the collaborator.

The following qualities are essential for the psychiatric nurse: acceptance of the patient as a human being; acceptance of *all* behavior as meaningful and as a response to a need; consistency with each patient over time; and conveyance of a feeling of warmth, acceptance, and genuine interest.

I. Communication Theory

A. Two types of communication
   1. Verbal includes all written and spoken messages.
   2. Nonverbal consists of behavior such as facial expression, position of the body, movement of the body, and respirations.

B. Function of the communication
   What does it accomplish?

C. Communication techniques
   1. Conveyance of a feeling of warmth, respect, genuineness, and empathy.
   2. Active listening—nurse attends to all that the patient has to say. Nurse does *not* impose her own agenda, but empathizes with what the patient is communicating. Nurse should not be a partial listener, should not be on the defensive, and should avoid giving advice. Be aware of the speaker's feelings and watch his non-verbal behavior.
   3. Nurse is non-judgmental and is accepting both in verbal and non-verbal behavior.
   4. Utilizes silence—allows time for patient to gather thoughts and feelings for verbal expression. Indicates acceptance of patient who is mute or withdrawn.
   5. Refrains from using "why" questions (they are difficult to answer) and questions that can be answered with a simple "yes" or "no."
   6. Open ended communication is utilized to allow patient to expand and provide information.
   7. Clarifies and explores topics when appropriate.
   8. Encourages exploration and description of feelings.
   9. Requests illustration to clarify a meaning.
   10. Provides a "mirror" for the patient
       a. "You appear angry."
       b. "I feel that you. . . ."
       c. Patient may then validate the observation or provide other information. Confirms or negates the nurse's perception.
   11. Rephrasing—in order to provide clarity for the therapist conversation can be rephrased, allowing the patient to validate the therapist's understanding or to provide more information.
   12. Reflecting—allows the therapist to make observations to the patient in regard to thoughts and feelings expressed and the congruency of the behavior on the part of the patient.
   13. Structuring in order to provide guidelines or create order.
   14. Offers a collaborative and cooperative relationship. The patient is an active partner in care.
   15. Uses appropriate self disclosure to build trust.
   16. Aids patient in evaluating significant others, experiences, and situations that provoke stress; enables problem solving.
   17. Summarizes each session; emphasizes important points, provides reality orientation for those with thought disorders, and serves as a method of terminating the session.

D. Barriers to communication
   1. Conveyance of the therapist's own feelings, such as anxiety, anger, and ambivalence toward the patient. It is the patient's needs and issues that are to be addressed.
   2. An appearance of being too busy or too stressed. Makes patient feel he should not bother the nurse.
   3. Using slang, jargon, or too much medical vocabulary. Be aware of economic, cultural, religious, and sexual implications during verbal interactions.
   4. Using "Band-aids" or glib statements, such as, "Don't worry. Everything is going to be just fine."
   5. Do not use trite expressions or clichés, such as "bummer," "awesome," or "Youth is wasted on the young."
   6. Judgmental or opinionated behavior.
   7. Expressing unnecessary approval.
   8. Expressing unnecessary disapproval.
   9. Advice giving; patients get plenty of advice from significant others. Provide opportunity for patient to do his own problem solving.
   10. Talking about personal experiences.
   11. Probing questions; therapist appears to be punitive.
   12. Misuse of confrontation; confrontation is a technique that must be carefully considered before being implemented.
   13. Not taking seriously the patient's feelings. This attitude invalidates the experience for the individual.
   14. Interpreting and analyzing patient's communication.
   15. Changing the subject; this implies disinterest on the part of the listener. Active listening precludes this from happening.
   16. Becoming defensive if patient states negative feelings regarding the physicians, the nurses, the treatment plan, or the hospital. Patient has a right to feelings, and they should not be negated.
   17. Ordering, directing, commanding, threaten-

ing, moralizing, and giving "shoulds and oughts."

II. Psychoanalytical Therapy

The nurse does not engage in psychoanalysis, but as a member of the interdisciplinary team, she should be cognizant of the techniques that are used. Also, a firm understanding of the concepts and the vocabulary is needed in order to interact appropriately.

A. Key concepts
   1. Free association—individual says whatever comes to mind, no matter how painful or seemingly irrelevant. Free association brings to light long repressed materials that will aid in awareness and will increase understanding.
   2. Dream interpretation—repressive forces are weakened during sleep and dreaming, so repressed material will surface in dreams.
      a. Manifest content—that material which is readily apparent to the dreamer.
      b. Latent content—that material which is disguised and symbolic to the dreamer.
   3. Analysis of resistance—at some point the analysand may resist—may show an unwillingness to talk about certain feelings, individuals, or events. Since the resistance keeps painful material from surfacing, the resistance must be analyzed. The material can then be brought forward and dealt with.
   4. Analysis of transference—transference occurs when the individual transfers feelings and attitudes onto the analyst that originated from a significant other. In response to these feelings, the analysand responds toward the analyst as he did toward the significant other.
   5. Counter-transference—the mixture of feelings that the therapist may have for the patient.

III. Person Centered Therapy

Major psychotherapy developed by Carl Rogers in the 1940s.

A. Primary objective of therapy—aid client in accepting and being himself.
B. Task of the therapist—be non-directive, noninterpretive, and listen attentively. Restatement of what the therapist hears is done in a non-judgmental manner.
C. Focus is on the client's present problems—not on past issues.
D. Unconditional positive regard, warmth, empathy, and genuineness are valued characteristics of the therapist.

IV. Behavior Therapy

Short-term therapy aimed at the individual who has not learned the skills necessary for coping with problems in living or the person who has acquired faulty coping patterns that are being maintained by reinforcement.

A. Primary objective of therapy is to change identified problem behavior.
B. Task of the therapist is to modify the behavior by manipulating environmental reward or punishment. Reinforcement should directly follow the desired behavior. The client should know what behavior is expected, what the reinforcement is, and why the reinforcement is given.
C. Focus is on an immediate problem caused by maladaptive coping behavior. The goal of therapy is to bring the desired responses under the control and self monitoring ability of the client.
D. Techniques
   1. Extinction—behavior will weaken and disappear if it is not reinforced.
   2. Systematic desensitization—used in cases where avoidance is the chief problem.
      a. By staying away from the anxiety provoking stimuli (e.g., snakes, elevators, or spiders), the anxiety is reduced.
      b. Client is taught to behave in a manner that is incompatible with anxiety while in the presence of the noxious stimulus.
      c. Joseph Wolpe's 3-pronged approach consists of relaxation training (one cannot be relaxed and anxious at the same time), the construction of hierarchies (a list of stimuli listed in rank order according to the amount of anxiety they provoke), and the desensitization procedure.
   3. Desensitization procedure
      a. Client implements previously learned relaxation techniques.
      b. Therapist directs client to imagine anxiety provoking scene while completely relaxed.
      c. When anxiety is experienced the session is terminated.
      d. Procedure is repeated until client can vividly imagine the most anxiety provoking scene in the hierarchy without experiencing anxiety.
   4. Aversion therapy—behavior is modified through the use of punishment.

a. A drug such as disulfiram (Antabuse), which makes an individual physically ill if they drink alcohol, is an example.
b. Electric shock administered after the undesired behavior occurs is utilized as well.
c. In order for this therapy to be effective the punishment must be appropriate and understood by the client, it must be delivered *every* time the undesired behavior occurs, and it must be delivered *immediately* after the undesired behavior occurs.

5. Positive reinforcement—good response is elicited to this technique in institutional settings. The reinforcement must be something that the individual wants or likes.
   a. Response shaping—every time the desired behavior occurs a reinforcement is forthcoming. (Child picks up toys and puts them away and is reinforced with a piece of candy.)
   b. Modeling—a therapist, a significant other, teacher, or a friend models the desired behavior for the client. Client, in turn, mimics the behavior. All of us are continually learning new, desirable behavior in this manner.
   c. Token economies—tokens (a form of positive reinforcement) are given when desired behavior occurs. Tokens can then be exchanged for something the individual values or desires. For the hospitalized patient the exchange might be for the privilege to leave the unit, a pass to walk around the neighborhood for a defined period of time, or a weekend visit home.
6. Behavior contracting—therapist and client agree on behavioral changes to be made and identify exactly which behavioral changes are to be exhibited by the client and how they will be rewarded. This contract is often in writing and signed by client and therapist.
7. Assertiveness training—for people who cannot "speak up" in an interpersonal situation owing to previous conditioning or lack of role modeling. Useful when the lack of appropriate assertiveness can be traced to maladaptive anxiety in interpersonal situations.
8. Biofeedback training—processes thought to be involuntary have been demonstrated to be modifiable by the operant and classical conditioning learning procedures. Migraines, asthma in children, and high blood pressure are some of the physiological responses that can be altered with this procedure.

V. Cognitive-behavioral Therapy

Based on the belief that cognitions (thoughts) influence both our motivation and behavior. Using learning principles, the therapist aids the client in altering cognitions so that desirable behavior will result.

A. Rational emotive therapy (RET)

Originated by Albert Ellis.

1. Important concepts of therapy
   a. Client holds irrational beliefs. ("I must be loved by everyone for everything I do.")
   b. Irrational beliefs lead to self defeating behavior.
   c. Self defeating behavior leads to self devaluation.
2. Task of therapist
   a. Dispute the false beliefs using rational confrontation.
   b. Teach the client to identify and dispute the irrational beliefs.
   c. Assist client to change thoughts and behaviors.

B. Cognitive restructuring therapy

Developed by Aaron Beck for the treatment of depression.

1. Important concepts
   a. Depression results from negative beliefs about the self, the world, and the future.
   b. Beliefs are held by the client in spite of evidence to the contrary because of the following:
      (1.) The client *selectively* perceives the world as harmful and ignores evidence to the contrary.
      (2.) Client *overgeneralizes* to all situations on the basis of limited experiences.
      (3.) Client *magnifies* the undesirable event.
      (4.) "All or none" thinking—everything is terrible, and they are worthless.
2. Task of therapist and focus of therapy
   a. Therapist and client identify together the negative beliefs and false assumptions held by the client.
   b. Experiences are designed that will result in rewards for the client.
   c. Evaluation of the experiences by therapist and client.
   d. Client encouraged to monitor any underlying assumptions present that are leading to self defeating behavior.
   e. Client is taught to continually monitor cognitions and to challenge whether they are true or not.

VI. Family Therapy

The important concept in this therapy is that the "identified patient" is often "the tip of the iceberg" of a much larger family problem. In order for the patient to be "cured," the entire family must be treated.

A. Conjoint family therapy
   Developed by Virginia Satir.
   1. Focus of therapy
      a. Change the faulty communication among the family members.
   2. Task of therapist
      a. Therapeutic use of self on the part of the therapist encourages family members to inspect and evaluate communication, interactions, and relationships among the family members.
      b. Improve faulty communications, interactions, and relationships among the family members.

B. Structured family therapy
   Based on a systems approach developed by Salvadore Minuchin. Family systems therapy was first developed by Murray Bowen in the 1950s. Bowen assumes that the family system is more important in the formation of abnormal behavior than the individual.
   1. Focus of therapy
      a. Family is a system.
      b. Present interactions among the family members.
      c. Change the context of the family.
   2. Task of the therapist
      a. Use of self as a "change medium" to alter the interactions among family members.
      b. Is an active participant but is *not* directive.

VII. Milieu Therapy

The milieu is everything that impacts upon the psychiatric inpatient. Milieu therapy is the theoretically based manipulation of the patient's environment in order to effect change in the behavior and personality of the individual.

A. Objective of the therapy
   1. Limit setting for the patient who is in need of it.
   2. Learning the basic social skills of:
      a. Assertion
      b. Vocation
      c. Recreation

B. Task of the nurse therapist
   1. Focuses with the patient on problem solving.
   2. Rehabilitation.

C. Focus or assumptions of the therapy
   1. Patients do have healthy parts to their personalities.
   2. Patients do have strengths.
   3. Patients can constructively influence the course of their own treatment.
   4. Patients can constructively influence the course of another patient's treatment.
   5. Consistent, constant therapeutic involvement by the staff personnel is essential.
   6. *All* staff personnel can impact on the patient in a therapeutic manner including maids, custodians, and desk clerks.

VIII. Group Therapy

Groups have 2 basic needs or goals: completion of a task or the satisfaction of the psychosocial or emotional needs of the members.

A. Irvin Yalom's therapeutic aspects of groups
   1. Imparting information and advice.
   2. Instillation of hope.
   3. Universality; others are experiencing the same thoughts and feelings.
   4. Corrective reenactment of primary family group. Members can alter learning experiences obtained earlier from their families.
   5. Development of social interaction techniques.
   6. Imitative behaviors—role modeling by others increases the behavioral repertoire of the individual.
   7. Interpersonal learning—interacting with more than one individual; opportunity to decrease distortions regarding interpersonal relationships.
   8. Existential factors—members aided by the group to deal with meaning of their own existence.
   9. Catharsis—an opportunity to freely express feelings that may not have been expressed previously.
   10. Group cohesion.
   11. Altruism—an opportunity for a group member to aid another by sharing part of himself.

B. Types of groups
   1. Informal—no formalized structure of task, e.g., in patient and staff groups that organize spontaneously in the hospital setting.
   2. Family—(see Family Therapy.)

3. Sensitivity training—increases self awareness, understanding of group process, and awareness of one's own behavioral effect on the group.
4. Therapeutic groups—prevention of emotional turmoil is the primary goal of this group. Education is a secondary goal. A self help group is an example of a therapeutic group.
5. Psychotherapy group—primary goal is the treatment of emotional stress and disorder using the group setting and the group process. A group is a good tool to teach interpersonal relating. More risk for the individual because more than one person is involved.

C. Stages of groups
1. Pregroup—decisions are made during this phase regarding who is the therapist (or leader), what is the purpose of the group, who will be members, and will the group be open (available to new members during the life cycle of the group) or closed (available *only* to the original selected and screened members).
2. Initial phase—the first few meetings of the group, when the members become comfortable with each other and delineate the "work" of the group, have been divided into 3 stages by Yalom.
   a. Orientation stage
      (1.) The group works to gain consensus on issues of task, confidentiality, goals, meeting times, and security.
      (2.) Members decide during these first few meetings what their own roles will be and how comfortable they will feel making disclosures in the early life of the group.
      (3.) Dependence upon the therapist or leader will surface at this time.
   b. Conflict stage
      (1.) Control, power, and authority are the issues that arise.
      (2.) Sub-groups may form within the group, and the leader's authority may be questioned.
      (3.) Hostility may be directed toward fellow members or the leader. Leader should provide safety and encourage anger to be vented.
      (4.) Members learn that conflict can bring about resolution of problems and personal and group growth.
   c. Cohesive stage
      (1.) After resolution of the conflict stage, the members feel a strong affinity toward one another.
      (2.) They are able to freely disclose information and more intimate sharing will occur.
3. Working phase
   a. Group is concerned primarily with task completion.
   b. Members actively work toward their own therapeutic goals.
   c. Leader facilitates the work of the members.
   d. Problem solving and resolution are the key components.
   e. The amount of self disclosure that occurs during this time will be relative to how much the individual trusts fellow members and how "safe" the group is.
4. Termination phase
   a. This concept is introduced during the first phase of the group, and it should be built in as part of the "work" that the members will accomplish.
   b. Termination is often a very traumatic issue, and the group termination offers a way to experience "saying good-bye" in a "safe" place.
   c. The leader is available to provide leadership and role modeling if necessary. Behaviors that may be elicited at this time are denial, regression, anxiety, and a strong feeling of accomplishment.

DIAGNOSTIC AND STATISTICAL MANUAL (DSM) OF MENTAL DISORDERS III CLASSIFICATION

Utilization of these diagnostic categories provides the interdisciplinary team (made up of psychiatrists, psychologists, nurses, and social workers) with a common vocabulary when discussing individuals. It also provides for consistency of approach when structuring a diagnosis or conducting research and collecting statistical data on the various disorders.

I. Five Axes of the DSM III

A. Axis I—clinical syndromes.
B. Axis II—personality disorders.
C. Axis III—physical disorders and conditions.
D. Axis IV—severity of psychosocial stressers.
E. Axis V—highest level of functioning in past year.

This outline will focus on Axis I and Axis II.

A. Axis I
  1. Disorders usually first evident in infancy, childhood, or adolescence.
  2. Organic mental disorders
  3. Substance use disorders
  4. Schizophrenic disorders
  5. Paranoid disorders
  6. Psychotic disorders not classified elsewhere.
  7. Neurotic disorders
  8. Affective disorders
  9. Anxiety disorders
  10. Somatoform disorders
  11. Dissociative disorders (or hysterical neuroses, dissociative type).
  12. Psychosexual disorders
  13. Factitious disorders
  14. Disorders of impulse control not classified elsewhere.
  15. Adjustment disorders
  16. Psychological factors affecting physical condition.

B. Axis II
  1. Personality disorders
    a. Paranoid
    b. Schizoid
    c. Schizotypal
    d. Histrionic
    e. Narcissistic
    f. Antisocial
    g. Borderline
    h. Avoidance
    i. Dependent
    j. Compulsive
    k. Passive-aggressive
    l. Atypical, mixed, or other personality disorder.
  2. Specific developmental disorders
    a. Developmental reading disorder
    b. Developmental arithmetic disorder
    c. Developmental language disorder
    d. Developmental articulation disorder
    e. Mixed specific developmental disorder
    f. Atypical specific development disorder

ABNORMAL (MALADAPTIVE) BEHAVIOR

I. Childhood and Adolescent Disorders

The clinical picture of the child may differ quite a bit from that of the adult. For example, the schizophrenic child exhibits delusions and hallucinations less often than the adult. Also, the underlying problem may be masked by behavior contrary to what one might expect. The depressed child may be irritable, may have temper tantrums, and may show low tolerance for frustration. In older children, depression might be masked by "acting out," e.g., taking drugs, running away from home, or becoming a delinquent.

A. Unsocialized disturbance of conduct

More common among boys than girls.

  1. Clinical picture—overt or covert hostility, disobedience, physical and verbal aggressiveness, destructiveness, lying, stealing, temper tantrums, quarrelsomeness, and vengefulness.
  2. Etiology—rejection, harsh and inconsistent discipline, and often an unstable marital relationship characterize the family environment. Parents are often emotionally unstable or sociopathic; therefore, no consistent guidance or genuine affection is given from the parent to the child. *Rejection* is the key factor.
  3. Therapeutic interventions
    a. Modify the home environment for the child.
    b. May have to remove child from family of origin and place in foster home.
    c. Utilization of behavior modification techniques.
      (1.) Teach parents how to control behavior of child through use of positive reinforcement of desirable behavior and punishment for undesirable behavior.
      (2.) Change in child's behavior may, in turn, change parent's attitude and behavior toward child.
      (3.) Parents (mothers in particular) can be taught assertiveness in order to effectively interact with their child and implement positive reinforcement or punishment, or both.

B. Anxiety and withdrawal
  1. Clinical picture
    a. These children are oversensitive, have unrealistic fears, have pervasive feelings of inadequacy, have sleep disturbances and a fear of school, and are shy and timid.
    b. Children experiencing anxiety become overdependent, while withdrawn children retreat from the scary world and into themselves.
  2. Etiology
    a. Constitutionally the child is more sensitive than the "average" child.
    b. Child has had traumatic experiences, such as illness, accident, or loss of significant

others; child feels helpless and inadequate.

c. An overanxious parent reinforces the child's cognition that he is inadequate to deal with life experiences.

d. Failure of a parent to provide adequate role modeling and guidance for child's development.

e. Poor interpersonal relationship experiences; more often than not the encounters have been unpleasant or unrewarding.

3. Therapeutic interventions

a. Foster constructive interpersonal relationships in the school.

b. Behavior modification techniques.

(1.) Teach appropriate assertiveness.

(2.) Provide positive reinforcement for appropriate social behavior.

(3.) Provide pleasant and constructive experiences in which the child can feel competent and develop feelings of adequacy.

C. Autism

1. Clinical picture

a. Occurs more often in boys than in girls, often apparent in the very first weeks of life, and occurs in all socioeconomic, ethnic, and family patterns.

b. Infant apart and aloof from parent. Baby is never "cuddly," never smiles, never looks around at surroundings, and does not seem to need or want contact with any other human being. Difficulty in relating to other people.

c. Poor language function; an absence of speech or severely restricted speech.

d. Echolalia—the constant repetition of a word or phrase.

e. Self stimulation in the form of headbanging, rocking, or spinning that may continue for extended periods of time.

f. May become obsessively attached to an object such as a rock, a hairbrush, or a light switch.

g. Obsessed with maintaining "sameness." Any familiar situation that is changed (for instance, rearranging the furniture in the family room) can result in a temper tantrum or a long crying spell.

h. Has a blurred, undifferentiated sense of self.

2. Etiology

a. A possible inborn defect that precludes the processing of incoming stimuli and the ability to relate it to the world around it.

b. Parents of autistic children do not seem to have demonstrably different personality characteristics than parents of "normal" children.

3. Therapeutic interventions

a. Warm and loving acceptance of the child accompanied by positive reinforcement for adaptive behavior.

b. Structural therapy that increases amount and variety of stimuli to enhance child's awareness of self and surroundings and child's relationship to the environment.

c. Highly structured formal schooling.

d. Behavior therapy to reduce self destructive behavior. Contracts are negotiated with parents in order for them to become treatment agents so that new behaviors can be generalized to the home setting. Parents reinforce "normal" behavior.

4. Prognosis is unfavorable. Less than 25% of the treated children achieve marginal adjustment.

D. Delinquent behavior

Child is behaving in an antisocial manner (theft, destruction of property, and violence against people).

1. Etiology

a. Personal pathology

(1.) Brain damage or mental retardation.

(2.) Neuroses or psychoses, or both.

(3.) Psychopathic traits (impulsive, defiant, resentful, lack of feelings of guilt or remorse, unable to learn from previous experience).

(4.) Pathogenic family patterns ("broken" homes, parental rejection or faulty discipline, psychopathic parental models)

(5.) Relationships with undesirable peers.

(6.) Sociocultural factors.

(a.) Feelings of alienation and rebellion.

(b.) "Social rejects"—those who drop out of school, do not work, and so forth.

(c.) Gang cultures built on delinquent behavior.

(7.) Unusual stress, such as trauma of death of parent, divorce disrupting family life, and discovery of adoption.

2. Therapeutic interventions

a. Juvenile institutions and training schools afford child the chance to learn about themselves and others, develop work skills, and further their education. May be able to receive psychological counseling on an individual and group basis. Behavior

therapy used in these settings in order to extinguish undesirable behavior and reinforce adaptive responses.
   b. Probation with close supervision within their own communities.
3. Special problems
   a. Child's inability to seek assistance.
   b. Children living in pathogenic families.
   c. Parents needing treatment as well as children.
   d. Parents can be used as "change agents" for their children.
   e. Placing children outside of the family if necessary.
   f. Early intervention crucial if the problem is not to become acute.
   g. Drug therapy with children should be used with great caution since we do not know, at this point in time, what effect the long-term use of medications has on growth and development. Careful assessment must be made in order to determine whether the child needs medication for actual anxiety or because he is mentally retarded; or whether the child is simply hungry, bored with the school's curriculum, or unhappy in a crowded classroom.

Nursing Assessment

The nurse should utilize a formal theoretical framework regarding normal childhood growth and development. Theories of Freud, Erikson, or Sullivan should be utilized as theoretical yardsticks. The nurse goes on to collect biopsychosocial data on the family as well as on the child. The developmental stage of the child also needs to be kept in mind as the assessment proceeds so that the child is addressed at the appropriate level. The child should be assessed in a holistic manner, and the data gleaned will relate to the biological, psychological, social, cultural, and spiritual aspects of the child's life as well as the environment and the family interactions that make up the child's world. Analysis of the child's difficulty will be followed by a nursing diagnosis that addresses the child's dysfunctional behaviors, which in turn leads to a plan of care and nursing interventions. The plan will be implemented, and the outcome evaluated.

II. Organic Mental Disorder

Symptoms and behavior are due to brain dysfunction and can be the result of a primary disease of the brain; a systemic illness, such as meningitis; a disturbance in circulation, such as that due to arteriosclerosis; or a toxic substance, such as alcohol or drugs. Organic brain syndrome (OBS) is one of the *primary* factors in the etiology of dysfunctional behavior, judgment, and intellectual achievement in children as well as in adults, including older adults.

A. Prevalence—number of individuals affected is growing due to increased life expectancy, sophisticated procedures that prolong or save the life of the brain injured, and procedures that sustain the life of those who would have died a quarter of a century ago.
B. Description is of disorder that arises in an individual with no previous history of such dysfunctions. There will be disruption in one or all of the following functions: perception, cognition, and emotion.
C. Etiology
   1. Organic, chemical, or physical destruction within the brain.
   2. Sensory monotony (e.g., repetitive noises).
   3. Sensory deprivation, such as in an intensive care unit.
   4. Sensory overload.
   5. Sleep and dream deprivation.
   6. Immobilization due to illness.
   7. Anxiety that the patient finds overwhelming.
D. Organic mental disorders
   1. Alzheimer's disease
      a. Rapid degeneration beginning at age 40 to 50 years.
      b. Onset gradual; individual evidences physical and mental slowing, begins withdrawing socially, becomes less alert, is intolerant to new ideas or changes in routine.
      c. As disease progresses, the individual has impairment of memory for recent events, becomes personally untidy, may have periods of agitation and confusion, and judgment may be impaired.
      d. At the terminal stage, the patient is reduced to a vegetative state.
   2. Huntington's chorea
      a. Genetically determined degenerative disease of the nervous system.
      b. Occurs in individuals between the ages of 30 and 50 years.
      c. The behavior (involuntary and irregular twitching and jerking movements) is accompanied by mental deterioration.
      d. Death occurs within 10 to 20 years.
      e. The physical manifestations may be evident several years before any neurological evidence can be demonstrated.
   3. Arteriosclerotic brain syndrome
      a. "Hardening of the arteries"; plaque accu-

mulates on the lining of the blood vessels, leading to inflexibility of the vessels and clogging of the arteries. This occurrence can lead to insufficient blood flowing to the brain or can lead to a rupture of the vessel and leakage into the brain.

b. Softening of the affected brain tissue results from the impaired nutrition to the brain cells.
c. Usually occurs after the age of 55 years and seems to be more common among people in lower socioeconomic groups.
d. First admission to a hospital usually occurs between the ages of 70 and 75 years.
e. 50% of the cases are of sudden onset with symptoms of clouding of consciousness; disorientation to time, place, and person; incoherence; and often hemiplegia.
f. Convulsive seizures may precede, occur at the same time, or occur after the acute attack.
g. Symptoms may last from days to months.
h. Onset may be gradual, with patient displaying symptoms such as weakness, fatigue, dizziness, depression, deficit in recent memory, slowing of activities, and loss of zest for living.
i. As symptoms progress in severity, the individual is hospitalized and may be increasingly more irritable and suspicious and may have some poorly organized persecutory delusions.
j. Concentration and intellectual functioning are impaired, and interest in the world and in others is markedly reduced.
k. Patient's initiative is impaired as is judgment.
l. Depression may be present due to the individual's perception of their failing physical and mental faculties.
m. This patient population is at high risk for suicide attempts.
n. Three key causal factors are as follows:
   (1.) Biological—possible genetic factor, diminished nourishment to the brain.
   (2.) Psychosocial—how well an individual responds to the stress of acknowledging the process of his own aging.
      (a.) Role of the pre-psychotic personality: undesirable personality traits, such as rigidity, suspiciousness, obsessive-compulsive traits, and poor adaptability to change, bode ill for the adjustment capabilities of the individual during this period of life.
      (b.) Stressors characteristic in old age: retirement and reduced income; fear of becoming an invalid; fear of death; loss of loved ones and friends and the loneliness that results.
   (3.) Sociocultural conditions—treated by society, family, and employers as undesirable and unnecessary; not treated with dignity; often not allowed to be personally responsible and therefore feel unimportant.

E. Nursing Process
   1. Assessment
      a. Physical examination and health history
      b. Comprehensive drug history
      c. Diagnostic testing
      d. Mental status examination
   2. Nursing diagnosis
      a. Sensory-perceptual alterations
      b. Thought process alterations
      c. Impaired verbal communication
      d. Ineffective individual coping
      e. Self care deficit
   3. Therapeutic interventions

      Based on the assessment findings for each individual and the nursing diagnosis that is made from the assessment.

III. Substance Abuse

Abuse of alcohol and drugs is a given in this country today. With this fact in mind, the nurse should stand ready to assess for signs of intoxication or withdrawal, or both, in *all* areas of clinical practice.

A. Definition of terms
   1. Intoxication is specific to the substance ingested and results in change in affect, level of consciousness, thought processes, cognition, and central nervous system functions.
   2. Withdrawal is specific to the substance that has been abused; produces a noticeable physiological effect when use of the substance is ceased or the amount ingested is decreased. The symptoms will stop if use of the substance is resumed.
   3. Tolerance occurs after repeated use of any given substance and results in more and more of the substance needing to be ingested in order to achieve the desired effect.

B. Three criteria (DSM III) for pathological substance use
   1. Pattern of pathological use as evidenced by intoxication throughout the day, inability to cut down or stop, blackouts, and overdose.

2. Impairment in social or occupational functioning.
3. Duration of use at least 1 month.

C. Alcohol abuse

1. Etiology
   a. Genetic and biological theories; one study found that sons of alcoholics were *4 times more* likely to become alcoholics than sons of nonalcoholics whether they were raised by their own parents or by nonalcoholic foster parents.
   b. Cultural variations from country to country.
   c. E. M. Jellinek's "disease" model—alcoholic is sick.
   d. Moral theory—alcoholics suffer from lack of will power.
   e. Psychodynamic theory embraces the notion that early developmental conflicts result in personality characteristics common in the alcoholic. Alcoholism is thought to be a manifestation of depression, or of an oral dependent personality. Alcoholics are more insecure and have lower self-esteem than nonalcoholics.
2. Clinical picture
   a. Abusers of alcohol can be found among patients in medical-surgical units and emergency rooms as well as psychiatric units. Careful observation on the part of the nurse is imperative.
      (1.) Slurred speech, staggering gait, impulsive behavior, loss of coordination, euphoria, and possible irritability may be signs of inebriation.
      (2.) Smell of alcohol.
3. Nursing assessment
   a. Must distinguish between alcohol intoxication, diabetic coma, and amphetamine abuse with small quantity of alcohol intake.
   b. During intake interview be direct but utilize open ended questions to assess for drinking pattern: how much, how often, interference with family life or social relationships, and interference with work or school.
   c. Secure a physical measurement for alcohol level in blood.
   d. Remain alert for withdrawal symptoms 24 hours after cessation of drinking. Delirium tremens characterized by hallucinations needs to be treated as a serious medical emergency.
   e. Cognitive and emotional aspects: frequent blackouts; no memory of the events during the time the person was drinking and intoxicated. Denial is used as a defense mechanism not only by the patient but by the family as well. Depression is often present and is not the precipitant but the *result* of the alcoholism. Does patient become defensive or vague when answering questions regarding alcohol consumption? Patient may present as anxious, complaining of a general feeling of anxiousness, insomnia, and "morning shakes."
4. Therapy

   Utilizing a multidisciplinary approach seems most effective. Program must be individualized to meet the needs of each unique patient.
   a. Objective—physical rehabilitation, abstaining from drinking, cognitive realization on the part of the alcoholic that life can be rewarding and problems in living can be coped with without alcohol.
   b. Measures used.
      (1.) Medical detoxification with therapeutic medications given to ensure safety and provide as much physical comfort as possible.
      (2.) Group therapy available for the alcoholic, the spouse, and the children; offers learning experiences to provide new coping strategies. Family therapy may be appropriate in some instances.
      (3.) Social interventions provide "bridges" for the recovered alcoholic to former interpersonal relationships and to the workplace.
      (4.) Behavior therapy involves use of aversive measures, such as medication and electric shock.
      (5.) Alcoholics Anonymous (also Al-Anon and Al-Ateen for the family).

D. Drug abuse

1. Etiology consists of same possible causes as those for alcohol abuse.
2. Categories
   a. Barbiturate, sedatives, and hypnotics. This category includes Seconal, phenobarbital, Amytal, Tuinal, Doriden, meprobamate (Miltown or Equanil), Quaalude, Placidyl, chloral hydrate, and the benzodiazepines, such as Valium, Librium, Dalmane, Ativan, and Serax. Clinical presentation is similar to alcohol intoxication: staggering gait, slurred speech, possible euphoria or irritability, and impaired judg-

ment. Withdrawal from the drug presents a clinical situation very similar to that of withdrawal from alcohol.

b. *Cannabis.* Drugs include marijuana, hashish, and hash oil. Intoxication, a delusional disorder, abuse, and dependence can result from use of this drug. Clinical presentation includes red eyes, dryness of mouth, substantial increase in heart rate, distinctive smell from smoking the drug that clings to hair and clothing, and increased appetite. Individuals may become passive, withdrawn. Smoking more than 2 to 3 "joints" each day can result in chronic passivity and loss of interest in school, work, and interpersonal relationships. Cognitively, the individual may feel that time has slowed down and may experience a sense of pleasure that can progress to euphoria. Perception of his surroundings may be heightened (color, sound, and touch may be more intense), and at the same time the individual may feel out of touch with his surroundings.

c. Cocaine and amphetamines. Addiction to these substances seems to come about because of the pleasure that the user experiences when indulging in them. People can become "hooked" on amphetamines that are prescribed by a physician for weight loss. Clinically in small doses, only mild physical symptoms occur; a small increase in pulse rate or blood pressure, perhaps dilated pupils. In chronic users, a runny nose may be present due to irritation of the nasal passages from "snorting" the substance. These people present as energetic, and the nurse may have to differentiate between what is substance abuse and what is possibly manic or hypomanic behavior and symptomatology.

d. Hallucinogens. This category includes LSD, PCP, psilocybin, peyote, and mescaline. Abuse of these agents is defined under the DSM III; a pattern of pathological use, impairment in social and occupational functioning, and duration of at least 1 month. A causative factor may be the subculture in which these agents are used, but "bad trips" and "flashbacks" in one individual and not in another have no explanation at the present time. Clinical picture varies from few physical signs and symptoms with LSD intoxication to nystagmus, ataxia, garbled speech, and hypertension with PCP. It is important to note that users of PCP behave in unpredictable ways and may be belligerent, impulsive, and extremely aggressive and combative. Catatonic excitement or withdrawal may occur, and there is a definite inability on the part of the abuser to understand the spoken word or to communicate intelligently. The user of PCP may also become violent.

3. Nursing diagnosis

   Will be formulated after assessment of physical and cognitive signs.

   a. Ineffective individual coping.
   b. Alteration in thought processes.
   c. Sensory-perceptual alterations.

4. Treatment
   a. Similar to that of alcohol.
   b. Medical support should be given throughout the withdrawal phase.
   c. Group and family therapy may be appropriate.
   d. Halfway houses where the individual can learn new coping skills and new social skills in a strictly monitored environment may be of benefit.

IV. Schizophrenia

A group of disorders that involves the withdrawal from interpersonal relating, the distortion of reality, and the disturbance of thought processes, emotions, and perceptions.

A. Etiology
   1. Genetic factors.
   2. Biochemical factors; the "dopamine hypothesis" posits that there is an excess of dopamine at synaptic sites in the brain.
   3. Neurophysiological factors; normal attentional and informational processes are disrupted, resulting in the cognitive and perceptual distortions found in schizophrenics.
   4. Psychosocial factors
      a. Early psychic trauma and increased vulnerability.
      b. Pathogenic parent-child and family interactions.
         (1.) "Schizophrenogenic" mothers and fathers.
         (2.) Severe, chronic, and destructive marital interactions on the part of the parents of a child at risk for schizo-

phrenia; Theodore Lidz researched this aspect.

(3.) Faulty communication of Gregory Bateson's "double bind" theory.

(4.) Personal authenticity is undermined. Often the actions and statements of the person who becomes schizophrenic are disqualified by one or more members of the family.

5. Faulty learning and coping; defense mechanisms such as denial, projection, and introjection are used in an exaggerated and maladaptive manner.
6. Problems with social role; it has been postulated that the schizophrenic creates a unique social role to escape from social demands and expectations that are destructive.
7. Stress and decompensation; severe life stress may cause a schizophrenic breakdown.

B. Symptoms of schizophrenia; may have an insidious onset or an acute, sudden onset.

1. Eugene Bleuler's Four A's, consisting of blunted affect, loose associations, autism, and ambivalence.
2. DSM III criteria
   a. Disorganization of a previous level of functioning.
   b. Language and communication are disturbed, and neologisms may be coined (a formal thought disorder).
   c. Delusions of varied content.
   d. Poor sorting of sensory perceptions.
   e. Affect is blunted or clearly inappropriate.
   f. Lacks a clear sense of personal boundaries and sense of self; not motivated or unable to direct and carry out a course of action.
   g. Motor disturbances may be present.
   h. Anhedonia (an inability to derive pleasure from anything or anyone).

C. Types of schizophrenia

1. Undifferentiated—this type and the paranoid type are the most common forms that patients suffer who present to inpatient psychiatric units. This form of the disease is increasing in incidence. Delusions, hallucinations, and a thought disorder may be present. The disorder does not fit into any of the other categories.
2. Paranoid—once, about 50% of the hospital admissions for schizophrenia were of this type. Its incidence is decreasing. Severe difficulty with interpersonal relationships is present accompanied by suspiciousness; absurd and illogical delusions that are extremely well organized; feelings and notions of persecution that are often directed toward family or friends, or both; delusions of grandeur, often accompanied by auditory or visual hallucinations; and dangerous behavior resulting from the hallucinations. Patient will not be as profoundly regressed or deteriorated as in other forms of chronic schizophrenia.
3. Catatonic—Patient may exhibit either extreme withdrawal or great excitement.
   a. Withdrawal—mute; patient may remain motionless and rigid in a fixed position for hours. Echopraxis (imitating actions of others) or echolalia (repeating words or phrases in a stereotyped fashion) may be present; may move from catatonic to excited stage very quickly.
   b. Excitement; patient may become violent.
4. Hebephrenic (disorganized)—much less common than the other forms; a more severe disintegration of the personality and occurs at an earlier age. Signature behavior of this type includes emotional indifference, infantile behavior, a silly smile, and shallow and inappropriate laughter; may giggle childishly and use similar sounding words (clang associations) repetitiously.
5. Schizoaffective disorder—a variety of symptoms are exhibited. Poor reality testing may be accompanied by delusions and hallucinations. Also present are symptoms of an affective disorder. One may discern manic or depressed behavior.

D. Nursing assessment

Consists of eliciting the aforementioned signs and symptoms of the various types of schizophrenia. Mental status examination should include data regarding any impairment in cognition, any disturbance in perception, and any problems in relating to others (psychosocial difficulties). Disorganized behavior and a deterioration in daily functioning, delusions or hallucinations, and flat or inappropriate affect are also important findings.

E. Nursing diagnosis

Based on findings during the assessment.

1. Fear (hypervigilance).
2. Impaired verbal communication.
3. Sensory-perceptual alterations.
4. Ineffective individual coping.
5. Self care deficit.
6. Alterations in thought processes.

F. Nursing interventions

1. Be judicious in the use of touch with such a patient. Be aware of his personal boundaries and that invasion of personal space can result in panic for this individual. Reassure that safety (from the threatening delusional system or hallucinations) will be provided.

2. Be prepared to spend quiet time with the silent, avoidant patient, allowing time for the patient to learn to trust and share thoughts. Clarify confusing communication with the patient. If messages are unclear request an explanation or a definition of terms if neologisms are part of the patient's speech.
3. Provide your own reality based perceptions to counteract any sensory-perceptual alterations that the patient may be experiencing. Acknowledge that the hallucinations seem very real to the patient and are probably very uncomfortable, but present reality to him.
4. After a therapeutic relationship has been established, nurse and patient together can determine where coping mechanisms are lacking in the patient's life and work on short-term and long-term goals that will enhance the patient's coping strategies.
5. During the acute phase the nurse may need to constantly remind the patient of daily grooming needs. If the patient is completely withdrawn the nursing staff may have to attend to most of the patient's activities of daily living until the patient can begin assuming responsibility. Constant, non-punitive reminders will be necessary during the acute phase.

G. Medications
1. Phenothiazines such as chlorpromazine (Thorazine), fluphenazine (Prolixin), thioridazine (Mellaril), and trifluoperazine (Stelazine).
   a. Side effects include oversedation, akathisia, Parkinson's syndrome, dystonia, orthostatic hypotension, impotence, photosensitivity, weight gain, menstrual irregularities, and potentiation of other drugs and alcohol.
   b. Complications include tardive oral dyskinesia (which is irreversible) and possible seizures.

H. Other therapeutic interventions
1. Electric shock therapy; quite effective in relieving psychotic states.
2. Behavior modification; token economies or positive reinforcements in the form of tokens that can be earned by the patient in payment for adaptive and healthy behavior (making the bed, showering, shaving, and playing a game with other people). These tokens can then be exchanged for something that the individual wants, such as a trip to the canteen, a walk outdoors with members of the staff, or a visit home. Limit setting can also be done for the patient in the home or in the hospital.
3. Milieu therapy—patient interacts with all individuals (including janitors and maids) on the inpatient psychiatric unit. Learns social skills, learns how to relate interpersonally with a broad spectrum of the population, and is oriented by those in the setting to what is reality and what is not.
4. Group therapy enables patient to do problem solving with fellow patients and staff regarding interpersonal issues, work-related issues, and issues regarding discharge and compliance with medication regimen.
5. Family therapy—for discussion of issues regarding medications, use of alcohol by the patient, and any behavior modification that the family can carry out.

V. Major Affective Disorders

Approximately 25 million Americans will suffer a severe depressive episode sometime during their lives. It appears that the major depressive disorder is on the increase while the bipolar disorder is on the decrease. Affective disorders are characterized by a disturbance in mood. Extreme elation or depression are exhibited.

A. Major depressive disorder
1. Etiology
   a. Psychoanalytical—Freud postulated that depression is "anger turned inward."
   b. Cognitive theory—Aaron Beck postulates that the individual's beliefs and interpretations of events are distorted, and these distortions underlie the depression.
   c. Learned helplessness theory—a cognitive approach developed by Martin Seligman. There are 2 types of people, the internals (assume responsibility for what happens to them) and the externals (attribute their success or failure to some global, uncontrollable event). It is the externals who are likely to become depressed since they feel that they are helpless to change things.
   d. Medical-biological theory—a deficiency of catecholamines, particularly norepinephrine, is associated with depression. Conversely, an excess of catecholamines may be associated with mania.
   e. Genetic influence—recent research indicates a possible 20% predisposition for depression among children of a depressed parent.
   f. Environmental stresses—failure at a job or work; failure at school; loss (of another

human being, a body part, or a bodily function); lack of resources; guilt; loneliness (in the elderly); competition for jobs and college acceptance; the complexity of modern living; a financial "squeeze" (particularly for the elderly during inflation); and the role confusion for both women and men, especially since the issues of the Women's Liberation Movement and the Equal Rights Amendment have been raised.

g. Holistic theory—a variety of the aforementioned theories may be implemented to explain the etiology of the individual's illness. Each person is unique, and no one theory can be utilized for every patient.

h. Pharmacological agents can precipitate a change in mood. Drugs the nurse should assess for include steroids, alcohol, barbiturates, oral contraceptives, cocaine, marijuana, antidepressants, and amphetamines.

2. Symptoms

Sad facies, low mood, anhedonia, sleep disturbance, loss of motivation, loss of interest, feelings of hopelessness, suicidal wishes, and appetite changes (either eating less with a resultant weight loss or eating more with a weight gain). Psychomotor retardation as evidenced by slow speech, slow and shuffling gait, and slow thought processes is often present. Preoccupation with thoughts about self and bodily functions prevalent. Appearance may be disheveled and poor eye contact is maintained. Agitation in form of pacing and hand wringing may be observed. Person will isolate himself from others and reduce social activities.

3. Nursing assessment

Observe individual for aforementioned signs and symptoms, and utilize assessment questions for sleep pattern, eating habits, and social behavior.

4. Nursing diagnosis

Based on findings during nursing assessment.

a. Disturbance in self concept (feels guilty and worthless).
b. Ineffective individual coping.
c. Dysfunctional grieving (denial of the loss or prolonged grieving).
d. Alteration in nutrition.
e. Sleep pattern disturbance.
f. Self care deficits.

5. Nursing interventions

a. Nurse and patient together set a long-term goal of patient's developing a more realistic self concept. Realistic self appraisal of what and whom the patient *really* is is very important in enhancing the patient's self respect and self esteem.

b. Nurse and patient working together determine the areas of the patient's life that are being ineffectively handled. What is hampering the patient from moving forward? Teach patient ways to handle stress, or aid patient in learning constructive outlets of feelings of anger, guilt, anxiety, and loss. Provide for assertiveness training if applicable.

c. Help the patient identify any and all losses that have not been grieved. Encourage the individual to mourn appropriately, and provide support during this time. Reassure that grieving is a natural and normal process that everyone who suffers a loss must attend to.

d. Determine patient's particular likes and dislikes regarding food. Provide small portions, give between meal feedings, and arrange for high protein, high calorie supplements if necessary. Special foods from home may entice the patient to eat. Sitting with the patient provides a social atmosphere that may improve nutritional intake and indicates that the nurse is interested in his welfare.

e. Disrupted sleep patterns or difficulty falling asleep can be aided by the following:
   (1.) Assure that the patient gets enough exercise during the day.
   (2.) Provide an opportunity for a leisurely warm bath before bedtime.
   (3.) Offer a glass of warm milk.
   (4.) Give a back rub.
   (5.) Spend time with the patient for some quiet conversation to mull over the day's events and provide closure.

f. If agitation is present, schedule regular meeting times with the patient to demonstrate acceptance and unconditional positive regard. The meetings also provide time for the patient to ventilate. During agitated periods the patient can be guided into activities that provide an outlet for excess energy.

g. Self care deficits
   (1.) If the patient has severe psychomotor retardation the nurse will need to assist in activities of daily living.
   (2.) Gentle reminders (combing of hair, brushing of teeth, putting on make-

up) may need to be accompanied by physical assistance on the part of the nurse, if appropriate. Safety needs must be provided for in the case of severe psychomotor retardation as well. Some of these patients could set themselves on fire with careless use of smoking materials; in case of an emergency evacuation of the unit, the staff would need to assist patients in their removal to a safe place.

6. Medications
   a. Tricyclics include amitriptyline (Elavil), doxepin (Sinequan), imipramine (Tofranil), and protriptyline (Vivactil); side effects are dry mouth, blurred vision, drowsiness, and constipation.
   b. Monoamine oxidase inhibitors (MAO inhibitors) such as isocarboxazid (Marplan), phenelzine sulfate (Nardil), and tranylcypromine sulfate (Parnate); patient *must* refrain from ingesting foods containing tyramine (aged cheese, alcohol) because the side effect of hypertensive crisis may result.
7. Other therapeutic interventions
   a. Electric shock therapy
      (1.) The mechanism that makes it efficacious is unclear.
      (2.) It has value for those who are severely depressed and are at risk for suicide, and those who are catatonically withdrawn.
   b. Cognitive therapy stresses the need for realistic self understanding, a realistic frame of reference and pattern of values, and more effective coping techniques.
   c. Behavior modification
      (1.) Behavior incompatible with depression is positively reinforced.
      (2.) Depressive behavior is ignored, and healthy behavior is acknowledged.
   d. Family therapy
      (1.) Depression impacts on every member of the family not just the patient.
      (2.) Behavior modification can be taught to members of the family in order to reinforce healthy and adaptive behavior and ignore maladaptive behavior.
8. Suicide
   a. 75% of all persons committing suicide are depressed at the time.
   b. Incidence is twice as high among college students as it is among young people not in college.
   c. Rates are higher among divorced, widowed, and single people than among those who are married.
   d. Rates are higher for unskilled laborers and psychiatrists, lawyers, dentists, and psychologists.
   e. The peak ages are 25 to 44 years.
   f. There has been a sharp increase in rates among adolescents and young adults.
   g. *Suicide rates among the 1st 10 causes of death in most Western countries, including the United States.*

Nursing Assessment

The Lethality Scale supplied by the Los Angeles Suicide Prevention Center (see Coleman) is a guideline, along with nurse's assessment (steps 11 to 14).

(1.) Suicide potential greater if individual is male and over 50 years of age.
(2.) Suicide potential is greater if individual has following symptoms:
   (a.) Sleep disturbances
   (b.) Depression
   (c.) Feelings of hopelessness
   (d.) Alcoholism.
(3.) Stress
   (a.) Loss of a loved one through death or divorce.
   (b.) Loss of business or employment.
   (c.) Increased responsibilities.
   (d.) Serious illness.
(4.) Greater suicide potential if there is a sudden onset of symptoms, a recurrent outbreak of similar symptoms, or a recent increase in longstanding maladaptive traits.
(5.) Suicide potential is greater if the plan is well organized, clear and detailed, and the method is extremely lethal, such as shooting, jumping, and hanging.
(6.) Higher suicide potential if person has no family or friends, or if they are unwilling to help.
(7.) Greater potential if the individual has a history of prior suicide attempts, or if the individual has a history of depression or repeated threats of suicide.
(8.) Greater suicide potential if there is chronic, debilitating illness.
(9.) No communication between the in-

dividual and relatives, or the relatives reject efforts by the individual or health professionals to reestablish communication, increases suicide potential.

(10.) Suicide potential greater if significant other is defensive, rejecting, punishing, or denies the need for help.

(11.) Direct questioning of the person as to whether they have ever had thoughts of harming or killing themself.

(12.) Do they *now* have thoughts of harming themselves?

(13.) What is causing him pain now?

(14.) How was the situation coped with in the past?

Nursing Interventions

(1.) If the energy level has increased for this patient (the psychomotor retardation is lifting), he is at greater risk for carrying out a suicide plan. He now has enough energy *to plan* a lethal suicide act and enough energy to *carry it out*. If the patient is on an "open" unit a move to a more secure unit may be in order to provide for physical safety. Suicide precautions or suicide watch should be instituted for the patient who has a concrete plan and the energy to carry it out.

B. Bipolar disorders

Bipolar disorders or manic-depressive illness are distinguished by at least one manic episode. There are 3 classifications: depressive, manic, and mixed (patient may exhibit both episodes of depression and elation).

1. Etiology
   a. Heredity—research by Kallman in 1958 found that genetic predisposition does play a role.
   b. Biochemical factors or catecholamine hypothesis; there is evidence of altered brain chemistry in all 3 types of bipolar disorders. Treatments such as electric shock therapy, antidepressant drugs, and lithium therapy influence the metabolism of the amines.
   c. Psychosocial factors
      (1.) Role modeling of family members as they cope with stress. Child learns to cope in the same manner.
      (2.) Severe stress, such as death of a loved one, failure in an important interpersonal relationship, or a severe setback in school or work can trigger the disorder.
      (3.) Defense strategy or a "flight into reality" for the manic; otherwise, the depression that would ensue would be intolerable.
2. Symptoms of mania include elation, flightiness, overactivity, ceaseless talking and visiting, may spend money recklessly, poor moral restraint, may become sexually provocative or act out sexually in an inappropriate manner. Poor judgment and no insight into own condition. As the mania progresses may become easily irritable, violent, and increasingly obscene in their language and behavior. Their thoughts progress so rapidly that flight of ideas and pressured speech occur, and patient may verbalize a desire to "slow down my mind."
3. Nursing assessment

   Observe patient for aforementioned signs and symptoms. Ask direct questions regarding eating and sleeping patterns prior to admission as well as any eccentric behaviors that may have been indulged in, e.g., giving away money, investing in "get-rich-quick" schemes.
   a. Delusions, hallucinations, and overtly aggressive or suicidal activities may accompany the mood disorder, which correspond to the depression or elation.
   b. Must distinguish between schizophrenia and bipolar disorder.
      (1.) There is a gradual deterioration of the schizophrenic, whereas the person with bipolar disorder functions well socially and at work after an episode.
      (2.) The family history is positive for an affective disorder and alcoholism; this is not true for the schizophrenic.
4. Nursing interventions
   a. The milieu may prove to be too stimulating for the manic patient, and he should be allowed to have "time out" in his own room. If the patient cannot provide for a quiet time, the nurse should firmly (nonpunitively) direct the patient to the room for some quiet time.
   b. If inappropriate behavior begins to escalate, medication should be given promptly and p.r.n.
   c. A careful watch over the patient's funds should be kept. Patients in the manic

phase have been known to plan grandiose parties or excursions for the entire unit. They may also involve other patients in grand travel schemes following their discharge.

d. If the patient is unable to sit still through an entire meal, small frequent feedings may be a better intervention. Liquid intake must be carefully assessed. It is not unusual for these patients to forget to eat and drink. A high protein, high calorie supplemental feeding may be indicated for the patient who has had a dramatic weight loss.

e. The patient may be so out of control that he eats everything in sight and forages from other patient's trays. Firm, nonpunitive limit setting would be in order here.

f. For the patient who intrudes upon another patient's personal space, or the staff's personal space, social guidelines must be established and enforced. Entry into other people's rooms, or the use of their personal possessions, is not negotiable.

g. Sleep patterns must be monitored, and the patient encouraged to stay in bed at night. These patterns also indicate when the medication is beginning to take effect.

5. Medications

a. Lithium carbonate is the treatment of choice; it is given orally, in daily divided doses until a therapeutic serum level of 0.5 to 1.5 mEq/L is attained. Side effects include fine tremor of the hands, nausea, vomiting, diarrhea, thirst, fatigue, and weight gain. Signs of toxicity may occur after 1.5 mEq/L is reached and include sluggishness, lethargy, fine tremor, ataxia, slurred speech, anorexia, vomiting, and diarrhea. The toxic condition can result in the death of the patient. Blood samples should be drawn every 3 to 5 days to determine when a therapeutic range is attained and to prevent toxicity.

6. Other therapeutic interventions

a. Behavior modification is used to help patient regain or remain in control if inappropriate behavior is escalating.

b. Group therapy; for planning about discharge and learning about importance of compliance with lithium therapy. Bipolar disorder can be controlled by lifelong intake of lithium carbonate, but the individual often stops the medication once he feels well.

c. Family therapy; for teaching the family the importance of the patient's compliance with the medication regimen and the need for periodic blood level checks. Family should also be taught the signs of toxicity.

VI. Anxiety Disorders

Subjectively, the individual experiences feelings of dread, apprehension, and alarm. There may be no identifiable precipitant for the feelings, but the discomfort that is experienced leads the person to react in a variety of ways, which he hopes will alleviate the uncomfortable feelings. The individual is rendered dysfunctional when anxiety leads to coping patterns that render the individual ineffectual and unable to carry out daily activities. Major defense mechanisms used to defend against anxiety are repression, conversion, dissociation, reaction formation, undoing, displacement, and projection.

A. Etiology

1. Behavioral theory—modeling; child learns to be anxious from a tense and nervous parent.
2. Learning theory: anxiety is a conditioned response to a particular stimulus.
3. Psychoanalytical theory—anxiety results from inability to cope with "dangerous" impulses. Repression is used, particularly to handle anger, so that person can remain loved, secure, and accepted; anxiety provoking decisions and any risk taking that could jeopardize security can result in extreme anxiety.
4. Biological theory—recent research indicates that there can be actual cardiac problems in people diagnosed with anxiety disorders and panic attacks. Research also shows that there is a definite connection between physiological functions and anxiety, but researchers cannot, at this time, state categorically that anxiety is caused by biological functions.

Generalized Anxiety Disorder

A. General anxiety

1. Tense, worried, uneasy but often unable to say why; difficulty making decisions; intolerable to them if they make a mistake; insomnia; may be diaphoretic and have sweaty palms; may have elevated blood pressure and increased heart rate (particularly in situations that provoke anxiety).
2. If one cause for worry is solved the individual goes on to find another source of concern and then another.

3. Individual may appear hypervigilant, scanning the room for possible problems or threats to self.

B. Panic attacks
  1. Person may seem to be having a coronary; symptoms occur suddenly, reach high intensity for a short period of time, and then subside.
  2. Palpitations, shortness of breath, diaphoresis, faintness, and a sense of impending catastrophe may appear as symptoms.
  3. The experience is a terrifying one for the individual and anyone with him, and medical assistance may be sought.
  4. Patient calms down after administration of sedatives and reassurance by medical personnel.
  5. The attacks are self limiting and will subside without further medical assistance.
  6. Nursing assessment
     a. Nurse should collect data relating to the biopsychosocial functioning of the individual.
     b. Any of the aforementioned symptoms should be assessed as well as social functioning.
  7. Nursing diagnosis
     a. Fear of a specific object or situation; or a pervading, nonspecific sense of dread.
     b. Ineffective individual coping.
     c. Physical symptoms.
     d. Disturbance in self concept, "I'm not the person I used to be."
  8. Medications
     a. Minor tranquilizers, Benzodiazepines, such as Librium, Serax, Tranxene, and Valium.
     b. Side effects include drowsiness, ataxia, possible confusion (particularly in the elderly), headache, dizziness and vertigo, and lethargy.
     c. *There is a high potential with these drugs for physical dependency.*
  9. Other therapeutic interventions
     a. Individual psychotherapy; the emphasis is on greater self understanding and knowledge of what the problem is. Focus is on a realistic appraisal of life situations and effective and adaptive coping behaviors. An example is Hildegarde Peplau's problem solving approach. Encourage patient to do the following:
        (1.) Identify anxiety as such.
        (2.) Connect relief giving patterns he uses to relieve his anxiety.
        (3.) Provide descriptive data of situations; interactions that immediately precede onset of anxiety.
        (4.) Formulate from the data the probable cause for the anxiety.
     b. Behavior therapy is quite effective.
        (1.) Systematic desensitization used for the anxiety disorders.
        (2.) Cognitive therapy may be used to change the individual's inner thoughts and beliefs, which in turn influences the behavior.
     c. Family therapy may be appropriate if a pattern of family behavior is keeping the individual "sick."

C. Obsessive-compulsive disorder

Obsessions are persistent and repetitive thoughts that an individual cannot seem to stop. The compulsive component is the repetitive behavior that the person engages in which relieves anxiety but causes dismay to the person performing it. This disorder is considered to be maladaptive because it causes distress to the person and is an exaggerated or irrational behavior that reduces the flexibility and capabilities of the individual involved. Often work, school, and social relationships are interfered with.
  1. Etiology
     a. Reaction formation—thoughts or behaviors are substituted for those that are causing anxiety, fear, or guilt.
     b. Guilt and fear of punishment (Lady Macbeth's compulsive hand washing to get rid of guilt).
     c. Assurance of order and predictability for an individual who views the world as a hostile place.
  2. Nursing assessment and diagnosis
     (See assessment and diagnosis under general anxiety and panic attacks.)
  3. Therapeutic interventions
     a. Cognitive
        (1.) Therapist facilitates discrimination between real and imagined threats and works with individual to respond in a more selective and adaptive manner to situations.
        (2.) Therapist enables individual to accept "bad" feelings or desires as something that everyone has at one time and to integrate those feelings into the self.
     b. Behavioral
        (1.) Ignoring the unwanted, ritualistic behavior and rewarding the healthy, adaptive behavior.

D. Phobic disorder

A phobia is an exaggerated, persistent fear of an object or place. The perceived danger is magnified out of proportion to the actual seriousness. The classic clinical symptom in a phobic individual is the avoidance of whatever it is that is feared. Anxiety ensues if the person attempts to approach the feared object. Symptoms then will range from mild uneasiness to a full-fledged panic attack.

1. Etiology
   a. Psychoanalytical theory
      (1.) A defense against threatening aggressive or sexual impulses.
      (2.) A displacement of anxiety from a feared person or object that *cannot* be avoided onto one that *can*.
   b. Behavioral theory
      (1.) Behavior is conditioned, and avoidance is learned and can be unlearned.
2. Nursing assessment and diagnosis. (See assessment and diagnosis under heading for general anxiety and panic attacks.) Particular attention would be paid to avoidant behavior; when, where, and how long it has occurred.
3. Therapeutic interventions
   a. Individual psychotherapy enables individual to gain insights into the symbolic reasons for the avoidant behavior. However, insight is usually not enough to change the behavior.
   b. Behavioral therapy utilizes guided imagery, flooding, and systematic desensitization techniques with good success.

Somatoform Disorders

A. Hypochondriasis

Neurotic behavior is manifested by physical complaints for which no organic cause can be found. Individual has unrealistic fear of disease and is preoccupied with functions of the body, particularly the digestive system. Detailed records of bowel movements and food ingested may be kept.

1. Etiology
   a. Overemphasis on bodily functions in early life.
   b. Maintenance by positive reinforcement. Significant others offer sympathy and attention to the individual; "secondary gains," such as these, reinforce the maladaptive behavior.
2. Therapy; patient is very resistant; anxiety is only kept at bay while the "symptoms" persist. The individual is loathe to give them up.
3. Nursing interventions
   a. Short-term goals
      (1.) Provide appropriate aids for relief of acute physical symptoms.
      (2.) Utilizing Peplau's approach in identifying anxiety, aid the patient in recognizing feelings and then connecting those feelings to how the body feels when these emotions are present.
      (3.) Nurse and patient working together will focus on the self-esteem of the patient and how personal growth can be accomplished, i.e., what would the patient like to be able to do and how are the symptoms stopping this from happening?
      (4.) Nurse sets limits on how long the patient can talk about the symptom and contracts with the patient to relax and talk about other topics.
   b. Long-term goals
      (1.) For the patient to be independent enough to argue.
      (2.) For the patient to be assertive for what he wants without resorting to physical symptoms to achieve control of anxiety or of significant others.

B. Psychogenic pain disorder

Similar to hypochondriasis in that no physical cause for the pain can be determined, or the reported severity of the pain is out of proportion to the physical etiology.

1. Etiology
   a. Overemphasis on bodily functions in early life.
   b. Faulty learning early in life that illness or pain, or both, is a means of escaping potentially unpleasant situations.
2. Therapeutic interventions
   a. Patient is very resistant.
   b. Nursing interventions are the same as those for somatoform disorders.
   c. Behavioral therapy utilizes positive reinforcement for adaptive behavior, and extinction procedures to stop the pain related behaviors.

C. Conversion disorder

Loss of function or control of part of the body that has no organic pathology. The physical incapacity allows the individual to escape an anxiety provoking situation. Symptoms may be sensory (blindness, deafness), visceral (pseudopregnancy), or motor (inability to walk, paralysis). A *belle indifference* is present in that the individual does not seem concerned about the dysfunction. Symptoms can be removed under hypnosis.

1. Etiology
   a. Personalities of such individuals are usually dramatic and histrionic.
   b. Symptoms are a means of escaping a threatening, anxiety producing (sometimes life threatening, as during a war) situation.
2. Therapeutic interventions
   a. Remove anxiety provoking agent if possible.
   b. Hypnosis will remove the symptoms.
   c. Individual psychotherapy to change the life style and promote adaptive behavior.
   d. For specific nursing interventions see hypochondriasis.

Dissociative Disorders

A. Psychogenic amnesia and fugue

The amnesia occurs in response to a stressful situation that other people would deal with more effectively (the death of a close relative, for example). Material is repressed but will surface spontaneously or under hypnosis. There is no organic pathology. The fugue state encompasses both an inability to remember *and* a flight from one's environment, which may last for days, months, or even years.

1. Etiology
   a. Conscious repression of unacceptable material.
   b. Behavior may be a learned pattern of avoidance of anxiety provoking situations.
   c. Personality of individual is often immature, highly suggestible, and egocentric.
2. Therapeutic interventions
   a. Watchful waiting and possible spontaneous recall.
   b. Hypnosis to bring the repressed material to the surface where it can be dealt with in the presence of a therapist.
3. Nursing interventions

   Same as for hypochondriasis.

B. Multiple personalities

Rare in clinical practice; two or more distinct, well-formed personalities within one individual. These personalities may relate with one another; one may be conscious and the dominant personality.

1. Etiology
   a. Many of these individuals have been sexually abused during childhood.
   b. Behavior is a mechanism whereby conflicts (such as sexual preoccupation) can be resolved by having several personalities indulging in behavior that would ordinarily be repressed, thereby decreasing anxiety.
2. Therapeutic interventions
   a. Hypnosis—in the relaxed state, the multiple personalities may emerge, paving the way for psychotherapy.

VII. Personality Disorders

These disorders are the result of immature and distorted personality development, resulting in maladaptive behavior that impairs functioning. Individuals often do not relate well with others and can cause problems for people who interact with them.

A. Etiology
   1. Heredity—there is no scientific evidence linking a predisposition or a constitutional tendency toward any of the personality disorders.
   2. Psychosocial factors are not yet established.
   3. Sociocultural factors are not yet established.

B. Types
   1. Paranoid

      Suspicious, hypersensitive, rigid, argumentative, tends to blame others for own mistakes or failures, suspects others of bad intentions toward him.
   2. Schizoid

      Lack of ability and interest in developing social relationships; classed as "loners."
   3. Schizotypal

      Seclusive, avoidant, oversensitive, superstitious thinking but *is* in touch with reality; displays odd behavior; speech and thinking similar to the schizophrenic but to a less severe degree.
   4. Histrionic

      Dramatic, often seductive, immature, and easily excitable; are dependent, helpless, self centered, and vain.
   5. Narcissistic

      Self absorption and an exaggerated sense of self importance; are grandiose and expect special treatment from those around them; have a strong sense of entitlement; exploit others and disregard feelings and rights of others.

6. Antisocial

   Violates the rights of others in an aggressive manner; has no remorse or feelings of wrongdoing. Person may also be charming, intelligent, and capable of carrying out elaborate "con" games.
7. Borderline

   Impulsive, angry, sees people and situations as all bad or all good; manipulative with staff and in relationships with others; are unstable enough to have short psychotic-like episodes.
8. Avoidant

   Unlike the schizoid, this person would like to relate with others. Reluctance to encounter rejection, ridicule, or criticism precludes this from happening. Low self esteem and loneliness result.
9. Dependent

   Lack of self confidence and feelings of helplessness make these people dependent upon others. They can function if they do not have to be alone.
10. Compulsive

    Excessive concern for rules, order, and efficiency; insist that everything be done *their* way; rigid, inhibited, overly conscientious, unable to relax and have fun. Often much time is paid to trivial details that are extremely time consuming.
11. Passive-aggressive

    Anger and hostility are vented in an indirect manner, such as pouting, "forgetting," being intentionally inefficient; often resentful of those in authority.

C. Characteristic symptoms
1. Problems with interpersonal relationships.
2. Do not "own" their problems, rather they blame fate, bad luck, or other people for their dysfunction.
3. Individuals are manipulative, unconscionable about immoral or illegal conduct; no qualms about hurting others.
4. Though the behavior is maladaptive and dysfunctional, it is repeated over and over again.
5. Assume no responsibility for their behavior; blame is projected onto someone or something else.
6. Do not seek therapy on their own; have little motivation to change and are difficult to engage in a therapeutic relationship.

D. Nursing assessment
1. Individual is usually not a reliable source of information, since he sees himself as blameless.
2. Discussion with a significant other, or a former significant other, may be necessary to elicit the dysfunctional behavior pattern.
3. Nurse assesses for the behaviors, as listed, for each of the disorders.

E. Nursing diagnosis

   Utilization of Kim and Moritz taxonomy is useful here.

Ineffective Individual Coping

1. Impaired social functioning
   a. Violation of social rules and norms.
   b. Lack of participation in organizations, activities.
   c. Relinquishment of social and role responsibilities.
2. Impaired relationships with significant others.
   a. Suspicious, aloof, mistrustful of others.
   b. Inability to develop or maintain close relationships.
   c. Demanding, dependent in relationships.
3. Impaired occupational functioning
   a. Inability to maintain employment.
   b. Difficulties in employment setting.
4. Impaired cognitive abilities
   a. Impaired problem solving.
   b. Impaired judgment and insight.
5. Impaired emotional responses
   a. Lack of emotional responses.
   b. Impaired control of anger, temper.
   c. Demanding, overreacting responses.
   d. Hypersensitivity

F. Therapy
1. Extremely difficult to engage in therapy. The person may become dependent on the therapist, others may utilize the therapy to act out either during the sessions or following the sessions.
2. Responds best in situations in which they cannot leave the treatment setting, e.g., prisons, inpatient psychiatric units.
3. Insight therapy not appropriate; utilizing the approach that the individual must change his behavior is sometimes advantageous.

G. Nursing interventions
1. For those who would act out, firm limit setting and a thorough orientation to the rules of the unit are necessary when the patient is first admitted.
2. For the patient who has strong dependency needs, the nurse and patient together work on the patient's initiating own daily care, being responsible for adequate intake of

nourishing foods, ridding self of the "shoulds" and "oughts" of others and aiming for self approval instead, and learning to deal with his own feelings, particularly anger, without resorting to maladaptive behavior.

VIII. Psychosomatic Disorders

Psychological factors play a major role in the causation of these illnesses. Stress and a predisposition to that particular illness are necessary before a psychosomatic disorder occurs.

A. Etiology

Stressful situations arouse a negative response; the emotional arousal continues because the stressor has not been adequately dealt with, and physiological impact upon one or more organs occurs.

1. Genetic factors

   Behavior may be a hereditary predisposition toward a particular disorder; may also be learned behavior, i.e., everyone in a particular family has peptic ulcers.
2. Differences in autonomic reactivity

   Person may always react to stressors with an elevated blood pressure, tightening of the neck muscles, and so forth.
3. Weakness in a particular organ that makes it vulnerable to stress.
4. Personality characteristics (the high achiever and perfectionist prone to migraines).
5. Inadequate coping mechanisms to deal with stressors.
6. Stressful interpersonal relationships.
7. Pathogenic family patterns in childhood.
8. Conditioned responses reinforced by secondary gains.

B. Psychosomatic patterns

1. Peptic ulcer
2. Heart attack
3. Hypertension
4. Anorexia nervosa
5. Bulimia
6. Asthma (in children)
7. Eczema

C. Therapeutic interventions

1. Nurse provides support for patient's physical needs and is non-judgmental.
2. Nurse and patient working together determine what kind of stressors may be precipitants for the disorder. Utilizing Peplau's approach, the nurse and patient determine what the alarm reaction is (e.g., a tightening of the gut), what the defensive reaction is (e.g., a pain in the gut that results in the patient leaving the scene because he is ill), and the resultant pathological reaction (e.g., a peptic ulcer).
3. Nurse and patient together assess what the patient's adaptive capacity is.
4. Minor tranquilizers may be used to decrease tension.
5. Dietary restrictions or special diets may be prescribed.
6. Behavior modification techniques, such as extinction or differential reinforcement, may be used to unlearn autonomic responses.
7. Biofeedback—individual learns to monitor and control body's responses.

Psychiatric Nursing Bibliography

Arieti, S. & Brody, E. B. (1974). *American Handbook of Psychiatry.* New York: Basic Books.

Arieti, S. (1974). *Interpretation of Schizophrenia.* New York: Basic Books.

Armstrong, S. W. (1983). Thought Disorders of Psychiatric Patients. *In* Burd, S. F., and Marshall, M. A. (eds.). *Some Clinical Approaches to Psychiatric Nursing.* London: MacMillan Company.

Arnold, H. (1976). Working with schizophrenic patients: The four A's. *American Journal of Nursing, 76*:941–943.

Authier, J., Authier, K. & Lutey, B. (1979). Clinical management of the tearfully depressed patient: Communication skills for the nurse practitioner. *Journal of Psychiatric Nursing and Mental Health Services,* 17:34–41.

Barry, P. D. (1984). *Psychosocial Nursing Assessment and Intervention.* Philadelphia: J. B. Lippincott.

Beck, A., Rush, A. J., Shaw, B. & Emery, G. (1979). *Cognitive Therapy of Depression.* New York: Guilford Press.

Beck, A. T. (1967). *Depression: Causes and Treatment.* Philadelphia: University of Pennsylvania Press.

Beck, A. T. (1971). Cognition, affect, and psychopathology. *Archives of General Psychiatry, 24*:495–500.

Beck, C. M., Rawlins, R. P. & Williams, S. R. (1984). *Mental Health-Psychiatric Nursing.* St. Louis: C. V. Mosby Co.

Bell, J. (1977). Stressful life events and coping methods in mental illness and wellness behaviors. *Nursing Research, 26*: 136–141.

Bluhm, J. (1981). When you face the alcoholic patient. *Nursing,* 2:71–73.

Boettcher, E. & Alderson, S. (1982). Psychotropic medications and the nursing process. *Journal of Psychiatric Nursing and Mental Health Services, 20*:12–16.

Carser, D. (1981). Primary nursing in the milieu. *Journal of Psychiatric and Mental Health Services,* 2:35–41.

Coleman, J. C., Butcher, J. N. & Carson, R. C. (1984). *Abnormal Psychology and Modern Life.* Glenview: Scott, Foresman and Company.

Davis, S. (1963). Toward a Study of Silence. *In* Burd, S. F. and Marshall, M. A. (eds.). *Some Clinical Approaches to Psychiatric Nursing.* New York: Macmillan Company.

Devine, B. (1981). Therapeutic milieu/milieu therapy: An overview. *Journal of Psychiatric Nursing and Mental Health Services,* 3:20–24.

Diagnostic and Statistical Manual of Mental Disorders, 3rd ed. (1980). Washington, D.C.: American Psychiatric Association.

Diran, O. (1976). You can prevent suicide. *Nursing, 76*:60–64.

Drake, R. E. (1975). Disruption and loss model. *Perspectives in Psychiatric Care, 13*:163–169.

Earle, A., Lynn, F., Manaser, J. & Selby, M. (1979). The role of the psychiatric nurse in the rehabilitation of the schizophrenic patient. *Journal of Psychiatric Nursing and Mental Health Services, 8*:16–23.

Evans, D. L. (1982). Explaining suicide among the young: An analytical review of the literature. *Journal of Psychosocial Nursing and Mental Health Service, 21*:9–15.

Feldman, L. (1976). Goals of family therapy. *Journal of Marriage and Family Counseling*. April, 103–113.

Field, W. E. & Ruelke, W. (1973). Hallucinations and how to deal with them. *American Journal of Nursing, 73*:638–640.

Floyd, G. J. (1975). Nursing management of the suicidal patient. *Journal of Psychiatric Nursing and Mental Health Services, 13*:23–26.

Frederick, C. J. (1973). The role of the nurse in crisis intervention and suicide prevention. *Journal of Psychiatric Nursing and Mental Health Services, 11*:27–31.

Frost, B. E. (1970). The active leader in group therapy for chronic schizophrenic patients. *Perspectives in Psychiatric Care, 8*:268–272.

Frost, M. (1975). Schizophrenia-1: Diagnosis and prognosis. *Nursing Times, 71*:328–332.

Frost, M. (1975). Schizophrenia-3: Delusions and hallucinations. *Nursing Times, 71*:431–433.

Frost, M. (1975). Schizophrenia-4: Aggressives and natural isolates. *Nursing Times, 71*:471–475.

Fuchs, C. & Rehm, L. (1977). A self-control behavior therapy program for depression. *Journal of Consulting and Clinical Psychology, 45*:206–215.

Gerace, L. (1981). Phenomenon of early engagement in family therapy. *Journal of Psychiatric Nursing, 19*:25–38.

Gillies, D., & Alyn, I. (1976). Psychosocial Assessment and Intervention. In *Patient Assessment and Management by the Nurse Practitioner*. Philadelphia: W. B. Saunders, 150–158.

Goodwin, D. W. (1979). Alcoholism and heredity: A review and hypothesis. *Archives of General Psychiatry, 36*:57–61.

Goren, S. (1979). A systems approach to emotional disorders of children. *Nursing Clinics of North America, 14*:457–465.

Grace, H., Layton, J. & Camilleri, D. (1981). *Mental Health Nursing: A Socio-Psychological Approach*, 2nd ed. Iowa: William C. Brown Company, 150–158.

Greenberg, W. C. (1982). The multiple personality. *Perspectives in Psychiatric Care, 20*:100–104.

Grollman, E. A. (1971). *Suicide: Prevention, Intervention, Postvention*. Boston: Beacon Press.

Hagerty, B. K. (1981). Obsessive-compulsive behavior: An overview of four psychological frameworks. *Journal of Psychiatric Nursing and Mental Health Services, 19*:37–39.

Hagerty, B. K. (1984). *Psychiatric-Mental Health Assessment*. St. Louis: C. V. Mosby Co.

Hare, A. & Boles, R. (1965). *Small Groups: Studies in Social Interaction*. New York: A. A. Knopf.

Harmon, T. M., Nelson, H. V. & Hayes, S. (1980). Self-monitoring of mood versus activity by depressed clients. *Journal of Consulting and Clinical Psychology*, February, 30–38.

Harris, E. (1981). Psychotropic drug therapy. *American Journal of Nursing, 81*:1303–1334.

Hein, E. C. (1973). *Communication in Nursing Practice*. Boston: Little, Brown and Company.

Hickey, B. (1983). Transitional relatedness and engaging the regressed borderline client. *Journal of Psychiatric and Mental Health Services, 21*:27–35.

Hough, G. S. (1976). Behavioral approach to alcoholism. *Nursing Clinics of North America, 11*:507–516.

Hunn, S., Mirana, C., Malgneaux, U. and Warshaw, C. (1980). Nursing Care of Patients on Lithium. *Perspectives in Psychiatric Care, 18*:214–220.

Jacob, M. S. & Sellers, E. M. (1977). Emergency management of alcohol withdrawal. *Drug Therapy, 2*:28–34.

Jacobson, A. (1980). Melancholy in the 20th century: Causes and prevention. *Journal of Psychiatric Nursing and Mental Health Services, 18*:11–21.

Jellinek, E. M. (1952). Phases of alcohol addiction. *Quarterly Journal of Studies in Alcohol, 13*:673–684.

Jellinek, E. M. (1960). *The Disease Concept of Alcoholism*. New Haven, Connecticut: Hillhouse Press.

Jorn, N. (1982). Regression in a case of multiple personality disorder. *Perspectives in Psychiatric Care, 20*:105–110.

Jourard, S. M. (1971). *The Transparent Self*. New York: D. Van Nostrand Company.

Kalman, M. (1982). Responding to a suicidal patient. In M. Miller (ed.) *Suicide Intervention by Nurses*. New York: Springer Publishing Company.

Keidel, C. C. (1983). Adolescent suicide. *Nursing Clinics of North America, 18*:323–332.

Kernberg, O. (1975). *Borderline Conditions and Pathological Narcissism*. New York: Aronson Publishing Company.

Kerr, N. (1980). Anxiety: Theoretical considerations. *Perspectives in Psychiatric Care, 18*:28–36.

Kicey, C. (1974). Catecholamines and depression: A physiological theory of depression. *American Journal of Nursing, 74*:2010–2020.

Kim, M. & Moritz, D. A. (1982). *Classification of Nursing Diagnosis*. New York: McGraw-Hill Book Co.

Knapp, M. (1972). *Nonverbal Communication in Human Interaction*. New York: Holt, Rinehart, & Winston.

Knowles, R. (1981). Handling depression by identifying anger. *American Journal of Nursing, 81*:968.

Knowles, R. (1981). Handling anger: Responding vs. reacting. *American Journal of Nursing, 81*:2196.

Kucera-Bozarth, K. (1982). Compliance with lithium regimens. *Journal of Psychiatric Nursing and Mental Health Services, 20*:11–15.

Kurose, K., Anderson, T., Bull, W., et al. (1981). A standard care plan for alcoholism. *American Journal of Nursing, 81*:1001–1006.

Laing, R. D. (1960). *The Divided Self: A Study of Sanity and Madness*. London: Travistock Publications.

Lazaroff, U. A. (1963). Nursing Interventions when the Patient Says "Should". In Burd, S. F. and Marshall, M. A. (eds.), *Some Clinical Approaches to Psychiatric Nursing*. New York: Macmillan Company.

Lewis, L. W. (1975). Hidden alcoholic: A nursing dilemma. *Nursing, 5*:20–30.

Lidz, T., Cornelison, A., Heck, S. & Terry, P. (1957). The intrafamilial environment of schizophrenia patients: Marital schism and marital skew. *American Journal of Psychiatry, 114*:241–248.

Lidz, T., Fleck, S. & Cornelison A. (1965). *Schizophrenia and the Family*. New York: International Universities Press.

Lidz, T. (1976). *The Person*. New York: Basic Books.

Lion, J. R. (1981). *Personality Disorders: Diagnosis and Management*. Baltimore: Williams and Wilkins.

Lipkin, G. B. & Cohen, R. G. (1973). *Effective Approaches to Patients' Behavior*. New York: Springer.

Loomis, M. E. & Horsley, J. A. (1974). *Interpersonal Change: A Behavioral Approach to Nursing Practice*. New York: McGraw-Hill Book Co.

Mahler, M. (1974). Symbiosis and individuation. *Psychoanalytic Study of the Child, 29*:89–106.

Masterson, J. (1981). *The Narcissistic and Borderline Disorders: An Integrated Developmental Approach*. New York: Brunner-Mazel.

Maynard, C. K. & Chitty, K. K. (1979). Dealing with anger: Guidelines for nursing intervention. *Journal of Psychiatric Nursing and Mental Health Services, 6*:36–41.

Minuchin, S. (1974). *Families and Family Therapy*. Cambridge: Harvard University Press.

Murray, J. (1974). Recipient participation in determining psychiatric treatment. *Nursing Research, 23*:325–333.

Murray, R. B. & Huelskoetter, M. M. W. (1983). *Psychiatric/Mental Health Nursing*. Englewood Cliffs, New Jersey: Prentice-Hall.

O'Connell, R. A. (1982). A review of the use of electroconvulsive therapy. *Hospital and Community Psychiatry*, *33*:469–473.

Parks, S. (1966). Allowing physical distance as a nursing approach. *Perspectives in Psychiatric Care*, *4*:31–35.

Pattison, E. (1965). Treatment of alcoholic families with nurse home visits. *Family Process*, *4*:75–94.

Ramshorn, M. (1970). The group as a therapeutic tool. *Perspectives in Psychiatric Care*, *8*:104.

Ray, O. (1978). *Drugs, Society, and Human Behavior*. St. Louis: C. V. Mosby Co.

Reubin, R. (1979). Spotting and stopping the suicide patient. *Nursing 79*, *9*:82–85.

Roberts, S. L. (1978). *Behavioral Concepts and Nursing Throughout the Life Span*. Englewood Cliffs, New Jersey: Prentice-Hall.

Rogers, C. R. (1980). *A Way of Being*. Boston: Houghton Mifflin Company.

Satir, V. (1972). *Peoplemaking*. Palo Alto, California: Science and Behavior Books, Inc.

Schneider, F. (1980). Depression characterized by the inability to grieve. *Patient Counseling and Health Education*, 2:161–169.

Schroder, P. (1979). Nursing intervention with patients with thought disorders. *Perspectives in Psychiatric Care*, *17*:32–39.

Seligman, M. E. P. (1975). *Helplessness*. San Francisco: Freeman.

Schwartzman, S. (1975). The hallucinating patient and nursing intervention. *Journal of Psychiatric Nursing and Mental Health Services*, *13*:23–26.

Shaw, B. F. (1977). Comparison of cognitive therapy and behavior therapy in the treatment of depression. *Journal of Consulting and Clinical Psychology*, August, *45*:543–551.

Smoyak, S. (1975). *The Psychiatric Nurse as a Family Therapist*. New York: John Wiley & Sons.

Stuart, G. W. & Sundeen, S. J. (1983). *Principles and Practice of Psychiatric Nursing*. St. Louis: C. V. Mosby Co.

Sundeen, S. J., Stuart, S. W., Rankin, E. & Cohen, S. (1976). *The Nurse Client Interaction: Implementing the Nursing Process*. St. Louis: C. V. Mosby Co.

Swanson, A. (1975). Communicating with depressed persons. *Perspectives in Psychiatric Care*, *13*:63–67.

Tishler, C. L., Lent, W. J. & McKenry, P. C. (1980). Assessment of suicidal potential in adolescents. *Journal of Emergency Nursing*, *6*:24–26.

United States Department of Health, Education and Welfare. (1981). *Fourth Special Report to the U.S. Congress on Alcohol and Health*. Washington, D.C.: United States Government Printing Office.

Vaillant, G. E. & Milofsky, E. S. (1979). The etiology of alcoholism. *American Psychologist*, *37*:494–503.

Wahil, A. (1981). Nursing therapy and the assessment of families. *Journal of Psychiatric Nursing*, *19*:30–35.

Watson, J. P. (1974). The treatment of anxiety. *Nursing Mirror*, *138*:72–73.

William, J. & Wilson, H. (1982). A psychiatric nursing perspective on DSM-III. *Journal of Psychosocial Nursing and Mental Health Services*, *20*:14–20.

Wilson, H. S. & Kneisl, R. (1980). *Psychiatric Nursing*. Reading, Massachusetts: Addison-Wesley.

Wollersheim, J. P. (1974). The assessment of suicide potential via interview methods. *Psychotherapy: Theory, Research, and Practice*, *11*:222–225.

Wolpe, J. (1973). *The Practice of Behavior Therapy*, 2nd ed. Elmsford, New York: Pergamon Press, Inc.

Yalom, I. (1975). *The Theory and Practice of Group Psychotherapy*. New York: Basic Books, Inc.

Section

PSYCHIATRIC NURSING PRACTICE QUESTIONS

1 • The capacity for reacting with anxiety to a potentially dangerous situation has survival value for the individual in that it serves as a:

1. Power source.
2. Fictive force.
3. Action deterrent.
4. Protective signal.

2 • Freud stated that all neurotic processes are developed in an attempt to avoid:

1. Reality.
2. Anxiety.
3. Responsibility.
4. Aggression.

3 • An anxiety reaction is basically a response to:

1. Change in libidinal energy.
2. Loss of ego control.
3. Increased repressive forces.
4. Shift in object cathexis.

4 • Normal anxiety differs from fear in that the stimulus for anxiety is:

1. An easily observable external threat to security.
2. Not immediately available to the conscious mind.
3. A more serious threat to one's social welfare.
4. Completely unrelated to one's life situation.

5 • Sullivan defined anxiety as:

1. A sign that self esteem had been endangered.
2. An inevitable part of every interpersonal relationship.
3. A phenomenon evoked by a situation of autonomy.
4. Disguised guilt arising from the use of security operations.

6 • According to Sullivanian theory, anxiety develops as a result of:

1. Innate biological drives that create overwhelming demands of action.
2. Persistent asynchronism between personal and social moral values.
3. Inability to avoid those social situations that bring punishment.
4. Distorted perception of others' evaluations of one's worth.

7 • According to Sullivan's concept of an anxiety continuum, complete absence of anxiety would be known as:

1. Euphoria.
2. Mirth.
3. Detachment.
4. Ecstasy.

8 • According to Sullivan's concept of an anxiety continuum, an extremely high level of anxiety is known as:

1. Fear.
2. Panic.
3. Agitation.
4. Tremor.

9 • Sublimation can most accurately be defined as:

1. Substitution of a similar goal for one that is being blocked.

2. Adopting the ideas, feelings, and behavior of another idealized person.
3. Finding a socially acceptable expression for one's id impulses.
4. Escaping painful situations through recourse to daydreams and fantasies.

10 • Repression can be best understood as:

1. The barring of unacceptable id impulses from consciousness.
2. The resumption of behavior typical of an earlier development level.
3. The conscious forgetting of one's acts, impulses, or desires.
4. Maintenance of a trait in the unconscious by expression of its opposite.

11 • Fantasy consists of:

1. A sensual experience for which no external stimulus exists.
2. Imaginary construction of scenes and events through memory manipulation.
3. Misinterpretation of a sensual stimulus through inattention.
4. Providing varied and inconsistent accounts of past events.

12 • Identification is achieved through the use of which of the following defense mechanisms?

1. Fixation.
2. Projection.
3. Sublimation.
4. Introjection.

13 • Anxiety results when the security of the ego is threatened by:

1. Failure of significant others to fulfill one's expectations concerning their behavior.
2. Danger that repressed desires and feelings will break through to consciousness.
3. Confrontation with an object or problem that one has been unable to master.
4. A gradual and steady elevation in one's moral percepts or ideal aspirations.

14 • The symptoms of an anxiety reaction differ from those of the other classic psychoneuroses in that the symptoms of an anxiety reaction:

1. Give no indication of the nature of the underlying conflict.
2. Are less apt to produce a severe degree of conscious discomfort.
3. Are so sufficiently entrenched as to be inaccessible to treatment.
4. Tend to be less closely related to one's view of himself.

15 • A crisis differs from more usual stress situations in that following a crisis, one is more apt to demonstrate:

1. A change in the level of psychological functioning.
2. A decrease in the number of defense mechanisms used.
3. An improvement in the ability to face adversity.
4. A severe decline in self confidence and trust in others.

16 • Crisis intervention therapy can be categorized in Gerald Caplan's theory of levels of disease prevention as:

1. Primary prevention.
2. Secondary prevention.
3. Tertiary prevention.
4. Quaternary prevention.

17 • Which of the following statements best describes Caplan's concept of tertiary level of disease prevention?

1. Reducing the incidence of affective disorders in the community.
2. Reducing the duration of psychotic illnesses in the community.
3. Understanding treatment philosophies and related therapeutic interventions.
4. Reducing impairment resulting from mental illness in the community.

18 • The nurse and a patient with an anxiety disorder are working together. The patient states, "You don't know what it's like to feel that you're suffocating." What response should the nurse make to facilitate therapy?

1. "When were you suffocating?"
2. "No, I guess I don't."
3. "Tell me how you feel."
4. "Suffocating? What do you mean?"

19 • During a one-to-one interaction with a patient who had suffered a panic attack the patient says, "When I had that attack I thought I was dying." What response by the nurse would be most therapeutic now and pave the way for further therapeutic work?

1. "You thought you were dying?"
2. "What made you think that?"
3. "Then what did you do?"
4. "Describe how you felt."

20 • Neurotic symptoms develop in response to unconscious

1. Anxiety.
2. Guilt.
3. Hostility.
4. Conflict.

21 • An obsessive-compulsive neurosis is characterized by:

1. The expression of unconscious conflict through physiological disturbances.
2. The absence of voluntary activity and a tendency to extreme negativism.
3. The presence of fixed, systematized, and well-concealed delusions.
4. Compelling, repetitive, and stylized patterns of behavior and ideation.

22 • An obsession is:

1. A pathologically persistent, repetitive, and unwelcome thought.
2. A clouding of consciousness with the production of illusions.
3. An exaggerated concern over one's physical health and well-being.
4. Interpretation of all events as being significantly related to oneself.

23 • Compulsion is best defined as:

1. A group of repressed, emotionally charged ideas that influence behavior.
2. The development of a desirable trait to disguise its undesirable opposite.
3. The morbid and irresistible urge to repeat a defensive act again and again.
4. The automatic tendency to oppose and resist what is suggested by others.

24 • The nurse would discover during interaction with an obsessive-compulsive patient that the patient's attitude toward his own ritualistic behavior is:

1. The feeling that the behavior is reasonable, productive, and protective.
2. Understood to be related to underlying feelings that precipitated it.
3. Recognized as unrealistic, but the ability to control it is out of the patient's hands.
4. One of great enjoyment that is derived from the highly structured activities in which the patient engages.

25 • Unconsciously, rituals are perceived by the person as:

1. Trivial time passers.
2. Dramatic declarations.
3. Secret signals.
4. Magical manipulations.

26 • According to Erikson's theory of psychosocial development the obsessive-compulsive person is one who struggles with the alternating attitudes of:

1. Trust versus mistrust.
2. Autonomy versus shame and doubt.
3. Initiative versus guilt.
4. Industry versus inferiority.

27 • When the nurse is developing the initial care plan for an obsessive-compulsive patient, she should be aware that all *but which one* of the following behaviors are typical of a patient with this syndrome?

1. Frugality.
2. Obedience.
3. Hoarding.
4. Avoidance.

28 • The difference between regression and fixation is:

1. Fixation is a return to an earlier level of development for gratification.
2. Fixation is the fear of an object that carries no realistic threat to welfare.
3. Fixation is the persistence of pre-genital interest into later psychosexual development.
4. Fixation is the loving of one's self excessively, to the exclusion of heterosexuality.

29 • An obsessive-compulsive individual differs from a phobic individual in that the obsessive-compulsive:

1. Attempts to avoid those objects that elicit fright.
2. Converts fears into various physical symptoms.
3. Actively protects himself from what is feared.
4. Effectively represses the conflicts and experiences no fear.

30 • Reaction formation can best be understood as:

1. Emphasizing a strong point to cover up a feeling of inadequacy or failure.
2. Keeping one of a pair of ambivalent attitudes unconscious by expressing the opposite.
3. The barring from conscious awareness of unwanted emotions, memories, or impulses.
4. The shifting of an emotion to a less dangerous object than that causing the emotion.

31 • Isolation can be defined as:

1. Determination of consciously acceptable reasons for one's actions, wishes, or shortcomings.
2. Withdrawal into extreme passivity in order to protect oneself from painful emotions.
3. A regressive thought process in which problems are solved by the use of fantasy.
4. Defensive separation of feelings and impulses from the reality of an event.

32 • Undoing can best be understood as:

1. Opposition to direction by using contrary behavior.
2. Avoidance of an anxiety-provoking situation or thought.
3. Neutralization of and atonement for anxiety-ridden acts.
4. Reversal of feelings by turning interests inward.

33 • In psychoneuroses other than obsessive-compulsive neurosis, which of the following defense mechanisms is most frequently used to protect the ego against unacceptable impulses?

1. Regression.
2. Repression.
3. Sublimation.
4. Denial.

34 • Which of the following is *not* an important concept of psychoanalysis?

1. Free association.
2. Transference.
3. Token economy.
4. Resistance.

35 • In psychoanalysis, insight may best be defined as the:

1. Extent of the patient's genuine understanding of the origins and unconscious dynamisms of his behavior.
2. Phenomenon of sudden awareness when a thought is first linked with its related strong emotion.
3. Awareness of those thought process that are determined by genetic control mechanisms.
4. Therapist's ability to distinguish factual from fantasized content in the client's free association.

36 • Which of the following methods has *not* been successful in treatment of obsessive-compulsive neurosis?

1. Behavior therapy.
2. Milieu or systems therapy.
3. Electroconvulsive therapy.
4. Supportive psychotherapy.

37 • During hospitalization the nurse would work with the obsessive-compulsive patient toward increasing:

1. Self esteem.
2. Self control.
3. Self examination.
4. Self denial.

38 • Which of the following statements is *untrue* regarding the use of electroconvulsive therapy?

1. Effective because it fulfills the patient's needs for punishment to expiate strong guilt feelings.
2. Effective in the treatment of severe depression, mania, and catatonic states.

3. Neurophysiological or biochemical mechanisms involved in its efficacy remain unexplained.
4. Complications are minimal, and the risk of death extremely low.

39 • The basic concept underlying the cognitive theory of depression that Aaron Beck postulates is:

1. The individual's beliefs and interpretations of occurrences are distorted.
2. The depressed person can be helped by medication directed toward clearing up his thought processes.
3. Anger is depression turned inward.
4. It is a disruption in activity that occurs when positive reinforcement is withdrawn.

40 • Which of the following statements refers to the psychoanalytic theory of depression?

1. Loss of a love object.
2. Helplessness in the face of uncontrollable stress.
3. Disruption of defense mechanisms supporting the ego.
4. Decrease in ego integrity.

41 • During assessment of a woman diagnosed with reactive depression (precipitated by the loss of a young child), the nurse would be particularly interested in:

1. The manner in which she had resolved previous losses.
2. The characteristics of her superego, id, and ego.
3. The degree of ambivalence toward the lost love object.
4. Her relationship with the child.

42 • Ambivalence is best defined as:

1. Unusual strength or persistence of an unpleasant feeling or impression.
2. The ability to change one's attitude when confronted with meaningful evidence.
3. The tendency for a feeling to remain below the level of consciousness.
4. The coexistence of conflicting emotions toward an object or person.

43 • In evaluating for change in the depressed patient the nurse would observe for *all but which one* of the following?

1. Eating, elimination, and sleeping patterns.
2. Interactions with patients and staff.
3. How many family members have visited.
4. Facial expressions, posture, and gestures.

44 • Which of the following is *not* a nursing intervention that would be implemented for a suicidal patient?

1. Assessing the suicidal potential of the patient by asking if he is thinking about taking his life.
2. Administering a tricyclic. They are fast acting and will cause the depression to lift.
3. Eliciting a short-term "no suicide" contract with the patient.
4. Moving to a more secure unit (locked) if the patient is on an open unit.

45 • A dependent personality implies which of the following?

1. A tendency to exaggerate the importance of sensual needs.
2. Cunning is employed in order to persuade others to his viewpoint.
3. Continuous seeking of support and protection from others.
4. Inability to verbalize needs clearly and directly.

46 • A depressed patient has refused to eat several meals. The appropriate interventions on the part of the nurse include *all but which one* of the following?

1. Provide frequent small feedings and between meal nourishment.
2. Deliver the meal tray, cut the meat, and butter the bread.
3. Suggest that the patient begin by eating the bread.
4. Place a glass of milk in the patient's hand and guide it to his mouth.

47 • A depressed female had been looking unkempt and disheveled for the past week. This morning she arises, takes a bath, puts on an attractive dress, and combs her hair before coming to breakfast. What is the appropriate therapeutic nursing response?

1. "Why how you've changed! I see you've got a pretty new dress. You must be getting better."

2. "Now that you've demonstrated that you can bathe and dress yourself, we hope you'll maintain a good appearance."
3. "As long as you were getting yourself dressed up this morning, why didn't you put on some lipstick and powder?"
4. "I see that you got up early, took a bath, combed your hair and put on a fresh dress before coming to breakfast."

48 • The family is an example of which of the following types of groups?

1. Primary
2. Secondary
3. Artificial
4. Intimate

49 • Which of the following statements is an accurate description of family interactions?

1. Roles within the family are explicitly defined and relatively unchanging.
2. The behavior of each family member is affected by that of every other.
3. Family life protects its members against conflict and anxiety.
4. The emotional climate of the family remains relatively the same through time.

50 • During the acute stage of mania, the predominant feeling would appear to be that of:

1. Freedom.
2. Elation.
3. Joviality.
4. Ecstasy.

51 • Which of the following would the nurse *not* expect to elicit from a hypomanic patient?

1. Unstable mood.
2. Pressured speech.
3. Increased motor activity.
4. Auditory hallucinations

52 • Symptoms of mania include *all but which one* of the following?

1. Flight of ideas.
2. Loose associations.
3. Grandiosity.
4. Religiosity.

53 • Dynamically, manic behavior is an attempt on the part of the patient to avoid consciously recognizing and experiencing feelings of:

1. Depression.
2. Hostility.
3. Euphoria.
4. Acceptance.

54 • The care plan for management of the acute phase of mania might include *all but which one* of the following?

1. Removing the patient to his room in order to decrease stimuli.
2. Provision of exercise, such as riding an indoor bike to dissipate excess energy.
3. Providing for the safety of the patient and the other patients in the milieu.
4. Allowing the patient to make unlimited phone calls on the psychiatric unit's phone.

55 • Rapport can be most accurately defined as:

1. Mutually advantageous give and take between participants in a meaningful relationship.
2. Unqualified acceptance of the ideas and attitudes of an unfamiliar person.
3. Willing submergence of one's own needs to the preferences of another person.
4. Loss of one's own individuality through conscious identification with another.

56 • A male patient is admitted to a hospital with acute mania. He is treated immediately with lithium carbonate and thorazine. As his acute manic phase began to subside, he began to give away his furniture, his car, and other valuables. Would a bill of sale or deed signed by him while he is hospitalized be considered a legal document?

1. No, because he is being treated in a psychiatric hospital.
2. No, because he is being treated with psychotropic medications that can cloud judgment.
3. Yes, because he still has all his civil rights.
4. Yes, because no one can be stopped from selling property that is rightfully his.

57 • Which of the following is *not* true? Patients can be committed to a hospital if:

1. They have been proved to be dangerous to self or to others.
2. They are unable to care for themselves at home.
3. They are unable to differentiate time, person, and place.
4. Inpatient treatment is more beneficial than outpatient treatment.

58 • Which of the following methods would *not* be appropriate for the nursing management of a manic patient's acting out and manipulative behavior on the unit?

1. Increasing both the thorazine and lithium carbonate dosages.
2. Writing out and enforcing limits set on the patient's behavior.
3. Spending extra time with the patient, regardless of the behavior.
4. Rejecting him when he disobeys or is loud in public.

59 • The manic patient may have difficulty sleeping, sometimes sleeping no longer than 2 or 3 hours at a time. In attempting to alleviate the insomnia, the nurse might do *all but which one* of the following?

1. Give a warm glass of milk at bedtime.
2. Encourage the patient to take a warm bath.
3. Provide an evening of quiet activity.
4. Allow the patient to remain up and watch T.V. if he awakens.

60 • In talking to a patient during the acute phase of mania the nurse should:

1. Raise voice pitch and intensity in order to claim the patient's wandering attention.
2. Refer chiefly to the feelings conveyed rather than to the verbal content expressed.
3. Refute or modify any erroneous statements as soon as the patient expresses them.
4. Attempt to explore the motivations for behavior by direct questioning.

61 • A manic patient learned that she could irritate her primary nurse by describing her as tomboyish, and she frequently referred to the nurse in that fashion. What approach to the problem should the primary nurse adopt?

1. Tell the patient that she is sensitive to comments concerning her femininity.
2. Promise to provide extra privileges when the patient learns to curb her comments.
3. Recognize that the patient is mentally ill and that her opinions are not valid.
4. Remain non-judgmental and respond without anger or retaliation.

62 • *All but which one* of the following are basic emotional tasks for the young adult?

1. Achieving independence from parental controls.
2. Identifying with a peer group of one's own sex.
3. Establishing intimate relationships outside the family.
4. Establishing a personal set of values.

63 • Which of the following disturbances in interpersonal relationships most often predisposes to the development of schizophrenia?

1. Faulty family atmosphere and interaction.
2. Absence of a parent of the opposite sex.
3. Extreme competition with authority figures.
4. Lack of participation in peer groups.

64 • According to Bateson's double-bind theory, which of the following causes schizophrenia to develop?

1. Conflict between self love and other love in relationships.
2. Discordance between the primary context and metacontext.
3. Dyssocial patterning prominence during late adolescence.
4. Reaction to a severe, universal state of anxiety.

65 • The psychopathology of schizophrenia typically includes *all but which one* of the following?

1. Regressive withdrawal to infantile behavior of omnipotence and rage.
2. Loss of ego strength with consequent inability to perceive reality.
3. Impaired sense of identity together with confusion of the sexual role.
4. Regression to anal stage of behavior with obsessive thoughts and compulsive behavior.

66 • Which of the following best summarizes the functions of the ego?

1. Supplementation.
2. Compromise.
3. Analysis.
4. Synthesis.

67 • In order for the child to develop a healthy ego, he must:

1. Relinquish his early infantile expectations of magical wish fulfillment.
2. Establish firm boundaries between his mother and his "self."
3. Interrelate with warmly affectionate parental and sibling figures.
4. Find free expression of his physical and emotional drives.

68 • Which of the following is most apt to induce regression of the ego to a fantasied union between the self and the mother?

1. Wish frustration.
2. Overgratification.
3. Harsh discipline.
4. Rigid control.

69 • According to Erikson, the child's first social achievement should be to:

1. Smile when his mother and father talk to him or stroke his face and lips.
2. Trust his mother to meet his needs for nutrition, affection, and protection.
3. Deposit his urinary and fecal excretions in an appropriate container.
4. Utter vocal sounds to express sensations of physical and emotional pleasure and pain.

70 • Regression can be most accurately defined as:

1. Resumption of behavior typical of an earlier level of development.
2. Banishment of unacceptable wishes or ideas from conscious awareness.
3. Unconscious symbolic efforts to eradicate a previous painful experience.
4. Turning of interest inward to total preoccupation with the self.

71 • Denial can best be understood as:

1. Unconscious refusal to recognize unwelcome thoughts and wishes.
2. Keeping one trait unconscious by conscious expression of its opposite.
3. An action designed to atone for an unacceptable act or impulse.
4. Offering justification for one's undesirable or unacceptable behavior.

72 • Typical features of schizophrenia are:

1. Denial of external reality, depression, substitution of fantasy for reality, and blunted and distorted affect.
2. Denial of external reality, disturbances in thought processes, substitution of fantasy for reality, and blunted or distorted affect.
3. Overinvestment in self, depression, substitution of fantasy for reality, and blunted and distorted affect.
4. Disturbances in thinking processes, denial of reality, depression, and substitution of fantasy for reality.

73 • Bleuler's Four A's of schizophrenia include:

1. Loose associations, blunted or inappropriate affect, ambivalence, and autism.
2. Amorphism, loose associations, blunted or inappropriate affect, and ambivalence.
3. Amoral behavior, loose associations, blunted or inappropriate affect, and ambivalence.
4. Alliterative behavior, loose associations, blunted or inappropriate affect, and ambivalence.

74 • The schizophrenic's tendency to distort personal experience can be expected to result in:

1. Disharmony in thought and feeling and flatness of affect.
2. Ease in social interaction and decrease of repressed instincts.
3. Narcissism and decrease of repressed instincts.
4. Hypochondriasis and flatness of affect.

75 • Delusions and hallucinations serve the functions of *all but which one* of the following?

1. Fulfilling unacceptable wishes.
2. Preventing overt depression.
3. Externalizing overwhelming guilt.
4. Reducing anxiety and fear.

76 • Use of delusional thinking signifies that the patient is:

1. Eager to excuse his behavior to friends and relatives.
2. Aware of his unusual vulnerability to external attack
3. Unable to differentiate between thoughts and external reality.
4. Unusually perceptive of the feelings and intentions of others.

77 • Phenothiazine tranquilizers are extremely effective psychotropic agents used in the treatment of schizophrenia. Which of the following reflects accurate teaching from the nurse to a person receiving this drug?

1. "You may experience decreased libido."
2. "Your blood pressure will increase."
3. "You should not drive an automobile."
4. "Your drug is an experimental drug."

78 • Benzotropine mesylate (Cogentin) might be administered to treat a specific side effect of the phenothiazine tranquilizer. If used for such purpose, Cogentin would be given to:

1. Stimulate cerebral cortical glial cells.
2. Counteract extrapyramidal, pseudoparkinsonism symptoms.
3. Stimulate smooth muscle of blood vessels.
4. Counteract muscle weakness of the extremities.

79 • Tardive dyskinesia can best be defined as *all but which one* of the following?

1. An irreversible side effect of antipsychotic medications.
2. Characterized by buccolinguomasticatory triad of head, jaw, and facial movements.
3. Characterized by choreiform movement of the extremities,
4. A temporary manifestation that can be relieved by small doses of the benzodiazepines (Librium, Valium).

80 • The nurse's chief goal in planning care for a schizophrenic patient should be:

1. Interpreting his speech and behavior.
2. Directing his activity on the ward.
3. Anticipating and satisfying his needs.
4. Providing a warm human experience.

81 • The therapeutic relationship between nurse and patient differs from a social relationship in that the former is characterized by:

1. Reciprocity of need expression and gratification.
2. Satisfaction of the emergent needs of the patient.
3. Major personality reconstruction of one participant.
4. Concern with the latent meanings of behavior.

82 • As the nurse works with the patient in planning for discharge and follow-up care, *all but which one* of the following are important to keep in mind?

1. The plans of the interdisciplinary team are most important.
2. The patient's goals and objectives need to be verbalized.
3. The nurse needs to weigh the cost-benefit to the patient when addressing placement.
4. It may take 2 or more hospitalizations before the patient can concur with the "healthy" discharge plan.

83 • Which of the following is *not* a characteristic of a therapeutic relationship?

1. The nurse is responsible for goal direction of the communication.
2. The nurse recognizes her own needs but concentrates on the patient's needs.
3. The nurse and patient examine and modify their behavior as indicated.
4. The nurse maintains a façade of professionalism and never self discloses.

84 • Communication can best be understood as:

1. The transmission of ideas from sender to receiver with little or no distortion.
2. Involvement of 2 or more persons in a reciprocal exchange of information.
3. Establishment of rapport and sympathy between persons through oral or written language.
4. Mutual interchange of ideas in which the opinions of all participants are modified.

85 • One week after the patient's admission, the nurse has established a therapeutic relationship with a schizophrenic 25-year-old male. During one of the interactions the patient lapses into a long silence, crosses his legs, and swings his foot rapidly back and forth. In order to be most therapeutic at this point the nurse should:

1. Comment that the patient seems anxious.
2. Direct his attention to the activities of nearby patients.
3. Switch to a completely different topic of conversation.
4. Touch his knee in a gently restraining fashion.

86 • According to Sullivan, this patient's anxiety would be:

1. Interpersonally created and interpersonally reduced.
2. Precipitated by identifiable current stressors.
3. Short lived and completely self limited.
4. Evoked only by analytical techniques.

87 • In describing the pathogenesis of schizophrenia, Sullivan theorized that:

1. The individual avoids assumption of unwanted adult responsibilities by adopting irrational, irresponsible behavior.
2. The individual forfeits his independence and forms a symbiotic union with his mother in order to avoid anxiety.
3. The individual labors under such a burden of intrapsychically generated stimuli that his poorly developed ego is overwhelmed.
4. The individual is confronted with psychosocial development tasks that he cannot master, and he protectively retreats to fantasy.

88 • An increase in the level of the schizophrenic's anxiety during the first few days of hospitalization would render the patient:

1. More receptive to the hospital staff's direction and control.
2. Intractable to treatment and incapable of communication.
3. Less able to focus attention on the reality of the situation.
4. More insightful concerning the illness and the need for care.

89 • After working with a schizophrenic female, age 35 years, for 2 months the primary nurse began to think that although she had initially been helpful, her relationship with the patient had not yielded the fullest possible therapeutic result. Upon recognizing this possibility she should carry out *all but which one* of the following?

1. Review the process recordings of the verbal and nonverbal communications with the patient.
2. Seek guidance from a nurse specialist or psychiatrist regarding the relationship.
3. Formulate a new or reaffirm the original approach to the patient, as indicated.
4. Terminate relationship with the patient, and reassign her to a different nurse.

90 • In preparing the patient for hospital discharge it would be particularly important that the nurse structure interactions in order to provide:

1. Advice concerning typical post-discharge problems and their solutions.
2. Instruction regarding proper dosage of the prescribed medications.
3. Opportunity for gradual termination of their relationship.
4. Approval of patient's efforts to achieve health and maturity.

91 • The nurse should begin the process of terminating the relationship with the patient when:

1. The treatment relationship is initiated.
2. When negative feelings are aroused by the patient.
3. The nurse believes that the patient perceives the nurse as a parent.
4. The patient seeks to terminate the relationship.

92 • The danger of drug addiction is greatest among which of the following?

1. Lawyers.
2. Salesmen.
3. Athletes.
4. Physicians.

93 • In which of the following occupational groups is habituation to amphetamines most common?

1. Obese housewives.
2. Aging secretaries.
3. Reserved teachers.
4. Aggressive salesmen.

94 • Marijuana use differs from heroin addiction in that:

1. Marijuana use is accompanied by increasing tolerance to the drug.
2. Marijuana abuse develops in neurotic rather than in psychotic individuals.
3. Dependency on marijuana is psychological rather than physical.
4. Addiction to marijuana can only be broken by gradual withdrawal.

95 • *All but which one* of the following drugs can produce an hallucinogenic effect?

1. Amphetamine.
2. Phenobarbital.
3. Marijuana.
4. Lysergic acid diethylamide.

96 • Methadone is useful in treatment of heroin addiction as a result of its tendency to:

1. Increase the electric potential across the myoneural junction.
2. Stimulate repair of the myelin sheath of the central nerve fibers.
3. Correct fluid and electrolyte imbalance in brain tissue.
4. Eliminate drug hunger and block the physiological effects of heroin.

97 • Which of the following is a disadvantage of methadone treatment for chronic heroin dependency?

1. Methadone causes blunting of intellectual functions.
2. Methadone produces many dangerous side effects.
3. Methadone is addicting, and addicts dislike its effect on them.
4. Continually increasing doses of methadone are required for control.

98 • Which single factor would have the greatest influence on the success or failure of an addict's treatment program?

1. The nurse's attitude toward drug addicts.
2. The drugs prescribed by the physician.
3. Significant other's understanding of the problems.
4. The addict's desire to change his habits.

99 • Which of the following aspects of a drug rehabilitation program would be most difficult for the addict?

1. Alleviating the symptoms of drug withdrawal.
2. Finding an economically satisfying job.
3. Eliminating the psychic dependence on the drug.
4. Reestablishing family and community relationships.

100 • The approach that would be most therapeutic in dealing with the addict would be one in which the patient could perceive the nurse as:

1. Permissive.
2. Protective.
3. Controlling.
4. Straightforward.

Answer Sheet for Psychiatric Nursing Practice Questions

1. 1 2 3 4
2. 1 2 3 4
3. 1 2 3 4
4. 1 2 3 4
5. 1 2 3 4
6. 1 2 3 4
7. 1 2 3 4
8. 1 2 3 4
9. 1 2 3 4
10. 1 2 3 4
11. 1 2 3 4
12. 1 2 3 4
13. 1 2 3 4
14. 1 2 3 4
15. 1 2 3 4
16. 1 2 3 4
17. 1 2 3 4
18. 1 2 3 4
19. 1 2 3 4
20. 1 2 3 4
21. 1 2 3 4
22. 1 2 3 4
23. 1 2 3 4
24. 1 2 3 4
25. 1 2 3 4
26. 1 2 3 4
27. 1 2 3 4
28. 1 2 3 4
29. 1 2 3 4
30. 1 2 3 4
31. 1 2 3 4
32. 1 2 3 4
33. 1 2 3 4
34. 1 2 3 4
35. 1 2 3 4
36. 1 2 3 4
37. 1 2 3 4
38. 1 2 3 4
39. 1 2 3 4
40. 1 2 3 4
41. 1 2 3 4
42. 1 2 3 4
43. 1 2 3 4
44. 1 2 3 4
45. 1 2 3 4
46. 1 2 3 4
47. 1 2 3 4
48. 1 2 3 4
49. 1 2 3 4
50. 1 2 3 4
51. 1 2 3 4
52. 1 2 3 4
53. 1 2 3 4
54. 1 2 3 4
55. 1 2 3 4
56. 1 2 3 4
57. 1 2 3 4
58. 1 2 3 4
59. 1 2 3 4
60. 1 2 3 4
61. 1 2 3 4
62. 1 2 3 4
63. 1 2 3 4
64. 1 2 3 4
65. 1 2 3 4
66. 1 2 3 4
67. 1 2 3 4
68. 1 2 3 4
69. 1 2 3 4
70. 1 2 3 4
71. 1 2 3 4
72. 1 2 3 4
73. 1 2 3 4
74. 1 2 3 4
75. 1 2 3 4
76. 1 2 3 4
77. 1 2 3 4
78. 1 2 3 4
79. 1 2 3 4
80. 1 2 3 4
81. 1 2 3 4
82. 1 2 3 4
83. 1 2 3 4
84. 1 2 3 4
85. 1 2 3 4
86. 1 2 3 4
87. 1 2 3 4
88. 1 2 3 4
89. 1 2 3 4
90. 1 2 3 4
91. 1 2 3 4
92. 1 2 3 4
93. 1 2 3 4
94. 1 2 3 4
95. 1 2 3 4
96. 1 2 3 4
97. 1 2 3 4
98. 1 2 3 4
99. 1 2 3 4
100. 1 2 3 4

Section

ANSWERS AND RATIONALES FOR PSYCHIATRIC NURSING PRACTICE QUESTIONS

1. (4) The function of anxiety is to warn the person of impending danger—the fight-flight response. Unlike a drive for hunger or sex, anxiety is produced initially by external causes and not by internal tissue conditions. Later, the individual's previous experiences together with his internal sensations provoke his anxiety.

2. (2) Freud described 3 types of anxiety: reality, neurotic, and moral. Reality anxiety is fear of real danger in the environment. Moral anxiety is fear of conscience. Neurotic anxiety is the fear that instincts will get out of control and result in punishment of the individual. Neurotic anxiety is more a fear of punishment than of the impulse expression that results in punishment from the world (parents, authorities, and friends).

3. (2) Anxiety reaction (or neurosis) occurs when the ego is unable to regulate drives or impulses. If the ego development is supported early in life and environmental factors do not overly intensify the drives, the ego is able to maintain control of drives and impulses.

4. (2) Fear is a recognized, external threat of danger. Signal anxiety is produced intrapsychically (perhaps "unconscious recalling"). Individuals become aware of tension but are not immediately aware of its origin.

5. (2) According to Sullivan, anxiety is a product of interpersonal relationships. Originally it is transmitted from mother to child, and later in life by threats to one's security.

6. (3) To avoid anxiety, the individual adopts protective measures over his behavior, i.e., punishment can be avoided by conforming to his parents' wishes. These security measures form the self system, and anxiety is controlled unless these situations of punishment or threat (may be due to inconsistency in the environment) cannot be avoided.

7. (1) Absence of anxiety (euphoria) occurs as fears dissipate. Euphoria is an exaggerated sense of well-being accompanied by carefree behavior.

8. (2) Panic is extreme anxiety, with "blind fear" of disapproval and marked disorganization of behavior.

9. (3) An example of sublimation is that of someone who becomes a surgeon or psychiatrist not for altruistic reasons, but rather to heal by special powers or to satisfy curiosity and a quest for omnipotence. Sublimation does not result in complete satisfaction.

10. (1) For example, a person may fail to see something that is in plain sight because perception of it is repressed. A person may become sexually impotent because of fear of sex impulses. Repressed content or impulses may be symbolically displaced (rebellion against father displaced to other authority figures).

11. (2) When our reality experiences are too painful, we reconstruct the world in fantasy as we would like it to be. We deny reality

and escape time and space; thus, "facts" are what we wish them to be.

12. (4) Introjection is the fantasized reincorporation of an object or person into the person's own ego or superego. A widow may unconsciously attempt to "regain" her dead husband by displaying some of his remembered characteristics.

13. (2) When large amounts of impulses, fears, or thoughts are repressed, the ego expends much energy in keeping thoughts in the unconscious. If the ego becomes weakened, this repressed material "threatens" to become conscious, and anxiety (a signal of impending danger) results.

14. (1) The symptoms in anxiety reaction are almost classic and include palpitations, dyspnea, and unbearable tension. However, these symptoms manifest themselves for a variety of underlying reasons.

15. (1) When a crisis is handled well, the individual's mental stability is maintained and there is return to the precrisis level of functioning or better.

16. (1) Crisis intervention properly instituted prevents a temporary decompensation from becoming a permanent disability. An example of secondary prevention is caring for an alcoholic during delirium tremens. Tertiary prevention applied to an illness is the rehabilitation phase.

17. (4) The impact of illness of any type on a community can be great. The impairment is not only in loss of life and loss of financial gain but in failure to reach potential in education, family integrity, inventiveness, and security.

18. (3) The best response is to ask the patient to describe the feelings and associate them with the crisis (the precipitant) that preceded the feelings.

19. (4) The nurse should request expansion of the comment until the patient can express the feelings that occurred. Later the patient could be helped to develop new methods to prevent these feelings from being immobilizing.

20. (4) Conflict is defined as the coexistence of 2 opposing goals or motivations. These incompatible needs produce anxiety, and behavior becomes hesitant, vacillating, and seemingly maladaptive (i.e., neurotic). Thus, conflict has a major role in the etiology of neuroses.

21. (4) Highly specialized and ritualized behavior is most characteristic of obsessive-compulsive reaction. The purpose of the behavior is to ward off the anxiety engendered by underlying conflict.

22. (1) An obsession is a persistent, conscious desire or idea recognized as irrational by the individual. Obsessions are conscious expressions of unconscious, conflicted wishes.

23. (3) In accordance with a persistent idea, a defensive act is carried out despite some conscious rejection by the individual.

24. (3) Although the behavior is recognized as unrealistic, the compulsive acts are carried out on pain of anxiety if they are not performed. Persons with many modes of self expression can withstand conflict to a greater extent than those whose repertoire of responses is limited.

25. (4) The rituals of the obsessive-compulsive person are seen as magical manipulations, the intent of which is to decrease intrapsychic tension.

26. (2) Erikson suggested stages of psychosocial development to parallel Freud's stages of psychosexual development. "Autonomy versus shame and doubt" corresponds roughly with Freud's anal phase.

27. (4) Avoidance would be probable in the phobic patient. Frugality, obedience, and hoarding are typical behaviors that can also be observed during the psychosexual anal stage of personality development.

28. (3) Fixation is the persistence of the behavior characteristic of one phase into the next phase of psychosexual development. This "holding over" implies arrested development. Regression is the resumption, under stress, of behaviors typical of an earlier phase.

29. (3) A phobia is a morbid dread of something. It is generally unconscious and may be immobilizing if the individual must be exposed to the dreadful object. Compulsive acts are designed to combat (or undo) what the person fears.

30. (2) Reaction formation is a common defense mechanism in obsessive-compulsive reaction. The conflict can be reduced by ex-

pressing consciously only one of a pair of ambivalent attitudes or goals.

31. (4) Isolation is also a way to express only one part of a conflict. In isolation, feelings (i.e., anxiety) are defensively separated from the act or impulse.

32. (3) Undoing combats anxiety development by repetitive actions designed to offset some other act or impulses.

33. (2) Repression is an unconscious defense mechanism whereby painful, anxiety producing thoughts are kept out of conscious awareness. Dissociative reactions and conversion reactions are examples of neuroses in which repression is a prominent feature.

34. (3) A token economy is a mechanism utilized in implementing a behavior modification program.

35. (1) Insight (understanding of behavior) in itself requires ego strength, and further ego strength is required to enable the patient to act constructively on these insights.

36. (3) Behavior modification therapy is the application of learning principles to change maladaptive behavior. Supportive psychotherapy is a treatment approach in which the personality is strengthened, and insight into the unconscious conflicts is not imposed. Milieu therapy is treatment through specific changes in the environment. Electroconvulsive therapy is used to relieve symptoms of patients suffering the most severe forms of depression or schizophrenia who are not responding to other interventions.

37. (1) Increasing self esteem is a goal for any patient. When anxiety is high, self esteem is lowered.

38. (1) Its efficacy in treating severe depression, mania, and catatonic states has been well documented, as have the minimal complications and risk of death. The reason why it works has yet to be fully determined.

39. (1) Beck's research gives evidence that the depressed individual does not interpret things in the same way that the non-depressed individual does.

40. (1) The loss of a love object, whether it be a person, place (such as a home), or work can result in reactive depression according to psychoanalytical theory.

41. (1) Of special significance will be how well this woman has handled loss in the past.

42. (4) Ambivalence often involves the coexistence of love and hate for the same person.

43. (3) The number of visitors would not be so important, but the patient's response to them would be.

44. (2) Tricyclics take up to 3 weeks to act. The patient will be relieved to share this burden with the nurse and reveal exactly what thoughts and plans are in mind. A "no suicide" contract is feasible over the short term, especially if suicidal plans are vague and not lethal. For a more lethal plan the patient should be moved to a locked unit. If already on a locked unit, suicide watch or precautions should be implemented by staff.

45. (3) Dependent persons continually seek directions about what to do, think, and feel. They need support and protection.

46. (1) Reducing the burden of making simple decisions and actively helping to meet nutritional needs are indicated. The nurse should remember that the patient's refusing to eat has significant meaning. It is a way for the patient to express anger toward the self and toward others.

47. (4) Her behavior is noted and commented on. She may not be ready to be well even if she is making progress toward mental health. Asking her to maintain this level of grooming may be a burden, and telling her to put on lipstick and powder indicates that she did not do enough to please you.

48. (1) The family is a primary group, other groups are considered secondary. "Artificial" and "intimate" are not official terms used to classify groups.

49. (2) The family is an interactional unit or system in which the behavior of each family member is affected by that of every other.

50. (2) Ecstasy is a mild word for the intensity of feeling that some persons in a manic state express. The underlying feeling, however, is aggression.

51. (4) Auditory hallucinations are not present, but a labile affect, pressured speech accompanied by flight of ideas, and increased motor activity should be expected.

52. (2) Loose associations are one of Bleuler's Four A's. They are found in schizophrenia not in manic-depressive disorder.

53. (1) It is thought that manic and depressive episodes are 2 variations of a similar illness. Some patients who have manic reactions also have histories of depressive episodes.

54. (4) Decreasing the stimuli may help prevent the patient's inappropriate behavior from escalating any further. He and the other patients must be kept safe from any hostile or destructive acts he might wish to engage in, and safe, healthy ways to dissipate excess energy should be encouraged as long as he is not physically depleted. For the manic patient the permission to make unlimited phone calls could amount to hours on the phone, precluding other patients from making calls or receiving them.

55. (1) Mutual advantageous give and take implies an interpersonal relationship in which each participant feels a noncompetitive sharing or compatibility.

56. (3) In most states people do not lose their civil rights when admitted to a unit designed to treat persons who are mentally ill. If the patient is deemed mentally incompetent (which is not a simple procedure), power of attorney may be given to another.

57. (3) Being antisocial or not being oriented to time, place, and person does not constitute grounds for institutionalization.

58. (4) Initially the medication dosage may be increased and later gradually decreased as a therapeutic lithium level is established. Limiting the behaviors and giving attention are indicated. Manic individuals need someone who can remain objectively calm or neutral in the midst of the chaos that can be generated in an acute manic state. The nurse's role is to provide a stabilizing force.

59. (4) The first 3 interventions have demonstrated efficacy in aiding sleep. To allow the patient to remain up and active once awake rewards and reinforces the poor sleeping pattern.

60. (2) The feelings behind the words are most important at this time. It is important to clarify the intent and to be certain that the nurse understands the patient's communication.

61. (4) The right approach is to remain non-judgmental, but this is very hard to carry out. Patients sometimes have an uncanny sense of our most vulnerable spots.

62. (2) Identifying with a peer group of the same sex is a task of the adolescent years.

63. (1) Disturbed communication in family interactions and atmosphere contribute to the development of schizophrenia. Needs are not met owing to the inconsistency in family interacting.

64. (2) According to Bateson, when there is discord between the primary context and the metacontext, schizophrenia develops.

65. (4) This psychopathology is not indicative of schizophrenia. Rather, it is indicative of a neurotic response to anxiety.

66. (4) The main function of the ego is to test reality, or as listed here, synthesize. Synthetic function of the ego is the ability to form wholeness. It therefore is the ability to maintain the functions necessary for the adaptations in life (e.g., withstand stress, solve problems, and develop coping mechanisms).

67. (1) Each of us has positive and negative parts of our personality, and each is inevitably expressed. We cannot predetermine in childhood to express only the positive, nor can we develop a healthy ego by free expression of all drives. The ego is developed primarily in the first year of life but continues growth throughout life. As conflict is encountered, the infant is found to develop a differentiated personality to cope with this conflict and to recognize himself as an individual. Thus, the ego begins to emerge, and magical wish fulfillment is given up. The mother is a source of satisfaction and dissatisfaction. The resolution of conflict results in strengthening of the ego.

68. (2) Overgratification, i.e., prolonged and consistent meeting of all perceived or anticipated needs, does not allow the individual to experience and resolve sufficient conflict to result in ego growth.

69. (2) Basic trust versus basic mistrust is the 1st of 8 stages of man's psychosocial development outlined by Erikson. The infant's task is to learn trust of self, trust of others, and trust in the environment.

70. (1) Regression is a major defense mechanism of the ego that can be observed in operation every day.

71. (1) Denial of internal and external reality contributes significantly to the development of symptoms observed in schizophrenia.

72. (2) Depression is not one of the classic features of schizophrenia.

73. (1) The classic Four A's of schizophrenia are associative looseness (loss of logical thinking), affect (blunting and distortion of affect), ambivalence, and autism (overinvestment in self, preoccupation with fantasy, and denial of reality).

74. (1) Distortion of reality leads to disharmony of thought and feeling, and therefore to flatness of affect.

75. (2) As bizarre as delusions and hallucinations may seem to be, they are necessary to the patient's psychic economy in that they serve as protective functions for the faltering ego.

76. (3) Although delusional thinking represents a distortion of reality and an inability to differentiate between thoughts and external reality, it nevertheless reveals a residue of the individual's experiences.

77. (3) In some patients, this type of drug causes extrapyramidal reactions (e.g., tremor, akathisia).

78. (2) Benztropine mesylate has an atropine-like action and is used along with levodopa to treat Parkinson's disease.

79. (4) At the present time this serious side effect of antipsychotic medication is irreversible. There is no known cure.

80. (4) Although the nurse should attempt to provide a warm human experience that is not to imply a rapidly developed, interpersonal relationship oozing with acceptance and sanction. Schizophrenic patients typically are withdrawn and rejecting of people.

81. (2) Therapeutic and social relationships differ, and the aim of a therapeutic relationship is to meet the needs of selected patients. If, however, the nurse should become extremely anxious while interacting with a patient, it would be advisable for her to retreat, seek the reason for the anxiety, and return to the patient later.

82. (1) The plans of the interdisciplinary team may be the "healthiest" discharge option for the patient, but unless this is also the goal of the patient it will all be for nought. It may take many hospitalizations before the patient can come to the realization that his needs would best be met by solutions other than his own.

83. (4) Carl Rogers states that for a therapist to be effective several qualities need to be present: warmth, genuineness, unconditional positive regard, and empathy. A facade of professionalism, with no self disclosure (if appropriate) would not meet these requirements.

84. (2) Communication does not require that opinions be modified, only that there is a reciprocal exchange of information.

85. (1) During very early contacts with the patient (when he was incoherent) this comment would have been useless. However, after a relationship with a modicum of trust is established, pointing out anxious behavior can result in identification of people, situations, or thoughts that are causing the anxiety.

86. (1) Anxiety, according to Sullivan, results from our interactions with significant others, and causes a reduction in self esteem.

87. (2) Sullivan's description of the etiology of schizophrenia is congruent with his hypothesis that anxiety is interpersonally engendered. As in the formulations of other theorists, schizophrenic behavior has as its purpose the avoidance of anxiety (or protection of the ego).

88. (3) Sullivan stated that as the anxiety level increases, the breadth of one's span of interest narrows, and if the anxiety is extreme enough, focus is entirely on the self.

89. (4) It is quite conceivable that we are not maximally effective with all patients. We experience plateaus where no progress is evident. The first 2 steps show how to evaluate whether or not a different approach is indicated.

90. (3) It is crucial that patients be prepared long in advance for the termination of the relationship. No one feels satisfied when a significant person leaves abruptly.

91. (1) At the onset of a nurse-patient relationship,

it is therapeutic to establish the appropriate temporal limits of the interaction.

92. (4) Physicians are in a high risk group for drug addiction, because the practice of medicine is a high stress occupation, and the availability of drugs is commonplace.

93. (1) In recent years amphetamines were used to facilitate weight reduction, but the complications were so great that their use in the treatment of obesity is now rare.

94. (3) Dependency on heroin is high both physically and psychologically. The physical dependence potential in marijuana is unknown. It has moderate psychological addicting properties.

95. (2) LSD commonly produces hallucinations. Marijuana and amphetamines do so in extremely high doses.

96. (4) The preferred treatment is to relieve the affective state that provoked the addiction. This method is not always possible, so others are instituted (i.e., methadone). The addict is given methadone to produce a physiological state that permits him to be socially functional. Methadone is given in dosages of 10 to 20 mg daily and gradually increased over a period of 4 weeks until the desired effect is achieved.

97. (3) Some researchers think that methadone is as addicting as heroin, but the effects on the body are not as harmful. However, addicts dislike the effects of methadone.

98. (4) Although it is true that the addict's desire to alter the behavior and its consequences is most influential in this change, he cannot do so until he feels some degree of self reliance and self confidence. The key person in enabling the change in life style is the addicted individual. Others encourage and support the move toward abstinence.

99. (3) Physiological dependence (withdrawal symptoms) cease within 1 week to 10 days, but psychological dependence may continue indefinitely.

100. (4) A matter-of-fact, straightforward application of minimal standards for conduct is helpful. It is important not to sanction unacceptable behavior, but it is equally important not to retaliate for such behavior.

PART TWO

Comprehensive Examination

Section 1

COMPREHENSIVE EXAMINATION

Wendy Smith is a 28-year-old gravida 1 para 0 who comes to the hospital in early labor. She is at 39 weeks' gestation and tells the nurse that her bag of waters has ruptured, and the fluid was dark colored.

1 • The nurse performed Leopold's maneuvers in examining Wendy. Abdominal palpation revealed a soft rounded mass in the fundus, irregular lumps or nodules on Wendy's right side, and a hard prominence on Wendy's right side above the symphysis pubis. The most accurate assessment of fetal position would be:

1. Left occiput anterior.
2. Right occiput posterior.
3. Right sacrum posterior.
4. Left sacrum anterior.

2 • In this fetal position, the nurse would most likely find the fetal heart tones:

1. Below the umbilicus on the mother's left side.
2. Below the umbilicus on the mother's right side.
3. Above the umbilicus on the mother's right side.
4. Above the umbilicus on the mother's left side.

3 • Under which of the following conditions is passage of meconium normal during the process of labor?

1. Face presentation
2. Transverse lie presentation
3. Breech presentation
4. Left occiput anterior presentation

4 • After delivery, the physician cuts the umbilical cord. Before the infant is given to the mother to hold, the nurse should carry out the following actions. Which action should be performed first?

1. Confirm identification, and apply bracelet.
2. Examine the infant for abnormalities.
3. Dry the infant, and place it in a warm environment.
4. Instill silver nitrate solution into the infant's eyes.

5 • Although the mechanism that initiates labor is unclear, it is thought that *all but which one* of the following may contribute to initiation of labor?

1. Decreased placental production of progesterone.
2. Increase in fetal activity.
3. Uterine response to overdistention.
4. Maternal production of oxytocin.

Rachel, a 2-month-old infant, has been brought to the Cardiac Clinic by her mother for the 1st time. She had an appointment 4 weeks ago, but her mother did not see the necessity of coming in earlier. She explained that the reason she came in now was that the infant was "getting bluer" when she cried. The doctor had explained to her after delivery that Rachel had a heart problem but that "sometimes it goes away by itself," and therefore she decided to go home and not worry.

Rachel weighed 5 lb 2 oz at birth; she lost 7 oz during the first 2 days. The mother was discharged after 48 hours, but the infant remained hospitalized for a total of 5 days to regain her birth weight. The infant now weighs 7 lb 11 oz, which puts her at the 5th percentile. Rachel eagerly takes her feedings but tires very quickly and stops nursing. Her mother added that she thought Rachel had trouble breathing sometimes and that this also seemed to be getting worse.

This infant is poorly nourished and irritable, lying still on the examining table, mildly dyspneic. Palpation over the precordium reveals a thrill, and cardiac auscultation at the 4th, 5th, and 6th intercostal spaces at the left sternal border reveals a high, harsh murmur heard throughout systole. When crying, Rachel shows visible cyanosis.

Rachel has apparently developed Eisenmenger's syndrome in which her original left to right shunt has now become a right to left shunt due to progressive increase in pulmonary vascular resistance.

The infant was admitted with plans for a cardiac catheterization as soon as she gains a little more weight.

6 • Assessment of a 2-day-old infant with ventricular septal defect would reveal all of the following *except*:

1. X-ray of the heart is normal.
2. EKG is normal.
3. Heart murmurs are heard.
4. Color of skin is cyanotic.

7 • Two-month-old Rachel is hospitalized with a provisional diagnosis of ventricular septal defect. While she is waiting for cardiac catheterization, the nurse will be alert for signs of cardiac decompensation. One of the signs is:

1. Diaphoresis when feeding.
2. Resting heart rate of 160 beats/min.
3. Severe respiratory distress while lying flat.
4. Cyanosis during deep sleep.

8 • The primary goal in preparing Rachel for surgical procedures should be:

1. To provide adequate nutrient intake.
2. To provide sensory stimulation.
3. To help her develop a sense of trust.
4. To help her develop her neuromuscular skills.

9 • Rachel's mother was encouraged to hear that her daughter's condition was now stabilized after the cardiac catheterization. All of the following are signs of stabilization *except*:

1. Her blood pressure at the wrist, using the flush technique, is 68 mm Hg.
2. The affected extremity is now cool to touch.
3. Her pulse, distal to the catheterization site, is now strong.
4. Dressing is clean.

10 • In ventricular septal defect, initially the blood is shunted from:

1. Left to right.
2. Right to left.
3. The aorta to the pulmonary artery.
4. The left atrium to the right atrium.

Oscar Crown, 55 years old, had a 5-year history of hypertension, which had been treated with hydrochlorothiazide, when he suffered a stroke during an altercation with a neighbor. On admission to the emergency room of a nearby hospital, he was comatose. Following a brain scan, which revealed a large left hemisphere lesion, and a spinal puncture, which revealed increased pressure and bloody spinal fluid, Mr. Crown was diagnosed as having suffered an intracerebral hemorrhage. Following administration of 420 ml of 25% mannitol solution intravenously, Mr. Crown slowly regained consciousness and was found to have right hemiplegia and expressive aphasia.

11 • In planning nursing interventions to maximize Mr. Crown's independence in self care following recovery from his stroke, the nurse should give highest priority to which aspect of his care?

1. Training Mr. Crown in left handed grooming and dressing activities.
2. Assisting Mr. Crown to ambulate using a walker.
3. Encouraging Mr. Crown to communicate with others in written form.
4. Supervising Mr. Crown in digital removal of stool from the rectum.

12 • Which of the following nursing measures should be instituted to prevent development of right arm deformities during Mr. Crown's rehabilitation period?

1. Supporting the right arm in a cloth sling during all waking hours.
2. Placing a rolled cloth in the right hand and securing it with bandage.
3. Full range of motion of shoulder, elbow, wrist, and fingers thrice daily.
4. Maintaining the right forearm and hand in a volar splint continuously.

13 • Which of the following nursing measures should be instituted to protect Mr. Crown from typical post-stroke lower extremity deformities?

1. Place a restraining sheet over his thighs, and tuck it in tightly under both sides of the mattress.

2. Teach Mr. Crown to press his feet against a footboard anchored between the end of the mattress and the foot of the bed.
3. Place a rolled blanket under both knees and a rubber donut under both heels.
4. Encase his feet in padded boots, and place a sandbag along the lateral aspect of his right thigh.

14 • While caring for Mr. Crown following his recovery from coma, the nurse observed that he consistently neglected to eat several of the foods on his meal tray. This observation should lead the nurse to:

1. Test Mr. Crown's peripheral vision by means of the direct confrontational test.
2. Request the dietitian to provide Mr. Crown with 5 rather than 3 meals each day.
3. Arrange for Mrs. Crown to be present at meal time to feed Mr. Crown.
4. Ask Mr. Crown whether there are certain foods that he dislikes or is allergic to.

15 • Which intervention by the nurse would be most helpful in facilitating restoration of Mr. Crown's speech function?

1. Directing him to write out his requests and responses until voluntary speech patterns return.
2. Providing practice in identifying objects verbally by pointing to and naming each object and having the patient repeat the name.
3. Circumventing his word finding problems by anticipating his needs and asking questions that he can answer either "Yes" or "No."
4. Providing him with books and magazines to read silently as a means of reacquainting himself with word structure and meaning.

Rose Hershey, 55 years old, was 20-lb overweight, with a 15-year history of NPH insulin–controlled diabetes when she was admitted to the hospital with gangrene of the right foot. Following a diagnostic work-up, which revealed markedly impaired circulation to both legs, Mrs. Hershey underwent a right, below-the-knee amputation with conventional delayed prosthetic fitting.

16 • In order to minimize Mrs. Hershey's psychological discomfort following surgery, it would be important for the nurse to initiate discussion of which of the following topics during pre-operative preparation?

1. The desirability of requesting pain medication for even minimal amounts of post-operative discomfort.
2. The possibility of experiencing phantom sensation referrable to the amputated leg segment.
3. The necessity for Mrs. Hershey to integrate her prosthetic leg into her total body image and self concept.
4. The advisability that Mrs. Hershey decrease her expectations of herself in order to accept dependence on others.

17 • The preferred means for reducing edema in Mrs. Hershey's stump on the 2nd day following amputation would be to:

1. Elevate the stump on rubber covered pillows.
2. Raise the foot of the bed frame.
3. Lift the foot of the bed onto wooden blocks.
4. Suspend the stump in a sling attached to an over-the-bed frame.

18 • After surgery Mrs. Hershey should be supervised in which of the following bed exercises to prepare for walking with crutches?

1. Pulling herself to sitting position with a rope tied to the foot of bed.
2. Raising and lowering her left leg while keeping the knee extended.
3. Kneading a sponge rubber ball between palms and fingers of both hands.
4. Using her palms to push herself up from a prone position.

19 • Observation of which of the following symptoms should lead the nurse to suspect that Mrs. Hershey is experiencing an insulin reaction?

1. Lethargy, rapid bounding pulse.
2. Diaphoresis, weakness, tremor.
3. Flushed, dry, hot skin.
4. Thirst, air hunger, sweet breath odor.

20 • In assisting Mrs. Hershey with grooming and dressing, the nurse should plan her morning care to include which of the following?

1. Checking the skin of her stump, and applying lotion to the suture line before the lower extremities are dressed.
2. Applying Band-Aids or Steri-Strips to hold the skin flap edges in approximation before covering the wound with a gauze dressing.

3. Rewrapping the stump with an elastic roller bandage before Mrs. Hershey moves from the bed to the wheelchair.
4. Massaging the stump with rubbing alcohol in order to remove skin bacteria and toughen the tissues for weight bearing.

The rural community in which Dolly Handmacher grew up was 15 miles from the small town in which she completed high school, worked as a secretary for 4 years, and met and married her husband. Dolly had been the oldest of 3 children but had felt distant from her parents and siblings. She had been a lonely, naive child. Although her controlling mother frequently warned Dolly about the dangers of close contact with boys and with public toilet fixtures, she had given her no sex instruction. Dolly's father, grandfather, and uncle, it was rumored, had all been guilty of marital infidelity. Dolly entered marriage feeling that sex was dirty, that men were untrustworthy, and that she had been soiled by her awkward experimentation with premarital sexual experiences.

Early in their marriage Dolly's husband Fred, a factory foreman, noted his wife's extreme personal fastidiousness. One day he came home from work to find that the water in the toilet had backed up, flooding the bathroom floor and soaking through the kitchen ceiling. After Dolly had thoroughly cleaned the bathroom and kitchen, she had spent hours scrubbing her body and clothing, feeling that she had been contaminated by the contents of the toilet. Following this event Dolly developed a number of compulsive washing rituals, with which her husband sometimes cooperated in an effort to reduce her persistent fear of contamination.

By means of these rituals Dolly managed to control her anxiety and to maintain the appearance of a conventional, efficient housewife for 9 years. One year after the birth of their first child, Dolly's husband was promoted to the position of plant supervisor, which required that he become more socially active than formerly. The demands of child rearing and increased socializing left Dolly less time for her compulsive cleaning routines, and she developed insomnia, irritability, and even more time consuming rituals. Finally, her husband persuaded her to see a psychoanalyst, whose therapy helped reduce her anxiety for a period of 1 year. Then Dolly became confused, had difficulty remembering the proper sequence of her routines, and began to experience suicidal thoughts. Shortly thereafter her psychiatrist hospitalized her for psychological testing and more intensive treatment.

21 • Which of the following nursing assessments upon Dolly's admission to the unit is the most crucial in planning interventions?

1. Whether she continues to have suicidal thoughts and the likelihood that she might act on these thoughts.
2. What kind of compulsive rituals she now engages in and how much of her day is devoted to them.
3. Determination of early childhood traumatic experiences that might have led to this admission.
4. Evaluation of how she perceives her roles as wife and mother and the feelings each role invokes.

22 • The most therapeutic nursing intervention for Dolly after admission would be to:

1. Assure the patient of a united approach from the nurses.
2. Provide the patient a portable timer with a long ringing bell.
3. Discuss the patient's schedule of activities for the day.
4. Make a list of the patient's compulsive rituals for reference purposes.

23 • In order to plan the patient's care the nurse must accept the fact that Dolly does not recognize:

1. That she is a human being separate and independent from other persons.
2. Either the cause for her symptoms of the concomitant secondary gains.
3. The therapeutic abilities of the various members of the treatment team.
4. The degree to which her rituals interfere with the activities of living.

24 • Shortly after she entered the hospital Dolly began to increase her ritualistic washing at bedtime, to the point that she was losing several hours of sleep. Which action by the nurse would *not* be therapeutic?

1. Talk with her to determine the cause of her bedtime anxiety.
2. Remind her to begin washing rituals early to ensure adequate sleep.
3. Limit the amount of time that Dolly may spend on her washing rituals.

4. Ignore her washing activities, and make no comments about them.

25 • Dolly's behavioral rituals serve the purpose of:

1. Blocking delusions and hallucinations from awareness.
2. Providing temporary and partial relief from her anxiety.
3. Drawing attention and approval from significant others.
4. Increasing the inhibitory powers of her super ego.

Mrs. Nora Sams was examined at the Prenatal Clinic at 28 weeks' gestation with the following physical symptoms: blood pressure of 160/90 mm Hg, proteinuria 1+, generalized edema, frontal headaches, and weight gain of 10 lb in 1 month.

26 • Which of the following is usually the *first* sign of pre-eclampsia?

1. Excessive weight gain.
2. Elevation of blood pressure.
3. Frontal headaches.
4. Progressive ankle edema.

27 • Mrs. Sams was sent to the hospital for immediate admission. Without waiting for a physician's order the admitting nurse should carry out all *but which one* of the following actions?

1. Examine the patient for amount and distribution of edema.
2. Place the patient to bed in a four bed ward.
3. Measure the patient's weight.
4. Obtain a urine specimen for measurement of protein level.

28 • In preparing a room for Mrs. Sams' admission the nurse should provide all *but which one* of the following (in addition to the equipment of a standard hospital unit)?

1. Urinary catheterization tray
2. Cloth restraints
3. Suction equipment
4. Intravenous infusion equipment

29 • Mrs. Sams' fluid intake and output should be carefully measured because:

1. Oliguria would indicate a serious complication.
2. Fluid intake should be limited to 1000 ml/24 hr.
3. Sudden diuresis could precipitate a convulsion.
4. Urine output of less than 100 ml every 4 hours would indicate need for magnesium sulfate.

30 • Mrs. Sams' postpartum care should be based on the fact that:

1. Convulsions may occur during the 1st 48 hours following delivery.
2. After delivery an immediate and complete recovery is assured.
3. Chronic renal damage will be suffered as a result of pre-eclampsia.
4. Convulsions will be experienced during any subsequent pregnancy.

Three-year-old Jimmy was brought to the emergency room of a hospital by his parents around 7:00 P.M. The receptionist at the front desk took one look at the child's condition and led them immediately to the emergency room area.

Initial assessment revealed a severely dyspneic child with audible wheezing and occasional weak coughing. Jimmy appeared flushed with circumoral pallor; he appeared exhausted and was lying limp in his father's arms. Vital signs were a temperature of 100°F (R), apical pulse of 106/min, and respirations of 36/min. Both parents appeared harried; the mother explained that the attack began over 2½ hours ago but that she had to wait for her husband to get home from work to bring them to the hospital.

Jimmy had not been ill, and he was perfectly healthy all morning. Later in the afternoon, the mother decided to open the window since the weather had been warm. She noticed a slight breeze that she felt was refreshing. Shortly after she went into the kitchen to do some work, she heard Jimmy cough a couple of times but since he continued playing, she ignored the coughing. When she returned to Jimmy about 10 minutes later, she found him sitting on the floor "trying to catch his breath." As she watched, wondering what to do, dyspnea continued to worsen. Jimmy had had a similar attack of dyspnea 6 months earlier but that episode subsided without medical intervention, and the mother thought this one would also subside by itself. When Jimmy became worse and was obviously having trouble catching

his breath, she became alarmed and called her husband at work.

In the emergency room, epinephrine, 0.15 ml of 1:1000 aqueous solution, was ordered and immediately administered subcutaneously. There was no improvement in Jimmy's condition after 20 minutes, and another dose was given. After the 2nd dose, his breathing improved slightly. He was admitted to the pediatric floor for further medication and treatment.

31 • Your nursing plan for Jimmy should be based on which of the pathophysiological changes in asthma?

1. Bronchospasms.
2. Laryngospasms.
3. Cardiomegaly.
4. Atelectasis.

32 • You note that Jimmy has characteristic wheezing respirations. Wheezing occurs:

1. On inspiration and is due to excessive bronchial secretions.
2. On expiration and is due to partial bronchial obstruction.
3. Only at night when the attack is most severe.
4. When the bronchioles and trachea are totally obstructed.

33 • Keeping the child well hydrated is an important nursing activity. All liquids should be given warm or at room temperature. Iced drinks should be avoided because they:

1. Suppress cough reflexes.
2. Act as gastrointestinal irritants.
3. Trigger bronchospasms.
4. Tend to lower blood pressure.

34 • You are aware that one of the side effects of epinephrine Jimmy was given in the emergency room is:

1. Decreased blood pressure.
2. Skin rash on the trunk.
3. Hematuria.
4. Tachycardia.

35 • Long-term care of the asthmatic child should include all of the following *except*:

1. Early recognition of the onset of acute symptoms by parents.
2. Identification of precipitating factors.
3. Resignation by the parent that they have a severely handicapped child.
4. Incorporating lung exercises into play activities.

Roy Marble, a 68-year-old farmer, suffered an inter-trochanter fracture of the right femur, with overriding of fragments, as a result of a fall. He was transported by ambulance to a nearby hospital where the fracture was treated on the following day by open reduction and internal fixation. For a short time following surgery, both of Mr. Marble's lower extremities were encased in light weight boot casts that were connected at the ankles with a horizontal bar.

36 • In planning for Mr. Marble's care immediately following admission to the hospital, the nurse should assemble which of the following equipment?

1. Stockinette, sheet cotton, and plaster bandage for cast application.
2. Over-the-bed frame, spreader apparatus, and canvas sling for pelvic suspension.
3. Thomas half ring, moleskin, spreader board, ropes, pulleys, and weights for leg traction.
4. Clear plastic inflatable splint for supporting and immobilizing the leg.

37 • If the recovery room nurse observes that Mr. Marble's right foot is cold and pale and shows slow capillary refill following nail compression, she should take which of the following actions?

1. Elevate the entire length of the right leg on firm pillows.
2. Wrap the exposed foot loosely in a towel, and cover the leg with a blanket.
3. Take the patient's vital signs, and check the hip dressing for evidence of hemorrhage.
4. Summon the surgeon to examine the extremity and evaluate the patient's condition.

38 • On Mr. Marble's first post-operative day, the surgeon ordered that the patient be allowed to get out of bed and sit in a chair. In preparing to assist Mr. Marble with this activity it would be most important for the nurse to:

1. Provide a low, soft, well-upholstered chair to protect Mr. Marble from skin pressure injury during sitting.
2. Question the surgeon to determine whether weight bearing is permitted on the operated leg.
3. Schedule Mr. Marble's move from bed to chair immediately before a meal or before visiting hours.
4. Adjust the bed frame to the lowest possible position before Mr. Marble swings his legs over the edge of the bed.

39 • Following removal of Mr. Marble's casts, which of the following nursing interventions should be used to prepare him for progressive ambulation?

1. The nurse should move his hips, knees, and ankles through full range of motion thrice daily.
2. Encourage him to perform all self care and move about freely and frequently in bed.
3. Direct him to actively flex and extend both hips and knees against resistant force applied by the nurse.
4. Instruct and supervise him in such isometric exercises as gluteal setting and quadriceps setting.

40 • Which of the following precautions should be taken in turning Mr. Marble to bathe his back and relieve pressure on his buttocks?

1. Flex the right hip at a right angle to improve his balance.
2. Turn him toward the side of the operated hip.
3. Maintain the right leg in abduction.
4. Prevent flexion of the right knee.

Louis Rossi, a 57-year-old car salesman with a history of 40-pack years of cigarette smoking and heavy alcoholic intake, sought medical attention for increasing hoarseness and a persistent cough. When endoscopy and biopsy revealed a malignancy of the left true vocal cord and of the left pharyngeal wall, a total laryngectomy and radical neck resection were performed.

41 • In selecting pre-operative interventions to enhance Mr. Rossi's post-operative recovery, the nurse should give highest priority to which of the following?

1. Informing him concerning the effects of smoking, voice strain, and alcoholism in etiology of pharyngeal and laryngeal malignancy.
2. Encouraging him to discuss at length his fears of the surgical procedure and its consequences.
3. Describing the types and amounts of foods and liquids to be included in a high protein, high carbohydrate, high vitamin diet.
4. Demonstrating the procedures for tracheostomy care and nasogastric tube feedings on an anatomical model.

42 • For the 1st 2 to 3 hours following laryngoscopic examination, the nurse should check Mr. Rossi for which of the following as evidence of complications of the procedure?

1. Increasing lethargy and somnolence.
2. Diminished breath sounds in the upper lobes.
3. Regurgitation of food and fluids.
4. Restlessness and shortness of breath.

43 • Mr. Rossi developed an infection of his neck wound post-operatively. A major nursing responsibility throughout his postoperative period would be to summon the physician on observation of which of the following indicators of serious complication?

1. Loss of the sense of smell or impairment of the sense of taste.
2. Inability to speak after removal of the tracheostomy tube.
3. Appearance of bright red blood on the neck dressing.
4. Dysphagia on resumption of oral feedings following removal of nasogastric tube.

44 • During his early post-operative period, Mr. Rossi experienced frequent coughing spells, during which large amounts of mucus were expelled through the tracheostomy tube. In applying suction to Mr. Rossi's tracheostomy tube, the nurse should observe which of the following guidelines?

1. Apply suction to the tracheostomy tube on an hourly basis to prevent drying of accumulated secretions.
2. Apply suction for no longer than 5 seconds at a time and oxygenate the patient between applications of suction.

3. Keep the suction catheter immersed in antiseptic solution between applications of suction.
4. Cover the catheter air vent so as to apply suction during both catheter insertion and withdrawal.

45 • In cleaning Mr. Rossi's tracheostomy tube the nurse should observe which of the following safety precautions?

1. Remove the inner and outer tubes as a unit in order to minimize trauma to the tracheal mucosa.
2. Lock inner and outer tubes together securely, and cleanse the lumen by inserting H_2O_2 soaked applicators.
3. Remove the inner cannula, soak it in soapy water for 5 minutes and in alcohol for 5 minutes, and air dry it for 10 minutes before replacement.
4. While one nurse supports the tracheal faceplate and the back of the patient's neck, a second nurse should change or adjust the neck tapes supporting the tube.

During his early childhood years, Irving Gold's parents had described him as a timid, sensitive boy who had frequent nightmares. Following each bad dream his mother would comfort him, but his father was disappointed by his son's unmanly fearfulness. During adolescence, Irving had been shy in the company of women and had experienced numerous somatic symptoms and acute attacks of guilt as a consequence of his masturbation.

During medical school, Irving was aloof toward his classmates. His mother discouraged him from socializing with other young people by carefully screening his phone calls and by insisting that he study at home rather than at the university library. In spite of his mother's open objections, he married at 30 years, after a very short courtship.

After he had completed his medical education, his residency, and had undertaken private practice with an older, well-known cardiologist, Dr. Gold accepted an appointment as director of the cardiac physiology laboratory of a private hospital. His research in cardiac physiology was reported widely in the professional literature and won him the admiration of his medical colleagues.

When he was 38 years old, and following the birth of his second child, increasing concern about financial responsibilities caused Dr. Gold to leave his position as a full-time hospital medical staff member to enter private practice. At the same time he accepted an appointment as an associate professor of internal medicine at the state university in order to satisfy his teaching interests.

During his first months in private practice, Dr. Gold became increasingly agitated and worried about his work. He confided to his wife that he was afraid of being sued for malpractice and doubted his ability to earn money to support his growing family. Although he had been an interested and affectionate father toward his older son, he demonstrated marked antipathy toward his newborn son, claiming that the birth of this child had precipitated his present financial problems. At about the same time, he expressed fear that his fellow physicians at the university had instigated a plot to discredit his research and deprive him of his faculty position. At his wife's suggestion he consulted a private psychiatrist to whom he devulged his fear of making a serious diagnostic error and his guilt concerning his inability to be perfectly honest in telling his patients the true nature and significance of their illnesses. He expressed concern, too, about his increasing consumption of alcohol, his insomnia, and his growing discomfort in face-to-face conversations with people.

Finally, Dr. Gold cancelled the appointments of his private patients, failed to appear for his scheduled lectures in the medical school, and spent his time in bed at home, refusing to see anyone but his wife. When he was told that his older son had undergone emergency surgery for acute appendicitis, he evidenced no concern for the child's welfare. His wife called her husband's psychiatrist, who convinced Dr. Gold to enter a private psychiatric hospital for treatment.

On admission to the hospital, Dr. Gold was ataxic, uncommunicative, and suspicious. He refused to eat, avoided contact with other patients, and displayed an arrogant, contemptuous, and hostile attitude toward patients and personnel. The psychiatrist made a diagnosis of schizophrenic reaction, paranoid type, and decided to treat Dr. Gold with psychotherapy, family therapy, and trifluoperazine (Stelazine).

46 • Which of the following would *not* be implemented as part of the initial care plan for Dr. Gold?

1. Ongoing assessment to determine if he has auditory hallucinations.
2. Meeting with him for a specified amount of time according to a prearranged schedule.

3. Offering reassurance freely.
4. Helping him to analyze what brought about his hospitalization.

47 • Which of the following would be the most effective broad question for the nurse to use in initiating conversation with Dr. Gold?

1. "Have you any family here in the city?"
2. "What would you like to talk about today?"
3. "Have you become accustomed to the hospital?"
4. "Are you beginning to feel any better?"

48 • The most favorable prognostic signs for Dr. Gold would include the following:

1. An immediate response to the Stelazine, his marital status, and his high level of functioning.
2. An immediate response to the Stelazine, his organized delusional system, and his paranoia.
3. A gradual response to the Stelazine, decline in his hostility, and an increased appetite.
4. A gradual response to the Stelazine, his good family relationships, and decreased paranoia.

49 • The communication pattern in Dr. Gold's original family was probably one in which he was frequently:

1. A witness to obscure intellectual debates between his scholarly elders.
2. The recipient of much confusing information with multiple or contradictory meanings.
3. The target of much sensual language that engendered sexual fantasies.
4. An observer of confrontations between an aggressive mother and a passive father.

50 • Goals of family therapy for Dr. Gold and his family should include which of the following?

1. Finding a different family scapegoat.
2. Reinforcing the family's double bind.
3. Correcting his distorted perceptions of his needs.
4. Role playing deviant behavior patterns.

Baby boy Johnson is 24 hours old. His respiratory rate is 80/min, his skin color is yellow, and his reflexes are intact. His blood type is O positive.

51 • The nurse could rule out physiological jaundice as the probable cause of Baby Johnson's yellow skin color because:

1. Physiological jaundice is extremely rare.
2. Physiological jaundice doesn't occur in type O positive babies.
3. Physiological jaundice doesn't usually develop until the 3rd day of life.
4. Severe hyporeflexia occurs in conjunction with physiological jaundice.

52 • All *but which one* of the following is characteristic of kernicterus?

1. Depressed Moro reflex.
2. Yellow-brown stools.
3. Whiny, high pitched cry.
4. Refusal or regurgitation of food.

53 • In view of Baby Johnson's symptoms, which laboratory test would be performed to diagnose his disorder?

1. Direct Coombs' test.
2. Blood typing.
3. IgA titer.
4. HB_sAg titer.

54 • Which of the following blood type combinations is most likely to produce hemolytic disease of the newborn?

1. O-negative mother and A-positive father.
2. A-positive mother and A-negative father.
3. O-negative mother and B-negative father.
4. O-positive mother and O-negative father.

55 • Baby Johnson's condition rapidly worsened, so an exchange transfusion was ordered. The primary reason for an exchange transfusion would be to:

1. Foster conjugation of circulating bilirubin.
2. Replace destroyed red blood cells.
3. Dilute circulating maternal antibodies.
4. Increase circulating blood volume.

Laura Moore, a 9-year-old girl with spastic cerebral palsy, is a patient on the pediatrics floor 3 days post-operatively from heel-cord lengthening surgery. Her recovery has been uneventful, and she has been going to physical therapy twice daily to maintain her skeletal alignment. Her discharge is scheduled in 4 days.

Laura's perinatal history indicates that she was born prematurely at 34 weeks and had an Apgar score of 6 at 5 minutes. No resuscitation was necessary, although she had a weak cry. She was discharged at 5 weeks, weighing 5 lb 4 oz. Mrs. Moore noticed that Laura had some difficulty with sucking and feeding, but she did not become alarmed because her daughter gained weight steadily.

When Laura was close to 5 months of age, it occurred to Mrs. Moore that Laura was not doing many of the things her older daughter had done at the same age, such as reaching for a toy, rolling over, and bearing some weight on her legs. She assumed that since Laura was a premature baby, her motor activities were just slower. Mrs. Moore waited a couple more months, but the child's motor skills had not improved at all.

After discussing this problem with several of her friends, Mrs. Moore decided to bring Laura to the clinic where a physician made a tentative diagnosis of spastic cerebral palsy and had Laura hospitalized. Subsequent test results confirmed this diagnosis, and Mrs. Moore has been taking care of her wheelchair bound daughter ever since that time with regular visits from the public health nurse. Laura attends an Easter Seal day school 5 days a week.

56 • Mrs Moore tells you that no one was aware that Laura had cerebral palsy until she was approximately 7 months of age. Physical signs of cerebral palsy do not manifest themselves in infants until approximately 2 to 4 months of age because of the following reason:

1. Muscles of infants under 4 months of age are not fully developed.
2. Cortical control of movement does not occur until after the infant is approximately 2 to 4 months of age.
3. The motor nerves of infants under 4 months of age are not fully developed.
4. The cerebral lesion that causes cerebral palsy has not reached the critical size.

57 • Physical examination of Laura done at the time of her initial diagnosis at 7 months of age would probably demonstrate all *but which one* of the following?

1. Showing preference for using the right hand.
2. Stands flat-footed with feet apart.
3. Stiff and "resisting" when being held.
4. Persistent tongue thrust.

58 • Physical examination of Laura now at 9 years of age gives you all of the following information *except:*

1. Arms abducted at shoulders, elbows flexed, hands fisted.
2. Extreme dorsal flexion of feet.
3. Tight and shortened muscles.
4. Poor control of coordinated motion.

59 • Because of Laura's difficulty with swallowing, her mother had been cradling her to use gravity flow to help Laura swallow. During Laura's hospitalization for heel cord surgery, the nurse determined that this method of feeding was not particularly successful. Consequently, she advised Mrs. Moore that another, possibly more effective, method for feeding Laura would be to:

1. Put her in a reclining chair.
2. Put her in a flexed, sitting position.
3. Place her arm at her side.
4. Keep her neck extended.

60 • Laura's speech is garbled, and although she has speech therapy twice a week, there is much more her mother could do at home to enhance her speech training. She can do the following:

1. Force the child to use her lips and tongue in eating.
2. Place food directly on the child's tongue.
3. Encourage the child to use her teeth to scrape food off spoon.
4. Speak to the child in normal tone and normal speed.

When 40-year-old Mary Forman's physician discovered a lump in Mary's left breast during a routine physical examination and a breast biopsy revealed adenocarcinoma, a radical mastectomy was performed. Because several axillary nodes were found to contain malignant cells, Mrs. Forman was treated with several cycles of 5-fluorouracil, methotrexate, and cyclophosphamide after her mastectomy wound was completely healed.

61 • Which of the following measures should be taken by the recovery room nurse to check Mrs. Forman for hemorrhage from the chest wound?

1. Loosen the chest pressure bandage to examine the incision directly.
2. Examine the color of Mrs. Forman's conjunctiva and nail beds for increasing pallor.
3. Abduct Mrs. Forman's left arm to shoulder level to facilitate inspection of the dressing.
4. Run her hand under Mrs. Forman's left side to check the condition of the lower bed linen.

62 • Which of the following interventions should the nurse use to prevent or decrease edema of Mrs. Forman's left arm following surgery?

1. Application of an ice bag or cold pack to the inner aspect of the upper arm.
2. Elevation of the left arm on pillows with the wrist higher than the elbow and the elbow higher than the shoulder.
3. Gently massage the left hand, forearm, and upper arm for 5 minutes 3 times a day.
4. Apply a sling to maintain the arm in adduction and the elbow in flexion.

63 • Which of the following nursing interventions should be employed to protect Mrs. Forman from post-operative muscle contracture deformities?

1. Maintain Mrs. Forman's arm in functional position through use of splints.
2. Encourage Mrs. Forman in finger wall climbing and arm pendulum exercises of her left arm 3 times daily.
3. Passively move all of Mrs. Forman's joints through full range of motion twice daily.
4. Direct Mrs. Forman to perform isometric exercises of upper and lower arm muscles.

64 • In teaching Mrs. Forman how to avoid long range complications of her surgical procedure, the nurse should emphasize the importance of:

1. Utilizing her right, rather than her left arm for dressing and grooming activities.
2. Cautioning other caregivers to use her right, rather than her left arm to take blood pressure or give hypodermic medications.
3. Avoiding the use of lotions or hand creams to soften the skin of the left hand and arm.
4. Refraining from elevating her arms above shoulder level in performing household tasks.

65 • On one of Mrs. Forman's clinic visits during the 6th month following mastectomy, her white blood cell count was found to be 2800/mm^3. The clinic nurse should take which of the following actions?

1. Question the patient closely to determine whether she has recently suffered an upper respiratory infection.
2. Hold the patient's ordered doses of 5-fluorouracil and methotrexate, and notify the patient's physician.
3. Obtain a "clean catch" urine specimen, and send it to the laboratory for culture and sensitivity tests.
4. Palpate the patient's cervical, axillary, and inguinal regions to detect the presence of enlarged lymph nodes.

Emma Turek was 40 years old and had been treated with ibuprofen for rheumatoid arthritis when she was admitted to the hospital with her 3rd exacerbation of acute, severe hand, elbow, knee, and ankle inflammation. The ibuprofen was discontinued, and she was given a short course of indomethacin to relieve her acute joint symptoms. She was then started on monthly intramuscular injections of gold thioglucose.

66 • In coordinating the efforts of all unit nurses who contribute to Mrs. Turek's care, her primary nurse should include which of the following care orders on her Kardex care plan?

1. Keep upper and lower extremities elevated on pillows and completely immobilized in prescribed rest splints.
2. Encourage self care in grooming, dressing, feeding, and toileting, offering as little nursing assistance as possible.
3. Discourage patient's use of assisting devices in order to minimize socially handicapping illness-related behavior.
4. Apart from scheduled diagnostic tests and medical treatments, allow patient to decide the time for all nursing care activities.

67 • During Mrs. Turek's exacerbation of acute joint inflammation, the nurse should institute which of the following precautions to minimize subsequent joint deformity?

1. Place Mrs. Turek in prone position for ½ hour, 3 times a day.
2. Maintain Mrs. Turek in low Fowler's position with feet against a footboard.
3. Keep a rolled towel under Mrs. Turek's knees to prevent hyperextension.
4. Move all Mrs. Turek's joints through full range of motion twice daily.

68 • After Mrs. Turek's joint inflammation has subsided and she is referred to physiotherapy for joint protection exercises, the nurse can best facilitate her response to physiotherapy interventions by:

1. Relieving Mrs. Turek of responsibilities for her bathing, grooming, and transfers in the nursing unit in order to conserve her energy.
2. Encouraging Mrs. Turek to spend her free time in the nursing unit in repeatedly practicing her physiotherapy exercises.
3. Placing Mrs. Turek in a room with another patient with rheumatoid arthritis and engendering rivalry between the two regarding rehabilitation progress.
4. Scheduling Mrs. Turek's activities so that her meals, bathing, toileting, and therapies are interspersed with rest periods.

69 • Because Mrs. Turek was underweight, she was given a high protein, high carbohydrate, high vitamin diet, but she sent most of the trays back to the kitchen with half of the food uneaten. Which of the following interventions should be undertaken to maximize Mrs. Turek's nutrition during hospitalization?

1. Plan for a relative to be present during mealtime to assist her to eat the foods served.
2. Request that the dietitian visit her daily during meal time to explain principles of good nutrition.
3. Request that her family prepare her favorite dishes and serve her these foods rather than the ordered diet.
4. Arrange for her tray to be served first and removed last, to provide her with more than usual time to complete the meal.

70 • In preparing Mrs. Turek for self care following hospital discharge, the nurse should instruct the patient that she should report which of the following symptoms as a possible indication of toxic reaction to the intramuscular injection of gold thioglucose?

1. Easy bruising and punctate hemorrhages.
2. Nausea and anorexia.
3. Muscle spasms and tremors.
4. Progressive deafness.

Lydia White had been widowed for 10 years and lived alone in a small house on the corner of her son's farm. A wiry, energetic 75-year-old woman who enjoyed reading, sewing, entertaining, and housework, Lydia lived comfortably on income from her well-chosen investments. Her only complaints were loneliness and occasional morning headache and dizziness.

Knowing that Lydia had had influenza, her granddaughter stopped by to visit one morning. Lydia was wandering aimlessly about the kitchen in her nightgown and greeted her visitor with, "Is that you, George? Is it time to go?" Lydia's granddaughter put her to bed, called her grandmother's physician, and stayed with her for the next few days. After a week of bed rest, Lydia recovered from her respiratory infection and became oriented to her surroundings, but had difficulty in remembering names, dates, and recent events and had to grope for once familiar words. She began to disregard her appearance, failing to wash her body and clothing as often as she had been accustomed to doing. She stopped cleaning house, and she preferred snacking on cookies, candy, canned milk, and cereal to cooking regular meals. Her worried family took her to her physician, who determined that Lydia's blood pressure was elevated and ordered antihypertensive medications. Lydia forgot to take the drugs just as she frequently forgot to eat.

Lydia fell while getting out of bed one morning and was left with temporary aphasia, confusion, and weakness of her right arm and leg. She was hospitalized briefly, was found to have suffered a cerebrovascular thrombosis, and with her son's consent was transferred to a nursing home for care. Upon arrival in the institution Lydia demonstrated only slight loss of physical strength, but marked fatigue, irritability, confusion, and obstinancy. During her first few months in the home, Lydia had several outbursts of temper in response to the staff's efforts to restrain her from walking about at night, entering other patients' rooms; and running away from the institution.

71 • In planning nursing care for Lydia the nurse should recognize that which of the following are psychological tasks of old age?

1. Maintaining old interests and planning for the future.
2. Becoming as self supporting as one's health permits.
3. Avoiding social withdrawal, inflexibility, and despair.
4. All of the above.

72 • One morning Lydia greeted the nurse with, "I'm going to take my driver's test today." Which response would be most therapeutic?

1. "What makes you think that you want to take a driver's test today?"
2. "I think you've forgotten. You've sold your car and don't drive now."
3. "Why don't you spend the day watching television in the reception room?"
4. "Don't you remember that you lost your driver's license for poor eyesight?"

73 • Assessment of Lydia by the nurse will probably reveal all *but which one* of the following?

1. Greatest impairment of recall for past events.
2. Impairment of judgment and comprehension.
3. Impairment of appropriate affect.
4. Marked impairment in regard to time of day or week.

74 • The nurse can most effectively minimize Lydia's disorientation by:

1. Keeping a night light burning throughout the hours of darkness.
2. Directing her daily to recite the names of her relatives and friends.
3. Restricting her visitors to the immediate family only.
4. Restricting all of her activities to her room.

75 • A fundamental requirement of therapeutic care for Lydia would be:

1. Removal of all externally induced irritation.
2. Providing a well-regulated mode of life.
3. Reconstruction of her personality patterns.
4. Substitutions of new interests for old.

John Christopher, 18 years old, has enrolled in college. Although he has had severe acne for several years, he has refused to see a physician, relying instead on various remedies suggested by his friends. However, with the prospect of meeting a new group of people in college, and since his acne was no better, John finally decided to seek medical attention. Mrs. Christopher was surprised when John asked her to accompany him, particularly since he had not asked his mother's company since his junior high school days.

The physician found acne covering most of John's face, shoulders, and upper chest in varying morphology—papules, pustules, nodules, and cysts as well as old scarring. John informed the physician that he had been vigorously scrubbing his face with soap at least 4 times a day, and he had been trying to eat less french fries and pizzas. The physician explained the pathophysiology of acne to John and his mother, and outlined a plan of therapy to be followed for the next 3 months.

76 • You are helping John analyze factors that could be related to the development of his severe acne. All of the following factors should be seriously considered *except:*

1. Most of his paternal uncles had severe acne as adolescents.
2. His acne is worse in the winter, especially after he spends a day skiing.
3. His acne usually worsens while he's cramming for a test in school.
4. Dairy products cause inflammation of his acne.

77 • There are various acne therapies available for John. The physician has given John several options for treatment. All of the following are treatments John can consider *except:*

1. Dermabrasion.
2. Antibiotics.
3. Ultrasound.
4. Peeling agents.

78 • John has difficulty understanding how the deliberate production of erythema and desquamation could eventually improve his appearance. You explain the following benefits of erythema and desquamation:

1. Toxic material in the pus is eliminated faster from the comedo.
2. It reduces the compaction that produces the comedo.
3. It helps tighten the comedo within the duct.
4. It slows down the rate of turnover of the epithelium that lines the follicular duct.

79 • The nurse discussed factors that *could exacerbate* the condition of acne. Before John leaves the clinic, the nurse asks him to review these factors with her. He made one error, which was the following:

1. Use of comedo extractor.
2. Exposure to excessive warmth and humidity.
3. Skiing all day in his nylon outfit.
4. Secondary bacterial invasion.

80 • The nurse is introducing John to the proper use of tretinoin (Retin A) cream. All of the following are proper steps *except:*

1. Apply ½ hour after washing face.
2. Use very small amounts.
3. Apply medication just after dinner.
4. Leave medication on for 30 minutes, then wash off.

Willie Hale, an emphysematous 60-year-old man with a 40-year history of smoking, was admitted to the hospital for treatment of bacterial pneumonia subsequent to an episode of influenza. Following sputum culture and sensitivity tests, the causative organism was identified as Streptococcus pneumoniae, *and the patient was treated with low flow O_2 by nasal cannula, ultrasonic nebulization, postural drainage, isoetharine (Bronkosol) inhalations, and cephalosporin intramuscularly.*

81 • In order to decrease Mr. Hale's energy expenditure and increase his comfort, the nurse should schedule his care procedures so that:

1. Isoetharine inhalations are administered 20 minutes before postural drainage.
2. Postural drainage is instituted 20 minutes before meal time.
3. Ultrasonic nebulization is instituted 20 minutes after postural drainage.
4. Cephalosporin injections are administered 20 minutes after meals.

82 • Care should be taken to maintain Mr. Hale's O_2 flow no higher than the ordered 3 L/min in order to:

1. Avoid eliminating the patient's hypoxemic respiratory stimulus.
2. Prevent drying and irritation of the respiratory mucosa.
3. Minimize retinal degeneration due to O_2 toxicity.
4. Discourage multiplication of respiratory tract pathogens.

83 • The nurse could probably increase Mr. Hale's respiratory efficiency by which of the following interventions?

1. Maintaining him in side-lying position to foster drainage of tracheobronchial secretions.
2. Instructing Mr. Hale to exhale slowly and evenly against pursed lips while contracting his abdominal muscles.
3. Applying an abdominal binder to improve diaphragmatic ascent during expirations.
4. Splinting Mr. Hale's lower rib cage during paroxysms of coughing to prevent intercostal muscle strain.

84 • In evaluating Mr. Hale's response to drug therapy, the nurse should observe him for which of the following as a manifestation of toxic response to cephalexin (Keflex)?

1. Deafness
2. Purpura
3. Jaundice
4. Diarrhea

85 • In preparing Mr. Hale for self care following discharge, the nurse should advise him to:

1. Install a humidifier in his home and workplace to liquify and facilitate removal of bronchial secretions.
2. Reduce the number of cigarettes smoked each day by half to decrease irritation of bronchial mucosa.
3. Use aerosolized deodorants to remove cooking odors, paint fumes, and industrial pollutants from the home.
4. Remain at home during the winter influenza season to avoid contracting acute respiratory tract infections.

Matt Oakes, 68 years old, was found to have adenocarcinoma of the rectum on a routine physical examination. Following confirmatory biopsy of the tumor mass and a complete preoperative work-up, an abdominoperineal resection of the rectum and a single-barreled left colostomy were performed.

86 • After informing Mr. Oakes that his tumor was malignant, the surgeon obtained written consent for the planned surgical procedure. In deciding the type and amount of information to give Mr. Oakes about his forthcoming operation, the nurse should:

1. Review his medical history to determine the extent of his previous surgical experience.
2. Ask Mr. Oakes what he would like to know about the planned surgical operation.

3. Query Mr. Oakes' wife concerning his usual response to illness and other stressful events.
4. Consult nursing references and hospital policies to determine information needed by patients in Mr. Oakes' situation.

87 • If the surgeon permits, which of the following pre-operative nursing measures would probably be most helpful in assisting Mr. Oakes to cope with the stress of his impending surgery?

1. Taking Mr. Oakes on a tour of the operating room, the recovery room, and the surgical intensive care unit to expose him to selected personnel and equipment to be involved in his post-operative care.
2. Demonstrating the procedures of colostomy irrigation and colostomy bag application on an anatomical model while Mr. Oakes observes and assists with the procedures.
3. Arranging for a completely rehabilitated colostomate to visit Mr. Oakes for the purpose of answering his questions about the operation and its consequences.
4. Providing Mr. Oakes with the address, telephone number, contact representative, and list of patient services provided by the local chapter of the American Cancer Society.

88 • In planning for Mr. Oakes' care during his first few days of hospitalization, the nurse should anticipate that he will receive which of the following drugs pre-operatively?

1. Ferrous sulfate
2. Neomycin
3. Morphine
4. Bisacodyl

89 • If it becomes apparent that Mr. Oakes will require colostomy irrigations, the nurse should advise him to:

1. Prepare a quart of mild soapy water at body temperature for use as an irrigating solution.
2. Perform the irrigation in arising to establish bowel emptying when he will be most likely to be at home.
3. Perform the irrigation while sitting on the toilet or commode to utilize a position that facilitates defecation.
4. Insert the irrigating catheter as far as possible into the bowel to prevent leakage of irrigating solution before catheter removal.

90 • In planning the health teaching that will be needed to prepare Mr. Oakes to care for himself following hospital discharge, the nurse should take into consideration the fact that:

1. Since constipation is common following colostomy of the descending colon, Mr. Oakes will require daily colostomy irrigations.
2. Since bowel resection decreases transit time, Mr. Oakes' left colon contents will be liquid, and colostomy irrigation will be unnecessary.
3. Since feces in the descending colon are normally solid, Mr. Oakes may achieve normal bowel function by irrigating every 2 or 3 days.
4. Even a patient whose colostomy could be regulated on diet alone should irrigate regularly to prevent stenosis of the stoma.

William Ranger was 42 years old but everyone called him "Billy." The only son and youngest child of a wealthy small town lumberman, he had studied business administration in college and had returned to his home town, married the banker's daughter, and taken a job as an agent in a real estate firm. Mr. Ranger was tall, slender, and good looking. He talked a lot, and engagingly, of his philosophy, feelings, and plans to anyone who would listen.

Mr. Ranger first drank alcohol in his parents' home. He consumed 4 to 5 drinks per weekend in high school and continued to drink in college and during his army service in Europe. Following the war his consumption of alcohol increased as he struggled to support his growing family. Although his wife objected to his drinking, she made escuses for him when drunkenness kept him from business appointments. Finally, Mr. Ranger disgraced himself and his firm with a display of intoxication, profanity, and belligerence in a contract closure meeting and was fired. His humiliation and remorse led to a week-long bout of heavy and continuous drinking in a nearby town. At the end of his spree he wrecked his car and was arrested for drunken driving, vagrancy, and creating a public disturbance.

During hospitalization for possible head injuries following the accident, Mr. Ranger developed delerium tremens, for which he was treated with sedatives, tranquilizers, and vitamins. When he returned to his home, his wife and teen-age children urged him to join Alcoholics Anonymous.

A member of that organization came to the home to explain their program to Mr. Ranger, but he refused to participate, stating that he could quit drinking anytine he wanted to. A year later, after a series of short-term jobs and long-term binges, Mr. Ranger recognized his inability to manage his problems alone and sought help from a community mental health center.

In his initial screening interview with the psychiatrist, Mr. Ranger revealed strong feelings of guilt and remorse concerning his drinking, resentment toward his strong and capable wife on whom he was dependent, ambivalence toward his domineering mother on whom he was still emotionally dependent, and fear of his successful and distant father. It was decided that Mr. Ranger would be accepted into the center's alcoholic treatment program and would be treated in group psychotherapy.

91 • Upon Mr. Ranger's admission following his accident the nurse should assess for *all but which one* of the following:

1. Malnutrition
2. Cross addiction
3. Extrapyramidal side effects
4. Confabulation

92 • In constructing a treatment plan for Mr. Ranger the nurse would operate on the principle that:

1. All alcoholics have the same underlying personality structure but differ in their physical response to alcohol.
2. All alcoholics have similar personality patterns but differ markedly in intelligence, potential, and drive.
3. All alcoholics have a common problem but differ considerably in their underlying personality patterns.
4. Alcoholics differ in so many respects that no single treatment method is widely applicable to them.

93 • Mr. Ranger said to the nurse therapist "You can't make me stop drinking!" Which response of the nurse reflects the most helpful attitude?

1. "I know I can't. You have to do it by yourself."
2. "That's true, but with help you will, won't you?"
3. "With such an attitude you will never stop drinking."
4. "What makes you think I want to control your behavior?"

94 • The nurse therapist could be most helpful to Mr. Ranger by:

1. Supporting him in his plans for working out his problems.
2. Advising him concerning methods for avoiding the temptation to drink.
3. Protecting him from disappointment from his family and coworkers.
4. Deterring him from the tendency to indulge in unhealthy thinking.

95 • In evaluating Mr. Ranger's progress the nurse would assess for which of the following?

1. His denial that he is an alcoholic.
2. His short-term goals for this hospitalization.
3. His coping mechanisms for abstinence from alcohol.
4. All of the above.

Items from Comprehensive Examination Section 1 That Address the Various Steps of the Nursing Process

Item Number	Assess	Analyze	Plan	Implement	Evaluate	Item Number	Assess	Analyze	Plan	Implement	Evaluate
1		x				49		x			
2	x					50			x		
3		x				51		x			
4				x		52	x				
5		x				53			x		
6	x					54		x			
7					x	55		x			
8			x			56		x			
9					x	57	x				
10		x				58	x				
11			x			59			x		
12		x				60				x	
13		x				61	x				
14	x					62		x			
15				x		63				x	
16			x			64				x	
17				x		65		x			
18				x		66			x		
19					x	67				x	
20			x			68				x	
21	x					69		x			
22				x		70					x
23			x			71			x		
24				x		72		x			
25					x	73	x				
26	x					74				x	
27				x		75			x		
28			x			76		x			
29					x	77					x
30			x			78				x	
31			x			79					x
32	x					80				x	
33				x		81			x		
34					x	82				x	
35		x				83		x			
36			x			84					x
37					x	85			x		
38			x			86				x	
39		x				87		x			
40				x		88			x		
41		x				89				x	
42					x	90				x	
43	x					91	x				
44				x		92			x		
45				x		93		x			
46			x			94				x	
47				x		95					x
48					x						

Answer Sheet—Section 1

No.	1	2	3	4
1.	‖	‖	‖	‖
2.	‖	‖	‖	‖
3.	‖	‖	‖	‖
4.	‖	‖	‖	‖
5.	‖	‖	‖	‖
6.	‖	‖	‖	‖
7.	‖	‖	‖	‖
8.	‖	‖	‖	‖
9.	‖	‖	‖	‖
10.	‖	‖	‖	‖
11.	‖	‖	‖	‖
12.	‖	‖	‖	‖
13.	‖	‖	‖	‖
14.	‖	‖	‖	‖
15.	‖	‖	‖	‖
16.	‖	‖	‖	‖
17.	‖	‖	‖	‖
18.	‖	‖	‖	‖
19.	‖	‖	‖	‖
20.	‖	‖	‖	‖
21.	‖	‖	‖	‖
22.	‖	‖	‖	‖
23.	‖	‖	‖	‖
24.	‖	‖	‖	‖
25.	‖	‖	‖	‖
26.	‖	‖	‖	‖
27.	‖	‖	‖	‖
28.	‖	‖	‖	‖
29.	‖	‖	‖	‖
30.	‖	‖	‖	‖
31.	‖	‖	‖	‖
32.	‖	‖	‖	‖
33.	‖	‖	‖	‖
34.	‖	‖	‖	‖
35.	‖	‖	‖	‖
36.	‖	‖	‖	‖
37.	‖	‖	‖	‖
38.	‖	‖	‖	‖
39.	‖	‖	‖	‖
40.	‖	‖	‖	‖
41.	‖	‖	‖	‖
42.	‖	‖	‖	‖
43.	‖	‖	‖	‖
44.	‖	‖	‖	‖
45.	‖	‖	‖	‖
46.	‖	‖	‖	‖
47.	‖	‖	‖	‖
48.	‖	‖	‖	‖
49.	‖	‖	‖	‖
50.	‖	‖	‖	‖
51.	‖	‖	‖	‖
52.	‖	‖	‖	‖
53.	‖	‖	‖	‖
54.	‖	‖	‖	‖
55.	‖	‖	‖	‖
56.	‖	‖	‖	‖
57.	‖	‖	‖	‖
58.	‖	‖	‖	‖
59.	‖	‖	‖	‖
60.	‖	‖	‖	‖
61.	‖	‖	‖	‖
62.	‖	‖	‖	‖
63.	‖	‖	‖	‖
64.	‖	‖	‖	‖
65.	‖	‖	‖	‖
66.	‖	‖	‖	‖
67.	‖	‖	‖	‖
68.	‖	‖	‖	‖
69.	‖	‖	‖	‖
70.	‖	‖	‖	‖
71.	‖	‖	‖	‖
72.	‖	‖	‖	‖
73.	‖	‖	‖	‖
74.	‖	‖	‖	‖
75.	‖	‖	‖	‖
76.	‖	‖	‖	‖
77.	‖	‖	‖	‖
78.	‖	‖	‖	‖
79.	‖	‖	‖	‖
80.	‖	‖	‖	‖
81.	‖	‖	‖	‖
82.	‖	‖	‖	‖
83.	‖	‖	‖	‖
84.	‖	‖	‖	‖
85.	‖	‖	‖	‖
86.	‖	‖	‖	‖
87.	‖	‖	‖	‖
88.	‖	‖	‖	‖
89.	‖	‖	‖	‖
90.	‖	‖	‖	‖
91.	‖	‖	‖	‖
92.	‖	‖	‖	‖
93.	‖	‖	‖	‖
94.	‖	‖	‖	‖
95.	‖	‖	‖	‖

Section 2

COMPREHENSIVE EXAMINATION

The nurse has agreed to teach a class on contraception to a group of women in the community. The age range of the group members is from 18 to 40 years.

1 • In constructing her plan for the class the nurse should be aware that many factors influence whether or not a woman will elect to use contraceptives and the type of contraception chosen. Which of the following could be expected to have the *least* effect on a woman's contraceptive choice?

1. Culture background
2. Religious beliefs
3. Perceived costs
4. Availability of abortion

2 • In discussing the basal body temperature method of birth control, the nurse should counsel the group that basal body temperature:

1. Should be measured rectally, within a few minutes of arising from sleep.
2. Shows marked diurnal-nocturnal differences during the woman's infertile period.
3. Drops slightly, then increases from 0.5 to 1° F at the time of ovulation.
4. Decreases steadily from the end of menstruation to a stable low level at mid-cycle.

3 • In differentiating the effects of various contraceptive methods the nurse should explain that most oral contraceptive pills prevent pregnancy by:

1. Suppressing the development of ova within the graafian follicle.
2. Destroying the ovum during its transit through the fallopian tube.
3. Preventing uterine implantation of the fertilized ovum.
4. Destroying sperm within the vagina and uterus.

4 • All *but which one* of the following are frequent side effects of oral contraceptives?

1. Weight gain
2. Nausea
3. Breast tenderness
4. Calf pain

5 • During the contraception counseling session, the nurse discusses the use of the diaphragm. She should advise group members that:

1. Water soluble jelly should be used to lubricate the diaphragm for insertion.
2. The diaphragm should be inserted at least 3 hours before intercourse to ensure sealing of the cervical os.
3. The woman should douche and remove the diaphragm immediately after intercourse.
4. The diaphragm should be left in place for 8 hours following intercourse.

Cindy, an 11-month-old infant, was admitted to the pediatric unit from the emergency room with a diagnosis of pneumonia. Medical history and clinical signs suggested a bacterial pathogen, and she was started on I.V. methicillin. Subsequently, sputum culture identified staphylococcus *as the pathogen. History taken from the father, who accompanied the infant, indicated that Cindy had had a mild upper respiratory infection for several days with nasal discharge and infrequent unproductive cough. He did not think her illness was serious, and if anything, he felt she was getting better. However, on the 4th day of her cold, she suddenly developed chills, a rectal temperature of 104° F, and appeared quite ill and listless. Although she was given acetaminophen (Tylenol), her respirations soon became shallow and rapid. The father then brought her to the emergency room while the mother remained home with the other children.*

6 • On assessing Cindy, the nurse would probably find all of the following clinical signs *except:*

1. Rapid, shallow breathing.
2. Fever of 103° F.
3. Sternal retractions.
4. Increased breath sounds over the involved lobe.

7 • When the etiological pathogen was identified as *Staphylococcus*, the nurse went to the drug reference to reacquaint herself with the side effects of semisynthetic penicillins, such as methicillin, nafcillin, and oxacillin. She knew one of these drugs would be used because:

1. Semisynthetic penicillins resist inactivation by staphylococcal penicillinase.
2. Semisynthetic penicillins cost less to the patient.
3. Semisynthetic penicillins produce no toxic effects in children.
4. Semisynthetic penicillin dissolves faster in a solution and is therefore safer to use than other antibiotics.

8 • In caring for Cindy, you should do all of the following *except*:

1. Place on strict bed rest.
2. Carefully restrict all fluids.
3. Postural drainage.
4. Place in mist tent.

9 • Cindy has been kept on continuous intravenous fluid to prevent dehydration. The result of the following activity will assist you in determining her hydration status.

1. Asking her if she wants a drink of water.
2. Comparing today's respiratory rate with that of yesterday's rate.
3. Assessing her skin and mucous membranes.
4. Measuring her girth.

10 • Maintaining fluid balance is an important nursing activity to prevent dehydration. In order to decide whether you will be able to start fluids orally or not, you should assess the child's

1. Urine output.
2. Respiratory rate.
3. Skin turgor.
4. Peripheral blood return after blanching.

Ed Ridgely, 60 years old, consulted a urologist because of inability to void. Catheterization yielded 500 ml of cloudy, foul smelling urine, and cystoscopy revealed prostatic enlargement. Mr. Ridgely was hospitalized, and a transurethral prostatectomy was performed.

11 • It would be especially important for the nurse to position Mr. Ridgely for the cystoscopic examination so as to prevent which of the following complications?

1. Ligamentous injury due to neck hyperextension.
2. Hypoventilation due to pressure of abdominal viscera on the diaphragm.
3. Circulatory obstruction due to compression of popliteal vessels.
4. Dropfoot due to inversion and plantar flexion of the feet.

12 • Both pre-operatively and post-operatively, an indwelling catheter was used to protect Mr. Ridgely against bladder injury due to overdistention. Which of the following precautions should be taken to protect Mr. Ridgely from complications arising from the catheter's presence?

1. Prevent tissue trauma from accidental dislodgment of the catheter by taping the catheter to the abdomen while Mr. Ridgely is supine.
2. "Milk" the catheter and drainage tubing in the direction of the collection bag to loosen mucus and clots from the catheter.
3. Refrain from manipulating the catheter-external meatus junction so as to prevent irritation and contamination of the urethral mucosa.
4. Attach the drainage collection bag to the bed's side rail so the patient can request personnel to empty the bag when full.

13 • As a result of his age, spinal anesthesia, and possible post-operative complications of transurethral resection of the prostate, the recovery room nurse should monitor Mr. Ridgely closely for which of the following problems during the immedate post-operative period?

1. Pneumonia
2. Seizures
3. Shock
4. Aspiration

14 • In planning for Mr. Ridgely's care on the operative and 1st post-operative day, the nurse should anticipate that he will require which of the following interventions?

1. Frequent turns from supine to side-lying to prone positions to prevent stagnation of urine in the renal pelvis and bladder.
2. Frequent irrigation of the catheter to remove blood clots and prevent urinary obstruction and bladder distention.
3. Passive range of motion of all lower extremity joints to prevent contracture deformities and joint anklyosis.
4. Elevation of the knees to foster venous return blood flow.

15 • In preparing Mr. Ridgely for self care following hospital discharge, the nurse should advise him to:

1. Eliminate bran and bulk foods from the diet to minimize rectal pressure against the prostate bed.
2. Limit fluid intake during afternoon and evening hours in order to minimize nocturia.
3. Avoid vigorous exercise and heavy lifting for 4 to 6 weeks following surgery.
4. Drink a glass of wine or beer at bedtime to ensure muscle relaxation and restful sleep.

Forty-five-year old Tom Kemper had been hospitalized several times for treatment of cirrhosis secondary to chronic alcoholism. Finally, he was admitted to the emergency room of the county hospital after vomiting a large quantity of bright red blood. Following control of bleeding with iced saline irrigations, gastroscopy revealed that a ruptured esophageal varix was the source of bleeding. A Sengstaken-Blakemore tube was inserted to prevent further bleeding, and a blood transfusion was given to restore blood volume.

16 • Which order on Mr. Kemper's written nursing care plan would be most effective in minimizing the skin problems to which he is predisposed?

1. Use an over-the-bed cradle to protect patient from the weight of upper bed linen.
2. Clip and file and the patient's fingernails so as to keep them short, smooth, and clean.
3. Provide a daily tub bath or shower, using an antibacterial sudsing cleanser.
4. Keep a cellulose-cotton absorbent pad under the patient's hips at all times.

17 • Shortly following his admission to the hospital, Mr. Kemper's physician ordered that the patient be given enemas until returns are clear and that lactulose and neomycin be started. The nurse should inform Mr. Kemper that the purpose of these interventions is to:

1. Put the bowel at rest and decrease secretion of gastrointestinal enzymes while oral feedings are withheld.
2. Decrease his abdominal distention so as to improve ventilatory efficiency and decrease hypoxia.
3. Remove blood and bacteria from the intestine in order to prevent bacterial production of ammonia.
4. Minimize the risk of peritoneal contamination in the event of peptic ulcer perforation.

18 • Which of the following nursing interventions should be used to protect Mr. Kemper from serious complications arising from the use of the Sengstaken-Blakemore tube?

1. Frequent oropharyngeal suction to remove pooled secretions and to prevent aspiration.
2. Simultaneous hourly deflation of the gastric and esophageal balloons, with slight advancement and retraction of the tube to prevent its adherence to mucosa.
3. Turning the patient from left to right side-lying position so as to facilitate suction of gastric contents.
4. Deflation of the gastric balloon during changes in the patient's position to prevent mucosal erosion.

19 • Which of the following devices should be kept in plain view at Mr. Kemper's bedside while the Sengstaken-Blakemore tube is in place?

1. Hemostat
2. Scissors
3. Tourniquet
4. Padded tongue blade

20 • Because Mr. Kemper's esophageal bleeding was controlled by balloon tamponade and he did not develop hepatic encephalopathy, he was discharged and placed on a 2000 calorie, high protein, low sodium diet and advised to avoid alcoholic intake in any form. When the diet was explained to him, Mr. Kemper confided that he would be unable to follow the order because he had a poor appetite. Which advice by the nurse would be likely to improve his compliance with the diet prescription?

1. "Take a small drink of coffee or tea before mealtime to whet the appetite."
2. "Limit the drinking of fluid with meals so as to increase the appetite for solid food."
3. "Eat 5 small meals rather than 3 large meals each day."
4. "Eat the carbohydrate and fatty foods first and protein foods last to ensure adequate intake of calories."

James Daring, age 28 years, is hospitalized upon court order following a drunken brawl in a local tavern. He is belligerent and irritable, and states that he is not to blame for the altercation. A history elicited from his mother who accompanies him reveals the following data.

James had done well in school until he was 11 years old. At this time he began to act out during school sessions, and his grades began to deteriorate. By the age of 12 years, he was skipping school several times a week and was failing most of his subjects. His mother found him smoking marijuana several times in the basement of their home. On one occasion he was sent home from school because he reeked of alcohol, and 3 times in 1 week he was sent home for instigating fights on the school grounds.

By the time James was 18 years old, he had been arrested 3 times for petty theft, and he was lying and conning to get what he wanted and to extricate himself from trouble. He had no close friends and used people to achieve his own purposes. If they failed to provide what he needed he moved on to someone else. At the age of 19 years, he was arrested for armed robbery and sentenced to 2 years in jail. Upon release from prison he returned home to live with his parents. He refused to look for work and spent his days and nights "with the boys, drinking, getting high, and having sexual relations with a different woman every night." His mother is not positive, but she believes that he is probably dealing in street drugs since he seems to have a never-ending supply of money to support himself. His mother states that it is difficult to deny him anything because he is so charming and likeable. It troubles her, however, that he is unable to see that he is responsible for what has happened to him, and that he seems to have no conscience—he never feels remorse about the people he hurts by his actions.

Further assessment by the psychiatrist reveals no symptomatology that would suggest schizophrenia or manic-depressive illness, and tests done previously within the school system reveal that James has an I.Q. of 120. A diagnosis of antisocial personality is made.

21 • In order to establish a therapeutic relationship with James the nurse should be aware that:

1. James will become dependent and look to the nurse for much of the decision making regarding his stay in the hospital.
2. James may become manipulative in order to achieve his own ends and may become angry if the nurse insists on remaining within the boundaries of the treatment plan.
3. James will probably be charming, easy to develop a relationship with, and compliant with the treatment plan that is developed by the interdisciplinary team.
4. James will be slow to develop a relationship with the nurse and will require short working sessions between nurse and patient.

22 • Mr. Daring begins to manipulate various staff members and has made some inappropriate sexual remarks to several of the nurses. In designing a care plan for Mr. Daring which of the following would *not* be an important part of the nursing process?

1. Assessment of the management problem he presents.
2. Planning a limit setting intervention unique to the patient's needs.
3. Avoidance of patient if he becomes sexually intrusive.
4. Enforcing the limit setting on any unacceptable behavior.

23 • Which of the following would *not* be part of the nursing interaction with James?

1. Helping him analyze what has brought about his hospitalization.
2. Utilizing unconditional positive regard and genuineness.
3. Providing guidelines for his behavior with female nursing staff.
4. Encouraging short-term goals for this hospitalization.

24 • Mr. Daring's pathophysiology may manifest itself in all *but which one* of the following ways?

1. The use of charm to get what he wants from staff.
2. Angry outbursts if his plans are thwarted.
3. Manipulation of several or all members of the staff in order to achieve his desires.
4. Being able to learn from past experiences and change his behavior.

25 • During the one-to-one interaction between Mr. Daring and his nurse he says to her: "I'm tired of me always talking about myself. You're so pretty. What's a sweet little thing like you doing working in a place like this?" The nurse's best response would be:

1. "I enjoy my work here. Let's get back to what we were just discussing."
2. "Mr. Daring, we are not here to talk about me."
3. "I've always wanted to be a psychiatric nurse. All in all this is a great place to work. Don't you like it here?"
4. "We need to work on your problems, Mr. Daring. You will be going home soon."

Judy Marvin, whose pregnancy has just been confirmed, was referred to the High Risk Prenatal Clinic by her internist. She has been diagnosed as having Class I heart disease and is to be followed during her pregnancy by both a perinatologist and a cardiologist. She is tearful and worried about her ability to carry her fetus to term and deliver it normally.

26 • The most common cause of valvular heart damage in the young adult as:

1. Poor childhood nutrition.
2. Congenital heart defects.
3. Rheumatic heart disease.
4. Repeated urinary infections.

27 • In order to protect Judy from complications of her illness, the nurse should be aware that all *but which one* of the following are apt to precipitate congestive heart failure in the pregnant woman with valvular damage?

1. Uncontrolled infection
2. High carbohydrate diet
3. Emotional stress
4. Lack of exercise

28 • At which point during gestation will Judy be at greatest risk for development of congestive heart failure?

1. 8 weeks
2. 12 weeks
3. 20 weeks
4. 30 weeks

29 • In planning for Judy's perinatal care the nurse should be aware that which of the following interventions would be *contraindicated* during labor?

1. Maintaining her in semi-recumbent position during labor.
2. Monitoring her vital signs at 10 to 15-minute intervals during labor.
3. Describing the purpose and procedure of regional anesthesia to her.
4. Urging her to bear down during delivery of the infant.

30 • The care that Judy receives during the 1st 48 hours post-partum should include all *but which one* of the following?

1. Encourage generous fluid intake.
2. Elevate the head of the bed.
3. Apply elastic stockings.
4. Assist the patient to ambulate.

Roger White, a 4-year-old child with moderate generalized edema, is lying apathetically in bed; his mother is sitting at his bedside looking worried. She tells you that she feels guilty about Roger's illness because the physician had told her that his disease probably was the result of impetigo he had a couple of weeks ago. She felt that had she taken better care of his impetigo, he would not have developed acute glomerulonephritis (AGN). She explained further that Roger's older brother also had impetigo, but he remains healthy.

Other than a few remnants of healing impetigo on his face, Roger was perfectly healthy until 2 days ago. Roger woke up in the morning feeling irritable, and his face was puffy, especially around the eyes. He refused breakfast that morning, which was most unusual. While Mrs. White was contemplating calling the pediatrician, Roger came to inform her that his urine was the color of "Coke." Roger was seen by the pediatrician who ordered him hospitalized.

31 • Assessment of Roger would probably reveal the following clinical signs, which is typical of AGN?

1. Cyanosis of lips and nails.
2. Positive Brudzinski's sign.
3. Mild to moderate hypertension.
4. Pale, amber-colored urine.

32 • Roger is now in the acute edematous phase of illness, and you are aware that all *but which one* of the following activities should be used to monitor edema?

1. Since he is anorexic, give him access to all the orange juice he wants.
2. Weigh him daily.
3. Take his blood pressure frequently.
4. Initiate seizure precautions.

33 • During Roger's hospitalization, your nursing activities should include:

1. Offering him a high protein diet.
2. Maintaining him at strict bed rest until day of discharge.
3. Weighing him every other day.
4. Offering him a diet with moderate sodium restriction.

34 • Roger is rapidly improving. You know this because:

1. His blood urea nitrogen concentration is increasing.
2. He is diaphoretic.
3. His edema is limited only to his extremities.
4. His blood pressure is 130/80 mm Hg.

35 • Hypertensive encephalopathy is one of the complications of A.G.N. Roger should be observed for symptoms of this complication, which include all *but which one* of the following?

1. Vomiting
2. Headache
3. Dizziness
4. Sudden increase in urinary output

John Powers, a portly 55-year-old man with a history of angina pectoris, which had been treated with nitroglycerin paste, was admitted to the hospital emergency room with agonizing substernal pain. When enzyme studies revealed elevations of LDH and CPK, and electrocardiography revealed abnormal Q waves, elevation of the ST segment, and occasional PVCs, he was admitted to the coronary care unit with a diagnosis of myocardial infarction. He was treated with bed rest, O_2 by nasal cannula, heparin I.V., warfarin (Coumadin) orally, and lidocaine I.V.

36 • If Mr. Powers should complain of substernal pain following admission to the coronary care unit, the preferred initial nursing intervention would be to:

1. Sit at the bedside and talk quietly with Mr. Powers in an effort to divert his attention and allay his anxiety.
2. Change Mr. Powers' position, give him a backrub, and place pillows so as to provide back support and maximize ventilation.
3. Increase the rate of O_2 flow through the nasal cannula from 4 to 8 L/min.
4. Administer an intravenous dose of the ordered morphine or meperidine (Demerol).

37 • If approved by the physician, which of the following nursing interventions could be expected to improve Mr. Powers' comfort and conserve his energy during his stay in the coronary care unit?

1. Bar all visitors from his bedside until he is transferred to the stepdown unit.
2. Turn off the arrhythmia alarm on his monitor during the night shift.
3. Assist Mr. Powers from the bed to a bedside commode in order to move his bowels.
4. Omit all bed making and bathing procedures unless the patient becomes incontinent of urine or stool.

38 • In monitoring Mr. Powers' response to treatment, the nurse should interpret which of the following physical findings as a possible indication of a serious complication of his myocardial infarction?

1. An excess of fluid output over fluid intake over a 24-hour period.
2. Detection of rales in the lung bases on chest auscultation.
3. Drowsiness, lethargy, and decreased frequency and duration of cough.
4. Elevation of oral temperature to 101° F orally.

39 • In monitoring Mr. Powers for the effects of drug therapy, the nurse should interpret which of the following as a possible indicator of an untoward drug effect?

1. Headache
2. Sore throat
3. White blood cell count of 18,000/mm^3
4. Cloudy urine

40 • In preparing Mr. Powers for self care following hospital discharge, the nurse should give him which of the following advice concerning optimum levels of physical activity?

1. No physical activity other than bathing, dressing, grooming, toileting, and feeding should be undertaken during the 1st week following discharge.
2. Recreational walking is permissible, but strenous activity, such as moving furniture or shovelling snow, is to be avoided.
3. Mr. Powers should be able to return to work in his office within 3 to 4 weeks following discharge from the hospital.
4. Mr. Powers and his wife may resume sexual activities immediately following his discharge from the hospital.

Bea Hoblet, a 22-year-old secretary, consulted her doctor with complaints of visual blurring, weakness, and urinary dribbling. Physical examination revealed nystagmus, hesitant speech, intention tremor, flexor spasiticity, and ataxic gait. Because Bea had experienced a similar episode of visual disturbance and incoordination several months before, following an influenza attack, a complete neurological work-up was performed, revealing elevated gamma globulin levels of the spinal fluid and delayed response on visual evoked response test. Bea was diagnosed as having multiple sclerosis and was hospitalized for treatment with ACTH, baclofen, bethanechol (Urecholine), and, later, physiotherapy.

41 • In order to evaluate Bea's response to therapy, the nurse should be aware that which of the following is a possible untoward effect of drug therapy?

1. An increase in muscle weakness due to administration of baclofen.
2. Marked loss of head, axillary, and pubic hair due to ACTH.
3. Constipation due to paralysis of smooth muscles by bethanechol (Urecholine).
4. Dehydration and weight loss due to combined effects of ACTH and baclofen.

42 • In order to elicit maximal support for Bea during the lengthy period of her rehabilitation, the nurse should inform her relatives that multiple sclerosis tends to produce which of the following psychological characteristics in its victims?

1. A steadily increasing depression as symptoms increase in severity.
2. Delusions of persecution with reference to the intentions of caregivers.
3. Sudden and unexplained outbursts of laughing and crying.
4. A tendency to exaggerate physical symptoms in order to control others.

43 • Which of the following devices should be employed to facilitate Bea's self care activities at this time?

1. Weighted eating utensils and plate guard.
2. Electric wheelchair with toggle stick drive.
3. Raised toilet seat.
4. Indwelling catheter.

44 • In preparing Bea for self care at home, the nurse should instruct her regarding the importance of:

1. Reducing her physical movements to a minimum so as to conserve energy for essential self care activities.
2. Using increasing visual monitoring to protect against skin trauma consequent to loss of pain and temperature sensation.
3. Limiting fluid intake during the evening hours in order to prevent urinary incontinence during sleep.
4. Scheduling all bathing, hygiene, and homemaking activities during morning hours to take advantage of peak energy levels.

45 • In order to protect Bea from injuries to which the tissue changes of multiple sclerosis predispose her, the nurse should include which of the following in Bea's predischarge health teaching?

1. Train her to use a thermometer to measure the temperature of bath water.
2. Suggest year-round use of sunglasses whenever she must be out of doors.
3. Advise her to avoid driving a car or operating motorized machinery.
4. Instruct her to carry a padded tongue blade in her pocket or purse.

Five days prior to hospital admission, 22-year-old Wade Hyskell developed swelling and pain of the inner aspect of the left elbow. Four days later he developed fever, chills, malaise, headache, and diarrhea. Even though he feared police arrest, he allowed his wife to take him to a general hospital.

On admission Mr. Hyskell stated that he had been a heroin addict for the past 2 years and had supported his increasingly expensive habit (currently $120.00 per day) by playing in a dance *band and by stealing. The examining physician noted an enlarged liver, fever, and tender, thickened veins on the dorsum of the left hand and forearm. Mr. Hyskell told the nurse that he was in the habit of taking 3 "fixes" of heroin a day and that he occasionally smoked a "joint," but that he no longer took amphetamines, to which he had been habituated some years before. He indicated that he had injected his last dose of heroin 5 hours before admission. The doctor restricted him to the unit and ordered blood, stool, urine, and throat cultures, a complete blood count, bed rest, chest x-rays, and an electrocardiogram.*

Six hours after admission Mr. Hyskell complained of rhinorrhea and abdominal cramps and threatened to leave the hospital, saying the methadone (10 mg orally q 12 h) which the admitting physician had ordered to relieve the withdrawal symptoms would not be effective. The following morning he refused breakfast but talked the aide into preparing a snack for him at 10:30 A.M. That same afternoon Mr. Hyskell requested a pass for "personal business reasons." His request was refused, and he was advised to remain in the hospital to be treated for possible viral hepatitis, type B, and to talk with the counselor from the local therapeutic community for the treatment of drug addiction. On the following day, Mr. Hyskell signed out of the hospital against medical advice saying, "This is something I just have to do."

Six months later, following a severe episode of viral hepatitis, type B, Mr. Hyskell presented himself to a therapeutic community for treatment of heroin addiction.

46 • The nurse may expect that, as a result of underlying personality characteristics, Wade will initially establish with her a relationship characterized on his part by:

1. Clinging dependence.
2. Approach-avoidance.
3. Concealed manipulation.
4. Passive aggression.

47 • Since he is apt to have difficulty with male-female relationships, therapeutic nursing interventions might be hampered, since he would tend to view the nurse as which of the following?

1. Seductive peer and mother figure.
2. Sexual object and mother figure.
3. Father figure and intellectual superior.
4. Mother figure and intellectual superior.

48 • From what is known of the psychodynamics of addiction the nurse should reason that Wade would probably derive greatest psychic satisfaction from which of the following activities?

1. Discussing theater.
2. Playing chess.
3. Collecting coins.
4. Smoking a pipe.

49 • As the nurse makes her assessment of Wade she should recognize that Wade, as a drug abuser, differs from a typical teen-age drug abuser in which of the following ways?

1. Physiologically he can no longer increase his heroin tolerance.
2. He can never recover his extreme socioeconomic loss.
3. His addiction has severely isolated him from his peer group.
4. His self identity is secure in that he no longer is an adolescent.

50 • As the nurse therapist and Wade work together, the chief goal would be to:

1. Prevent his use of heroin.
2. Increase his economic productivity.
3. Alter his response to stress.
4. Reshape and strengthen his superego.

Baby boy Samuels was admitted to the regular nursery unit. He is 2 days old, weighed 6 lb 4 oz at birth, birth was spontaneous, Apgar scores at birth were 9/9, and he has no gross abnormalities. The infant is being breast-fed.

51 • The nurse administered vitamin K to Baby Samuels, according to the physician's order, and the following precaution should be taken:

1. Administer the drug deep into a muscle using the Z-track technique.
2. Avoid application of pressure to the injection site following administration.
3. Pinch and lift the gluteal muscle before injecting the drug at a 90 degree angle.
4. Inject the drug at a 45 degree angle into the lateral muscle of the mid-thigh.

52 • Measurement revealed that Baby Samuels' head circumference is 34 cm, and his chest circumference is 32 cm. On the basis of these findings the nurse should:

1. Record the measurements on the infant's chart in routine fashion.
2. Notify the physician of evidence or congenital anomaly.
3. Summon the physician for an immediate physical examination.
4. Consult the mother's prenatal record for genetic history.

53 • It would be of critical importance for the delivery and nursery nurses to protect newborn baby Samuels against heat loss because:

1. Heat loss is accompanied by proportionate fluid loss.
2. Cold increases O_2 consumption and energy consumption.
3. Decrease in temperature increases heart rate and blood pressure.
4. Too rapid cooling would stimulate violent shivering.

54 • When Mrs. Samuels touches her nipple to her son's cheek he turns toward the nipple. This reaction is known as the:

1. Babinski's reflex.
2. Rooting reflex.
3. Moro's reflex.
4. Fencing reflex.

55 • Mrs. Samuels is concerned that her son is losing weight. Baby Samuels' expected postpartum weight loss would not exceed:

1. 8 oz
2. 10 oz
3. 12 oz
4. 15 oz

John Dudley is a 9-year old boy and currently in the 4th grade in school. He now is hospitalized on the pediatric floor; he is a happy, talkative, and cooperative youngster. According to his medical history, his mother took him to the pediatrician, relating that the school nurse called her 3 hours earlier saying that John had fallen to the floor during gym class and convulsed.

When the mother got to school, she found John in the nurse's office sleeping soundly; there was a quarter size hematoma on the right side of his forehead where he had apparently hit himself when he fell. After waiting for John to awaken, Mrs. Dudley took him directly to the pediatrician's office.

The mother was extremely upset and nervous, telling the doctor that John had never had convulsions before and she felt that, in all probability, some child had knocked her son to the floor.

The physician had the child hospitalized and ordered a CAT scan as well as an EEG. He explained to the mother that the reason he was hospitalizing John was that he wanted seizure precautions taken until diagnosis could be established.

The CAT scan findings were negative, but analysis of the EEG determined idiopathic grand mal seizures. The physician prescribed phenytoin (Dilantin) and phenobarbital; the process of appropriate dosage determination is now in progress.

56 • John's physician told John's mother that her son's type of epilepsy was idiopathic (unknown cause) rather than symptomatic (acquired). The etiology of John's epilepsy could be:

1. A genetic disorder.
2. Birth trauma.
3. Rubella (German measles).
4. Meningitis.

57 • The mother did not have information on the description of John's seizures, so the nurse called John's school to talk to his gym teacher who witnessed the occurrence. He would be apt to give the nurse the following information regarding John's tonic-clonic seizures:

1. John was able to resume gym activities after resting 45 minutes.
2. His arms and legs jerked back and forth the instant he fell to the floor.
3. He yelled for help during the convulsions.
4. John told his friend that he smelled a peculiar odor just before the seizures.

58 • The nurse is preparing John for diagnostic procedures ordered by his physician. She explains to John that the main purpose of these procedures is to determine:

1. How long he will have these seizures.
2. Genetic predisposition of the seizures.
3. The type of his seizures.
4. Whether his I.Q. will be affected.

59 • You know that with all possible seizure disorders, you should take seizure precautions. You should do all of the following for John *except*:

1. Use bed's side rails.
2. Put him in a room close to the nurse's station.
3. Pad all hard surfaces around his bed.
4. Keep emergency cart in his room.

60 • During discharge planning with Mrs. Dudley, you discussed various factors that could trigger John's convulsions. In reviewing these factors with her now, she lists the stimuli. They are all correct *except*:

1. Fatigue.
2. Dehydration.
3. Emotional stress.
4. Drinking a cold soft drink.

After months of chronic dyspepsia, John Gunderson, 58 years of age, consulted his physician with complaints of burning epigastric pain, nausea, and vomiting of a small amount of coffee ground–like material. Following discovery of a duodenal filling defect on upper gastrointestinal barium x-ray and a duodenal ulcer crater on gastroduodenoscopy, Mr. Gunderson was treated for 6 weeks with cimetidine (Tagamet). When he suffered a more serious episode of upper gastrointestinal bleeding several months later, a subtotal gastrectomy, gastrojejunostomy, and vagotomy were performed.

61 • On Mr. Gunderson's first hospitalization, his care needs could be best met by placing him in which of the following patient units?

1. A private room at the far end of the corridor on a medical-surgical unit.
2. A double room on a self care unit with a 25-year-old man being prepared for elective orthopedic surgery.
3. A 4-bed room next door to the patient's lounge on a medical unit.
4. A 3-bed room next door to the nurses' station on a surgical unit.

62 • When Mr. Gunderson was returned to the recovery room following subtotal gastrectomy, gastrojejunostomy, and vagotomy, a nasogastric tube had been inserted and was attached to a suction siphon. The nurse should take which of the following precautions in irrigating the nasogastric tube?

1. Instill no more than 30 ml of irrigant before aspirating the contents of the tube to avoid forcing mucus and clots into the stomach.
2. Use iced distilled water as an irrigant in order to constrict gastric vessels and minimize bleeding.
3. Inject a few ml of air through the tube before instilling the irrigant to loosen mucus and facilitate its removal.
4. Apply gentle force in instilling irrigant so as to avoid undue pressure against the suture line.

63 • During Mr. Gunderson's early post-operative period, which of the following observations by the nurse would indicate that the patient had recovered sufficiently to permit removal of the nasogastric tube?

1. Decline of temperature, pulse, and respirations to normal levels.
2. Return of normal sounds on auscultation of the abdomen.
3. Equivalence of daily fluid intake and output volumes.
4. Bowel movements of normal size and frequency.

64 • During Mr. Gunderson's 1st 2 to 3 postoperative days, which of the following nursing measures would be employed to prevent complications and promote physical comfort?

1. Frequent oral and nasal hygiene.
2. Maintaining the patient in left side-lying position.
3. Daily massage of back and extremities.
4. Elevating the foot of the bed.

65 • When the nasogastric tube was removed and Mr. Gunderson resumed oral feedings, he developed a "dumping syndrome" or flushing, sweating, palpitations, and dizziness after meals. In preparing Mr. Gunderson for discharge, the nurse should advise him that symptoms of "dumping" can be minimized by:

1. Avoiding drinking liquids with meals
2. Increasing intake of high carbohydrate foods.
3. Taking a short walk immediately after each meal.
4. Eating foods with little bulk or fiber content.

Willie Walker, a 60-year-old diabetic, sought medical attention for aching pain in his right calf. The pain was of 1 year's duration, was provoked by walking, and was relieved by rest. Physical ex-

amination revealed normal femoral pulses, diminished popliteal pulses, and absent tibial and dorsalis pedis pulses on the right. Arteriography revealed narrowing and tortuosity of the right femoral and popliteal arteries with apparently normal arteries in the lower leg and slight narrowing of the left femoral artery. The patient was admitted to the hospital for insertion of a femoropopliteal bypass graft on the right.

66 • Following Mr. Walker's arteriography procedure the nurse should employ which of the following measures to protect him from potential complications?

1. Elevating the fully extended lower extremities on pillows.
2. Comparing the calf circumference measurements of the two legs.
3. Checking the popliteal, posterior tibial, and dorsalis pedis pulses in both legs.
4. Maintaining the legs in abduction by placing a pillow between the thighs.

67 • On Mr. Walker's admission to the recovery room following surgery, the nurse should check his femoral, popliteal, posterior tibial, and dorsalis pedis pulses in his right leg in order to:

1. Determine the effectiveness of the operation in restoring circulation.
2. Obtain baseline data against which to evaluate subsequent findings.
3. Detect indirect evidence of bleeding from the site of the vascular anastamosis.
4. Gauge his blood pressure and state of hydration as an index of fluid balance.

68 • In addition to frequent checking of peripheral pulses, the recovery room nurse could ascertain the adequacy of arterial blood supply to Mr. Walker's leg by which of the following measures?

1. Assessing the skin temperature of his 2 feet by placing the dorsum of her hand against the dorsum of each foot.
2. Determining the interval of time between elevating his leg at a 45 degree angle and his perception of calf pain.
3. Determining the degree of pedal edema by finger indentation of the tissue and observing the time needed for the pit to disappear.
4. Observing the time required for color to return to the nailbed following release of toenail compression.

69 • In preparing Mr. Walker to care for himself at home, the nurse should warn him of the dangers of self medication with which of the following types of drug?

1. Headache anodynes
2. Sinus remedies
3. Gastric antacids
4. Bulk producing laxatives

70 • In teaching Mr. Walker proper foot care measures, the nurse should advise him to:

1. Apply alcohol to the feet after bathing to reduce skin bacteria and prevent infections.
2. Place a hot water bottle at the feet on cold, winter nights to prevent reflex vasoconstriction.
3. Avoid going barefoot even in the house, and avoid the use of soft slippers.
4. Elevate the foot of the bed on blocks to prevent or relieve pedal edema.

Eva Kowalski was 28 years old when her father left home to escape the nagging of his extremely religious and demanding wife. Eva, her father's favorite, grieved over his departure, but her sense of duty to her mother kept her from following him. Shortly thereafter, on her way to work at a large business machine corporation, Eva suffered an acute attack of palpitations, dizziness, and shortness of breath, which subsided spontaneously within a few minutes. Fearing serious heart disease, Eva consulted an internist who was unable to find evidence of any anatomical or physiological disorder.

Eva returned to work but continued to suffer occasional attacks of palpitations and shortness of breath and to worry about having heart disease. She gradually became unable to enjoy any of her usual activities. During the next 6 months Eva's mother urged her to marry the young office coworker whom she had been dating. Somewhat unenthusiastically Eva set the date for the marriage, but 3 days before the wedding she suffered a severe attack of palpitations and shortness of breath. Remembering the internist's assurances that there was nothing wrong with her heart and lungs she decided that she must be losing her mind and went for help to a nearby community mental health center.

Eva told the community mental health nurse who interviewed her that she was afraid that she was losing control and that she must have help to keep from acting irrationally. Eva also told the nurse that she had almost died of pneumonia during infancy and had suffered repeated at-

tacks of asthma throughout childhood, during which her overly protective mother had become even more solicitous concerning her welfare. Eva described herself as having been a superior student in both high school and business school. She had held a responsible position in the business machine corporation for 8 years, had had several promotions, earned a substantial salary, and was well-liked by her coworkers. However, she now felt inadequate in her work and did not, she said, "really enjoy life." She is tired a great deal of the time, and her palpitations and shortness of breath keep her house bound when she is not at work.

71 • The nurse is using Hildegard Peplau's approach to nursing intervention with an anxious patient. Which of the following would be the *first* step in helping Eva understand and learn to cope with anxiety.

1. Encouraging Eva to identify her feelings as those of anxiety.
2. Encouraging Eva to connect her patterns of behavior to her anxiety.
3. Encouraging Eva to provide descriptive data of what has immediately preceded the onset of her feelings.
4. Encouraging Eva to deduct the probably cause of her anxiety.

72 • In determining whether Eva's reaction to anxiety is neurotic or psychotic, the nurse will be guided by the fact that neurotic anxiety is:

1. Based on realistic fears.
2. Disproportionate to its cause.
3. Accompanied by delusions.
4. Incapable of reduction.

73 • In evaluating Eva's progress the nurse will look for changes in:

1. Fatigue, delusions, and hallucinations.
2. Fatigue, fears, and physical complaints.
3. Fatigue, rejection, and dissociation.
4. Flight of ideas, illusions, and disorientation.

74 • During therapy Eva was presented with the idea that her physical symptoms were an expression of her feelings. Eva replied, "I have to express myself that way." Which response would be most helpful?

1. "Why must you express yourself through physical symptoms?"
2. "I see that you feel strongly about this."
3. "What feelings do you need to express?"
4. "Is that the best way of expressing yourself?"

75 • In attempting to formulate plans for her future, Eva said, "I don't know. I liked my job. But I can't go back there now, can I?" Which response would be most appropriate?

1. "What do you think?"
2. "What have you done?"
3. "You like working there?"
4. "You have to do something."

Sally Sims is a 14-year-old girl who is being seen in the Scoliosis Clinic for the first time. History indicates that Mrs. Sims initially believed something was wrong with her daughter about 6 months ago. She had been cautioning her daughter to "stand up straight" because she had noticed that the hem of her dresses and skirts always hung lower on one side. When this observation continued over a period of 6 months or so, Mrs. Sims asked Sally to undress so that she might see what the problem was. On examination, she noticed that Sally was "leaning over" to one side.

She contacted the Pediatric Clinic staff where Sally had been given all of her immunizations, and they suggested that Mrs. Sims contact the Scoliosis Clinic. Physicians in the clinic found a moderate lateral curvature of her thoracic spine that did not disappear on flexion of the trunk. They ordered a Milwaukee brace to be worn 23 hours a day with prescribed exercises to be done daily. Both Mrs. Sims and Sally were informed by the physician that the brace was a conservative treatment and that if the brace was not successful in realigning the vertebral column, surgery would be a definite possibility.

76 • Assessment of Sally's spine indicated that the scoliosis was structural rather than nonstructural. Assessment of structural scoliosis will reveal the following:

1. There is a convexity in the lumbar vertebrae.
2. It is difficult to visualize the scapulae.
3. There will be a rib hump.
4. There will be 2 dimples, each lateral to the spine in the lumbar area.

77 • The nurse will include Sally when she develops the care plan. In caring for an adolescent, the nurse should consider the following in regard to Sally:

1. She will not need a peer group while in the hospital.
2. She will feel more comfortable relating to younger children while in the hospital.
3. She will still need contact with a peer group from home.
4. She will quickly renounce her peer group.

78 • Sally has been put into traction prior to surgery. She is extremely angry and has become uncommunicative. Which of the following is the most likely cause for her anger?

1. Sally is forced to assume a dependent state.
2. Her coping mechanisms are not firmly established.
3. Her hormonal changes tend to interfere with her ability to heal properly.
4. She is certain to respond poorly to pain.

79 • A patient in traction needs careful observation for neurological impairment. The following sign will alert the nurse to a possible neurological problem due to the traction:

1. Upper extremity hyporeflexia.
2. Nausea and vomiting.
3. Loss of lateral gaze.
4. Temperature over 102 degrees F.

80 • Sally has had surgery for Harrington rod insertion, and she now has a body cast. Cast care requires special attention, particularly in observing conditions of the skin and circulation. Which of the following is most suggestive of a potential problem?

1. Sensation of itching under the cast.
2. Patient states leg tingles and leg feels cool to touch.
3. Cast's surface feels damp 24 hours after application.
4. There is no pain.

Cora Peach, a plump 40-year-old mother of 5 children, was brought to the hospital emergency room with severe pain in her right upper abdomen and right shoulder and persistent vomiting. Physical examination revealed a hard, pear shaped mass in the right upper quadrant of the abdomen. A radiogram of the abdomen revealed several small irregular opacities in the right upper abdomen; an intravenous cholangiogram confirmed the diagnosis of cholelithiasis. A few days later, a cholecystectomy and common duct exploration were performed. Mrs. Peach was returned to the recovery room with a T tube and a soft rubber drain protruding from the right upper abdomen.

81 • The nurse should particularly emphasize which of the following topics during Mrs. Peach's pre-operative teaching?

1. Explanation of the purpose of post-operative use of the anti-embolism stockings.
2. Demonstration of the method for splinting the gallbladder incision during coughing and deep breathing.;
3. Teaching meditation procedures for control of post-operative pain and anxiety.
4. Explanation of the procedure and equipment for enteral or parenteral hyperalimentation.

82 • In writing a plan for Mrs. Peach's care during the first day or two following surgery, the primary nurse should direct the associate nurse to administer the doses of the prescribed narcotic liberally to prevent Mrs. Peach from:

1. Moving about too freely and dislodging the T tube.
2. Irritating her throat by excessive coughing.
3. Limiting her respiratory excursions in order to avoid pain.
4. Exerting strain on the incision by straining at stool.

83 • During the first several days following surgery, Mrs. Peach should spend much of her time in which position in order to minimize post-operative complications?

1. Supine
2. Trendelenburg
3. Prone
4. Low Fowler's

84 • Which of the following devices could be expected to aid Mrs. Peach's post-operative recovery by encouraging early mobilization following surgery?

1. Wheelchair
2. Walker
3. Single point cane
4. Abdominal binder

85 • During the 1st day following surgery, 200 ml of dark green fluid drained from Mrs. Peach's T-tube into the attached drainage bag. In evaluating this observation, the nurse should conclude that:

1. The sutures that closed the cystic duct have slipped, allowing bile leakage into surrounding soft tissues.
2. The incision into the common duct has broken open, permitting bile and blood to accumulate in the gallbladder bed.
3. Chronic cholecystitis has caused biliary cirrhosis, with distortion of the biliary drainage system.
4. Bile is temporarily blocked from transit to the duodenum by post-operative edema of the common duct.

Seventy-five-year old Roy Keeler consulted a vascular surgeon with complaints of brief episodes of visual loss and motor weakness. Findings of a carotid bruit on the left and evidence of platelet emboli on left funduscopic examination led to carotid and vertebral arteriography, which revealed 90% obstruction of the left carotid and 50% obstruction of the right carotid. A left carotid endarterectomy was performed.

86 • Mr. Keeler was returned to the recovery room following surgery with the following vital signs; Temperature of 99.6 degrees F rectally, pulse of 80/min; respirations of 20/min; and blood pressure of 120/88 mm Hg. For which of the following changes in vital signs, within the 1st 2 hours following surgery, should the recovery room nurse notify the surgeon?

1. Temperature elevation to 100.6 degrees F, rectally.
2. Pulse increase to 92/min.
3. Increase in respirations to 24/min.
4. Fall in blood pressure to 100/68 mm Hg.

87 • Development of which of the following during the first day or two following surgery should cause the nurse to alert the surgeon to possible embolization of a clot from the operative site?

1. Asymmetry of facial muscles.
2. Burning pain in the incision.
3. Sudden, severe chest pain.
4. Pain and tenderness in the calf.

88 • Which of the following post-operative problems should the recovery room nurse interpret as a possible indicator of serious post-operative complication of Mr. Keeler's neck surgery?

1. Diaphoresis
2. Thirst
3. Hoarseness
4. Lethargy

89 • Which of the following should be kept in plain view at Mr. Keeler's bedside during the 1st 12 to 24 hours following surgery?

1. Hemostat
2. Scissors
3. Tracheostomy tube and tray
4. Padded tongue blade

90 • On his discharge from the hospital, Mr. Keeler was told by his surgeon to take 600 mg of acetylsalicylic acid every morning with breakfast. In teaching him about self care at home, the nurse should explain that the purpose for the medication is to:

1. Relieve pain resulting from surgical trauma to neck tissues.
2. Decrease the risk of seizures by preventing temperature elevation.
3. Relieve inflammatory edema of neck tissues traumatized during surgery.
4. Reduce risk of carotid thrombosis by preventing platelet aggregation.

Victoria Clapper was 48 years old and in an acute manic state when her husband brought her to the inpatient psychiatric unit. Victoria's history, as conveyed to the psychiatrist by her husband, was as follows: when she was 4 years old her mother died; soon afterward her father married a younger woman, who had 5 children in the next 7 years; Victoria's stepmother relegated to Victoria much of the responsibility for the care of her step-brothers and step-sisters; but at the same time, her stepmother managed to keep Victoria at the periphery of the family life and its activity. A college scholarship enabled Victoria to leave home and study music immediately after she was graduated from high school. On being graduated from college she married Henry Clapper, a college chemistry professor, and took a position

as a high school music teacher in the small community in which her husband taught.

During the 6 months preceding her hospitalization Victoria first complained of a variety of somatic symptoms, then became exceedingly jealous of what she considered to be her husband's excessive attention toward his young female laboratory assistant. Finally, after 3 days of severe depression, Victoria made a vicious verbal attack on the judges who had failed to award her favorite pupil the 1st prize in a state music contest.

On admission to the hospital Victoria moved about restlessly, waving her arms in a threatening manner while loudly berating her husband, the hospital personnel, and the state music judges. She demanded to be released from "this jail" and cursed the nurse and psychiatrist who interviewed her. The psychiatrist described Victoria as a possessive and dependent person who feared rejection and abandonment who was in an acute manic state.

91 • Which of the following best describes the most suitable environment for Victoria during her acute mania?

1. A seclusion room with a large window.
2. A spacious room with few people in it.
3. A dayroom filled with other patients.
4. A well-lighted, 4-bed room.

92 • Which of the following nursing interventions would be most helpful to Victoria immediately following admission?

1. Providing a calm and safe environment.
2. Staying with her and talking to her.
3. Helping her to set limits on her behavior.
4. Administering medications as ordered.

93 • In order to convince Victoria that she will not be able to manipulate the hospital personnel as she has others, the nurse should:

1. Carefully explain how the nurse's relationship will differ from her superficial interactions of the past.
2. Give her a short clear definition of the limits that will be set on her behavior.
3. Outline the consequences of any attempt on her part to manipulate or exploit them.
4. Acquaint her with the complete health history that was obtained from her husband.

94 • At 1:00 A.M. one night during her 2nd week of hospitalization, Victoria rushed up to the nurse's station and demanded that her therapist come to the ward immediately to write an order giving her a pass. Which should be the 1st response by the nurse?

1. "Okay, Victoria, go to the dayroom and wait. I'll call him immediately."
2. "Victoria, you are just being difficult. You know that I cannot do that."
3. "Your request is unreasonable, and I will not call your doctor now."
4. "You must be very upset to want a pass immediately."

95 • Lithium carbonate was prescribed upon Victoria's admission to the hospital. Toxic effects would be most apt to appear if the blood level of the drug were to exceed:

1. 0.08 to .12 mEq/L.
2. 0.8 to 1.2 mEq/L.
3. 8.0 to 12.0 mEq/L.
4. 80 to 120 mEq/L.

Items from Comprehensive Examination Section 2 That Address the Various Steps of the Nursing Process

Item Number	Assess	Analyze	Plan	Implement	Evaluate	Item Number	Assess	Analyze	Plan	Implement	Evaluate
1	x					49	x				
2				x		50			x		
3				x		51				x	
4					x	52	x				
5				x		53				x	
6	x					54	x				
7		x				55					x
8				x		56		x			
9					x	57	x				
10	x					58				x	
11		x				59				x	
12		x				60					x
13					x	61		x			
14				x		62				x	
15				x		63					x
16			x			64				x	
17				x		65				x	
18		x				66					x
19		x				67	x				
20				x		68	x				
21		x				69		x			
22			x			70				x	
23		x				71		x			
24		x				72		x			
25				x		73					x
26	x					74				x	
27		x				75				x	
28	x					76	x				
29			x			77			x		
30				x		78		x			
31	x					79					x
32					x	80					x
33				x		81		x			
34					x	82			x		
35					x	83				x	
36		x				84		x			
37				x		85					x
38					x	86					x
39					x	87					x
40				x		88					x
41					x	89			x		
42				x		90				x	
43		x				91			x		
44				x		92		x			
45				x		93				x	
46		x				94				x	
47		x				95					x
48					x						

Answer Sheet—Section 2

1. 1 2 3 4
2. 1 2 3 4
3. 1 2 3 4
4. 1 2 3 4
5. 1 2 3 4
6. 1 2 3 4
7. 1 2 3 4
8. 1 2 3 4
9. 1 2 3 4
10. 1 2 3 4
11. 1 2 3 4
12. 1 2 3 4
13. 1 2 3 4
14. 1 2 3 4
15. 1 2 3 4
16. 1 2 3 4
17. 1 2 3 4
18. 1 2 3 4
19. 1 2 3 4
20. 1 2 3 4
21. 1 2 3 4
22. 1 2 3 4
23. 1 2 3 4
24. 1 2 3 4
25. 1 2 3 4
26. 1 2 3 4
27. 1 2 3 4
28. 1 2 3 4
29. 1 2 3 4
30. 1 2 3 4
31. 1 2 3 4
32. 1 2 3 4
33. 1 2 3 4
34. 1 2 3 4
35. 1 2 3 4
36. 1 2 3 4
37. 1 2 3 4
38. 1 2 3 4
39. 1 2 3 4
40. 1 2 3 4
41. 1 2 3 4
42. 1 2 3 4
43. 1 2 3 4
44. 1 2 3 4
45. 1 2 3 4
46. 1 2 3 4
47. 1 2 3 4
48. 1 2 3 4
49. 1 2 3 4
50. 1 2 3 4
51. 1 2 3 4
52. 1 2 3 4
53. 1 2 3 4
54. 1 2 3 4
55. 1 2 3 4
56. 1 2 3 4
57. 1 2 3 4
58. 1 2 3 4
59. 1 2 3 4
60. 1 2 3 4
61. 1 2 3 4
62. 1 2 3 4
63. 1 2 3 4
64. 1 2 3 4
65. 1 2 3 4
66. 1 2 3 4
67. 1 2 3 4
68. 1 2 3 4
69. 1 2 3 4
70. 1 2 3 4
71. 1 2 3 4
72. 1 2 3 4
73. 1 2 3 4
74. 1 2 3 4
75. 1 2 3 4
76. 1 2 3 4
77. 1 2 3 4
78. 1 2 3 4
79. 1 2 3 4
80. 1 2 3 4
81. 1 2 3 4
82. 1 2 3 4
83. 1 2 3 4
84. 1 2 3 4
85. 1 2 3 4
86. 1 2 3 4
87. 1 2 3 4
88. 1 2 3 4
89. 1 2 3 4
90. 1 2 3 4
91. 1 2 3 4
92. 1 2 3 4
93. 1 2 3 4
94. 1 2 3 4
95. 1 2 3 4

Section 3

COMPREHENSIVE EXAMINATION

Mrs. Sage developed spontaneous and painless bleeding at 37 weeks' gestation. She had suffered no trauma and had had no other complications during her pregnancy. Her husband reported the bleeding by phone to the obstetrician, and the obstetrician advised Mr. Sage to bring his wife to the hospital immediately.

1 • In organizing resources for Mrs. Sage's care on hospital admission, the nurse should expect that which of the following measures will be performed *first* following Mrs. Sage's arrival at the hospital?

1. Sterile vaginal examination.
2. Venipuncture to obtain blood for typing and cross matching.
3. Insertion of an indwelling catheter.
4. Measurement of anteroposterior pelvic diameter.

Because ultrasonography revealed a low lying placenta, a diagnosis of placenta previa was made. Mrs. Sage was placed on complete bed rest and within a few hours her bleeding ceased.

2 • During the period of Mrs. Sage's enforced bed rest, which of the following interventions should be prohibited?

1. Monitoring of fetal heart tones.
2. Performance of digital rectal examination.
3. Elevation of the head of the bed.
4. Palpation of the uterine fundus.

3 • While the nurse was bathing Mrs. Sage on the day following her admission to the hospital, Mrs. Sage began to cry. The most appropriate nursing intervention would be to:

1. Ask Mrs. Sage why she is crying.
2. Request the physician to order a sedative.
3. Sit quietly with Mrs. Sage until the crying ceases.
4. Ask Mr. Sage to comfort his wife.

4 • After 3 days of bed rest, Mrs. Sage's condition changed suddenly. The nurse summoned the physician, reporting that Mrs. Sage was complaining of severe abdominal pain and lightheadedness, that her abdomen was rigid, that she was sweating profusely, and that her pulse was rapid and weak. Mrs. Sage's symptoms are suggestive of:

1. Onset of labor.
2. Supine hypotensive syndrome.
3. Severe eclampsia.
4. Abruptio placenta.

5 • While waiting for the physician to arrive, it would be most important for the nurse to:

1. Push oral fluids.
2. Monitor fetal heart tones.
3. Elevate the head of the bed.
4. Obtain a urine specimen for measurement of protein content.

Mrs. Allen, a 19-year-old mother, walked into the Pediatric Clinic of a large teaching hospital without an appointment carrying her 4-month-old daughter, Cassie. She indicated that her sister insisted that she bring her child to the hospital because the child "didn't look right." Mrs. Allen herself indicated that she didn't think anything was wrong with her baby.

Mrs. Allen was sullen, and when she took a seat in the waiting room, she placed Cassie in an empty seat next to her and proceeded to watch T.V. When she was finally called to see the physician, she picked up the infant, walked into the examining room, and handed the infant to the nurse without saying a word; she then took a seat in the corner of the room.

The infant's history was that of a full term baby, whose weight and length were 7 lbs 4 oz (3.3 kg) and 20 in (50.8 cm). No unusual problems occurred during pregnancy, labor, or delivery. Mother and child were discharged from the maternity floor after 2 days. Mrs. Allen had no infor-

mation on the infant's weight gain since she had not brought Cassie back to see a physician after discharge from the hospital. Cassie's mother gave no specific reason for this omission, and when asked, she merely shrugged her shoulders.

Cassie was being fed whole homogenized milk and baby cereal. Mrs. Allen explained that the formula recommended by the hospital was too expensive so she switched to whole milk. Cassie was a "fussy" eater, "hated" her cereal and, as a result, took her milk and ate her cereal irregularly and sporadically. The mother had no idea how much milk Cassie took in a 24-hour period or how much cereal she ate.

Mr. Allen is a truck driver who leaves home 3 to 4 days at a time, and Mrs. Allen spends most of her time watching T.V. and taking care of the baby. She said she was usually bored and depressed because she had no one she could talk to.

Physical examination of the infant revealed a somewhat rigid female with a pinched and expressionless look on her face. She weighed 10 lb 1 oz (4.6 kg) (4th percentile), and she was 22½ inches (57 cm) long (3rd percentile). Cassie's skin was dry and wrinkly, her eyes sunken in, giving the appearance of a wizened old lady. She was lethargic through most of the examination, occasionally emitting a weak cry.

The physician could find no obvious organic pathology and based on her abnormal height and weight for a 4-month-old infant, admitted her to ascertain the diagnosis of failure to thrive (nonorganic).

6 • A normal baby at 4 months of age should:

1. Be able to sit without support.
2. Locate sound by turning head to side.
3. Resist toy pull.
4. Grab for a toy out of reach.

7 • One of the primary objectives in planning Cassie's nursing care should be:

1. To make the mother realize that her child was starving.
2. To persuade the father that his involvement is absolutely essential.
3. To structure the factors in the environment for healthy psychosocial interactions.
4. To convince the family's relatives to take over the infant's care on weekends.

8 • Negative feeding patterns play an important role in the occurrence of nonorganic failure to thrive. When the nurse feeds the infant a different feeding pattern is implemented by:

1. Being persistent when the infant initially refuses feeding.
2. Adhering to "on-demand" schedule for feeding.
3. Singing happy songs to the infant while feeding.
4. Allowing the infant to determine the length of time required for the feeding.

9 • Mrs. Allen feels isolated and depressed most of the time, and she copes by watching TV all day long. In order to nurture the child back to health, the mother needs to acquire appropriate mothering skills. The nurse can help Mrs. Allen by:

1. Directing her to the latest text on growth and development.
2. Appealing to her maternal instincts.
3. Telephoning her at least once a week to ask how she is getting along.
4. Demonstrating some basic mothering skills and how to "mold" (i.e., positioning and posturing her body to make the infant more comfortable in her arms).

10 • The public health nurse visited the Allen's home to evaluate Cassie's progress. The nurse's report was essentially positive in that she found:

1. Two female relatives visiting Mrs. Allen.
2. Mr. Allen had changed jobs, and now he is home in the evenings.
3. There was good eye-to-eye contact between mother and infant.
4. The apartment was immaculate and sparkling clean.

Doris Bloch, a 26-year-old college teacher, had undergone craniotomy for removal of a cerebral astrocytoma, following which she received radiation therapy and chemotherapy. Because she was left with right hemiparesis and minimal cognitive deficits, her parents brought her to a rehabilitation facility for upgrading of functional skills. While a patient in the rehabilitation hospital, Doris was started on a daily dose of prednisone.

11 • Doris's illness will upset the Bloch family dynamics principally because it will interfere with Doris's achievement of which of the psychological tasks of young adulthood?

1. Accomplishment of physical and emotional independence from parents.
2. Establishment of a value system to guide personal decision making.
3. Selection of an occupational role and development of work-related skills.
4. Formation of affectional and sexual bonds to a member of the opposite sex.

12 • While caring for Doris, the nurse should monitor her closely for which of the following as a sign of dangerously elevated intracranial pressure?

1. Homonymous hemianopia
2. Loss of peripheral vision
3. Unilateral pupil dilation
4. Centrifugal scintillating scotoma

13 • When the nurse administered the first dose of prednisone, Doris asked, "What's this medicine? Are they giving me more chemotherapy?" Which response by the nurse would be most appropriate?

1. "This is a hormone that is intended to increase your resistance to infection."
2. "This is a substance to regulate the sodium and potassium levels in your blood."
3. "This is a medication to increase your muscle strength and physical endurance."
4. "This is a drug to prevent brain edema that might result from your tumor or its treatment."

14 • During Doris's stay in the rehabilitation facility the nurse should make which of the following adjustments in the patient's care to compensate for the loss of strength from the patient's disease and treatment?

1. Bathe, dress, feed, and toilet Doris so she can conserve her energy for occupational therapy and physiotherapy.
2. Schedule all occupational therapy and physiotherapy to take place in Doris's room, to eliminate need for transfers and wheelchair mobility.
3. Provide assistive devices to facilitate self care with minimal energy expenditure while maintaining independence in self care.
4. Allow Doris to cancel scheduled nursing, physiotherapy, or occupational therapy activities whenever she is fatigued.

15 • In teaching Mr. and Mrs. Bloch to care for their daughter following hospital discharge, the nurse should instruct them to report which of the following to the physician as a possible sign of tumor recurrence?

1. Hair loss
2. Easy fatigability
3. Muscular twitching
4. Moon face appearance

Della Hicks, 76 years of age, was brought to the emergency room of her local hospital; she was suffering rectal prolapse. After the prolapse was reduced, the physician performed a sigmoidoscopic examination, prescribed a daily dose of psyllium hydrophilic mucilloid (Metamucil), and advised a high fiber diet and high fluid intake. While the nurse was preparing Della for a proctosigmoidoscopic examination, Della asked "What is the doctor going to do now? Hasn't he already put the bowel back into place?"

16 • Which response by the nurse would be most appropriate?

1. "Everyone over 40 years of age should have an annual proctoscopic examination to check for rectal cancer."
2. "This examination has nothing to do with your present problem but must be performed on every hospitalized patient."
3. "This examination is needed to identify any bowel problems that may have predisposed to rectal prolapse."
4. "Only the external rectal prolapse has been corrected. Now the doctor must reduce the telescoped inner bowel."

17 • In providing Della with discharge instructions, the nurse should caution Della against:

1. Prolonged straining at stool.
2. Eating raw vegetables and fruit.
3. Use of rectal suppositories.
4. Application of commercial hemorrhoid remedies.

18 • The nurse should instruct Della that all *but which one* of the following would be suitable for inclusion in Della's diet?

1. Whole wheat bread
2. Apples, nuts, and raisins (Waldorf salad)
3. 100% bran cereal
4. Lettuce, tomatoes, and cucumbers (garden salad)

19 • In addition to taking Metamucil and increasing dietary fiber, the nurse should advise Della to do which of the following to prevent future episodes of rectal prolapse?

1. Take a hot sitz bath every evening.
2. Engage in regular daily exercise.
3. Eliminate coffee, tea, and colas from the diet.
4. Lie down for a short time following each meal.

20 • Della should be advised that, in the event of a subsequent rectal prolapse, her first action should be to:

1. Don a rubber glove, lubricate the index finger, and gently replace the prolapsed bowel.
2. Take a hot sitz bath to see whether the prolapsed bowel will reduce spontaneously.
3. Apply a sterile dressing and an ice pack over the protruding bowel.
4. Assume the knee-chest position and place a moist cloth over the prolapsed bowel.

Dr. Steven Dos, 55 years old, a professor of Greek literature at a nearby university, was brought to the admission center of a private inpatient psychiatric hospital by his wife of 30 years. Mrs. Dos denied any previous hospitalizations for her husband. One month ago a fire at the university destroyed the notes he had collected over a 10-year period during his sabbatical visits to Greece. It also consumed an unfinished manuscript that Dr. Dos had worked on for the past 6 summers. He had hoped to have the manuscript completed in 6 more months at which time he would submit it for publication. Mrs. Dos stated that his work meant everything to him and that his promotion as a tenured professor depended upon this work. There were no copies of the notes or the manuscript.

Since that time he had refused most meals, with a consequent weight loss of 16 lb. He spent most of each day in bed, refusing to get up and wash, shave, or dress himself. He had not left the house for the past 3 weeks. He was sleeping poorly and complained of early morning wakening. She fears at this time that he might take his own life, because he repeatedly states "There is no reason to go on. Everything that meant anything to me is gone."

He is unshaven, his hair is uncombed, and his clothes are disheveled. He sits slumped over in his chair with his head in his hands. He speaks slowly and in a whisper, and he is tearful when he says "Nothing will ever be the same again. I'm not the same person I was. I'm worthless. My life is over." He sees his situation as hopeless, and that he is powerless to influence the rest of his life.

The working diagnosis, which was confirmed by psychological testing, is major depression. A thorough physical examination reveals no abnormalities.

21 • There is indirect evidence that underproduction of which of the following chemical substances may cause a major depression?

1. Aminobutyric acid and vitamin B complex.
2. Acetyl coenzyme A and pyruvic acid.
3. Dexamethasone and ACTH.
4. Norepinephrine and serotonin.

22 • Which of the following attitudes of the nurse would be most helpful in overcoming any reluctance on the part of Dr. Dos to take his medications?

1. Firm kindness.
2. Rigid insistence.
3. Humble entreaty.
4. Gentle bantering.

23 • If Dr. Dos were to make a suicide attempt, during which phase of the hospitalization would it be most likely to occur?

1. Immediately after hospital admission.
2. At the point of his deepest depression.
3. When his depression begins to abate.
4. Shortly before hospital discharge.

24 • The interdisciplinary team's initial care plan for Dr. Dos included helping him achieve a positive, realistic self concept. In evaluating Dr. Dos the nurse should assess for all *but which one* of the following?

1. A degree of self esteem and self respect.
2. A feeling of acceptance by others.
3. A feeling of belonging.
4. A feeling of humility.

25 • The nurse should do which of the following when she observes Dr. Dos shivering in the corner of the dayroom?

1. Ignore his shivering in order to force him either to get a sweater or request one.
2. Get a sweater for him and, without comment, drape it over his shoulders.
3. Direct him to his room, instruct him to get the sweater and to put it on before he returns to the dayroom.
4. Comment to him that you have observed him shivering, and go with him to get a sweater.

Susan Josephson is a gravida 1 para 0 who is a known diabetic. She has received insulin since she was 10 years old. Although her pregnancy was unplanned, she has decided to continue the pregnancy. Susan has expressed concern over her ability to deliver a healthy child.

26 • In planning Susan's care the nurse should expect that:

1. Susan's insulin requirements will be highest during her 1st trimester.
2. Fetal macrosomatia will develop in response to Susan's increased water retention.
3. Repeated hospitalizations may be necessary to provide rest, determine fetal status, and decide mode of delivery.
4. Vaginal delivery will occur spontaneously at about 37 weeks of gestation.

27 • On Susan's visit to the physician at 16 weeks' gestation, a high level of glycosuria was discovered. At this point Susan's management should probably include:

1. A fasting blood glucose determination.
2. An oral glucose tolerance test.
3. An increase in insulin dosage.
4. Diet restrictions to decrease caloric intake.

28 • Susan became nauseated at 18 weeks' gestation and developed excessive vomiting. The primary concern in Susan's management at this time would be the possibility of:

1. Poor O_2 supply to the fetus.
2. Spontaneous abortion.
3. Development of ketoacidosis.
4. Occurrence of congenital anomalies.

29 • Susan's expected date of confinement would be more difficult to determine than that of a non-diabetic mother because diabetics have:

1. Irregular menses.
2. Smaller than normal babies.
3. Babies with larger than normal heads.
4. Less than normal weight gain.

30 • Although infants of diabetic mothers are frequently larger than normal, infants of some diabetic mothers are unusually small because of:

1. Hypoglycemia *in utero*.
2. Smaller than normal uterine size.
3. Fetal thyroid hyperfunction.
4. Atherosclerosis of the placenta.

Susan's baby was delivered at 37 weeks' gestation. He weighed 9 lb 6 oz, and his Apgar scores were 9/10 at birth. He was taken to the intermediate care nursery for observation.

31 • In examining Susan's infant for abnormalities, the nurse should be aware that all *but which one* of the following congenital anomalies tend to occur with increased incidence in infants of diabetic mothers?

1. Central nervous system anomalies.
2. Caudal regression syndrome.
3. Congenital heart defects.
4. Missing limbs.

32 • In planning for care of Susan's infant, the admitting nurse in the newborn nursery should be especially concerned about:

1. The amount of insulin given Susan during labor and delivery.
2. The infant's 1 minute and 5 minute Apgar scores.
3. The infant's early delivery date.
4. The infant's larger than normal body size.

33 • Susan's infant will be most susceptible to hypoglycemia at which of the following times?

1. 1 to 3 hours after birth
2. 8 hours after birth
3. 24 hours after birth
4. 48 hours after birth

34 • In assessing the condition of Susan's baby the nurse should interpret which of the following laboratory test findings as indicative of hypoglycemia?

1. Below 30 mg/dl in the 1st 24 hours of life and below 90 mg/dl after 3 days.
2. Below 30 mg/dl in the 1st 72 hours of life and below 45 mg/dl after 3 days.
3. Below 45 mg/dl in the 1st 24 hours of life and below 120 mg/dl after 3 days.
4. Below 45 mg/dl in the 1st 72 hours of life and below 120 mg/dl after 3 days.

35 • During his 1st 2 days of life, Susan's baby should be monitored closely for development of which of the following—as an indication of a possibly serious complication of his earlier than normal birth?

1. Regurgitation.
2. Shivering.
3. Babinski's reflex.
4. Muscular tremors.

Ina West, 55 years of age, consulted her physician with complaints of diarrhea and cramping lower left abdominal pain. When proctosigmoidoscopy revealed diverticulitis, the physician hospitalized Mrs. West and prescribed bed rest, liquid diet, docusate sodium (Colace), neomycin, and propantheline. Mrs. West's health history indicated a 3-year history of bowel problems.

36 • Development of which of the following symptoms should cause the nurse to suspect a severe complication of Mrs. West's illness?

1. Absent bowel sounds
2. Excessive flatus
3. Black stool
4. Increasing blood pressure

37 • Two days following hospital admission, Mrs. West suffered perforation of a sigmoid diverticulum, so a temporary transverse colostomy was created. On the 3rd post-operative day the surgeon opened the exteriorized bowel loop with electrocautery. In preparing Mrs. West for colostomy surgery, the nurse should make which adjustment in the usual pre-operative preparations?

1. Elevate the enema bag only slightly so fluid flows into the bowel under low pressure.
2. Permit the patient to drink clear liquids up to 2 hours before the operation.
3. Avoid shaving the abdomen to prevent lacerations that could later be contaminated with fecal drainage.
4. Arrange for a rehabilitated colostomate to talk with the patient about life style changes following colostomy.

38 • Which of the following nursing actions would significantly increase Mrs. West's comfort during opening of the bowel loop on the 3rd post-operative day?

1. Administering a dose of the ordered narcotic immediately before the cauterization.
2. Concealing the bowel loop from the patient's view during the procedure.
3. Providing adequate ventilation of the patient's room throughout the procedure.
4. Distracting the patient's attention by engaging her in conversation while the bowel is being opened.

39 • Six months following creation of the temporary colostomy, proctoscopic examination revealed that the lower bowel was healed, so the colostomy was closed and the proximal and distal colonic segments were anastomosed. After recovery from this 2nd surgery, what type of diet should Mrs. West be advised to eat?

1. Mechanically and chemically bland diet.
2. High protein, high fat, low carbohydrate diet.
3. High carbohydrate, low residue diet.
4. High fiber diet with increased fluids.

40 • At discharge, following her 2nd hospitalization, Mrs. West should be instructed to notify her physician in the event that she experiences which of the following symptoms?

1. Constipation
2. Diarrhea
3. Narrow or ribbon-like stools
4. Blood in the stool

While driving to work one day, a private duty nurse came upon a car that had jumped the curb and struck a light pole. Upon investigating the accident scene, the nurse found the driver, who was the sole occupant of the car, to be alive but dazed, and unrestrained by a seat belt.

41 • After hailing a passing motorist and asking him to summon the police and emergency medical services, the nurse's first action should be to:

1. Palpate the cervical spine for swelling and pain.
2. Ascertain whether the airway is clear of debris.
3. Examine the head, trunk, and extremities for evidence of hemorrhage.
4. Ask the patient to move each of his extremities in sequence.

42 • Upon questioning by the nurse, the driver of the wrecked car indicated that he had struck his head against the windshield on impact. The nurse observed no discoloration, swelling, or depression of the forehead, and no inequality in pupil size. On the basis of available information the nurse should assume that:

1. The driver's head injuries are confined to skin and subcutaneous tissues, without involvement of bone or brain tissue.
2. The driver has suffered a mild brain injury or concussion as a result of the blow to the head.
3. The patient is in no immediate danger of neurological dysfunction, but may develop post-traumatic epilepsy.
4. It is probable that the driver has suffered both a head and a spinal injury as a result of the impact.

43 • In preparing the accident victim for transport to the hospital, which of the following steps should be taken?

1. Slide the patient carefully from the driver's seat, lower him slowly onto a stretcher, and strap him securely before transport.
2. Allow the patient to move from the driver's seat at his own pace, providing assistance as necessary as he assumes a supine position on the stretcher.
3. While one person holds the patient's head erect and in a neutral position (not turned to the right or left), a 2nd person should lift him from the driver's seat to the stretcher.
4. The patient's head and trunk should be strapped to a short spine board while he remains in the driver's seat and before he is moved at all.

44 • On the victim's arrival at the hospital emergency room, the admitting nurse should question the police and emergency medical technician who accompany him concerning all *but which one* of the following?

1. The time, location, and circumstances of the patient's injury.
2. Whether the patient suffered unconsciousness following the accident.
3. Drugs and other treatments administered at the accident scene or on the trip to the hospital.
4. Underlying medical conditions that may influence the patient's response to treatment.

45 • Mr. Cohen, the accident victim, was discharged home to his wife's care after spending the night in the hospital. The nurse should instruct Mrs. Cohen to notify the physician or bring Mr. Cohen to the emergency room in the event that he experiences which of the following symptoms?

1. Dull headache
2. Increasing lethargy
3. Dizziness and vertigo
4. Ecchymosis of the forehead

Paul Cottin, age 25 years, arrived at the intake clinic via police escort accompanied by his mother. He was screaming and gesticulating wildly, seemingly responding to voices that only he could hear. "I have to kill them. God told me so. They're all evil. I'm Christ, you know. I do what my Father tells me to do."

History taken from his mother revealed that Paul had always had trouble in school and by the age of 15 years he had dropped out of school and tried his hand at working at various fast-food outlets. He had no friends and had difficulty getting along with his coworkers. He was usually fired after a month or two owing to tardiness (several hours late) and an inability to follow through with the demands of his job. His mother also reported that he had never had a girlfriend. At family functions he sat quietly for a while with other family members but usually retreated to his room and remained there, despite entreaties from his mother that he come and join the family.

He voluntarily joined the army at age 20 years and apparently functioned fairly well during that time. Upon discharge he had been unable to hold a steady job, had no friends, and took no interest in the opposite sex.

Approximately 3 weeks ago he began behaving in a bizarre fashion. His mother had to waken him and help him dress or he would never have made it to work. If left to himself his shoes did not match, his shirt would only be half buttoned, and the shirt tails would be hanging out. He would often forget to do the most elementary things such as brushing his teeth and combing his hair. There were many days when he could not remember how to get to work. He felt that people at work were trying to poison his food and that the police were watching his every move. He spent many sleepless nights, pacing the floor and talking to himself. His mother reported that he "sees" his dead father, whom Paul says gives him advice. He had not eaten for the past week, and for the past 3 days he had become increasingly agitated, pacing and shouting that "I am the Son ... I will take care of everything."

The critical incident that brought him to the hospital occurred 1 hour prior to admission when he took his pistol outside and began threatening the neighbors. His admitting diagnosis is schizophrenia, undifferentiated type.

46 • Of primary concern to the nurse who assesses Paul upon admission to the unit is:

1. His relationship with his mother.
2. His nutritional status.
3. His ability to carry out activities of daily living.
4. His predisposition to violence.

47 • After completion of the nursing assessment of Paul's needs, the nurses outlined a plan for interacting with him on the unit. Their plan should include all *but which one* of the following?

1. Assigning one nurse to develop a therapeutic relationship with him.
2. Restricting him to the unit for several days until initial assessments are confirmed.
3. Structuring the milieu so that Paul has maximum interaction with other patients.
4. Administering his medication p.r.n. as ordered to help him regain some control and reintegrate.

48 • Paul's auditory hallucinations result from:

1. A tendency to distrust visual, tactile, and olfactory perceptions.
2. Overinvestment of libidinal energy in the hearing apparatus.
3. Increased hearing acuity developed during his time in the army.
4. Inability to distinguish memory traces from current sensory stimuli.

49 • Paul told the nurse that the editorial in the daily newspaper contained a coded message telling him that his hospitalization was being overseen by the President of the United States. This behavior indicates that he was experiencing:

1. Distortion of sensation.
2. Delusions of grandeur.
3. Ideas of reference.
4. Ideas of transference.

50 • The medication helped Paul to reintegrate his thoughts and behavior, and the nurse had established a therapeutic relationship with him. At this point the nurse and Paul sat down to update his care plan. Which of the following would take priority at this point in time?

1. Addressing issues such as when he will be leaving and where he will be going.
2. Setting short-term and long-term goals for this hospitalization.
3. Impressing upon him the importance of medication compliance after discharge.
4. Talking about family systems and what went wrong in the family for him.

Eight-month-old Billy Dillon has been brought to the pediatrician's office by his mother. She reports that "he is rubbing his ears again," is extremely irritable, is anorexic, and was up 4 times last night crying. He has a moderately severe upper respiratory infection with coughing and nasal discharge. She added that this is the 3rd flare-up of what she believes is a continuous ear infection; Billy had been given antibiotic therapy for 10 days on 2 previous occasions. Mrs. Dillon reports that Billy has had so many "colds" that she has lost count of the number.

Examination shows a bright red right tympanic membrane with bulging of the entire pars tensa with no visible landmarks and no mobility; his left tympanic membrane is moderately reddened with moderate bulging of the anterior and superior quadrants; and the short process can be seen. Light reflex is still visible in the anterior inferior quadrant. There is faint visibility of the short process. His temperature is 102°F, rectally.

The physician's diagnosis is acute suppurative otitis media. He prescribed ampicillin, stressing emphatically to the mother that the medication must be given to Billy for the entire 10 days no matter how well the child appeared to her.

51 • Otitis media is found much more frequently in children than in adults. The basis for this finding is the difference in the anatomy of the eustachian tube. Children's eustachian tubes differ from those of adults in the following way:

1. They lie more in an angle.
2. They are wider and longer.
3. The cartilage lining is undeveloped.
4. The cilia are undeveloped.

52 • In assessing Billy, you would expect to observe all *but which one* of the following?

1. Enlarged postauricular lymph nodes.
2. Enlarged cervical lymph nodes.
3. Rhinorrhea.
4. Bulging fontanelle.

53 • In your discussion with Mrs. Dillon, you pointed out the possibility of surgical intervention if this antibiotic therapy is unsuccessful. All *but which one* of the following factors will be considered in determining whether surgical intervention is necessary?

1. Risk of hearing loss.
2. Temperature of over 102°F.
3. Persistent and severe earache despite analgesics.
4. Worsening symptoms despite medical treatment.

54 • Some children retain fluid in their middle ear for months and even up to 2 years without any pain, fever, or discomfort. The factor most apt to account for this fluid retention is:

1. The fluid may be glue-like and would not pass down a normal sized eustachian tube.
2. The child is drinking too much liquid.
3. The child's kidneys are dysfunctional, causing fluid retention.
4. The child's lacrimal ducts are back-flowing into the middle ear.

55 • Billy has completed his 10 days of antibiotic therapy. The following finding indicates he has not recovered from otitis media.

1. A pearly grayish white tympanic membrane.
2. The malleus is visible.
3. The short process is visible.
4. The light reflex is scattered throughout the tympanic membrane.

Ronnie Manson, a six-year-old boy, is being admitted to the pediatric floor with the following findings made by his pediatrician: One week's history of irritability, tiredness, anorexia, weight loss of 3 lb, irregular fever, and pallor. During this time, he had 2 episodes of upper respiratory infection with fever and coughing. Ronnie's outstanding complaint has been aches and pains in the bones of his extremities.

Physical examination revealed lymphadenopathy, enlarged spleen and liver, bone tenderness, and ecchymosis of the skin and mucous membrane. The pediatrician has admitted Ronnie for diagnosis and ordered peripheral blood studies, bone marrow aspiration, and lumbar puncture. Results of bone marrow aspiration showed marked hypercellularity, greatly diminished fat globules and bone particles, and blast cells 65%. Analysis of the cerebral spinal fluid was negative. Laboratory findings were hematocrit value of 31%, hemoglobin concentration of 9.0 gm/100 ml, low white blood cell count, and low platelet count. Based on these findings, Ronnie was tentatively diagnosed as having acute lymphocytic leukemia and was scheduled to begin chemotherapy as soon as other work-ups could be completed.

56 • In discussing Ronnie's diagnosis with family members, it is important to indicate that a definitive classification of the child's leukemia cannot be made and that there is a possibility the diagnosis will be changed for the following reason:

1. Different pathologists may disagree concerning interpretation of a blood or marrow sample.
2. Sudden and complete remission of this disease is known to occur.
3. There are a variety of cell types, and the immature cells have not become differentiated enough to permit classification.
4. Affected school-age children have a tendency to change from the lymphoid type to the non-lymphoid type.

57 • Mrs. Manson was told by her friend that in leukemia healthy cells are "eaten up" by the leukemic cells. You discuss pathophysiology with Mrs. Manson, and give her accurate information by telling her that healthy cells are not "eaten up," but rather that they:

1. Are changed histologically by body enzymes when leukemia develops.
2. Migrate to other parts of the body to avoid being destroyed.
3. Become temporarily dormant.
4. Are destroyed because the leukemic cells compete with them for nutrients.

58 • All *but which one* of the following results from blast cells proliferating in the bone marrow?

1. Anemia.
2. Tendency to bleed.
3. Susceptibility to infection.
4. Iron deposition in the liver.

59 • During chemotherapy, immunosuppression becomes intense, exposing the child to a variety of infections. The nurse, therefore, should take all *but which one* of the following steps to protect this susceptible child?

1. Protective isolation.
2. Strict hand washing.
3. Immunization against rubella, rubeola, and mumps.
4. Restrict all visitors with any sign of infection.

60 • Soon after admission, you should prepare Ronnie and his parents for the various diagnostic procedures he must undergo. Prior to Ronnie's I.V. pyelogram, you discuss this procedure again to make certain that they understand the purpose of this test, which is:

1. To see whether the leukemic cells have invaded his kidneys.
2. To "flush out" the glomeruli in the kidneys.
3. To determine the functional status of the kidneys since some of the antileukemic medication will be excreted by the kidneys.
4. To instill antileukemic drugs into the kidneys.

Lee Perry, 60 years old, was brought to the physician by her husband, who reported that, over the past year, Lee had become increasingly lethargic and forgetful. Noting that Lee was slow to respond to questions and that her deep tendon reflexes showed delayed relaxation time, the physician sent blood samples for measurement of T_4, T_3, and thyroid-stimulating hormone (TSH). On the basis of laboratory test results, Lee was diagnosed as having primary hypothyroidism and was started on a daily dose of sodium levothyroxine (Synthroid).

61 • During health history taking and physical assessment of Mrs. Perry the doctor's office nurse should check the patient for which of the following, as evidence of a potentially serious complication of illness?

1. Hand tremor, nystagmus, and ataxic gait.
2. Angina, dyspnea, and tachycardia.
3. Flatulence, cramping, and diarrhea.
4. Urinary frequency, urgency, and dribbling.

62 • Which of the following diets would be best suited for Lee immediately following diagnosis of hypothyroidism?

1. High protein, high carbohydrate, high calorie diet.
2. Low protein, low sodium diet with low fluid intake.
3. Low calorie, high fiber diet with high fluid intake.
4. Chemically bland, low fiber diet with low fluid intake.

63 • Mr. Perry should be advised that during the first few days of Lee's therapy with sodium levothyroxine (Synthroid) she should be monitored for occurrence of which of the following, as an indication of an untoward effect of the drug?

1. Headache
2. Nausea
3. Tremor
4. Angina

64 • In preparing Mr. Perry to care for his wife following initiation of Synthroid therapy, the nurse should instruct him to expect his wife to experience:

1. Increased fatigue following physical activity.
2. Weight gain due to improved appetite.
3. Greater urinary output after 2 to 3 doses of Synthroid.
4. Nervousness and irritability during adjustment to increased T_4.

65 • In order to prevent unnecessary complications of her disease and treatment, Mrs. Perry should be advised to:

1. Wear a Medic Alert tag containing her diagnosis and Synthroid dose.
2. Avoid ingestion of high fiber and high residue foods.
3. Limit fluid intake to less than 1500 ml/day.
4. Avoid outdoor exercise during cold weather.

John Pine, 48 years of age, sought medical attention for sudden development of a swollen, red, painful joint at the base of his right great toe. Elevation of serum uric acid level, x-ray evidence of crystalline deposits in the inflamed joint, and finding of sodium urate crystals in synovial fluid aspirated from the inflamed joint led to a diagnosis of gout. Following 24 hours of bed rest and colchicine therapy, Mr. Pine's symptoms were relieved. Colchicine was discontinued, and probenecid was administered on a daily basis.

66 • Which of the following test results obtained during Mr. Pine's diagnostic work-up should the nurse interpret as suggestive of a potential complication of his illness?

1. White blood cell count of 13,800/mm^3.
2. Hematocrit value of 55%.
3. Serum creatinine concentration of 2.5 mg/dl.
4. Serum glucose level of 130 mg/dl.

67 • The nurse should utilize which of the following devices to increase Mr. Pine's comfort during hospitalization?

1. Rubber covered pillow
2. Bed cradle
3. Foot elevation
4. Abduction wedge

68 • Colchicine therapy is usually continued until joint symptoms are relieved or the patient develops symptoms of drug toxicity. The most common symptom of drug toxicity is:

1. Gastrointestinal irritation.
2. Eighth cranial nerve damage.
3. Loss of urine concentrating ability.
4. Obstruction of bile excretion.

69 • In addition to the prescribed probenecid, Mr. Pine should be encouraged to do which of the following to prevent possible complications of his disease?

1. Engage in 30 minutes of active exercise daily.
2. Maintain a daily fluid intake of 2500 ml.
3. Secure annual vaccinations against pneumonia and influenza.
4. Eliminate highly spiced foods from his diet.

70 • As part of his predischarge instruction, Mr. Pine should be taught to inform subsequent caregivers that he is receiving maintenance therapy with probenecid, as that drug potentiates the effects of all *but which one* of the folowing?

1. Penicillin
2. Sulfonamides
3. Indomethacin
4. Digitalis

Upon admission, 19-year-old Patti Lapin stands 5 ft 6 in and weighs 98 lb. Her hair is stringy, she wears no make-up, and her clothes hang on her small frame. This is her 4th admission—her 1st admission being at the age of 13 years. All have been for anorexia nervosa. She appears extremely malnourished, refuses food or liquid intake except water, and is panic-stricken over the fact that she will not be able to engage in her usual exercise routine—running 8 miles a day regardless of the weather followed by 2 hours of strenuous aerobic exercise.

Her family lives in an upper middle class suburb of a large city. Her mother is active in the community and seldom has time for Patti. Her father is a successful lawyer. Patti's father has a history of demanding perfection from his daughter. She has taken piano lessons since the age of 6 years, but in spite of many successful recitals she has never completely pleased him ("You misplayed several notes. Maybe next time you'll get it right."). She feels that no matter what she does it is never good enough for him. When she began to develop physically he began to tease her, and she felt ashamed of her budding womanhood. She began dieting in the hope that her breasts would remain flat and undeveloped. Her efforts culminated in what was to be her 1st hospitalization. She prefers to wear jeans and sloppy sweatshirts and has stated on occasion that she wished she were a boy.

Though Patti has the potential to be a good student, she had a record throughout high school of not turning assignments in on time or of doing haphazard work. Prior to her 3 hospitalizations she had disengaged from her friends, taken part in no social activities, and spent most of her free time in her room. Nonetheless, she managed to be admitted to a small college with a fine academic reputation. The 1st quarter went well. She pledged a prestigious sorority, made many new friends, and had her 1st date. Her grades were average. During Christmas vacation her father informed her that until she was ready to make straight A's she could not return to college. It was at this point that she began her restricted intake of food and began her strenuous exercise regimen. She refused phone calls from her friends and isolated herself in her room.

Her admitting diagnosis is anorexia nervosa. A complete physical examination is done upon admission.

71 • The nursing assessment of Patti includes all *but which one* of the following?

1. Starvation related to refusal to eat.
2. Compulsive physical activity in order to maintain control of weight.
3. Distorted body image related to anxiety over sexual development.
4. Intense fear of separation-individuation.

72 • Patients such as Patti are usually very good at bartering to get what they want. Which of the following would be an example of the nurse-patient being involved in a barter that would be beneficial?

1. In return for eating all of the food on her tray Patti is allowed to have off the unit privileges.
2. In return for not engaging in ceaseless exercises in the middle of the room Patti may spend the day in her room.
3. In return for eating all of the food on her tray she may exercise in the day room as long as she likes.
4. In return for interacting with at least 1 patient in the day room she only needs to eat ½ of the food on her tray.

73 • Which of the following would probably be the first thing that alerted her parents that something was wrong?

1. Her lack of interest in school and her social withdrawal.
2. Her docile behavior and her lack of interest in food.
3. The fact that she was never diagnosed as physically ill.
4. The manipulative behavior she employed to avoid food.

74 • Which one of the following interventions would the nurse most certainly be responsible for?

1. Behavior modification.
2. Individual therapy.
3. Family therapy.
4. Group therapy.

75 • In evaluating healthy behaviors evidenced by Patti the nurse would assess for all *but which one* of the following?

1. Documented increase of food intake.
2. Documented decrease of exercise.
3. Documented acts of submissive behavior.
4. Documented increase of interpersonal interactions.

This is Eric Porter's 9th hospitalization on the same floor for sickle cell vaso-occlusive crisis. He was 1st admitted to this floor as a 6-year-old youngster, but he has had multiple admissions during the past 2 years. Due to his repeated admissions to this floor, he considers most of the nursing personnel as his friends. He is accustomed to the routine and is thoroughly familiar with the treatment modality given patients with sickle cell crises.

Eric was diagnosed as having sickle cell anemia at 18 months of age when he experienced hand-foot syndrome. He was seen in a neighborhood clinic, and when his mother was told that there was no cure for sickle cell anemia, she took him home, and eventually the edema of his hands and feet receded without treatment. Over the past years, he has had numerous vaso-occlusive crises. His mother was able to care for him in some cases but at other times, hospitalization was required due to the severity of pain.

Eric Porter is a poorly developed, poorly nourished black male who appears much younger than his chronological age of 15 years; he appears to be around 12 years of age. He is lying in bed with the covers over his head, moaning and complaining of pain in his knees and back. He has just been given acetaminophen with codeine phosphate (Tylenol with Codeine No. 3), which he is to receive p.r.n., every 3 to 4 hours. He is receiving 5% glucose I.V. for hydration. He informs the nurse that his parents will be visiting this evening, and in the meantime he wants to be left alone.

76 • According to Eric's mother, his frequency of hospitalization during the past 2 years relates to his non-compliance. Eric is anxious to "be just like his friends" and overextends himself in various extracurricular and social activities. In your discussion with Eric, he identified certain steps he can take to lessen his hospitalization. One of the things he can do is:

1. Ask his brother to do all his chores at home.
2. Cut back school attendance to 3 times weekly.
3. Seek medical attention for even the slightest infection.
4. Go on a vegetarian diet.

77 • You are reviewing with Eric and his mother all of the factors that could predispose to vaso-occlusive crisis. All of the following are predisposing factors *except*:

1. Dehydration.
2. Infection.
3. Strenuous physical exercise.
4. Diet high in sugar content.

78 • Eric has developed an ulcer on his right leg, and he tells you that it just suddenly appeared one morning. You explain the sickling phenomenon and tissue necrosis as:

1. "The sickled cells have formed a tourniquet-like band around the circumference of your right leg and cut off the circulation."
2. "Sickling of cells results in sluggish blood flow and lack of oxygen to tissues."
3. "You will soon outgrow these sickling episodes."
4. "Teenagers have more of a tendency for sickling than younger children."

79 • Eric has several cousins who are preschoolers. Their mother would like to know what type of diagnostic test would be the most definitive for sickle cell anemia. You give Eric all the information about diagnosis so that when the aunt visits, he will be able to give his aunt correct information. The test that gives the most definitive result is:

1. Peripheral stained blood smear.
2. Sickledex.
3. Mantoux's test.
4. Hemoglobin electrophoresis.

80 • According to the theory of Erikson, adolescents are in the stage of developing a sense of identity. In what developmental task would Eric normally be expected to be involved?

1. He is establishing identity within a group.
2. He is establishing a gender role identification with the appropriate sex parent.
3. He is establishing who he is in relation to others.
4. He is establishing himself as a distinct individual.

John Kent, 52 years of age, was brought to the doctor by his wife who reported that, over a period of several months, John had shown progressive anorexia, weight loss, weakness, and fatigue. Noting a blue-black discoloration of Mr. Kent's oral mucosa, the physician ordered 24-hour urine collection for determination of 17-ketosteroids and 17-hydroxycorticosteroids, measurement of plasma cortisol levels, and an ACTH stimulation test. Test results led to a diagnosis of primary adrenocortical hyposecretion or Addison's disease. The patient was treated with daily oral doses of hydrocortisone, 20 mg, and fludrocortisone, 0.1 mg.

81 • Immediately following his admission, Mr. Kent's visitors should be screened so as to eliminate any who:

1. Would be likely to comment on his changed appearance.
2. Might bring him gifts of food or drink.
3. Are suffering communicable infectious diseases.
4. Are themselves victims of chronic endocrine disorders.

82 • Until onset of fludrocortisone effect, the nurse should encourage Mr. Kent to:

1. Increase fluid intake to 2500 ml/day.
2. Remain on complete bed rest.
3. Turn, cough, and deep breathe every hour.
4. Avoid intake of highly salted foods.

83 • Which of the following should the nurse interpret as an expected result of Mr. Kent's hormone replacement therapy?

1. A decrease in his pulse rate to normal levels.
2. A steady increase in his body weight.

3. A slow increase in his serum potassium levels.
4. A decrease in his temperature during the afternoon to normal.

84 • In preparing Mr. Kent for self care following hospital discharge, the nurse should stress the importance of regular medical follow-up as a result of the:

1. Possibility that the Addison's disease is temporary and that his hormone replacement can be discontinued later.
2. Need to adjust his medicine dosage during periods of infection, diarrhea, and profuse diaphoresis.
3. Likelihood that Mr. Kent will develop additional endocrine diseases in the future.
4. Probability that androgen replacement therapy will be needed when normal mineralocorticoid levels have been restored.

85 • As part of his predischarge instruction, Mr. Kent should be advised to carry which of the following with him at all times?

1. Hard candy
2. Padded tongue blade
3. Urine testing tape
4. Syringe of hydrocortisone

Bill Dwyer, 57 years of age, consulted his physician with complaints of extreme weakness and fatigue. When a complete blood count revealed markedly increased red blood cells (8 million/mm³), slightly increased white blood cell count (15,000/mm³), and moderately elevated platelet count (350,000/mm³), a marrow biopsy was performed, revealing hyperplasia of red blood cells and granulocytic and platelet precursors. Mr. Dwyer was diagnosed as having primary polycythemia; a phlebotomy was performed with removal of 500 ml of blood; and the patient was treated with an intravenous dose of radioactive phosphorus (^{32}P).

86 • The nurse should protect Mr. Dwyer from untoward effects following phlebotomy by:

1. Applying povidone-iodine (Betadine) ointment and an occlusive dressing over the venipuncture site.
2. Withholding food for 4 hours and withholding fluid for 2 hours.
3. Directing the patient to sit up for 5 minutes before attempting to walk.
4. Refraining from subsequent blood pressure measurement in the phlebotomized extremity.

87 • Throughout hospitalization and on subsequent clinic or doctor's office visits Mr. Dwyer should be observed for evidence of all *but which one* of the following as possible complications of polycythemia?

1. Deep vein thrombosis
2. Congestive heart failure
3. Gout
4. Diabetes mellitus

88 • The nurse should avoid which of the following during Mr. Dwyer's care in order to protect him from unnecessary discomfort?

1. Forceful dorsiflexion of the foot.
2. Giving him a hot bath or shower.
3. Elevation of the head above 30 degrees.
4. Positioning him on his left side.

89 • During discharge instruction Mr. Dwyer should be impressed with the necessity for long-term follow-up for his disease, as the radioactive phosphorus that he received may produce which of the following sequela?

1. Sterility
2. Cataract
3. Myxedema
4. Leukemia

90 • In instructing Mr. Dwyer how to care for himself following hospital discharge, the nurse should emphasize the importance of which of the following activities?

1. Engaging in physical exercise on a daily basis.
2. Eating large quantities of protein and iron rich foods.
3. Limiting fluid intake during late afternoon and evening hours.
4. Immobilizing the joints in position of maximum function during bed rest.

Jonathan Williams is a 37-year-old unmarried electrician working for a telephone company. Two weeks ago he was promoted to foreman of his section. As he left the house the 1st day of his new position his hands began to shake, he was extremely nauseated, he was diaphoretic, and he experienced severe palpitations. While driving to work he felt that he would lose control of the car, and at times he did not recognize his surroundings—even though he had been driving the same route to work for the past 5 years. He had the inexplicable feeling that something terrible was about to happen, so he turned around and went back home. The symptoms disappeared once he was back in his own home. This went on for an entire week, and the symptoms became so severe that Mr. Williams now refuses to leave the house for any reason. The mere thought of going out to shop, to a movie, or to work sends him into a state of near panic. He fears that if the symptoms become severe enough he will have a heart attack.

Mr. Williams gives a history of being the youngest child in a family with 5 children. His parents were in their late middle years when he was born, and his mother told him that he was a "mistake." He states, "I know they wished I had never been born." His father was seldom home, and when he was he was gruff and unapproachable. His mother was always tired, and he has no recollection of either parent ever showing any affection or love toward him. His 2 older sisters were the "pets" of the family, and much attention, flattery, and praise were heaped upon them by the parents. In spite of his being the youngest child he was also the one that could be counted on to do work around the house that needed to be done. He was the "conscientious" one.

This is his 1st psychiatric admission. Upon examination his cognitive functions seem unimpaired, and his physical examination is non-remarkable. Diagnosis upon admission to the unit is anxiety disorder, agoraphobia (fear of open spaces).

91 • The therapeutic method that is the fastest and seems to have the best results with this type of disorder is:

1. Insight therapy.
2. Client-centered therapy.
3. Behavior therapy.
4. Psychoanalytic therapy.

92 • Which of the following would be the most appropriate activity for Mr. Williams' 1st excursion off of the locked unit?

1. A walk around the block with other patients and several staff members.
2. Off the ward privileges to the snack shop if he is accompanied by a staff member.
3. A walk in the hall outside of the unit to the soft drink machine accompanied by a staff member.
4. A pass home for the weekend.

93 • During his excursion off the unit Mr. Williams begins to experience anxiety. Which of the following would *not* be an appropriate intervention on the part of the nurse?

1. Help the patient identify the anxiety as such.
2. Aid the patient in identifying what it is that is making him anxious.
3. Encourage him to explore the relief-giving patterns he uses to cope with his anxiety.
4. Encourage him not to think about his distress and carry on with the outing.

94 • During the outing the nurse would primarily evaluate Mr. Williams for:

1. Changes in vegetative signs and tolerance for being off the unit.
2. Tolerance for being off the unit and interactions with others.
3. Interactions with others and changes in vegetative signs.
4. Physical and emotional response to being off the unit.

95 • Prognosis for Mr. Williams is:

1. Poor, because origin of the disorder is rooted early in psychosexual development.
2. Poor, because insight therapy will not be effective for this disorder.
3. Excellent, because once the disorder is treated and relieved it will not return.
4. Good, because there is no physical basis for the symptomatology.

Items from Comprehensive Examination Section 3 That Address the Various Steps of the Nursing Process

Item Number	Assess	Analyze	Plan	Implement	Evaluate	Item Number	Assess	Analyze	Plan	Implement	Evaluate
1			x			49		x			
2			x			50			x		
3				x		51	x				
4					x	52	x				
5		x				53					x
6	x					54		x			
7			x			55					x
8				x		56		x			
9				x		57				x	
10					x	58		x			
11		x				59				x	
12					x	60				x	
13				x		61	x				
14			x			62				x	
15					x	63					x
16				x		64			x		
17				x		65				x	
18				x		66					x
19				x		67				x	
20		x				68					x
21		x				69				x	
22				x		70				x	
23		x				71	x				
24	x					72		x			
25				x		73	x				
26			x			74				x	
27					x	75					x
28					x	76				x	
29	x					77				x	
30		x				78				x	
31	x					79		x			
32			x			80	x				
33	x				x	81			x		
34					x	82				x	
35					x	83					x
36						84		x			
37		x				85				x	
38				x		86				x	
39				x	x	87					x
40						88				x	
41	x					89	x				
42		x				90			x		
43				x		91		x			
44					x	92			x		
45		x				93					x
46	x					94					x
47			x			95		x			
48		x									

Answer Sheet—Section 3

1. 1 2 3 4
2. 1 2 3 4
3. 1 2 3 4
4. 1 2 3 4
5. 1 2 3 4
6. 1 2 3 4
7. 1 2 3 4
8. 1 2 3 4
9. 1 2 3 4
10. 1 2 3 4
11. 1 2 3 4
12. 1 2 3 4
13. 1 2 3 4
14. 1 2 3 4
15. 1 2 3 4
16. 1 2 3 4
17. 1 2 3 4
18. 1 2 3 4
19. 1 2 3 4
20. 1 2 3 4
21. 1 2 3 4
22. 1 2 3 4
23. 1 2 3 4
24. 1 2 3 4
25. 1 2 3 4
26. 1 2 3 4
27. 1 2 3 4
28. 1 2 3 4
29. 1 2 3 4
30. 1 2 3 4
31. 1 2 3 4
32. 1 2 3 4
33. 1 2 3 4
34. 1 2 3 4
35. 1 2 3 4
36. 1 2 3 4
37. 1 2 3 4
38. 1 2 3 4
39. 1 2 3 4
40. 1 2 3 4
41. 1 2 3 4
42. 1 2 3 4
43. 1 2 3 4
44. 1 2 3 4
45. 1 2 3 4
46. 1 2 3 4
47. 1 2 3 4
48. 1 2 3 4
49. 1 2 3 4
50. 1 2 3 4
51. 1 2 3 4
52. 1 2 3 4
53. 1 2 3 4
54. 1 2 3 4
55. 1 2 3 4
56. 1 2 3 4
57. 1 2 3 4
58. 1 2 3 4
59. 1 2 3 4
60. 1 2 3 4
61. 1 2 3 4
62. 1 2 3 4
63. 1 2 3 4
64. 1 2 3 4
65. 1 2 3 4
66. 1 2 3 4
67. 1 2 3 4
68. 1 2 3 4
69. 1 2 3 4
70. 1 2 3 4
71. 1 2 3 4
72. 1 2 3 4
73. 1 2 3 4
74. 1 2 3 4
75. 1 2 3 4
76. 1 2 3 4
77. 1 2 3 4
78. 1 2 3 4
79. 1 2 3 4
80. 1 2 3 4
81. 1 2 3 4
82. 1 2 3 4
83. 1 2 3 4
84. 1 2 3 4
85. 1 2 3 4
86. 1 2 3 4
87. 1 2 3 4
88. 1 2 3 4
89. 1 2 3 4
90. 1 2 3 4
91. 1 2 3 4
92. 1 2 3 4
93. 1 2 3 4
94. 1 2 3 4
95. 1 2 3 4

Section 4

COMPREHENSIVE EXAMINATION

Judy Trent was admitted to the labor unit at 18 weeks' gestation reporting that she had been bleeding heavily for 2 hours. There is no history of other pregnancy related problems and no history of trauma.

1 • While transferring Judy from the stretcher to the bed the 1st question that the admitting nurse should ask is:

1. "Is your bleeding accompanied by pain?"
2. "Did you have intercourse before the bleeding started?"
3. "Has anything like this happened before in this pregnancy?"
4. "Are you sure of your expected date of confinement?"

2 • Which of the following nursing actions should be implemented first in Judy's care?

1. Palpate the uterus for tone.
2. Perform Leopold's maneuvers.
3. Auscultate fetal heart tones.
4. Obtain a history and perform a physical examination.

3 • When the intern arrived on the unit, he requested that the nurse accompany him while he performed a vaginal examination. Which of the following would be the best response by the nurse?

1. "Mrs. Trent has been sedated. Can you come back later?"
2. "Mrs. Trent is bleeding heavily, so a vaginal examination is contraindicated."
3. "Please check with the patient's attending physician before examining her."
4. "Mrs. Trent is very anxious, so please approach her gently."

4 • The nurse should prepare a double delivery setup for this patient in the following area:

1. Labor room.
2. Birthing room.
3. Operating room.
4. Ward admitting or treatment room.

5 • Judy's physician made a diagnosis of threatened abortion. All *but which one* of the following are characteristic of threatened abortion?

1. Bright red bleeding
2. Mild cramping
3. Passage of tissue
4. Closed cervix

Tony, a 5-week-old infant, has been hospitalized with a diagnosis of pyloric stenosis. He is now on I.V. fluids and has a nasogastric tube for stomach decompression, awaiting pre-operative medication for surgery.

According to his mother, Tony began regurgitating portions of his feedings about 2 weeks ago; he usually regurgitated immediately after nursing, but occasionally he did this later. Initially she thought she had not burped him sufficiently, so she burped him more frequently during nursing. Despite this, emesis continued to increase in volume, and she also noticed that the vomiting became more forceful, "like a fountain." Tony became increasingly irritable and always appeared hungry, gnawing and sucking on his fist and eagerly nursing. In addition, the mother noticed that his usual 4 to 6 bowel movements were reduced to 1 or 2 a day.

Physical examination revealed an irritable but adequately nourished and developed infant, weighing 8 lb 10 oz (35th percentile) and measuring 21½ inches (50th percentile). Outstanding findings were an upper abdominal distention, an easily palpable olive shaped "tumor" felt in the epigastrium just right of the umbilicus, and a visible peristaltic wave moving from left to right. The skin appeared dry with decreased turgor. The rest of the physical examination was completely normal.

6 • Because of his persistent vomiting, Tony could have developed:

1. Metabolic alkalosis.
2. Metabolic acidosis.
3. Respiratory alkalosis.
4. Chronic diarrhea.

7 • Tony's pre-operative care will be directed primarily toward:

1. Preventing infection.
2. Keeping him quiet to prevent vomiting.
3. Restoring electrolyte balance.
4. Increasing his weight.

8 • The surgeon believes that Tony is now ready for surgery because the following laboratory values indicate electrolytes are balanced.

1. Sodium, 142 mmol/L; chloride, 100 mmol/L.
2. Sodium, 150 mmol/L; chloride, 112 mmol/L.
3. Sodium, 130 mmol/L; chloride, 90 mmol/L.
4. Sodium, 126 mmol/L; chloride, 88 mmol/L.

9 • The best feeding plan for Tony after pyloromyotomy should include:

1. Offering small amounts of thick cereal as soon as all vomiting stops.
2. Burping him after every ½ oz, then placing him on his left side after feedings.
3. Allowing him to go on a "demand" schedule for the 1st 48 hours post-operatively.
4. Offering small amounts of formula at frequent intervals, then placing him on his right side after feedings with his head slightly elevated.

10 • As part of discharge planning, you have discussed stages of infant development with Tony's mother. She is correct in telling you that by 8 weeks she will expect Tony to be able to:

1. Roll over.
2. Reach out for his favorite toy.
3. Hold his head up 45 degrees while lying on his stomach.
4. Feed himself a cracker.

Alice Trent, age 40 years, sought medical attention for paroxysms of sharp pain in the lower left cheek. Following a neurological work-up, Alice's problem was diagnosed as trigeminal neuralgia, and carbamazepine (Tegretol) and acetaminophen (Tylenol) were prescribed.

11 • In teaching Mrs. Trent about her prescribed medications, the nurse should caution the patient to watch for which of the following as a symptom of the toxic effect of carbamazepine?

1. Gum hypertrophy
2. Bleeding tendencies
3. Tinnitus
4. Diarrhea

12 • The nurse's discharge teaching for Mrs. Trent should include which advice concerning prevention of pain episodes?

1. Eat a liquid or semisolid diet in order to reduce chewing to a minimum.
2. Eliminate unnecessary talking and singing in order to avoid provoking pain.
3. Take ordered pain medication on a regular basis in order to raise the pain threshold.
4. Keep a diary to identify activities that trigger pain episodes, then avoid those activities.

13 • In preparing Mrs. Trent for self care at home the nurse should caution her against:

1. Wasting money on quack medicines and treatments.
2. Exposure to emotionally and physically stressful situations.
3. Social withdrawal and neglect of normal activities.
4. Exposure to persons with upper respiratory infections.

14 • The nurse should suggest which adaptation of personal hygiene measures to protect Alice from complications of her disorder?

1. Wash the face only once daily, using soap lathered hands rather than a wash rag.
2. Use cotton tipped applicators and tepid mouthwash rather than a toothbrush and toothpaste.
3. Take a daily tub bath rather than a shower to protect the face from water spray.
4. Use a dry powder rather than a shampoo to clean the hair so as to minimize scalp stimulation.

15 • Because carbamazepine was unsuccessful in controlling Alice's attacks of pain, percutaneous radiofrequency gangliolysis (electrical current to destroy nerves) was performed to eliminate her discomfort. Following Alice's recovery from the anesthetic, she should be assessed for:

1. Visual defects.
2. Loss of hearing.
3. Loss of facial touch sensation.
4. Disturbances of equilibrium.

Marie White, 21 years of age, was brought to the hospital emergency room with a self inflicted gunshot wound of the left anterior chest. On admission her pulse was 140, and blood pressure was 90/60 mm Hg. A sucking sound was evident as air was drawn into the anterior chest wound with each inspiration, and blood bubbled from the wound with each expiration.

16 • On Marie's admission to the emergency room, the nurse's first action should be to:

1. Question Marie concerning the type of gun and caliber of bullet responsible for the wound.
2. Undress the patient completely and examine her entire body, front and back, for the bullet exit wound.
3. Perform a venipuncture to obtain blood for typing and cross matching and to insert an intravenous line.
4. Apply several layers of petroleum jelly (Vaseline) gauze over the wound, and anchor the dressing with wide adhesive tape.

17 • After placing an occlusive dressing over Marie's sucking chest wound, the nurse's next action should be to:

1. Prepare equipment for emergency thoracentesis and water seal–type drainage.
2. Assess patency of the airway, adequacy of breathing, and efficiency of circulation.
3. Place Marie in the left side-lying position with the right arm supported on pillows.
4. Insert an indwelling catheter and nasogastric tube in preparation for surgery.

18 • The nurse can best determine whether either pneumothorax or hemothorax has caused mediastinal shift by:

1. Placing her outstretched hands over Marie's lower rib cage and comparing the amount of chest expansion on inspiration.
2. Percussing the left side of the chest to determine the size and location of the heart.
3. Palpating the trachea just above the suprasternal notch to detect evidence of deviation.
4. Auscultation of the second right intercostal space to detect evidence of the second heart sound.

19 • Which of the following findings would support a diagnosis of pneumothorax?

1. Crepitant rales in the lung bases.
2. Hyperresonance on chest percussion.
3. "Splitting" of the second heart sound.
4. Flatness to percussion from sternum to left mid-axillary line.

20 • When x-ray film and pleural tap results revealed a left pneumothorax and hemothorax, 2 chest tubes were placed in the left pleural space and connected to closed chest drainage. In order to ensure proper function of the closed chest drainage setup, the nurse should:

1. Seal and secure all connections between plastic tubing, glass rods, stoppers, and bottles with adhesive tape.
2. Keep the glass tubings in the water seal bottle well above the level of fluid in the bottle.
3. Caution Marie to breathe as quietly as possible to decrease air inflow into the pleural space.
4. Irrigate the chest tube with sterile normal saline to clear the tube of mucus and clots.

Rita Mason, age 22 years, is admitted to the hospital complaining of an inability to move her right arm. Her affect is calm, and her attitude almost indifferent. She denies any numbness, pain, or tingling in the arm. She gives the following history.

She and her husband married directly upon graduation from a Catholic high school. She was always an indifferent student and looked forward to making a home and raising a family. Their first child was born 10 months after their wedding, and 3 more children followed. The youngest child is an infant of 3 months. She states that they are "good" children, but that lately "I have been awfully nervous. I can't think straight, and I'm starting to have these awful feelings that I might hurt one of the kids. I see on television where someone has beaten—and maybe killed a kid—and I'm so afraid I'm going to lose control and maybe do the same thing. My husband says I'm crazy—that I never could do a thing like that—and that I should just forget about it. But lately I'm having terrible dreams that seem real, where I hurt the baby, or one of the older kids." At this point in her narrative she becomes anxious, shifting her feet and body and glancing nervously about. Her affect is one of worry and concern, and at one point she becomes tearful. She states that after the 2nd child was born she realized that 2 children would really be all that she could cope with at that time, but her religion does not allow for limiting the size of the family.

A complete physical work-up was done at admission, and no organic cause for the paralyzed arm could be found. A psychological and psychiatric work-up was done resulting in a working diagnosis of somatoform disorder, conversion type.

21 • Since the physical work-up results were negative for any physical etiology of Rita's inability to move her right arm, the most probable explanation for this phenomenon is:

1. Rita is malingering in the hopes that she can get a well-deserved rest in the hospital.
2. Rita is suffering from hypochondriasis resulting from having her children so close together.
3. Rita is utilizing illness as a means of reducing her anxiety.
4. Rita is suffering from neurasthenia, and a few days of rest will relieve the symptom.

22 • All *but which one* of the following signs and symptoms would the nurse expect to elicit from this patient?

1. Concern and worry over her inability to move her right arm.
2. A lack of concern, *la belle indifference*, regarding the conversion symptom.
3. A true inability on the patient's part to use the arm because the symptom is an unconscious defense.
4. Movement of the arm during sleep or while Rita is under hypnosis.

23 • In planning for the care of Rita the nurse should recognize that which of the following is true?

1. Rita's symptom is under voluntary control.
2. Rita will be concerned by her impairment.
3. Rita's symptom is a coping mechanism.
4. Rita has insight into her problem.

24 • Besides the paralysis of the arm which one of the following might the nurse expect to observe?

1. Rita will become defensive and angry if it is pointed out to her that she can move her arm while asleep.
2. Rita will be reluctant to undergo further examinations and will try to focus on issues other than her symptom.
3. There will be no atrophy or wasting away of the affected limb as would be expected if this were true paralysis.
4. Rita will have periods of great anxiety or fear regarding her inability to move her right arm.

25 • All *but which one* of the following is thought to be a causal factor in conversion disorder?

1. The presence of an unpleasant situation.
2. A desire to escape from a situation.
3. A conscious effort to reduce anxiety.
4. An unconscious effort to reduce anxiety.

Mrs. Barbara Cathlin was brought to the birthing room for an elective cesarean delivery. Mrs. Cathlin is anxious but fully cooperative, and her husband was permitted to remain with her during the cesarean birth. Mrs. Cathlin delivered a 7 lb 6 oz male infant whose Apgar scores were 9/9. The mother's post-operative recovery was unremarkable.

26 • During the early postpartum period Mrs. Cathlin should be checked for Homans' sign in order to detect the presence of:

1. Infection.
2. Edema.
3. Phlebitis.
4. Hemorrhage.

27 • Methylergonovine (Methergine) is sometimes given to mothers following cesarean delivery. The nurse should question administration of this medication to Mrs. Cathlin if she has a history of:

1. Postpartum hemorrhage.
2. Toxemia.

3. Diabetes.
4. Hyperemesis gravidarum.

28 • As a result of the physiological stress of surgery and the need for intensive post-operative recovery care, mothers who undergo cesarean delivery are unable to have their newborn infants with them as early and as frequently as mothers who have vaginal delivery. As soon as Mrs. Cathlin's condition permits, the nurse should arrange for her to hold her infant in order to facilitate:

1. Mother to infant emotional bonding.
2. Oxytocin production by the hypothalamus.
3. Movement of milk through the ductile system of the breast.
4. Instruction in infant care procedures.

29 • Mrs. Cathlin experienced difficulty in breast-feeding her infant. The nurse should encourage the mother to:

1. Bottle feed her infant until she is pain free and her incision is healed.
2. Experiment with various breast-feeding positions in order to find the one that is most comfortable.
3. Pump her breasts and give the breast milk to the baby in bottle feedings.
4. Avoid breast-feeding completely in order to conserve her energy for post-operative healing.

30 • On Mrs. Cathlin's 3rd postpartum day, she began to cry, saying, "I wish I had been able to go through labor so my baby could have been born the way that babies are supposed to be born." The most effective response by the nurse would be:

1. "I'll ask the doctor to explain why the cesarean birth was necessary."
2. "It's normal to feel disappointed now, but you'll feel better about it in a few days."
3. "You're upset because you didn't have a vaginal delivery. It seems hard to accept that your baby wasn't born in the usual way."
4. "Many of our mothers have cesarean births. I'll ask one of them to come in and talk with you about it."

Four-year-old Angela Foster's nursery school teacher first noticed that Angela was slowly but definitely becoming clumsier during the past several weeks. Even when Angela was alone and not hurried, she seemed to trip and bump into tables and chairs. When she mentioned this to Angela's mother, Mrs. Foster concurred with the teacher but added that she thought Angela was just going through a "clumsier" stage.

Mrs. Foster asked the teacher, however, about her daughter's recent behavior because at home she noticed that Angela was more irritable lately, cried easily, and was pickier than usual during her meals. The teacher mentioned that with 14 other children in the classroom, she didn't notice anything unusual about Angela's behavior.

Several days after the teacher talked to Mrs. Foster, Angela woke up in the morning and suddenly vomited. She lay in bed for awhile rolling her head from side to side, but in a short time she was sitting up and watching TV. That morning Angela refused to go to nursery school, whined and clung to her mother. When the child again vomited what little she had eaten for breakfast, Mrs. Foster decided to contact the pediatrician for an office visit.

After obtaining a medical history, the pediatrician performed a physical examination and found moderate bilateral papilledema, positive Babinski's sign, and hyperreflexia. On the basis of the history and physical examination, the physician decided to admit Angela to the pediatric unit. He explained to the mother that Angela will need several diagnostic tests, and the 2 important ones will be a CAT scan and an angiogram. The CAT scan revealed a moderate size tumor in the cerebellum, probably an astrocytoma; preparation is now in progress for an angiogram in preparation for surgery.

31 • Tumor invasion of the cerebellum manifests certain clinical findings. Physical assessment of Angela would probably reveal the following:

1. Head circumference at 80th percentile and out of proportion to her height and weight.
2. Sudden weight gain since hospitalization due to edema.
3. Poor muscle tone of her lower extremities.
4. Brisk pupillary reaction to direct light.

32 • The nurse has included parent teaching of the surgical procedure for brain tumor in her care plan for Angela. The following post-operative information will be discussed with the Fosters.

1. If Angela experiences no headache, she will be allowed to get up in 24 hours.
2. A lumbar puncture may be done.

3. Previous symptoms of headaches and neuromuscular problems will be eliminated.
4. If the incision is small, only that portion of the scalp will be bandaged.

33 • Despite being somewhat irritable at times, Angela is a bright, pleasant 4 year old. The nurse had developed age appropriate pre-operative teaching for Angela. With careful explanation she will understand the following:

1. Her cerebellum has changed in size and shape due to the tumor.
2. Activities in the operating room and the intensive care unit are different.
3. By wrapping a doll's scalp, she will know the type of dressing she will have.
4. The large syringe she saw lying on a table in the intensive care unit will *not* be used on her when she gets her "shot."

34 • Following infratentorial craniotomy, fluid intake is monitored closely since:

1. Swallowing causes increasing pain with headaches.
2. There is still danger of increased intracranial pressure due to cerebral edema.
3. There is always a possibility of renal involvement.
4. There is strong likelihood of inappropriate antidiuretic hormone secretion.

35 • The nurse had discussed lumbar puncture during teaching sessions with the Fosters. Evidence of Mr. Foster's comprehension of this procedure was obvious when the nurse overheard him explain the procedure to a visiting relative.

1. The procedure will be done in the operating room.
2. The procedure will be done every day for 3 days.
3. The procedure is to inject antibiotics to prevent infection.
4. The procedure is to analyze spinal fluid for tumor cells.

Marie Stott, 25 years of age, sought medical help for severe pain in the right ear, which developed during the course of a severe upper respiratory infection. Her temperature was 102° F, and Rinné's test revealed air conduction of sound to be less than bone conduction. Physical examination revealed an erythematous bulging eardrum, and purulent exudate could be seen in the external auditory canal. The physician diagnosed otitis media, ordered bed rest, oral erythromycin, acetaminophen for pain, and oral pseudoephedrine.

36 • In preparing Ms. Stott to care for herself at home, the nurse should instruct her to:

1. Pack the external auditory canal with cotton to prevent contamination of skin and clothing by purulent drainage.
2. Take the full number of erythromycin tablets prescribed, even if symptoms abate before all tablets have been consumed.
3. Blow her nose frequently in order to clear the nasopharynx and to keep the eustachian tube open.
4. Irrigate the external auditory canal with warm saline solution twice daily to remove purulent secretions.

37 • In addition to taking the prescribed erythromycin and pseudoephedrine, Ms. Stott should be advised to:

1. Cleanse the external auditory canal gently with cotton tipped applicators.
2. Perform Valsalva's maneuver several times each day.
3. Drop warm oil into the external auditory canal 2 times each day.
4. Keep the head inclined to the right when sitting or reclining.

38 • During discharge instruction, Ms. Stott should be advised to return to the physician if she experiences which of the following symptoms after 2 to 3 days of medicinal therapy?

1. Continuing drainage from the external auditory canal.
2. Weakness, fatigue, and anorexia.
3. Itching of the external auditory canal and pinna.
4. Increasing pain, hearing loss, and dizziness.

39 • In order to prevent complications of her illness, Ms. Stott should be advised to:

1. Avoid going out-of-doors until her symptoms are completely relieved.
2. Avoid swimming and washing her hair until approved by her physician.
3. Refrain from sleeping on her right side while there is drainage from the external ear.
4. Cleanse the right auricle twice daily with an alcohol soaked pledget.

40 • During Ms. Stott's later visits to the physician's office for follow-up care, the nurse should be alert for the patient's mention of which of the following symptom of complications from otitis media?

1. Toothache
2. Tinnitus plus vertigo
3. Dry mouth
4. Migraine headache

Ed Stern, 53 years of age, consulted his physician with complaints of constant low back pain and increasing fatigue. When x-rays revealed osteolytic (punched out) lesions of the vertebrae and skull, and electrophoresis revealed an immunoglobulin (Bence Jones protein) in the urine, a diagnosis of multiple myeloma was made. Mr. Stern was hospitalized for radiation therapy and chemotherapy with cyclophosphamide and prednisone.

41 • Which of the following nursing measures will be needed to protect Mr. Stern from a serious complication of his illness?

1. Complete bed rest
2. Fluids of 3000 to 4000 ml/day
3. Postural drainage T.I.D.
4. Reverse isolation

42 • Which of the following test results, obtained during Mr. Stern's diagnostic work-up, should the nurse interpret as a possible indicator of serious disease complication?

1. Serum calcium concentration of 10.2 mg/dl.
2. Platelet count of 75,000/mm^3.
3. Urine specific gravity of 1.011.
4. Fasting serum glucose concentration of 70 mg/dl.

43 • Which of the following devices should be provided to Mr. Stern to protect him from self injury during hospitalization?

1. Padded tongue blade
2. Posey's vest
3. Cloth mitts
4. Walker

Following radiation and chemotherapy Mr. Stern's pain was relieved, and he was discharged from the hospital. Six months later he was readmitted with lower extremity weakness and paresthesias. Diagnostic work-up revealed compression of the thoracic spinal cord by an extradural plasmocytoma. A laminectomy was performed, and the tumor was removed.

44 • Mr. Stern's post-operative care plan should ensure that:

1. He be immobilized in supine position until bony healing is complete.
2. He be maintained in prone position with bridging of bony pressure points.
3. His position be changed every 2 hours, using log rolling when turning.
4. He move about freely in order to prevent arthritis and contracture deformities.

45 • When it was determined that his spine was stable, Mr. Stern was transferred to a rehabilitation facility for upgrading of activities of daily living skills. Which action by the nurse would be likely to maximize Mr. Stern's progress in physiotherapy and occupational therapy?

1. Prompt administration of the prescribed analgesic as soon as he reports occurrence of pain.
2. Encourage Mr. Stern to repeat his physiotherapy and occupational exercises while on the nursing unit.
3. Assist Mr. Stern with bathing, dressing, and grooming to conserve his energy for physiotherapy and occupational therapy.
4. Urge Mr. Stern to match the accomplishments of another patient who has been fully rehabilitated.

Margaret Runyon, age 55 years, is admitted to the geropsychiatric unit of a nursing home. She is mute and rather untidy in appearance, and her husband (who accompanies her) states that she spends all day sitting in a chair staring at the wall. She has not read a newspaper in the last several years and is unable to fully understand the TV programs that she does watch. At meals she has to be reminded to eat, and she cannot remember what she had to eat the day before. She can carry on a conversation about happenings in the distant past but often forgets her children's names. At the age of 45 years, Margaret was brought to the attention of the family physician by her husband of 23 years after she began to behave in a way that was incompatible with her former activities. They met in college where she majored in biochemistry. She was a bright and vivacious member of a sorority, often doing volunteer work to raise funds for worthy organizations, and was elected president of the chapter her senior year. She graduated magna cum laude, landed a well-paying job immediately after graduation, and 1 year later he and she were married. Two children graced their marriage in the 1st 5 years, but Margaret seemed to have no problem adapting, easily combining the role of mother with that of a full-time professional.

After a full diagnostic evaluation, the working diagnosis is Alzheimer's disease, advanced stages.

46 • When Margaret first saw a physician at the age of 45 years her symptoms might have been all *but which one* of the following?

1. Gradual withdrawal from social activities that she once found pleasurable.
2. Becoming less alert, more "forgetful."
3. Agitation if her daily routine was changed.
4. A delusional system with some paranoia.

47 • All *but which one* of the following signs and symptoms would the nurse expect Margaret to reveal at this time?

1. Impairment of memory for recent events.
2. Poor grooming and attention to activities of daily living.
3. Impairment of judgment.
4. Delusional material about her family.

48 • In planning for Margaret's care the nurse would implement all *but which one* of the following?

1. Establish a helpful, trusting relationship.
2. Implement insight therapy.
3. Support and encourage family visits.
4. Encourage participation in social activities.

49 • When evaluating Margaret's progress the nurse would realistically hope for:

1. Participation in group sing-alongs twice a week.
2. Maintenance of reality contact through the use of unit schedules and a calendar in her room.
3. Self care with appropriate assistance.
4. All of the above.

50 • The nurse can expect which of the following regarding Alzheimer's disease?

1. Progression is rapid.
2. Age of onset is between the ages of 40 and 50 years.
3. It is irreversible and fatal.
4. All of the above.

Seven-year-old Gloria Russell has been transferred onto the regular pediatric floor from the pediatric intensive care unit (PICU) where she had spent 5 days. She was treated for meningococcus meningitis with ampicillin; for cerebral edema with steroids and mannitol; she received assisted ventilation, a cooling blanket for hyperpyrexia, and phenobarbital for 2 seizure episodes. Her condition has now stabilized, and her physician's orders for ventilation, cooling blanket, indwelling catheter, and phenobarbital have been discontinued. Her parents are at her bedside, expressing relief about their daughter's improvement and leaving the PICU. They are also amazed that Gloria has no recollection of events during the last 5 days.

The nurse reviews information from the history with Mrs. Russell. Gloria and her 2 younger brothers, 6 and 3 years of age, all had upper respiratory infections with coughing and nasal discharge. Mrs. Russell had treated her children "the usual way" keeping them home from school the first couple of days, giving acetaminophen (Tylenol) for elevated temperature, and insisting that they rest as much as possible. They all appeared to be getting better until 5 days ago when Gloria suddenly complained of a severe headache, had chills and fever, and vomited several times within an hour. Her condition rapidly worsened and by that evening, she had petechiae and purpuric rashes on her body, and she was barely responding to external stimuli.

Her parents took her to the emergency room of their small community hospital, but after spending 2 hours there where her condition deteriorated even further, she was transferred by ambulance to the PICU of this large teaching hospital.

51 • The Russells are puzzled because their daughter, Gloria, had only a mild case of upper respiratory infection before suddenly becoming critically ill with meningitis. The nurse and parents analyzed the course of Gloria's illness during the past week, and they now understand that the probable cause of their daughter's meningitis was:

1. A contaminated hot dog she ate at a picnic the weekend before.

2. Contracting bacteria from one of her brothers who was harboring the bacteria in his throat.
3. The bacteria from her nasopharynx invading her circulatory system.
4. Triggering by a tuberculin skin test, which she received at school.

52 • The Russells ask for information pertaining to Gloria's clinical manifestations. You explain that clinical manifestations are related to all *but which one* of the following?

1. Effectiveness of therapy for antecedent illness.
2. Age.
3. Type of organism.
4. Immunization history.

53 • One of the complications of bacterial meningitis is increased intracranial pressure. The nurse should be alert to all of the following signs *except*:

1. Papilledema.
2. Decreased pulse.
3. Decreased blood pressure.
4. Alteration in sensorium.

54 • Positioning a child properly in bed will minimize pain experienced by the child with meningitis. The child will be most comfortable in the following position:

1. A semi-Fowler's position.
2. A prone position.
3. A supine position.
4. A position using no pillow with head slightly raised.

55 • Lumbar puncture is carried out to analyze the cerebral spinal fluid for the effectiveness of antimicrobial therapy. Which finding would indicate that a significant number of bacteria are still present?

1. Decreased protein concentration.
2. Decreased glucose concentration.
3. Decreased white blood cell count.
4. Decreased CSF pressure.

Twenty-six-year old Jan Lake experienced weakness, fever, and night sweats 2 weeks following removal of an abscessed tooth. On physical examination her physician detected a loud systolic murmur at the apex. When this murmur changed in character and intensity on the following day, he ordered blood cultures, which revealed streptococcic septicemia. On the basis of medical history, physical findings, and laboratory results, a diagnosis of infectious endocarditis was made. The patient was hospitalized and treated with 10 million units of penicillin I.V. each day.

56 • In preparing Jan's Kardex care plan, her primary nurse should order which of the following to be assessed on a daily basis to detect a possible serious complication of the patient's illness?

1. Body weight
2. Abdominal girth
3. Calf circumference
4. Heart sounds

57 • Sudden development of which of the following would suggest a serious complication of Ms. Lake's endocarditis?

1. Migraine headache
2. Unilateral weakness
3. Skin rash
4. Hematemesis

58 • Which of the following nursing measures should be used to protect Ms. Lake from cardiac complications?

1. Provision of quiet diversionary activities.
2. Maintaining her in high Fowler's position.
3. Provide postural drainage 3 times a day.
4. Limit fluid intake to 1200 to 1500 ml/day.

59 • Throughout the course of her antibiotic therapy, all *but which one* of the following precautions should be taken?

1. Temperature measurement every 4 hours around the clock.
2. Frequent change of venipuncture site and intravenous fluid tubing.
3. Encourage liberal fluid intake from 2000 to 2500 ml/day.
4. Enforce complete bed rest in supine position with venipuncture arm immobilized.

60 • In preparing Ms. Lake for self care, the nurse should emphasize the necessity for:

1. Avoiding physical activity except that necessary for activities of daily living.

2. Receiving prophylactic antibiotics before, during, and after surgery and dental procedures.
3. Avoiding contact with children so as to lower the risk of contracting infectious diseases.
4. Sleeping with the head elevated on pillows and the head of the bed elevated on blocks.

John Louis, 35 years old, was brought to the hospital emergency room suffering nausea, vomiting, and right abdominal pain of 3 hours' duration. His oral temperature was 102° F, and his white blood cell count was 16,000/mm³. Physical examination revealed muscle guarding and rebound tenderness on the left side of the abdomen. A laparotomy was performed, and an acutely inflamed appendix was removed. He was returned to his room with a nasogastric tube in place and a soft rubber drain in the abdominal wound.

61 • As part of Mr. Louis' preparation for surgery the nurse should determine:

1. The exact duration of his abdominal pain.
2. The time of his last food intake.
3. The date of his last tetanus immunization.
4. His usual bowel emptying time and frequency.

62 • For the first few days following surgery, Mr. Louis should be observed for manifestations of peritonitis, which would include all *but which one* of the following?

1. Bradycardia
2. Hypotension
3. Shallow respirations
4. Abdominal distention

63 • Although Mr. Louis recovered quickly from anesthesia, ambulated a short distance on his 1st post-operative day, and had his nasogastric tube removed on his 2nd post-operative day, he developed tachycardia, fever, and abdominal distention. The physician diagnosed peritonitis, reinserted the nasogastric tube, started intravenous fluids, and ordered parenteral penicillin and clindamycin. On Mr. Louis's 6th post-operative day he summoned the nurse and complained that something in his abdomen had "broken loose," and a gush of liquid had soaked his wound dressing. On removing the dressing the nurse discovered that the edges of Mr. Louis' surgical wound had separated and a coil of intestine was protruding through the wound. The nurse's first action should be to:

1. Raise the patient's knees to decrease strain on the incision.
2. Don sterile gloves and gently replace the protruding tissue in the abdominal cavity.
3. Cover the open abdominal wound with a sterile, saline soaked dressing.
4. Redress the wound, and apply a scultetus abdominal binder.

64 • If Mr. Louis should develop peritonitis postoperatively, which of the following should be done to protect him from injury?

1. Elevate the bed's side rails.
2. Immobilize his arms with cloth restraints.
3. Apply an abdominal binder.
4. Place a bed board beneath the mattress.

65 • Nurses can decrease morbidity and mortality associated with appendiceal rupture by teaching the public to refrain from:

1. Swallowing apple seeds, grape seeds, and other such nondigestible matter.
2. Inserting a rectal suppository to prevent or relieve constipation.
3. Bending sharply forward while straining at stool.
4. Administering a laxative to relieve pain in the abdomen.

Three days ago Mark Williamson, age 35 years, went on a jealous rampage and chased his wife through the house with a revolver. She fled to the neighbor's house, and police were called to the scene. Fed up with his suspicions and his accusations, Mark's wife filed charges, and he was arrested. The judge ordered him to seek treatment at an inpatient facility because of the 6-year history of his verbal and physical harassment of his wife.

Upon admission Mark appears angry and belligerent. He states that he has been suspicious of his wife's behavior since the early days of their marriage. "You know, she was always buying new clothes. Looked real nice. Always had her hair done once a week, and lots of make-up. Now you know something had to be going on. I tried to catch her, but she's too smart for that. We get these phone calls at home. She tells me it's just a girlfriend, but I know better. She goes out during the day when she should be home cleaning house or something." Three or four times during the 6-year marriage she was late coming home to fix dinner, and "I roughed her up a little bit. We've got 3 kids, but who knows whose they are?" He admits to following her sometimes to see who it is that she is meeting, but he has never been able to catch her with anyone. He is envious of her recent promotion to assistant buyer for a large retail clothing store, and he thinks that his inability to negotiate a salary increase for himself was influenced by phone calls she made to his supervisors. In spite of the fact that his wife, his family, and their friends insist to him that she is a faithful and loving wife he is unshakeable in his belief that she is unfaithful.

Mr. Williamson denies auditory or visual hallucinations, and he does not appear to have any depressive or manic manifestations. He is an electrical engineer and has held the same middle management job with his firm for the past 10 years. The admitting diagnosis is paranoid disorder.

66 • The nurse can expect the following behavior from Mr. Williamson in the next few days:

1. Emergence of a definite thought disorder as he becomes less defensive and more comfortable on the unit.
2. A fixed delusional system that is unshakeable despite any evidence that can be produced to the contrary.
3. A loss of affect and signs of autistic behavior if medication is not started immediately.
4. A change in his belief system as psychotherapy is instituted and he gains insight into his own behavior.

67 • This hospitalization will be aimed at short-term interventions. Which of the following series of options would the interdisciplinary team consider for discharge planning with this type of patient?

1. Long-term hospitalization, a half-way house, or return to the family.
2. A half-way house, return to the family, or arrangements for Mark to live alone.
3. Long-term hospitalization, out-patient clinic, or a nursing care facility.
4. Long-term hospitalization, out-patient clinic, or a return to the family.

68 • The defense mechanism that Mr. Williamson is using is:

1. Denial.
2. Identification.
3. Projection.
4. Rationalization.

69 • Treatment for Mr. Williamson would include which of the following?

1. Major tranquilizers.
2. Unconditional positive regard and acceptance on the part of the nurse.
3. Marital therapy.
4. All of the above.

70 • Upon admission the nurse and Mr. Williamson sit down to work out a short-term care plan for him. Which of the following topics would probably *not* be considered?

1. Management of his anger.
2. His medication regimen.
3. Activities of the unit.
4. Post-discharge psychotherapy.

Mrs. Betty Johnson delivered a female infant weighing 7 lb 12 oz early yesterday morning. She has elected to breast-feed her infant. The mother and baby are doing well.

71 • Mrs. Johnson wants to breast-feed her baby, have rooming-in privileges around the clock, and assume care of the infant. Which behavior would signify that Mrs. Johnson has entered the "taking hold" phase of Reva Rubin's restorative process?

1. Relating details of the labor experience to friends.
2. Curling her hair and putting on make-up.
3. Asking the nurse to change her baby's diaper.
4. Giving her baby a bath.

72 • Mrs. Johnson's breasts are engorged. The nurse should instruct the mother to:

1. Wear a tight breast binder except when feeding.
2. Apply cold compresses before and after feeding.
3. Take pain medication every 4 hours.
4. Apply warm compresses before feeding.

73 • Mrs. Johnson should be advised that proper care of her nipples would include:

1. Daily cleansing with a water soaked cloth.
2. Cleansing with alcohol soaked pledgets.
3. Wearing plastic nipple covers.
4. Washing with soap and water before each feeding.

74 • Mrs. Johnson should be informed that the normal stools of a breast-fed infant are characterized by all *but which one* of the following?

1. May be eliminated after each feeding.
2. May be watery and curdy.
3. May contain small amounts of mucus.
4. May be dark and well formed.

75 • For women who decide not to breast-feed, an antilactogenic agent may be administered. Bromocriptine (Parlodel) is the drug of choice because it is non-hormonal in nature. The principal side effect of bromocriptine is:

1. Early resumption of ovulation.
2. Profuse diaphoresis.
3. Extreme thirst.
4. Ringing in the ears.

Sammie Olson, age 17 years, has been hospitalized by his physician for a protracted case of infectious mononucleosis. Sammie has been under his physician's care for the past 5 weeks, and although he had not been acutely ill at any time, neither has his condition improved to any significant degree. However, because of his long confinement, Sammie has begun to show signs of depression. The physician had him admitted primarily to rule out complications and also to remove him temporarily from a home environment that evidently has not been conducive to his recovery.

The physician had talked to Sammie's mother about Sammie's recuperation—his need for rest, his need for nourishing meals, the need to keep sick people away from him. But it seems that after his mother leaves for work, Sammie persuades his friends to visit him and, despite his fatigue, entertains his friends in his bedroom.

Examination of Sammie revealed a well developed and well nourished adolescent with a finding of hepatomegaly; lower border of liver edge palpated 1 cm below the costal margin on inspiration. He appeared extremely fatigued, and after removing his clothes, he flopped on the examining table thoroughly exhausted. Remaining physical findings were essentially negative. Laboratory results showed increased atypical mononuclear leucocytes and a positive heterophil agglutination test.

Sammie Olson refused to be engaged in conversation, choosing instead to answer questions with a shrug or a nod of his head. The only time he actually spoke was to inform the physician that he was hospitalized against his will.

76 • Infectious mononucleosis is characterized by symptoms that appear insidiously and never become particularly acute. The adolescent's usual *chief complaint* is the following:

1. He has lost his appetite.
2. He is unable to maintain his usual level of activity.
3. He is unable to sleep at night.
4. He has diarrhea and vomiting.

77 • The following body system is *primarily* affected in infectious mononucleosis:

1. Gastrointestinal system.
2. Renal system.
3. Lymphatic system.
4. Neuromuscular system.

78 • Sammie Olson was extremely angry about being hospitalized against his will primarily because he would be separated from his peers. In order to support this adolescent the nurse should include the following in his care plan:

1. Keep him busy with bedside activities to distract him from thinking about his friends.
2. Ask the family to have some family member continuously at his bedside.
3. Send him to occupational therapy twice a day to meet other patients.
4. Encourage him to keep in contact with his friends by telephone.

79 • The nurse realizes that adolescents have certain developmental tasks to attend to in order to maintain a sense of well-being. One of the tasks of adolescents is:

1. To establish a gender role identification.
2. To identify themselves as separate from their parents.
3. To see themselves as unique and separate from every other individual.
4. To seek approval from authority figures.

80 • Definitive diagnosis of infectious mononucleosis was made on Sammie Olson on the basis of his clinical manifestations and positive laboratory findings. The following titer of the heterophil agglutination test proved diagnostic:

1. 1:160
2. 1:140
3. 1:120
4. 1:100

Dot Giles, 40 years old, developed fever and severe diarrhea after returning from a trip through rural Mexico. When* Salmonella typhi *was isolated from blood culture, typhoid fever was diagnosed, and the patient was hospitalized and treated with chloramphenicol.

81 • During the acute phase of Dot's illness the nurse should monitor the patient closely for which of the following, as indicative of a serious complication?

1. Chills, fever, and headache.
2. Sudden, brief abdominal pain.
3. Bradycardia and lethargy.
4. Urinary and fecal incontinence.

82 • While caring for Dot, which of the following precautions should be used to prevent spread of typhoid fever to others?

1. Wash the hands thoroughly before leaving the patient's room.
2. Wear a gown and mask while working in the patient's room.
3. Wear a gown and gloves when disposing of feces or fecally contaminated objects.
4. Disinfect urine and stool with chlorinated lime before disposal into the hopper.

83 • Which of the following devices should be used to increase Mrs. Giles' comfort during the acute phase of her illness?

1. Circolectric bed
2. Ice bag
3. Over-the-bed cradle
4. Room deodorizer

84 • The nurse should employ which of the following measures during the acute phase of Mrs. Giles' illness in order to protect her from injury?

1. Keep the bed's side rails elevated at all times throughout the day.
2. Place her on an alternating pressure mattress or a water mattress.
3. Place a folded drawsheet over her thighs, and tuck it under the mattress on both sides.
4. Secure opposite upper and lower extremities to the bed frame with cloth restraints.

85 • During the first few days following her admission to the hospital, Mrs. Giles' nutritional needs should be met by:

1. Hourly administration of 3 oz of milk and cream mixture.
2. A high carbohydrate, high protein diet with increased liquid intake.
3. A high caloric diet that contains only high residue foods.
4. Administration of hyperalimentation fluids intravenously.

Nan Rose, 30 years of age, had experienced eyelid ptosis, dysphagia, progressive weakness, and increased fatiguability for several months before seeking medical attention. When an intravenous injection of edrophonium produced a prompt improvement in muscle strength and function, a diagnosis of myasthenia gravis was made and pyridostigmine was ordered.

86 • In planning Ms. Rose's care the following principle should be followed:

1. All physically demanding activities should be scheduled during the morning when she is well rested.
2. Greatest physical movement should be scheduled for afternoon when adrenocorticoid levels are highest.
3. Physically demanding activities should be scheduled for an hour or so following pyridostigmine administration.
4. Activity of large muscle groups should be discouraged to conserve limited energy for contraction of small muscle groups.

87 • Ms. Rose should be instructed that which of the following is a possible symptom of pyridostigmine overdose?

1. Tetany
2. Dry mouth
3. Tinnitus
4. Muscle weakness

88 • Ms. Rose should be monitored for which of the following as an indication of acute worsening of symptoms (myasthenic crisis)?

1. Abdominal cramps
2. Muscle tremor
3. Facial grimacing
4. Respiratory distress

89 • Which of the following diets would be best suited to Ms. Rose's needs if she continues to experience dysphagia?

1. High protein liquids
2. Soft, semisolid foods
3. Ground meats and shredded vegetables
4. Dry finger foods

90 • During her discharge instruction, Nan should be informed that which of the following is apt to increase symptoms of myasthenia gravis?

1. Antacids
2. Multivitamins
3. Antibiotics
4. Expectorants

Shirley Brenner, 35 years of age, was admitted 2 days ago to a medical unit. Her chief complaints are lack of appetite, fear of "eating the wrong thing," too many stools or too few (depending on which time of the day one speaks with her), and pains that radiate from the right upper quadrant of her abdomen to the left lower quadrant. She describes the pain as "pressure—pushing. If I don't eat it's not as bad."

Her medical history dates back to when she was 17 years of age. She had similar complaints at that time, although the symptoms appear to have been more severe. After 1 week in the hospital, and despite the fact that physiological tests revealed that Shirley was a healthy teenager, it was decided to do an appendectomy on the basis that she could be suffering from subclinical appendicitis. Upon examination post-operatively, the appendix was found to be normal.

Her parents remained quite concerned because immediately after discharge their daughter became frantic, "Hysterical with the pain," as her mother stated. Shirley and her parents changed physicians, and because of the pain (and what Shirley called "heat"), which was now localized in the upper right quadrant, a cholecystectomy was performed. The gallbladder was not diseased, no stones could be demonstrated, and Shirley's symptoms appeared immediately after discharge from the hospital.

Her parents have spent the last 17 years trying to find the appropriate physician who could intervene on Shirley's behalf. Countless medications have been tried—all to no avail. She attended college for 2 years, but left when the physicians in the health service made it clear that they thought she was malingering. Her parents welcomed her back to the family home. She has lived there ever since, holding a part-time job here and there, but spending much of any given week lying about the house consuming over-the-counter digestive aids. For the past 2 years she has kept a detailed daily record of all of her stools—frequency, color, amount, and consistency. This record she presented to the admitting physician.

Her appearance at this time is calm, but she does appear concerned about her physical condition. She states that her greatest fear now is that she has cancer.

A complete physiological work-up reveals no abnormalities or dysfunction in the abdominal area, and her blood and urine test results are within the normal range. The working diagnosis is hypochondriasis, and much against Shirley's protests, a psychological consult has been arranged.

91 • Nursing assessment would reveal that:

1. Shirley has no support group of peers.
2. Shirley has highly developed social skills.
3. Shirley does not wish to see her parents.
4. Shirley is reconciled to being on a psychiatric unit.

92 • Which defense mechanism has Shirley been using?

1. Sublimation.
2. Conversion.
3. Identification.
4. Rationalization.

93 • All *but which one* of the following is true regarding Shirley's symptomatology?

1. Primary gain is achieved by keeping her anxiety out of her awareness.
2. She receives secondary gains.
3. It provides a measure of control over others.
4. It is congruent with a fugue pattern.

94 • Shirley and the nurse plan some short-term goals that will enhance Shirley's life after discharge. Which one of the following would probably not be appropriate for Shirley?

1. Enrolling in some adult education courses at the university.
2. Processing events in Shirley's life and determining when she begins to experience anxiety.
3. Delineating what behaviors Shirley engages in when she feels anxious.
4. Leaving home and moving immediately into a studio apartment.

95 • In evaluating the nursing approach, the nurse would consider the following questions. Which of the 4 is the *least* important regarding Shirley?

1. Were her maladaptive responses reduced?
2. Did she gain insight into the origins of her illness?
3. Did she learn adaptive coping skills?
4. Were nursing interventions modified to fit her needs?

Items from Comprehensive Examination Section 4 That Address the Various Steps of the Nursing Process

Item Number	Assess	Analyze	Plan	Implement	Evaluate	Item Number	Assess	Analyze	Plan	Implement	Evaluate
1	x					49					x
2		x				50		x			
3			x			51		x			
4			x			52				x	
5	x					53	x				
6		x				54				x	
7			x			55					x
8					x	56			x		
9				x		57					x
10	x					58				x	
11					x	59				x	
12				x		60			x		
13				x		61	x				
14				x		62					x
15					x	63		x			
16		x				64		x			
17	x					65				x	
18	x					66		x			
19	x					67			x		
20				x		68		x			
21		x				69				x	
22	x					70			x		
23			x			71	x				
24					x	72		x			
25		x				73				x	
26	x					74	x				
27		x				75					x
28				x		76	x				
29				x		77		x			
30		x				78			x		
31	x					79	x				
32				x		80					x
33		x				81					x
34					x	82		x			
35					x	83		x			
36				x		84			x		
37				x		85				x	
38					x	86			x		
39				x		87					x
40					x	88	x				
41		x				89				x	
42					x	90				x	
43			x			91	x				
44			x			92		x			
45				x		93		x			
46	x					94			x		
47	x					95					x
48			x								

Answer Sheet—Section 4

1. 1 2 3 4
2. 1 2 3 4
3. 1 2 3 4
4. 1 2 3 4
5. 1 2 3 4
6. 1 2 3 4
7. 1 2 3 4
8. 1 2 3 4
9. 1 2 3 4
10. 1 2 3 4
11. 1 2 3 4
12. 1 2 3 4
13. 1 2 3 4
14. 1 2 3 4
15. 1 2 3 4
16. 1 2 3 4
17. 1 2 3 4
18. 1 2 3 4
19. 1 2 3 4
20. 1 2 3 4
21. 1 2 3 4
22. 1 2 3 4
23. 1 2 3 4
24. 1 2 3 4
25. 1 2 3 4
26. 1 2 3 4
27. 1 2 3 4
28. 1 2 3 4
29. 1 2 3 4
30. 1 2 3 4
31. 1 2 3 4
32. 1 2 3 4
33. 1 2 3 4
34. 1 2 3 4
35. 1 2 3 4
36. 1 2 3 4
37. 1 2 3 4
38. 1 2 3 4
39. 1 2 3 4
40. 1 2 3 4
41. 1 2 3 4
42. 1 2 3 4
43. 1 2 3 4
44. 1 2 3 4
45. 1 2 3 4
46. 1 2 3 4
47. 1 2 3 4
48. 1 2 3 4
49. 1 2 3 4
50. 1 2 3 4
51. 1 2 3 4
52. 1 2 3 4
53. 1 2 3 4
54. 1 2 3 4
55. 1 2 3 4
56. 1 2 3 4
57. 1 2 3 4
58. 1 2 3 4
59. 1 2 3 4
60. 1 2 3 4
61. 1 2 3 4
62. 1 2 3 4
63. 1 2 3 4
64. 1 2 3 4
65. 1 2 3 4
66. 1 2 3 4
67. 1 2 3 4
68. 1 2 3 4
69. 1 2 3 4
70. 1 2 3 4
71. 1 2 3 4
72. 1 2 3 4
73. 1 2 3 4
74. 1 2 3 4
75. 1 2 3 4
76. 1 2 3 4
77. 1 2 3 4
78. 1 2 3 4
79. 1 2 3 4
80. 1 2 3 4
81. 1 2 3 4
82. 1 2 3 4
83. 1 2 3 4
84. 1 2 3 4
85. 1 2 3 4
86. 1 2 3 4
87. 1 2 3 4
88. 1 2 3 4
89. 1 2 3 4
90. 1 2 3 4
91. 1 2 3 4
92. 1 2 3 4
93. 1 2 3 4
94. 1 2 3 4
95. 1 2 3 4

Section 1

COMPREHENSIVE EXAMINATION: ANSWERS AND RATIONALES

1. (1) Because the breech or soft part is in the fundus, the occiput must be the presenting part. Since the irregular nodules are on the mother's right, the fetal back must be on her left.

2. (1) With a vertex presentation, the fetal heart tones are most audible below the mother's umbilicus. In the left occiput anterior presentation, the fetal heart tones are generally heard best through the fetal back, which is toward the mother's left side.

3. (3) Pressure from the uterus on a presenting breech may provide enough force to empty the infant's rectum. In all other presentations, relaxation of the infant's anal sphincter and release of meconium are the direct result of fetal hypoxia or anoxia and are signs of an abnormality.

4. (3) The 1st nursing priority is to prevent undue temperature decreases, the 2nd is to check for abnormalities, and the 3rd is to identify the infant. The instillation of silver nitrate eye drops can safely be delayed for as long as 2 hours after birth.

5. (2) Increase in fetal activity is not thought to initiate labor. A decrease in progesterone levels, uterine overdistention, and maternal production of oxytocin all serve to initiate onset of labor.

6. (4) Since cardiac function during gestation is compensated by fetal circulation, early x-ray films may show a normal heart size. An EKG shortly after birth often reflects cardiac status *in utero*, and this finding also could be normal. Murmurs are rarely present in the neonate with cardiac defect because of the normally high pulmonary vascular resistance, which tends to equalize the pressure between the 2 ventricles.

7. (3) Respiratory distress while lying down is caused by increased blood flow to the heart and lungs from the extremities.

8. (1) One of the physical consequences of heart defects is growth retardation. This consequence is due to inadequate nutrient intake, feeding difficulties, and increased caloric requirements, resulting from tachypnea and tachycardia.

9. (2) Coolness of affected extremity may indicate vessel obstruction.

10. (1) Because of the higher pressure within the left ventricle, blood flows through the defect to the right ventricle.

11. (1) A cerebral hemorrhage in the middle cerebral artery distribution will probably result in greater upper extremity than lower extremity dysfunction. Therefore, Mr. Crown will probably experience greater return of lower extremity than upper extremity function on a spontaneous basis. Training him in left handed self care techniques would, therefore, greatly increase his independence. If given a stool softener and a diet high in roughage, most post-stroke patients regain normal bowel function, so there would be no need to teach Mr. Crown the technique for manual removal of stool from the rectum. Mr. Crown's non-functional upper right extremity would make it difficult or impossible for him to use a walker. Generally, patients with expressive aphasia regain speech function only through repeated speech practice; he should be encouraged to communicate through oral rather than written means.

12. (3) Typical upper extremity deformities that may result from a cerebrovascular accident are shoulder adduction, elbow flexion, wrist flexion, and finger flexion. The tendency for these contraction deformities can be minimized by active or passive movement of all joints in the involved extremity through full range of motion 3 times daily; by extending the arm, forearm, and wrist on pillows alongside the trunk when the patient is supine; by bandaging a hard plastic cone in the patient's hand; and by maintaining the wrist in extension through use of wrist splints for 2 hours at a time (alternating with 2 hours of splint removal to permit wrist movement). The involved arm should be supported by a sling to prevent shoulder subluxation only while the patient is ambulating, since a sling fosters shoulder adduction.

13. (4) Typical lower extremity deformities following cerebrovascular accident include external rotation of the hip, knee flexion, and plantar flexion of the ankle. These deformities can be minimized by placing a trochanter roll from the lateral femoral trochanter to the knee to maintain the leg in neutral position and by applying padded boots to keep the foot at a 90 degree angle with the lower leg. Pressure of the soles on a hard surface, like a footboard, stimulates plantar flexion, thereby enhancing the tendency for footdrop. A restraining sheet over the thighs might discourage knee flexion but would facilitate external rotation of the hip. A rolled blanket under the knee would encourage knee flexion contractures, and a rubber donut under the heel can cause pressure damage to tissue.

14. (1) A cerebrovascular lesion in the parietal or temporal lobe may damage the optic nerve radiations posterior to the optic chiasm, causing the patient to lose vision in the same half of the visual fields of both eyes (right or left homonymous hemianopsia). A lesion on one side of the brain produces a defect in the opposite side of the visual field. One manifestation of such loss in Mr. Crown would be his inability to see the food on the right side of his tray or his inability to see persons or objects to his right. The possibility of visual field loss should be investigated before exploring his food preferences or his need for smaller, more frequent meals. Restoration of Mr. Crown's self sufficiency in activities of daily living make it desirable that he feed himself, with assistive devices if necessary, rather than being fed by someone else.

15. (2) In Broca's or motor aphasia, the problem is primarily one of speech expression, and the patient may be unable to speak or communicate in writing (or both). To stimulate return of language function, the nurse should encourage the patient to speak, even though his efforts are hesitant, error prone, and frustrating to himself and others. In speaking for the patient (asking questions that can be answered monosyllabically), the nurse deprives the patient of needed practice. Simply reading verbal material or writing out his communications affords no opportunity to learn new methods of self cuing and speech stimulation.

16. (2) The majority of new amputees experience perceptions relating to the missing limb segment (itching, throbbing, and discomfort). Patients should be warned in advance that such sensations are possible so they will not conclude that they are losing their grip on reality.

17. (3) Post-operatively, the stump should be elevated on pillows for no longer than 24 hours because longer elevation of the stump predisposes to hip flexion contracture. Raising the foot of the bed or suspending the stump in a sling would likewise predispose to hip flexion contracture. By raising the foot of the bed on blocks, stump edema can be reduced while keeping the hips in a neutral or an unflexed position.

18. (4) To use crutches correctly, Mrs. Hershey must be able to extend her elbows and support her body weight on her palms, as she grips the crutch's hand bar. She should be helped to increase triceps strength (the triceps muscle extends and stabilizes the elbow). Pushing herself up from a prone position involves elbow extension and will strengthen the triceps.

19. (2) An insulin overdose, omission of a meal, vomiting of food, or overexertion all can result in hyperinsulinism or too large a supply of insulin to handle available blood

glucose. The symptoms of hyperinsulinism are headache, hunger pangs, weakness, dizziness, pallor, diaphoresis, tremor, anxiety, and irritability.

20. (3) In order to prepare a smoothly tapered stump for optimum prosthesis fitting, and to prevent pressure breakdown of skin over the weight-bearing surface of the stump, stump edema should be prevented by applying an elastic roller bandage to the stump while the patient is still supine, i.e., before she moves from bed to chair. Since the skin of the stump must be intact and tough to withstand pressure injury from the prosthesis, lotion (which softens the skin), alcohol (which dries and cracks the skin), and adhesive tape (which irritates and excoriates the skin) should not be applied.

21. (1) Of primary importance during the assessment is the question of whether there is suicidal ideation present. If there is, the nurse needs to know whether there is a clear plan and the lethality of that plan. Appropriate nursing interventions (admitting patient to a locked unit rather than an open one, placing patient on suicide precautions or suicide watch) must then be implemented.

22. (3) Through conversation and observation, the nurse can establish how much time is spent in compulsive acts. If the underlying conflict is intensified following hospitalization, the ritualistic behavior will increase and vice versa.

23. (2) The nature of the conflict and any secondary gain from the symptoms are out of Dolly's conscious awareness. Trying to force a change in behavior prior to achievement of insight by Dolly is nonproductive.

24. (2) Reminding Dolly to begin her rituals early in order that she may retire at a predetermined time is an inviting option; however, this suggestion is based on logic and implies control over the rituals. For the nurse to remind Dolly to begin her rituals possibly would be encouraging sick behavior. Determining the cause of the increase in anxiety at bedtime is the key to the nurse's intervention.

25. (2) Behavioral rituals help to avoid inexplicable anxiety that would arise if the impulse was not followed.

26. (1) A weight gain of more than 2 pounds per week is usually the first sign of pre-eclampsia. Headaches and hypertension usually develop later and are signs of severe pre-eclampsia. Ankle edema occurs in normal pregnancy and is not indicative of pre-eclampsia.

27. (2) Mrs. Sams should be placed in a private room in order to decrease the amount of external stimuli to which she will be subjected. Her weight on admission should be recorded as a baseline against which to determine the amount of fluid retention following initiation of treatment. Likewise, the amount and distribution of edema should be noted so that the effectiveness of treatment can be evaluated later. Mrs. Sams' urine will be examined for protein content in order to assess the seriousness of her condition.

28. (2) Restraints should not be applied to a patient with impending convulsions, lest the immobilization of extremities predispose to fractures during violent convulsive movements. Intravenous equipment may be needed for parenteral administration of certain drugs. An indwelling catheter may be required to ensure accurate measurement of fluid output. Suction equipment will be needed if the patient aspirates respiratory secretions during convulsions.

29. (1) Oliguria would suggest occurrence of renal shutdown. Diuresis would constitute a desired response to therapy. Fluid intake should be individualized according to the severity of the patient's condition. Since magnesium sulfate is primarily excreted in the urine, urinary output should be at least 30 ml/hr before magnesium sulfate is administered to minimize toxic response to the drug.

30. (1) There is always a possibility of post-partum convulsions in the pre-eclamptic patient, even if convulsions did not occur prior to delivery. However, following delivery, many previously pre-eclamptic patients show no evidence of permanent renal damage. Further, many patients who are pre-eclamptic during the 1st pregnancy are normotensive during subsequent pregnancies; one cannot predict that a pre-eclamptic woman will develop pre-eclampsia during all subsequent pregnancies.

31. (1) The mechanisms responsible for the obstructive symptoms of asthma are edema of the mucous membranes, bronchospasms, and accumulation of tenacious secretions.

32. (2) Because of the increased resistance in the airway, the child must force expiration through the partially obstructed lumen, resulting in the wheezing with expiration.

33. (3) Cold liquids can trigger reflex bronchospasm and should be avoided.

34. (4) The side effects of epinephrine are tachycardia, weakness, pallor, tremors, elevated blood pressure, and nausea.

35. (3) Parents of asthmatic children can decrease their children's stresses and their own stresses by encouraging their children to perform breathing exercises, by identifying and eliminating factors that precipitate attacks, by recognizing early acute symptoms, and by treating attacks promptly.

36. (3) Femoral fractures provoke severe muscle spasms that exert pull on bone fragments and disrupt bony alignment and may compress blood vessels so as to obstruct circulation. Usually, traction is applied pre-operatively to overcome muscle spasm, disengage bone fragments, and prevent additional soft tissue injury. A cast or splint would immobilize the bony fragments and prevent mechanical damage to soft tissues by bony projections but would not overcome muscle spasm. Pelvic sling suspension is used to immobilize pelvic rather than femoral fractures.

37. (4) Because edema may develop in the operated extremity and a plaster cast is inflexible, the cast can constrict limb vessels and obstruct arterial supply to the part. Impaired arterial circulation may cause any of the following symptoms; pulselessness, delayed capillary filling following pressure, pallor, coldness, and paresthesias. Since irreversible nerve damage and gangrene may result from impaired arterial circulation, a constricting cast must be removed immediately; therefore, the surgeon should be summoned whenever signs of arterial embarrassment are noted. Elevating the limb might reduce soft tissue edema but not rapidly enough to correct arterial obstruction. Placing additional covers on the limb will not warm the leg that is cold due to arterial obstruction. Vital signs and hip dressing should be checked frequently while the patient is in the recovery room, but the patient's symptoms indicate arterial insufficiency for which the surgeon should be notified immediately.

38. (2) Weight bearing too soon following open reduction of a fractured femur can break the fixation device and displace bone fragments; therefore, weight bearing is usually not permitted during the early post-operative period. Acute flexion of the hip, such as that produced by sitting in a low soft chair or arising from a low position, will strain the recently stretched joint capsule, predisposing to dislocation of the prosthesis or of the femoral head. Since elderly patients become confused when hurried, plenty of time should be provided for the patient's move from bed to chair; the move should not be attempted immediately before a scheduled activity such as meal or visiting hours.

39. (4) Isometric exercises, which consist of muscle contraction and increase in muscle tension without a change in muscle length, are effective in increasing muscle strength. Gluteal setting, or pinching the buttocks together so as to move the leg laterally, and quadriceps setting, or pushing the popliteal space against the mattress so as to lift the heel from the bed surface, will strengthen muscles that are involved in walking. Passive range of motion exercises preserve joint motion but do not increase muscle strength. Vigorous exercise or movement by the patient may cause him to adduct, externally rotate, or acutely flex the hip, any of which movements may dislocate the operated hip or weaken the nail and plate used for internal fixation.

40. (3) Since adduction, external rotation, and acute flexion of the hip may all create strain on the internal fixation device, the operated hip should be extended throughout the turn; the patient should be turned only to the unoperated side; and, while turning and while in the side-lying position, the operated leg should be maintained in abduction with pillows. While in the side-lying position, the operated knee can usually be flexed slightly to increase comfort and balance.

41. (2) Since free and complete expression of feelings tends to occur only when the patient has full speech ability, and loss of normal speech ability will diminish interpersonal communication for several weeks following

laryngectomy, the patient should be encouraged to freely ventilate his fears and concerns before surgery so he will have more energy to invest toward rehabilitation activities during the post-operative period.

42. (4) Possible complications of laryngoscopy include laryngeal edema and respiratory obstruction, the symptoms of which include restlessness, apprehension, and shortness of breath. Since the local anesthetic used to facilitate passage of the laryngoscope obliterates the gag reflex for 2 to 4 hours, the patient would not be allowed to eat or drink for 4 hours following the procedure in order to prevent aspiration.

43. (3) When radical neck surgery is complicated by wound infection, rupture of the carotid artery may occur. Since exsanguination could result from rupture of the carotid artery, observation of bright red blood on the neck dressing should lead the nurse to summon the physician while exerting direct pressure to the wound. Since laryngectomy would make normal speech impossible and since air would be inspired and expired through the tracheostomy rather than through the nose, loss of normal speech and smell are expected following the operation. Surgical disruption of laryngeal tissues would result in dysphagia following removal of the nasogastric tube and resumption of oral feedings.

44. (2) Suctioning removes gases as well as secretions from the lower air passages, and so it should be applied only during catheter withdrawal and should be limited to 5 seconds at a time, with intermittent aeration or oxygenation of the patient to prevent hypoxia. Since suction is of itself irritating to the trachea, it should be employed only when tracheal secretions are present, rather than on a regularly scheduled basis. A sterile catheter should be used for each episode of suction application and then discarded following use in order to prevent introduction of pathogens into the lower respiration tract.

45. (4) Since a paroxysm of coughing could cause dislocation of the tracheostomy tube during replacement or adjustment of neck tapes, one nurse should hold the tube securely in place while a second nurse replaces and ties the tapes. The outer cannula should never be removed from the tracheostomy by the nurse. The inner cannula must be removed from the outer to be cleaned, soaked in H_2O_2 to loosen crusts, disinfected, rinsed thoroughly, and replaced within 10 minutes to prevent obstruction of the outer cannula with secretions that result in difficulty in reinserting the inner cannula.

46. (4) Upon admission this type of patient would be hard pressed to analyze or synthesize information. Analysis of precipitating factors for hospitalization would come later, after the patient is better integrated.

47. (2) This is a broad opening remark that allows the patient privacy and distance and encourages him to converse on any topic he so chooses.

48. (1) An effective and immediate response to the psychotropic medication along with a strong support system and a high level of functioning before hospitalization bodes well for the paranoid schizophrenic. Slow response to the medication along with continued use of the paranoid delusional system would not.

49. (2) Confusing, contradictory, inconsistent communications in Dr. Gold's early family life possibly did not allow the development of a healthy ego or of defense mechanisms.

50. (3) Scapegoating and reinforcing deviant behavior patterns are to be avoided in family therapy. A situation in which one family member is identified as "sick" (schizophrenic) is an indication of the "illness" of the family as a unit. The distorted perceptions of reality and of needs should be identified, and alternative modes of gratification sought.

51. (3) Physiological jaundice occurs in 40 to 60% of term infants and commonly develops on day 3 of life. By definition, physiological jaundice never occurs during the 1st 24 hours following birth.

52. (2) Normal transitional stool is yellow brown in color. Depressed reflexes, a high pitched cry, and regurgitation of feedings are manifestations of the nerve cell damage that is caused by deposition of bile pigments in vital areas of brain tissue (kernicterus).

53. (1) The Coombs' test is used to demonstrate certain antigen-antibody reactions. It can detect the presence of maternal Rh-positive antibodies on the red blood cells of the fetus or neonate. IgA is an immunoglobulin that is found in colostrum and protects the new-

born against *Escherichia coli*. HB_sAg is the surface antigen of the virus that causes hepatitis B.

54. (1) Incompatibilities of the Rh factor occur when the mother is Rh negative, the father is Rh positive, and the fetus is Rh positive. Rh isoimmunization occurs when Rh-positive red blood cells enter the maternal circulation during a previous delivery, and the maternal body produces antibodies against the "foreign protein" of the Rh-positive cells. When this Rh-negative mother becomes pregnant with another Rh-positive fetus, the antibodies in the mother's blood cross the placenta and destroy the fetus's red blood cells.

55. (2) The exchange transfusion is performed to replace the infant's destroyed red blood cells with red blood cells that have not been coated with maternal antibodies.

56. (2) Since voluntary control of motor movement is not established until later in infancy, the clinical signs of cerebral palsy would not be evident in early infancy.

57. (2) Spasticity of the calf and plantar muscles causes her to stand on her toes.

58. (2) The primary problem in spastic cerebral palsy is that the muscles are in a state of continuous contraction with extreme plantar flexion.

59. (2) Children are best fed in a normal sitting position with the body flexed and arms brought forward on the table.

60. (1) In order to force the child to use her lips and tongue, place food at the side of the tongue, forcing her to move the tongue around her mouth. Also force the child to use her lips to remove food from the spoon rather than scraping it off with her teeth. Speak to her very slowly in order to increase her comprehension.

61. (4) Because the breast has an abundant blood supply, many vessels must be cauterized or ligated during radical mastectomy. The pressure dressing is applied both to prevent post-operative bleeding and to prevent subcutaneous accumulation of drainage, which would interfere with wound healing. Loosening of the pressure dressing would remove the hemostatic effect of compression. Wide or forcible abduction of the arm may disrupt ligatures and initiate bleeding during the immediate post-operative period. Nail and conjunctival pallor will develop only after considerable blood loss. If the chest wound were to bleed extensively, blood would be apt to run down the lateral chest wall and pool on the lower bed linen.

62. (2) Removal of axillary nodes and lymphatics interferes with lymph drainage from the arm until new lymph channels have an opportunity to develop. Since fluid flow is influenced by gravity, lymph flow can be facilitated through the reduced number of lymphatics by elevating the arm above heart level. Cold should not be applied to the arm, as it would constrict blood vessels and decrease blood flow. The part should not be massaged, as fluid filled tissues are easily damaged by pressure. A sling should not be used because adduction of the arm constricts the axilla and would further interfere with lymph flow through the remaining lymph nodes.

63. (2) Disuse of the left arm following surgery would facilitate fibrosis and shortening of ligaments and tendons, causing contracture deformities. To prevent such deformities, Mrs. Forman should be encouraged in active, rather than passive movement of both upper extremities. "Wall climbing" exercises encourage elbow extension and shoulder flexion. Arm swinging exercises loosen shoulder muscles and ligaments and strengthen accessory muscles of shoulder movement. Splinting the arm in functional position would encourage contracture of fibrous tissue structures. Isometric exercises would increase muscle strength without preserving joint motion.

64. (2) Surgical removal of axillary lymphatics diminishes protection against infection of arm tissues. Consequently, the arm must be protected from pressure, puncture, and other trauma. The patient should wear a Medic Alert bracelet indicating that the involved arm is not to be used for hypodermic injections, venipuncture, or blood pressure measurement. The patient should use both arms actively in self care so as to maintain muscle strength and joint mobility. Lotions and creams should be applied to the involved hand and arm to keep the skin from drying and cracking. Within a few days following surgery, Mrs. Forman should be encouraged to raise her arms higher and

higher above shoulder level in order to maintain full range of motion.

65. (2) One of the most serious toxic effects of chemotherapeutic agents is bone marrow depression, with reduction of circulating polymorphonuclear leukocytes. Generally, when the white blood cell count falls below $3000/mm^3$ (normal is 7000 to $10{,}000/mm^3$), the chemotherapeutic agent is withheld until the white blood cell count again rises above $3000/mm^3$. While Mrs. Forman's decreased white blood cell count would predispose her to infections of many types, monitoring her for the presence of a current respiratory or urinary infection would be less urgent than discontinuing the drug responsible for the leukopenia. Although some white blood cells (agranulocytes) are produced in lymph nodes, Mrs. Forman's leukopenia is more likely the result of chemotherapy-related marrow depression than replacement of normal lymphoid tissue with malignant cells.

66. (4) Because of repeated exacerbations and remissions of joint symptoms, the patient with rheumatoid arthritis feels a lack of control over her life. Allowing the patient to determine the time for arising, bathing, napping, toileting, retiring, and (if possible) eating allows her a measure of control over events and surroundings. Although rest splints are used to relieve pain by supporting involved joints in position of maximum function, the splints should be removed at intervals and the joints moved to (but not beyond) the point of pain to prevent fibrous ankylosis. During the phase of acute joint inflammation, the nurse should assist Mrs. Turek with care activities in order to conserve the patient's strength and minimize trauma to acutely inflamed tissues. Assistive devices are useful in permitting the patient the greatest possible independence while, at the same time, minimizing painful joint motion.

67. (4) Typical joint deformities of rheumatoid arthritis are flexion contractures and ankylosis of elbows, wrists, hips, and knees and flexion or extension contractures of fingers and ankles. To prevent such deformities, the patient should be positioned so that flexion of elbows, wrists, hips, and knees is discouraged, and hands and feet are maintained in a position of maximum function. Placing the patient in the prone position 3 times a day encourages hip and knee extension. Low Fowler's position fosters hip and knee flexion; foot pressure against a footboard fosters plantar flexion and knee flexion, especially when the patient is in Fowler's position. A towel under the knees encourages knee flexion. Moving patients with acutely inflamed joints through full range of motion causes destruction of the tissues of those joints.

68. (4) The goals of Mrs. Turek's exercise program will be to maintain motion in the affected joints and to prevent muscle atrophy. To achieve these goals she will be advanced from gentle passive motion of the joint to active movement of the joint in activities of daily living. Since one of the symptoms of rheumatoid arthritis is easy fatigability, the nurse should help conserve Mrs. Turek's energy by alternating scheduled activities and scheduled rest periods throughout the day. Relieving Mrs. Turek of all responsibility for self care in the nursing unit would encourage the attitude of passivity, which would jeopardize the success of rehabilitation efforts. Encouraging too frequent or too long exercises in the nursing unit might cause injury to already weakened joint structures. Stimulating competition with another arthritic patient predisposes one or the other to negative self evaluation and poor self image.

69. (4) Joint pain and limited upper extremity motion make eating difficult for the patient with rheumatoid arthritis, so additional time and energy are needed to consume each meal. If she is given extra time to complete each meal, she may be able to eat all of the food served to her. Having someone feed her would encourage passive dependence and diminish self esteem. The food brought in by family members may not provide the high calorie, high vitamin diet that she needs to gain weight.

70. (1) Gold compounds may cause dermatitis, bone marrow depression, and nephritis in some patients; therefore, a complete blood count and urinalysis are performed at each clinic visit, and the current dose of gold salt is withheld if toxic effects are evident.

71. (4) Nurses and other members of the health team too frequently direct their efforts to maintaining the status quo. Many aged persons are capable of developing new interests and friends and planning for the future.

72. (2) An out of context comment of this kind frequently catches us by surprise. A factual comment similar to "Lydia, you've forgotten; you decided to sell your car because you don't drive anymore" is almost always the best response. Exploring the comment is inappropriate, as is ignoring it. To remind Lydia of a loss (driver's license) and failing physical capacity may be truthful but perhaps a little blunt.

73. (1) The memory patterns for past events are well established, but recent events are forgotten. Chemicals necessary for placing a thought in the memory may not be available in sufficient quantity.

74. (1) Keeping a light burning will help Lydia orient herself in space. Requiring her to recite names would be demeaning. Stimulation by family, friends, and neighbors is helpful in maintaining orientation and interest.

75. (2) Provision of safety and consistency, in an environment with which Lydia has, or can gain, some familiarity, is indicated. The goal is not to reconstruct the personality, but to help Lydia and others to cope with her overt behavior.

76. (4) There is no evidence that any specific foods are a factor in acne.

77. (3) There is no concrete evidence that ultrasound treatment is of any benefit to acne.

78. (2) The effectiveness of erythema and desquamation is the result of increased rate of turnover of the epithelium that lines the follicular duct, which reduces the compaction that produces the comedo. When compaction is reduced, there is loosening of the comedo within the duct that facilitates its removal or shedding.

79. (1) Use of comedo extractor will not exacerbate the condition. If the comedo extractor is used properly, it will reduce the risk of future inflammatory lesions and scarring.

80. (4) The 1st week, medication is left on for 2 hours and then washed off. The next week, it is left on for 4 hours. From then on it is applied at bedtime and left on overnight.

81. (1) Since isoetharine is a sympathomimetic that has a bronchodilator effect, administering it 20 minutes before the postural drainage procedure will facilitate removal of bronchial secretions. Since postural drainage causes bronchial secretions to move toward the upper respiratory passages and stimulates coughing, administering postural drainage shortly before meals would be apt to interfere with appetite and digestion. Increased humidification, through ultrasonic nebulization, would best facilitate removal of thickened bronchial secretions if performed before, rather than after, postural drainage. Since intramuscularly injected cephalosporin has no direct effect on the lining of the gastrointestinal tract, the time of drug administration need not be planned with reference to the time of food ingestion.

82. (1) Patients with increased residual lung volume and air trapping have chronically elevated P_{CO_2} levels and therefore have lost the normal stimulus to the medullary respiratory centers (above normal arterial P_{CO_2}). In such patients, low P_{O_2} levels stimulate chemoreceptors in the aorta and carotid arteries, which send impulses to the respiratory center to increase the rate and depth of respiration. Although Mr. Hale's pneumonia has caused him to be hypoxemic, too great a rise in P_{O_2} level would eliminate his usual respiratory stimulus, and respiratory failure would result. Retinal damage due to O_2 toxicity occurs principally in infants and only at very high O_2 concentrations. Since Mr. Hale would be receiving humidified O_2 and ultrasonic nebulization therapy, his O_2 therapy should not produce drying of respiratory mucosa and thickening of secretions.

83. (2) Exhaling against pursed lips increases intraalveolar pressure, thereby preventing alveolar collapse during expiration, prolonging expiration, decreasing air trapping, and reducing residual air volume. These changes will improve oxygenation of the blood and increase CO_2 elimination. An abdominal binder would limit inspiration in the emphysematous patient whose fixed chest position makes it necessary for him to use abdominal muscles to assist ventilation efforts. Splinting the patient's lower rib cage would likewise limit air exchange in a patient whose chest movements are already limited. Frequent changes in position, rather than a static position in bed, would be needed to mobilize tracheobronchial secretions from the lower airways.

84. (4) The most frequent untoward effect of cephalexin is diarrhea, which probably results from imbalance of intestinal flora due to overgrowth of non-susceptible organisms. In a few patients, diarrhea is severe enough to require discontinuation of the drug. The drug is not known to cause 8th cranial nerve damage, marrow depression, or parenchymal liver cell damage.

85. (1) Providing additional humidity to ambient air will liquefy bronchial secretions and facilitate their removal by postural drainage exercises and effective coughing. The patient should be advised to stop smoking altogether rather than to decrease the number of cigarettes, as smoking paralyzes the respiratory cilia and interferes with movement of secretions from the lower respiratory tree. The patient should avoid contact with cooking odors, paint fumes, and the like, and deodorant also can provoke bronchospasm in sensitive individuals. Confinement to the home during the influenza season may be impossible and could interfere with the patient's exercise program. He should be protected against respiratory infections by annual vaccinations against influenza and pneumonia.

86. (2) Individuals differ in the type and amount of information needed to cope with illness- and treatment-related anxiety. Asking Mr. Oakes what he would like to know about the forthcoming operation allows him to control the amount of incoming information to be processed, as well as the source and timing. Although Mr. Oakes' medical history, his coping style, and nursing reference books would all provide useful health teaching cues, Mr. Oakes' expressed information needs should be the basis for pre-operative teaching.

87. (3) The patient with adequate physical and emotional strength may profit from an opportunity to talk with a recovered colostomate pre-operatively, in order to ventilate his concerns and seek first hand information from someone who has experienced a colostomy. If, following such an interchange, Mr. Oakes requests additional specific information about colostomy care, the nurse may provide him with pictures and posters illustrating colostomy irrigation and colostomy bag application or may allow him to handle and inspect colostomy supplies and equipment that will be used in his care. A tour of the operating rooms and recovery room is helpful to some patients, but would probably be less helpful than a visit with a rehabilitated rectal cancer patient.

88. (2) In order to decrease the risk of post-operative peritonitis due to spillage of intestinal contents during surgery, an intestinal anti-infective, such as kanamycin (Kantrex) or neomycin (Neocin), is given orally to reduce the bacterial count of the colon and to soften and decrease the bulk of the feces. Although Mr. Oakes may be anemic owing to blood loss from his tumor, the anemia would be treated with blood transfusion rather than with ferrous sulfate, which tends to cause constipation. The bowel would be emptied prior to surgery by giving a high calorie, low residue diet for several days rather than by administering a catharatic, such as bisacodyl that stimulates the colonic mucosa to initiate reflex peristalsis, which could have disastrous effects in a patient with a bowel obstruction. Mr. Oakes is not likely to experience severe pain pre-operatively, so he will not need morphine or other narcotics until after surgery.

89. (3) Since the squatting position is most conducive to defecation, fecal expulsion from the stoma will be facilitated if the patient assumes a sitting position on the toilet, with his feet elevated on a stool during colostomy irrigations. Warm tap water or saline is preferred as an irrigant, because a soap solution would irritate the intestinal mucosa. The irrigations should be carried out at the same time as the patient's preoperative bowel habit time, which may or may not be early morning. The irrigating catheter needs to be inserted only 2 to 6 inches in order to distend the colon sufficiently to stimulate evacuation. Inserting the full length of the catheter increases the possibility of bowel trauma or perforation.

90. (3) Although an ascending colostomy is hard to regulate and requires daily irrigation to minimize inappropriate emptying, a descending colostomy is relatively easy to regulate and requires irrigation every 2nd or 3rd day (if at all) to establish bowel regularity. Many patients with descending colostomy achieve bowel regularity and control through diet regulation alone.

91. (3) Extrapyramidal side effects are neurological reactions to phenothiazines, not alcohol. Malnutrition, cross addiction, and confabulation can be the result of long-term alcohol abuse.

92. (3) The majority of alcoholics have been found to have an underlying character trait of the passive-aggressive personality. Other alcoholics are compulsive, depressive, paranoid, or antisocial personalities.

93. (2) When Mr. Ranger defiantly states that the nurse can't control his behavior (drinking), he is correct but perhaps is conveying "I wish someone would make me stop drinking." The nurse's response is a "no-fight" position that confronts him, conveys the expectation that he will stop drinking, and challenges him to declare a nondrinking goal. The nurse also could have asked, "Do you want to stop drinking?"

94. (1) It is impossible to control the thoughts of another person or to protect him from disappointment. Since the temptation to drink is ever present to an alcoholic, advice on how to avoid it may be meaningless.

95. (4) If he is denying the fact that he is an alcoholic his prognosis for rehabilitation is not favorable for this hospitalization. His short-term goals and coping mechanisms for abstinence will foretell his probable success following discharge.

Section 2

COMPREHENSIVE EXAMINATION: ANSWERS AND RATIONALES

1. (4) Cultural background, religious beliefs, and the woman's perception of the disadvantages or costs of different contraceptive methods all influence the woman's contraceptive choice—by determining ideal family size and by determining the acceptability of various contraceptive devices. Availability of abortion is least likely to influence contraceptive choice.

2. (3) From 24 to 36 hours before ovulation the basal body temperature drops from 0.2 to 0.3° F. Within 24 to 48 hours following ovulation the basal body temperature rises from 0.5 to 1.0° F and remains slightly elevated until the day before the next menstrual period, when it drops to the lower level, which is characteristic of the 1st part of the cycle. Since sperm remains viable for 48 to 72 hours, and the ovum is capable of being fertilized for 48 hours, the woman's fertile period extends from about 48 hours before ovulation (perhaps 24 hours before the brief temperature drop) to 48 or 72 hours after onset of the temperature elevation.

3. (1) Oral contraceptive pills are combinations of estrogens and progesterone that block the production of luteinizing hormone releasing factor by the hypothalamus, which in turn prevents the surge of luteinizing hormone at mid-cycle that is essential for development of the ovum. The intrauterine device interferes with uterine implantation of the fertilized ovum; spermicidal foam destroys sperm in the vagina.

4. (4) Weight gain, nausea, and breast tenderness are all common side effects of oral contraceptive pills. Calf pain would suggest possible thrombophlebitis, a serious untoward effect of oral contraceptives, which results from increases in certain clotting factors.

5. (4) The diaphragm should be left in place for 8 hours following coitus to ensure destruction of sperm in the vagina. Spermicidal jelly, rather than water soluble jelly should be applied to the upper surface (cervical surface) of the diaphragm in order to provide a second mechanical barrier to the movement of sperm. The diaphragm should be inserted no more than 2 hours before intercourse to ensure potency of the spermicidal jelly, which covers the cervical os.

6. (4) In *Staphylococcus* pneumonia, there are early diminished breath sounds resulting from rapid accumulation of purulent fluid in the lung.

7. (1) Because *Staphylococcus* pneumonia is caused by penicillinase producing staphylococci, semisynthetic penicillins, such as methicillin, nafcillin, or oxacillin, are used.

8. (2) Fluid is not restricted in pneumonia. Due to high fever and rapid respirations, dehydration is always a danger.

9. (3) Body fluid loss reduces the circulating blood volume, which then affects skin and muscles. With dehydration, mucosa appears dry and skin turgor becomes poor, and with rehydration, mucosa appears moist and skin turgor returns to normal.

10. (2) Fluids are frequently administered intravenously rather than orally in pneumonia because with rapid, shallow breathing, there is always the danger of aspirating the liquid.

11. (3) In the elderly, the combination of prolonged immobility, knee flexion, and pressure against popliteal structures predisposes to stagnation of venous blood flow in the lower extremities, pressure injury to venous walls, and phlebothrombosis. To prevent such injury, the height and angle of the stirrups should be adjusted and the knee supports should be padded to support and immobilize the legs in abduction without popliteal pressure or hip and iliac strain. Since Mr. Ridgeley's upper body will be supine and horizontal, there will be no neck hyperextension or pressure of abdominal viscera against the diaphragm. The stirrup's footplate or foot sling will maintain the foot at right angles to the lower leg throughout the procedure, so dropfoot will not be a problem.

12. (1) Pressure of the catheter against the urethral wall may cause urethritis. If infection supervenes in an irritated urethra, a urethral fistula may develop and is most apt to occur at a point of acute urethral flexion, such as the penile-scrotal junction. By taping the catheter to the abdominal wall when the patient is supine, the urethral angle at the penile-scrotal junction is less acute, thereby reducing the risk of fistula formation. The external urinary meatus and adjacent catheter should be cleansed twice daily with antiseptic solution to remove crusted material and to prevent ascending urinary infections. For the drainage apparatus to function properly, the collection device must be positioned so urine can fall freely by gravity without obstruction, whether the patient is supine, sitting, or upright; therefore, the bag should not be suspended from the bed's side rail. The catheter should be kept patent by irrigation, not by "milking" the tube.

13. (3) Since the patient is not rendered unconscious by spinal anesthesia and vomiting is less likely following spinal than following general anesthesia, aspiration is not an expected problem. Neither spinal anesthesia nor prostatic surgery in itself predisposes to seizure activity. Although the patient is immobilized for some time during the procedure and immobility in the supine position fosters pooling of respiratory secretions, hypostatic pneumonia, if it occurs, would not develop rapidly enough to be evident immediately after surgery. Spinal anesthesia causes hypotension through paralysis of sympathetic vasomotor nerves. If the operation is lengthy, considerable blood may be lost during surgery, with consequent decrease in circulating blood volume and in blood pressure. In addition, several of the sedative-hypnotics that are administered pre-operatively to decrease anxiety and promote relaxation also decrease blood pressure.

14. (2) Frank bleeding from the prostatic bed may occur during the 1st 24 hours after surgery. Blood of arterial origin tends to clot and may block the catheter, obstructing urinary drainage and causing bladder distention, which, in turn, will strain the operative site and cause further bleeding. To prevent such obstruction, the catheter must be irrigated frequently. Although Mr. Ridgely's position should be changed at intervals to promote comfort and prevent skin pressure damage, the prone position would be likely to cause catheter obstruction. Contracture deformities and ankylosis require days and weeks to develop and are not a concern immediately after surgery, though active toe, ankle, knee, and hip exercises will prevent lower extremity venous pooling and thrombophlebitis. Knee flexion would predispose to intravascular clotting.

15. (3) Because Valsalva's maneuver during heavy lifting or straining at stool may increase intravesicular pressure enough to initiate bleeding from the prostatic bed for 4 to 8 weeks following surgery, heavy lifting and constipation must be avoided. A high bulk, high fiber diet with increased liquid and stool softeners are effective in preventing constipation. Alcohol in any form is to be avoided until surgical healing is complete because alcohol tends to irritate the inflamed prostatic bed and provokes bladder spasm.

16. (2) Patients with cirrhosis frequently experience pruritus, perhaps as a result of retention of bile salts and their deposition in skin tissues. The patient's fingernails should be kept short, smooth, and clean. He should be cautioned against scratching, as skin excoriations can easily be infected owing to the patient's poor nutritional status. The patient should be bathed without soap, as soap of any type would be irritating to the patient's hypersensitive skin. Unless the patient is incontinent or perspires profusely,

there is no need for a cellulose-cotton absorbent pad. The weight of upper bed linen would not cause skin irritation, although soap residue on the lower linen might irritate the skin of the back, elbows, and heels.

17. (3) Although the incidence of peptic ulcer is higher in alcoholics than in the general population, the cause of Mr. Kemper's bleeding is an esophageal varix. His abdominal distention is due to ascites rather than to distention of the bowel with feces and gas. Following a massive upper gastrointestinal hemorrhage, the bacteria normally present in the bowel break down the blood protein to form ammonia, which is absorbed into the blood. Since excessive blood ammonia causes disturbance of nervous tissue function (hepatic coma), enemas and cathartics are given to rapidly remove the blood from the gut, and neomycin is given to eradicate the intestinal bacteria responsible for ammonia production. No untoward effect results from intestinal enzyme secretion during periods of fasting.

18. (1) The Sengstaken-Blakemore tube is a triple bore tube with 2 balloons that provides a means for gastric suctioning, gastric tamponade, and esophageal tamponade. When the esophageal and gastric balloons are inflated, the patient cannot swallow his saliva, so frequent suctioning is needed to prevent aspiration of oral secretions. The patient should be maintained in low Fowler's position to facilitate respirations. Since movement or dislodgment of the tube could provoke variceal bleeding, since traction is exerted on the tube at the nares, and since inflation of the gastric balloon prevents displacement of the tube while it is subject to traction, neither balloon should be deflated without a physician's order.

19. (2) If the gastric balloon of the Sengstaken-Blakemore tube should rupture accidentally, the traction exerted on the tube could cause upward displacement of the tube, with obstruction of the airway by the esophageal balloon. In the event of such emergency, both balloons should be immediately deflated by cutting the outside tubing to both balloons.

20. (3) The cirrhotic patient with no signs of hepatic coma should receive a high protein diet to facilitate tissue and blood rebuilding. Therefore, protein is probably the most, rather than the least, important of the 3 basic food groups in Mr. Kemper's diet. Coffee or tea taken before a meal may decrease appetite, and a meal without liquids may render the food unappetizing. By serving 5, rather than 3 meals a day, and by decreasing the volume of each meal, the patient may be able to eat all food served.

21. (2) The antisocial personality does not become dependent on any one person. Rather, he uses an individual for his own needs and then moves on to someone else. Manipulation will be utilized by him if necessary to gain his own ends, and anger will replace his charming demeanor if he is blocked or thwarted.

22. (3) Assessment of the manipulative procedures James is using, plus the planning and enforcing of limit-setting interventions would be crucial to effective interventions. Avoidance of a patient does not help him deal with his inappropriate behavior.

23. (1) Analysis of why he has been hospitalized is grist for long-term psychotherapy. The antisocial personality has no insight into his own behavior.

24. (4) One of the key characteristics of the antisocial personality is the inability or unwillingness to profit from past experiences and use them as tools for changing behavior.

25. (1) This response acknowledges the patient's remarks, allows for minimal and appropriate therapist self disclosure, and utilizes the communication techniques of redirecting and refocussing the conversation.

26. (3) Rheumatic fever is characterized by inflammation of the endocardium, or heart lining, which causes fibrotic scarring of valve flaps and cordae tendineae, the fibrous cords that attach the valve flaps to the ventricular wall. Scarring of the valve flaps may cause either stenosis (narrowing) or insufficiency (widening) of the valve opening.

27. (4) Rest, rather than exercise, is needed by the pregnant woman with heart disease, since circulatory changes associated with pregnancy increase cardiac workload. Many high carbohydrate foods are also high in sodium, so a high carbohydrate diet may lead to weight gain as a result of both increase in fatty tissue and excess fluid retention. In either case, the increase in body weight elevates the cardiac workload.

28. (4) Maternal blood volume peaks at about 28 to 32 weeks' gestation, creating the greatest amount of cardiac strain and maximizing risk of congestive heart failure.

29. (4) During uterine contraction blood is expelled from the uterus into the circulation. Bearing down during a contraction increases the amount of blood that is expelled from the uterus into the circulation and increases cardiac workload. The amount of venous return flow to the heart can be decreased somewhat by maintaining the patient in semi-recumbent position. Caudal or epidural anesthesia is often used to eliminate labor pain, as pain is a stresser that may precipitate congestive heart failure.

30. (1) Immediately following delivery the cardiac patient is at high risk for congestive heart failure because delivery results in marked reduction of intra-abdominal pressure, fluid moves from extravascular spaces into the blood stream, and venous return flow to the heart is increased. Therefore, the patient should be maintained in low Fowler's position to decrease venous return flow. Elastic stockings should be applied, and the patient should be encouraged to ambulate to prevent venous thrombosis in the dilated lower extremity veins. Excessive fluid intake should be avoided, as it would increase intravascular volume and predispose to congestive heart failure.

31. (3) A child with acute glomerulonephritis (AGN) may appear pale, but there is no cyanosis. The urine is typically dark or cola colored due to the presence of erythrocytes. Obstruction of glomeruli by immune complexes causes reduction in glomerular filtration rate, retention of water and sodium, and ultimately hypertension. In rare cases, hypertension may be severe enough to cause convulsions. Brudzinski's sign (involuntary flexion of hips and knees on flexion of the neck in the supine position) is a sign of meningeal irritation, not cerebral edema.

32. (1) During the acute stages of AGN, fluid intake is monitored carefully. The glomerular capillary loops become dysfunctional owing to swelling and infiltration, reducing the capacity to form filtrate; this problem in turn results in generalized edema.

33. (4) Although a regular diet is allowed for most children, it should contain no added salt. The decreased plasma filtration results in retention of salt.

34. (2) Signs of improvement are an increase in urine output with diaphoresis, decreasing edema, and return of blood pressure to normal.

35. (4) Edema of the brain is caused by hyperfusion of the brain, and symptoms, such as vomiting, headache, and dizziness, are the result of increased intracranial pressure. Urine volume is decreased rather than increased, as a consequence of water and sodium retention.

36. (4) The anxiety produced by chest pain provokes the stress response and increases catecholamine levels, which increases myocardial O_2 demand; therefore, Mr. Powers' chest pain should be relieved immediately by administering the ordered narcotic, which is given intravenously to ensure effective absorption. Changes of position and opportunities to ventilate feelings will not relieve the pain of myocardial ischemia. An O_2 flow rate of 4 L/min by nasal prongs should provide sufficient oxygenation to prevent extension of the infarct if the patient remains at rest.

37. (3) Since Valsalva's maneuver stimulates the vagus and slows the heart rate, straining at stool is to be avoided following myocardial infarction. Consequently, the patient is given a stool softener and is encouraged to use a bedside commode rather than a bedpan for bowel evacuation. Turning off the alarm for a patient who is predisposed to life-threatening arrhythmia would deny him the protection for which he was admitted to the coronary care unit. Barring all visitors from Mr. Powers' bedside may cause him such anxiety as to increase his myocardial O_2 demand and increase the risk of arrhythmia. Unless the patient is extremely debilitated, the omission of hygiene measures would increase the patient's discomfort rather than decrease it.

38. (2) Complications of acute myocardial infarction include ventricular arrhythmias, congestive heart failure, and embolization of a mural thrombus. Symptoms of congestive heart failure include dyspnea, orthopnea, dependent edema, enlarged liver, distended neck veins, and basal rales. A slight excess of fluid output over fluid input might be insignifi-

cant or might reflect elimination of fluid that was retained due to an earlier excessive production of ADH. A mild temperature elevation is expected following infarction and reflects the inflammatory process that occurs within the myocardium. Lethargy and diminished cough are possible effects of lidocaine and morphine.

39. (4) The most dangerous toxic effect of warfarin (Coumadin) is hemorrhage from any site. Bleeding from the kidney or bladder may occur as microscopic, rather than gross hematuria. Microscopic hematuria causes the urine to have a cloudy appearance. In this patient, headache, unless severe, would seem to be an insignificant symptom that could safely be treated with a mild analgesic. Drying and irritation of pharyngeal tissues may result from O_2 flow or from mouth breathing. The white blood cell count is usually elevated between 10,000 and 20,000/mm^3 from 2 to 7 days following an infarction, reflecting inflammatory changes in the myocardium.

40. (2) On hospital discharge following myocardial infarction, the asymptomatic patient should resume some physical activity beyond personal hygiene and feeding activities, and walking is good exercise for such individuals. Because some coronary patients have type A personalities, they must be cautioned against strenuous muscular activity, which would increase myocardial O_2 demand and strain the infarcted myocardium. Usually, the patient should not resume sexual activity for 4 to 8 weeks following infarction since the blood pressure elevation during intercourse increases myocardial O_2 demand. The patient should not return to work, even part-time, for 8 to 10 weeks following infarction in order to avoid the physical and emotional stresses encountered during employment.

41. (1) Baclofen relieves flexor spasms of skeletal muscle in patients with multiple sclerosis, as a result of its ability to inhibit both monosynaptic and polysynaptic reflexes at the spinal cord level. Toxic effects of the drug include dizziness, easy fatigability, and muscle weakness; therefore, following initiation of the drug, Bea may experience accentuation of the weakness and fatigue caused by her primary disease process, and the drug dose may have to be reduced. ACTH causes hirsutism rather than hair loss; bethanechol stimulates rather than depresses smooth muscle contraction. Rather than dehydration and weight loss, both ACTH and baclofen cause fluid retention.

42. (3) In multiple sclerosis, rapid mood swings occur as a result of limbic system involvement. Rather than depression, hyperexcitability and inappropriate euphoria are frequently seen in multiple sclerosis, possibly due to denial of the nature and consequences of the disease. Variations in the patient's motor ability and coordination may cause family members to suspect the patient of malingering, but there is no evidence that such tendency exists or that multiple sclerosis patients are any more inclined toward paranoia than other types of patients.

43. (1) Bea's intention tremor and incoordination may cause a considerable amount of food to spill during meals. This problem can be minimized by providing a plate guard against which to scoop food onto a spoon or fork with weighted handles, to lessen erratic movements of the hands. Since bed rest is indicated for 2 to 3 weeks during treatment of an acute exacerbation and since multiple sclerosis patients should be kept as active as possible for as long as possible, an electric wheelchair would be contraindicated at this time. Because bethanechol (Urecholine) and a regular, every 2-hour voiding schedule may foster complete bladder emptying and relieve dribbling, an indwelling catheter should be postponed for as long as possible, so as to prevent bladder infections. Since Bea's hip flexion is not limited and the squat position fosters defecation, a raised toilet seat would not be used.

44. (2) Loss of pain, temperature, touch, and position sense renders Bea at increased risk of physical injury from a number of causes. Consequently, she should be taught to monitor the position and condition of her body parts and the objects with which they come into contact in order to prevent burns, cold injury, punctures, and lacerations. Because of spasticity, Bea is subject to flexion contractures, so all joints should be put through full range of motion daily, and Bea should be encouraged to remain active in self care and homemaking activities. Rather than scheduling all activities in the morning, they should be scattered throughout the day and alternated with rest periods to conserve energy. Since Bea is subject to bladder infections and constipation, she should have a liberal fluid intake throughout 14 to 16 hours of the day.

45. (1) Since multiple sclerosis often results in loss of pain and temperature sense in the extremities, Bea should be taught to prevent burns by measuring the temperature of bath water and to prevent cuts by watching her hands while using a knife or other sharp instrument. The visual problems associated with multiple sclerosis are the result of optic nerve demyelination and are not caused or aggravated by exposure to sunlight. Multiple sclerosis does not predispose to convulsions, so a padded tongue blade will not be needed. Unless permanent visual loss or incapacitating muscle weakness occurs, there is no reason to stop driving a car.

46. (3) Escape from responsibility and rejection of authority are typical of drug addicts. Wade's initial efforts in carving out his turf in the unit will be filled with manipulation. However, he later may become overly dependent on the nurse, a situation to be avoided.

47. (2) Avoidance of a dependent, mothering relationship is accomplished by making the patient feel secure and self reliant. Drug addiction may impair one's ability to relate in a close, interpersonal relationship but does not destroy one's appreciation of sex.

48. (4) If the psychodynamic etiology of Wade's drug addiction was nongratification of oral dependency needs, pipe smoking would be one means of providing oral satisfaction. The other activities listed are not viewed as gratifying oral needs.

49. (3) Teenagers often begin taking drugs to be included in their "in group." Because of Wade's living situation (married, age 22), his peer group would be different from that of the adolescent. It is important for him to participate in group psychotherapy, to help him relate to peers and to begin self examination.

50. (3) Wade probably developed a stimulus (anxiety, stress, problems) response (take drugs) type pattern to cope with life. Two approaches can then be employed to help decrease stress and anxiety and to alter his response to stress. Improving his ability to cope and decreasing drug administration are often followed by employment and general personality strengthening.

51. (4) The gluteal muscle is small, poorly developed, and extremely close to the sciatic nerve. The gluteal muscles do not develop sufficiently to serve as an intramuscular injection site until the child has been walking for some time. Therefore, the preferred intramuscular injection site in the neonate is the vastus lateralis muscle on the lateral aspect of the thigh. There is no reason to use the Z-track technique or to refrain from applying pressure to the injection site.

52. (1) Since, in the normal infant, the head circumference is about 2 cm greater than the chest circumference, it will be sufficient to record the measurements on the infant's chart. A head circumference less than 32 cm would suggest microcephaly. A head circumference that is 4 cm greater than the chest circumference would raise the possibility of hydrocephaly.

53. (2) Cold increases O_2 consumption by tissues, elevating cardiac workload during the difficult period of transition from intra-uterine to extra-uterine life. If the infant is unable to satisfy this increased O_2 need by breathing room air, there is a switch from aerobic to anaerobic metabolism, with accumulation of lactic acid in the tissues (metabolic acidosis).

54. (2) The normal neonatal rooting reflex consists of opening the mouth and turning the face toward anything that touches the cheek. This reflex should be utilized to orient the newborn infant to the breast in preparation for nursing. The Moro or startle reflex, which is also a normal neonatal reflex, is elicited by a loud noise or sudden motion. Following such a stimulus, the infant responds by initial trunk and limb extension, followed by symmetrical limb flexion and adduction (as if embracing). The tonic neck or "fencing" reflex is a normal neonatal reflex that is elicited by turning the supine infant's head to one side, whereupon the arm and leg of the side toward which the head is turned extend, and the opposite arm and leg flex. The Babinski's reflex, which is normal in infants but abnormal in adults, consists of dorsiflexion of the great toe and fanning of the 2nd, 3rd, 4th, and 5th toes when the sole of the foot is stroked.

55. (2) For a term infant of normal weight, a weight loss of 10% or less is acceptable during the early postnatal period. Baby Samuels weighed 6 lb, 4 oz, or 100 ounces at birth. Therefore, the infant could lose up to 10 oz of weight before a diagnostic work-up would be needed.

56. (1) Although by definition, the cause of idiopathic epilepsy is unknown, it may result from a genetic factor. Birth trauma, rubella, and meningitis are all acquired causes of epilepsy.

57. (4) Epilepsy is preceded by an aura in some children. In tonic-clonic seizures, the child loses consciousness immediately and experiences tonic contractions followed by clonic contractions.

58. (3) Diagnostic procedures such as the CAT scan, EEG, and echoencephalogram could give information about the type of seizures the child experiences and possibly determine the cause of the seizures. There is no procedure that could determine genetic factors, how long the child will have seizures, or potential I.Q.

59. (4) A hospitalized child with a history of convulsive seizures requires precautions to prevent physical harm during seizures. During the tonic phase, the child could become cyanotic for 15 to 20 seconds, but he is in no critical danger; breathing resumes automatically when the tonic phase ends. Therefore, there is no necessity for keeping an emergency cart in his room.

60. (4) Stimuli that could activate the hyperexcitable cells are physiological stimuli, such as abnormal blood glucose levels, dehydration with electrolyte imbalance, emotional stress, and endocrine changes. Drinking a cold soft drink would not be a sufficient physiological stimulation to trigger seizures.

61. (1) Since peristalsis and gastric acid secretion are increased by emotional tension, the peptic ulcer patient's environment should be kept as quiet, calm, and unhurried as possible, in order to facilitate mental rest. Since the noise level is usually high in both the nurses' station and in the patients' lounge, it would be unwise to assign Mr. Gunderson to a bed near either of these facilities. Since a young man who is being prepared for elective surgery is likely to receive many visitors and to be interviewed by various caregivers, Mr. Gunderson might have difficulty resting and sleeping in a room with such a patient. A private room, at the end of a hall, far removed from elevators, ward kitchen, nurses' station, patients' lounge, and linen and supply rooms should afford him the best opportunity for long, uninterrupted periods of quiet relaxation.

62. (4) For the first day or two following surgery, application of undue force against the gastrojejunal suture line by the catheter or irrigating solution might loosen sutures or dislodge clots and cause bleeding or peritonitis. Hence, the irrigating solution should be instilled gently. Normal saline, rather than distilled water should be used as an irrigant, since frequent water irrigations of the stomach could wash out enough electrolytes to upset the acid-base balance. About 100 ml of irrigant are required to aspirate the nasogastric tube adequately. Air should not be instilled through the tube as it would not clear the tube of mucus or clots and could distend the stomach, placing strain on the suture line.

63. (2) Manipulation of the intestine during surgery causes loss of normal peristalsis for 24 to 48 hours post-operatively. While peristalsis is absent, swallowed air and gastrointestinal secretions accumulate, distending the stomach and bowel and exerting pressure on the suture line. The nasogastric tube is used to remove secretions until peristalsis returns—manifested by bowel sounds and passage of flatus. Peristalsis usually resumes within 2 to 3 days after surgery, though vital signs may not be at pre-operative baseline values by then, and intake and output values may not be exactly balanced, since the body is still replacing intra-operative fluid losses. Normal bowel movements will not occur until the patient begins oral feeding.

64. (1) The presence of a nasogastric tube fosters mouth breathing and drying of the oral mucosa. Without oral food intake there is lack of stimulus to salivary glands, so parotitis may develop. To counter the tendency for oral infection and to decrease discomfort due to pressure of the nasogastric tube, the mouth should be cleaned of crusts and debris and lubricated frequently. The nares should also be cleaned and lubricated to prevent irritation by the tube. Although frequent changes in position and back rubs

should improve the patient's comfort, there is no therapeutic advantage to his lying on his left side, and massage of the extremities is contraindicated because of the possibility of mobilizing thrombi from the leg veins.

65. (1) Following a subtotal gastrectomy the reservoir function of the stomach is lost. When food in undigested form is dumped quickly into the jejunum, it creates a hypertonic intestinal content that draws in water from surrounding tissue spaces and blood vessels. The resulting fall in blood pressure produces shock-like symptoms. By limiting carbohydrates, eating several small dry meals, avoiding drinking fluids with meals, and lying down for a brief period following each meal, the patient can retard gastric emptying and reduce the volume of osmotically active particles that are delivered to the jejunum during each meal.

66. (3) Needle injury to the arterial wall at the dye injection site may cause thrombotic obstruction of the vessel. Since decreased blood flow through the already narrowed vessel could cause gangrene, peripheral pulses in the injected leg should be checked every hour for 8 hours. In a patient with diffuse peripheral arteriosclerosis, elevating the legs would decrease perfusion of the tissues and cause ischemic muscle pain. Unilateral lower extremity edema (which could be detected by comparing thigh or calf circumference in the 2 legs) would be more suggestive of thrombophlebitis than of arterial thrombosis. Maintaining the legs in abduction would not diminish the risk of femoral artery inflammation or thrombosis.

67. (2) One of the most serious complications following femoropopliteal bypass surgery is thrombosis of the graft, which results in obliteration of popliteal, posterior tibial, and dorsalis pedis pulses. If initially palpable pulses disappear within a few hours after surgery, the graft may have to be replaced. On the other hand, the presence or absence of distal pulses immediately following the operation does not confirm or refute the effectiveness of the surgery since some time is required to fully restore circulation in a previously ischemic vessel. Because distal pulses could be palpable even if there were blood loss from the vascular anastomosis, measuring the circumference of the limb would provide a more reliable indication of bleeding into soft tissues. Sphygmomanometer reading, stethoscope examination, electrocardiogram, and hourly urine output values would be more accurate indices of cardiac function and blood pressure than would peripheral pulse volume in a patient with peripheral arteriosclerosis.

68. (4) The capillary blanching or filling test consists of pressing a thumbnail against the fingernail or toenail, then quickly releasing the pressure. The normal response is blanching of the tissue under the nail with pressure, and return of normal pink color when pressure is released. In the limb with obstructed arterial circulation there is a delay in color return. The patient's leg should not be elevated post-operatively, since gravity-dependent reduction in arterial flow could have serious consequences. It is unlikely that Mr. Walker would have pedal edema, which results more frequently from venous than arterial disturbance. Testing the patient's skin temperature with the dorsum of the hand is, at best, a rough measure of temperature and circulatory efficiency.

69. (2) Most commercial sinus remedies and many commercial cold remedies, such as Neo-Synephrine, contain a vasoconstrictor, which would narrow lower extremity vessels, increasing tissue ischemia, so they should be avoided by a patient with peripheral arteriosclerosis.

70. (3) Since even minor foot trauma may lead to gangrene in the patient with peripheral arteriosclerosis, Mr. Walker should never go barefoot for fear of striking his foot against a piece of furniture or stepping on a sharp object. Leather, hard soled slippers would provide greater protection from an object falling on the foot than would soft cloth slippers. Lotion, rather than alcohol, should be applied to the foot, since the alcohol would dry the skin and cause it to fissure, thereby increasing the risk of infection. Direct heat should never be applied to ischemic tissues, as heat elevates the rate of tissue metabolism, increasing tissue need for O_2. Lower extremity arteriosclerosis, of itself, does not cause dependent edema, and elevating the foot of the bed would decrease arterial flow to the leg, so the patient would be apt to develop ischemic rest pain.

71. (1) The nurse and patient working together will first try to identify the feelings that Eva experiences as anxiety. Then the patient can identify which behaviors are utilized to deal with the anxiety. From that point, work would be done describing what immediately precedes the anxiety—a situation, a person—and finally the patient will try to deduct the probable cause of the anxiety.

72. (2) Neurotic individuals have a good ability to discuss reality, but their reactions to it may be disproportionate to the stimuli intensity.

73. (2) People suffering from neuroses usually complain of fatigue, fears, and somatic complaints—as did Eva. Delusions are not symptomatic of neurotic anxiety. Flight of ideas is present in the manic phase of bipolar disorder. Eva has not presented herself as disoriented.

74. (3) We frequently express our feelings in physical symptoms, but this action is seldom conscious. When Eva says, "I have to express myself that way," it would be most helpful for the nurse to determine if Eva can say which feelings she needs to express. The nurse could then help Eva express feelings and associate them with the current crisis.

75. (1) Patients who experience an episode of confusion or mental illness are at times reluctant to return to the same place of work. Usually this reluctance is unwarranted. Again, the principle here is to help Eva develop the ability to make her own decisions and to discuss dependence on others.

76. (3) When Sally bends over, observing her from directly behind will reveal a rib hump.

77. (3) Loss of peer group contact is a severe emotional threat to Sally because of loss of group status and group acceptance. She needs reassurance from her peer group in order to maintain her self confidence and self worth.

78. (1) It is difficult for a child at any age to be restricted, but this is particularly true of adolescents who have experienced independence for several years in various areas of their lives, particularly self help activities.

79. (3) In assessing patients in traction, attention is paid to cranial nerve functions and to deep tendon reflexes in the extremities. Loss of lateral gaze results from injury to cranial nerve C6. Hyperreflexia, paralytic ileus, and urinary retention are all potential problems.

80. (2) Circulation should not be impeded in any way by the cast. Temperature, color, and sensation should all be compared in all extremities, and there should be no pain, numbness, tingling, or edema.

81. (2) Mrs. Peach's obesity and high abdominal wound will make it difficult to cough postoperatively. However, hourly coughing and deep breathing during the early post-operative period will protect her from pneumonia. By teaching her to interlace her fingers and apply manual pressure over the wound dressing while coughing, the nurse can minimize the patient's discomfort and encourage effective bronchial toilet. Narcotics, rather than meditation techniques should be used to relieve Mrs. Peach's postoperative pain and encourage full lung expansion. Elastic stockings may be worn postoperatively, but their purpose can be explained at the time of application.

82. (3) The incision for gallbladder surgery is so high on the abdominal wall that wound pain, if not relieved, causes inhibition of ventilatory movement. Liberal administration of analgesics facilitates turning, coughing, and deep breathing, all of which will be required to prevent post-operative atelectasis and pneumonia. The T tube is sutured to the skin and secured to the dressing, so it is not likely to be dislodged by moving about in bed.

83. (4) Following cholecystectomy and choledochostomy, the patient should rest as often as possible in low Fowler's position so that any blood or bile that leaks from the cystic duct stump or common duct incision will drain into the pelvis—from which it could be more easily drained than from the subdiaphragmatic area. Prone, Trendelenburg, and supine positions would all encourage subdiaphragmatic accumulations of drainage.

84. (4) Because Mrs. Peach is obese, the provision of abdominal support through binder application should increase her comfort in ambulating and sitting in a chair. A wheelchair would enable her to move from her room to other hospital areas with ease but would discourage the ambulation needed to prevent peripheral phlebothrombosis, hypostatic pneumonia, and loss of muscle tone. Since Mrs. Peach experienced no disequili-

brium or loss of lower extremity strength, there would be no need for a cane or walker during ambulation.

85. (4) Following common duct exploration and stone removal, a T tube is placed, with short limb sutured into the common duct and long limb brought to the surface of the abdomen, to facilitate bile drainage during duct healing and to prevent leakage of bile into the peritoneal cavity due to increased pressure in the duct. During the 1st 24 hours, when the common duct is edematous due to surgical manipulation, from 200 to 300 ml of bile will drain from the T tube. The amount of drainage from the T tube decreases as the common duct heals, so that on the 7th to 10th post-operative day the tube can be removed.

86. (4) Following carotid endarterectomy, an adequate blood pressure must be maintained in order to ensure patency of the operated vessel. The 20 mm Hg drop in both systolic and diastolic pressure should be reported to the surgeon immediately so that cardiotonic or vasopressor (or both) drugs can be initiated as necessary to maintain cerebral circulation. The amount of temperature, pulse, and respiration increases could be accounted for by the patient's greater activity and anxiety as he recovers from the effects of the anesthetic.

87. (1) Since the carotid artery incision creates a roughened area of vascular intima upon which platelets and blood cells may accumulate and from which a clot could be released into the cerebral circulation, the patient should be closely monitored post-operatively for symptoms of embolization to the ophthalmic artery or a branch of either the middle cerebral or anterior cerebral artery. If such symptoms are observed, the surgeon must be notified immediately so he can assess the patency of the operated carotid artery. Incisional pain would not suggest clot embolization. Calf pain would be characteristic of thrombophlebitis, and sharp, sudden chest pain would suggest either coronary artery obstruction or pulmonary embolus.

88. (3) Because several of the cranial nerves traverse the neck and may be obscured by blood or sponges and injured by instruments used during the operative procedure, the patient should be monitored post-operatively for symptoms of cranial nerve injury, among which the more common are dysphagia and hoarseness due to vagal injury and shoulder sagging and scapular asymmetry due to injury to the spinal accessory nerve. Diaphoresis could result from the patient's temperature elevation. Thirst could be a response to operative blood loss or throat irritation by the endotracheal tube. Lethargy may result from the sedative that he received pre-operatively or the lingering effects of the anesthetic agent.

89. (3) Since the neck provides such a confined operative field, considerable trauma of surrounding neck structures may occur during carotid endarterectomy. Post-operative edema of these structures or hemorrhage from traumatized or improperly ligated vessels may obstruct the airway, causing respiratory insufficiency or asphyxia. Since rapidly developing edema or hemorrhage from a large vessel may cause sudden respiratory obstruction, a tracheostomy tube should be kept at the bedside for emergency use. A hemostat and scissors are usually included in a tracheostomy tray.

90. (4) Since many of the risk factors that led to Mr. Keeler's carotid arteriosclerosis and thrombosis can be assumed to still exist, and since there is evidence that low doses of aspirin prevent platelet aggregation, aspirin is administered on a daily basis to some patients following carotid endarterectomy to protect against cerebral embolization of a platelet thrombus from the carotid bifurcation. By hospital discharge, Mr. Keeler should no longer experience incisional pain and operative edema of soft tissues should have subsided.

91. (2) During an acute manic state, patients are physically active and need room to move about and express some of the "pressure" contained within the body.

92. (4) At times, use of medications (tranquilizers) is the best way to calm patients so that interpersonal communication is possible.

93. (2) Behavior of the manic person usually puts the staff in a defensive posture. To prevent this, it is useful to clearly establish the limitations on behavior based on the patient's needs. The patient needs to express

hostility, to be protected, and to feel security derived from knowing what to expect. Hence, the necessity of consistently applied limits.

94. (4) It is unrealistic to call the therapist at 1:00 A.M. unless this is part of a preplanned, preannounced treatment approach. The problem here is how to say "no" at the outset and not have an angry patient upsetting everyone on the unit. The first step is to ascertain why she is awake demanding a pass. Persons in a manic state do not respond well to direct commands but are easily distracted.

95. (2) The recommended oral dose is 300 mg. T.I.D. for maintenance. This dosage results in an appropriate blood concentration of 0.8 to 1.2 mEq/L.

Section 3

COMPREHENSIVE EXAMINATION: ANSWERS AND RATIONALES

1. (2) Since a vaginal examination may precipitate uncontrollable hemorrhage in a patient with placenta previa, the procedure should not be performed in a patient with a possible diagnosis of placenta previa (a common symptom of which is painless bleeding) until the blood has been typed and 2 units of cross matched blood have been readied for transfusion, in the event of massive bleeding.

2. (2) Since rectal examination may precipitate uncontrollable bleeding in the patient with placenta previa, a rectal examination should not be performed unless the patient is taken to a delivery room where a "double setup" has been readied to permit either a vaginal or cesarean section delivery. Since excessive maternal bleeding would compromise fetal circulation, fetal heart tones should be monitored frequently to detect signs of fetal hypoxia. The uterine fundus can be palpated to determine the degree of uterine muscle tone. The fundus is soft and relaxed unless labor has begun.

3. (1) It is necessary to know what Mrs. Sage is feeling in order to deal effectively with her emotional response to her situation. In asking Mrs. Sage why she is crying the nurse acknowledges awareness of Mrs. Sage's mood and signals her readiness to provide emotional support while Mrs. Sage ventilates her feelings. Administration of a sedative would only postpone Mrs. Sage's coping with her feelings. In asking Mr. Sage to comfort his wife the nurse would be delegating her responsibilities for emotional support of her patient.

4. (4) Although with onset of labor the uterine fundus becomes firm during contractions, the entire abdomen is not continuously rigid. In supine hypotensive syndrome a woman in the 3rd trimester suffers a fall in blood pressure on assuming the supine position, but she does not experience abdominal pain. In abruptio placentae, or premature separation of the placenta, the placenta is torn from its bed, causing bleeding. Accumulation of blood behind the placenta causes pain and produces an enlarged, firm uterus. Massive blood loss would produce shock, with profuse diaphoresis, rapid thready pulse, and falling blood pressure.

5. (2) Since massive blood loss due to placental separation causes maternal hypovolemia, shock, and fetal hypoxia, fetal heart tones should be closely monitored to detect worsening of fetal condition. Evidence of fetal distress would indicate need for cesarean section. It would be inadvisable to push oral fluids in a patient who is apt to require general anesthesia and major surgery within a short time, as vomiting and aspiration could occur. Elevating the head of the bed might further decrease the patient's already lowered blood pressure.

6. (2) At approximately 3 to 4 months of age the infant locates sound by turning the head to the side and looking in the same direction.

7. (3) Nursing care should be planned to establish healthy psychosocial interaction because findings show that the principal problem in nonorganic failure to thrive is disturbance in the relationship between the child and the principal caregiver.

8. (1) The infant's negative feeding pattern is an entrenched habit that is difficult to rectify and refusing feeding is part of the problem. Therefore, nurses must be gently persistent when the infant initially refuses feeding.

9. (4) Many mothers of failure-to-thrive children—especially adolescent parents—lack skills for relating to and caring for their children. Teaching the mother some basic skills related to care of her child could effect changes to improve the mother-child relationship.

10. (3) Children who fail to thrive because of nonorganic causes also generally fail to maintain eye contact. Therefore, if good eye contact is established between mother and child, progress toward healthy interaction is evidently being made.

11. (1) The personality changes and functional losses caused by the brain tumor and its treatment make it necessary for Doris to become physically and emotionally dependent upon her parents at precisely that life stage in which the individual's chief psychological task is to separate from his or her family of origin and to identify with his or her family of commitment. In having completed college and taught college for a couple of years, Doris had selected an occupational role and had acquired the necessary work skills to fulfill that role. Although Doris's illness has produced some cognitive losses, it is less certain that her disabilities will interfere with value identification or with heterosexual attachment than that they will force her into physical and emotional dependence upon her parents.

12. (3) When a supratentorial mass increases intracranial pressure to a severe degree, the cerebral peduncle may herniate through the tentorial notch, compressing the 3rd cranial nerve (oculomotor) and causing pupillary paralysis. Homonymous hemianopia is characteristic of stroke damage to optic nerve radiations behind the optic chiasm. Loss of peripheral vision is characteristic of glaucoma. Centrifugal scintillating scotoma, or sparkling colored lights, is characteristic of migraine headache.

13. (4) Fluid tends to leak from capillaries within the brain tumor into surrounding brain tissue. This cerebral edema causes symptoms by increasing intracranial volume. Radiation can cause brain inflammation, and the associated vasodilation would likewise increase intracranial pressure. Prednisone has an anti-inflammatory effect and decreases urinary excretion of sodium, thereby increasing fluid retention and edema. Prednisone lowers resistance to infection rather than increasing resistance. Without some knowledge of physiology, Doris would be unable to interpret the significance of prednisone's ability to regulate sodium and potassium levels. Although the adrenal corticosteroids tend to increase the patient's sense of well-being, they do not increase muscle strength per se. In fact, in high doses they decrease muscle strength by increasing protein catabolism.

14. (3) The objective for a rehabilitation program is to assist the patient to become as self sufficient as possible in activities of daily living. Therefore, the nurse should not "take over" all responsibility for Doris's bathing, dressing, toileting, and mobility. Neither should all therapies be performed in the patient's room, as that would deprive her of contact with other patients and the social stimulation to be derived from group activities. Since both the disease and its treatment will predispose Doris to fatigability, the nurse should not encourage Doris to cancel therapies when she is lacking in energy. Rather, assistive devices, such as a long-handled back washer, long-handled reacher, washcloth mitt, long-handled shoehorn, stocking stretcher, pants' hooks, and so forth, should be provided to enable Doris to provide self care with least possible expenditure of energy.

15. (3) A recurrence of tumor growth would cause increased intracranial pressure and, if the tumor involves the motor cortex or causes pressure on the motor cortex, may cause Jacksonian or focal convulsions, which often begin with twitching of fingers, toes, or lips on one side of the body and spread to involve other muscles on the same side. Doris and her family would have been taught that hair loss and fatigability are likely consequences of chemotherapy, that hair will grow back in 8 weeks following cessation of therapy, and that energy level will improve when red blood cell count increases following cessation of treatment. Moon face appearance is a common consequence of long-term adrenocorticosteroid therapy and results from fluid retention.

16. (3) A rectal tumor or polyp may cause a feeling of incomplete bowel emptying with defecation and thereby provoke the prolonged straining at stool that results in prolapse. Therefore, following reduction of prolapse, a proctosigmoidoscopy should be performed to identify rectal conditions needing treatment. Although it is true that all persons over 40 years of age should have an annual proctoscopic examination, there is another, more specific reason for Della's receiving the examination. The intussusception occurs in the rectosigmoid segment and is relieved when the prolapse is reduced.

17. (1) In a patient with laxity of perineal musculature, the most frequent cause of rectal prolapse is repeated and prolonged straining at stool. The patient should be encouraged to eat a diet high in fiber, i.e., one containing large quantities of fresh fruit, fresh vegetables, and whole grain. If dietary management and daily doses of psyllium hydrophilic mucilloid do not relieve constipation, a glycerine suppository may be used to facilitate defecation. Since multiple pregnancies predispose to rectal prolapse by weakening perineal muscles and to development of hemorrhoids, the patient with prolapse may also suffer hemorrhoids, for which a commercial remedy may yield some relief.

18. (3) The fresh apples, dried raisins, and nutmeats in a Waldorf salad would be desirable since all contain fiber, as do the lettuce, tomatoes, and cucumbers in the garden salad. Whole grains, as in whole wheat bread, are also good sources of fiber. However, 40%, rather than 100%, bran cereal would be preferred for Della, as 100% brain cereal causes fecal impaction in some elderly individuals with markedly decreased intestinal peristalsis.

19. (2) The greater mobility associated with regular physical exercise will increase peristalsis and prevent constipation, thereby eliminating the stimulus for straining at stool that causes rectal prolapse in susceptible individuals. A hot sitz bath might relieve the pain or itching of hemorrhoids but would not prevent rectal prolapse. Although excessive caffeine increases peristalsis in some individuals, increased peristalsis is not the cause of rectal prolapse. Lying down after a meal would decrease the effectiveness of the gastrocolic reflex in moving the stool into the rectum and stimulating the urge to defecate.

20. (4) Each rectal prolapse further weakens perineal and sphincter muscles and predisposes to subsequent prolapse. To avoid expensive and stressful trips to the emergency room or physician's office for reduction of rectal prolapse, the patient should assume the knee-chest position with a moist cloth over the protruding bowel. The forward fall of abdominal viscera in this position will often result in reduction of the prolapse. A hot sitz bath would cause increased engorgement of the extruded bowel, making it more difficult to reduce. Extreme cold would cause vasoconstriction, interfering with blood supply to the bowel wall. The patient should not try to forcibly replace the extruded bowel because of the possibility of perforating the traumatized bowel wall.

21. (4) Metabolism of neural tissue amines, such as serotonin and norepinephrine, has been reported as abnormal in selected areas of the brain in persons who are depressed. For this reason, monoamine oxidase (MAO) inhibitors, isocarboxazid and tranylcypromine sulfate (Marplan and Parnate), have been used in the treatment of depression.

22. (1) The nurse-patient interpersonal relationship is formed with 2 main objectives: (1) to allow expression of anger and feelings of defeat and (2) to improve self esteem. Depressed patients do not function well in a stress-filled environment. Selected routines must be altered to accommodate the patient while ensuring proper physical care (drinking, eating, grooming, and eliminating). Therefore, rigid insistence, humble entreaty, and gentle bantering are not useful. An attitude of firm kindness perhaps suggests that the nurse is strong enough to tolerate expressions of anger and loving enough to accept the patient who has hostile feelings.

23. (3) Depressed patients most frequently attempt suicide when they experience abatement of their depression. An episode of what may be termed "elation" should be viewed as a "red flag." This type of change may be an indication that decisions have been made to attempt suicide and a method to this end outlined.

24. (4) Feeling humble is not considered part of a positive self concept, although humility does allow the individual to make a more bearable impact on others than does arrogance.

25. (4) Nursing interventions are planned to meet patients' needs and to encourage as much learning and independence as possible. Associating the identified need with the need gratifier (e.g., need for warmth with provision of a sweater) is therapeutic.

26. (3) The pregnant diabetic patient should be informed that repeated hospital admissions may be required to regulate her diabetic condition, determine the status of the fetus, and decide the mode of delivery. In addition, Susan would also need to be hospitalized for treatment of any infections that develop during pregnancy. The diabetic patient's insulin requirements generally do not change during the 1st trimester, although they may increase during the 2nd and 3rd trimesters. Excessive fetal size is the result of fetal hyperglycemia and excessive insulin production by the fetal pancreas.

27. (2) An oral glucose tolerance test should be used to determine the degree of her diabetic control, as the test is a more reliable index of insulin-carbohydrate balance than is the fasting blood glucose determination. There is insufficient evidence at this point to warrant either a decrease in caloric intake (caloric intake should not be markedly reduced for fear of causing ketoacidosis) or an increase in insulin dosage.

28. (3) The primary concern arising from Susan's nausea and vomiting is the possibility that ketoacidosis may develop, which would be harmful to both mother and baby (ketonemia can cause irreversible central nervous damage in the fetus). Ketoacidosis during the period of organogenesis (4th to 8th weeks of gestation) would be more apt to cause congenital anomalies than ketoacidosis at 18 weeks of gestation. Susan has demonstrated no evidence of abortion, such as bleeding or cramping.

29. (1) Women with diabetes of long standing tend to have irregular menstrual cycles, which makes calculation of expected dates of confinement more difficult than for non-diabetic women. Since in older diabetics and in diabetics of long standing the fetus is at increased risk during the later weeks of gestation, planned delivery of the infant of a diabetic mother during the 37th week of gestation is a fairly common practice.

30. (4) In general, infants of diabetic mothers tend to be larger than normal because during late pregnancy, high levels of maternal blood glucose cause fetal hyperglycemia, which in turn stimulates the fetal pancreas to produce insulin. This excess fetal insulin acts as a growth hormone to the fetus. The combination of fetal hyperglycemia and fetal hyperinsulinism causes macrosomatia. However, infants of mothers whose diabetes is of long standing may be smaller than normal, as a result of atherosclerosis of placental vessels and resulting fetal malnutrition.

31. (4) Missing limbs are not typical congenital anomalies found in infants of diabetic mothers. However, central nervous system anomalies, such as anencephaly, microcephaly, and hydrocephaly; caudal regression syndrome, with sacral agenesis, shortened limbs, and hip deformity; and congenital heart defects may occur in infants of diabetic mothers if episodes of hyperglycemia and ketonemia occur during the period of fetal organogenesis (between the 4th and 8th week of intrauterine life).

32. (1) At delivery the infant is suddenly cut off from the high blood glucose supplied by the maternal circulation. If the mother was given increased insulin dosage during labor and delivery, some of that insulin, as well as insulin produced by the fetal pancreas in response to maternal hyperglycemia, would tend to produce infant hypoglycemia. Severe or persistent hypoglycemia in an infant would produce irreversible brain damage.

33. (1) Hypoglycemia is most apt to occur in the infant of a diabetic mother between 1 and 3 hours after birth. The high level of glucose in the infant's blood at the time the cord is cut falls rapidly as a result of the high metabolic rate of the newborn infant and the fact that his pancreas tends to overproduce insulin for several hours.

34. (2) A blood glucose level below 30 mg/dl during the 1st 72 hours of the infant's life and below 45 mg/dl after the 1st 3 days of life is diagnosed as hypoglycemia.

35. (4) "Early" hypocalcemia, or hypocalcemia in the 1st 2 postnatal days, is apt to occur in the preterm infant of a diabetic mother, perhaps as a result of parathyroid dysfunction associated with another endocrine imbalance. Symptoms of hypocalcemia include muscular twitching, tremors, and respiratory stridor.

36. (1) One of the most serious complications of diverticulitis is bowel perforation and peritonitis, which would result in shock and intestinal paralysis, with decreased blood pressure and lack of bowel sounds. Excessive flatus is a common symptom of diverticulosis. Black tarry stool indicates bleeding high in the gastrointestinal tract rather than bleeding low in the tract.

37. (1) Since the patient with diverticular disease frequently also suffers irritable bowel syndrome, and inflammation of the diverticula makes the bowel wall extremely friable, cleansing enemas should be gently administered to prevent bowel perforation. Preoperative skin preparation and fluid restriction would be the same as for any abdominal surgery. Since Mrs. West's colostomy will be temporary, there is less need to inform her of long-term life style changes.

38. (3) Since the bowel lacks sensory end organs, there will be no pain associated with cauterization of the bowel loop, but an odor of burning tissue will be present. Increased ventilation of the room will be needed to minimize or eliminate the odor. Deliberately blocking the patient's view of the procedure may increase anxiety, and unnecessary chatter may distract the surgeon and irritate the patient.

39. (4) Although there is still some controversy regarding the matter, most authorities believe that a high fiber diet, by increasing stool bulk, facilitates flow of feces through the bowel and discourages collection of feces in diverticula. A mechanically bland diet would contain little or no fiber, as would a low residue diet.

40. (4) Since diverticula are most apt to develop at those points where blood vessels traverse the bowel wall, diverticulitis may cause erosion of these vessels and hemorrhage, which can be massive and fatal. Therefore, the patient should notify her physician on seeing blood in the stool. Bowel irregularity, with either constipation or diarrhea, is characteristic of diverticulosis, and the patient should use a stool softener and high bulk diet to prevent constipation. Repeated bowel inflammation with healing and scarring often causes stenosis of the sigmoid colon, with narrow or ribbon-like stools.

41. (2) The first priority in the treatment of any emergency condition is establishment of an open airway, since hypoxia resulting from an obstructed airway will cause brain death in 3 to 5 minutes. To open a clogged airway it may be necessary to pull the jaw and tongue forward and insert a finger into the mouth to remove foreign material. When the airway has been cleared and respirations established, attention should be turned to circulatory function. The patient should be examined for heart rate, rhythm, and force, and evidence of hemorrhage (which should be controlled with direct pressure). When respiration and circulation have been restored, the patient should be examined for fracture and dislocation. All of these factors should be evaluated before attempting to move the patient.

42. (4) Any patient suffering head injury during a motor vehicle accident should be assumed to have a cervical spine injury as well as some degree of brain damage until both types of injuries have been ruled out. The lack of forehead indentation does not rule out the possibility of a linear skull fracture in the frontal or in other regions of the skull. In the case of either epidural (arterial) or subdural (venous) bleeding, hours and days, respectively, may elapse between the injury and symptoms of increased intracranial pressure, with cerebral herniation through the tentorium and evidence of 3rd nerve damage, such as pupillary dilation and fixation. Moving the patient with a cervical spine fracture could cause immediate cord transection and render an incomplete spinal cord injury a complete injury.

43. (4) Following a motor vehicle accident, the patient with a head injury should be assumed to have a cervical spine injury until proved otherwise. Since even slight movement can dislocate a cervical fracture and cause cord transection, the patient's head, neck, and trunk should be immobilized before removing him from the driver's seat.

44. (4) Both the police and the emergency medical technician would have obtained information about the time and circumstances of the accident in order to carry out their primary job responsibilities. The medical technician will have questioned the nurse and other bystanders as to whether the victim was unconscious after the accident and the type of care given the victim before the ambulance arrived during their assessment of the patient's condition. Since all these factors will influence the patient's condition and his response to treatment, the admitting nurse should record such information for later use by the medical team. Since the patient was dazed and was alone in the car, the medical technician will probably have no information about the patient's underlying health conditions other than that on a Medic Alert tag or wallet card, if either exists.

45. (2) Post-concussion syndrome includes severe headache, dizziness, vertigo, and fatigue, so these symptoms would be expected for several days or weeks following a blow to the head. It is also possible that a bruise might appear on Mr. Cohn's forehead, as a result of his head's having struck the windshield on impact. However, increasing lethargy is a common symptom of increasing intracranial pressure, which could result from a subdural hematoma and could lead to coma and death. The patient with lethargy should be returned to the physician or to the emergency room for follow-up care.

46. (4) Though his relationship with his mother may be important when discharge planning is begun, and his nutritional status and ability to care for himself are important in designing a care plan for Paul, it is imperative for the nurse to assess him for his potential for violence toward himself, other patients, or the staff. Safety for all is of the utmost importance!

47. (3) Maximum interaction with other patients would only serve to frighten Paul and maintain his present behavior. He would probably need to retreat to his room in order to decrease the stimuli of the new environment. An interpersonal relationship with a schizophrenic person is developed slowly over a period of time because the patient is withdrawn, distrustful, and communicates symbolically.

48. (4) Auditory hallucinations mean that the patient hears voices that do not exist externally or result from external stimuli but rather arise from internal stimuli. Hallucinations are projected conflicts and, as such, contain an element of frustration and anxiety.

49. (3) Delusions, such as ideas of reference, overcompensate for feelings of isolation through fantasies of being the focus of universal attention (hence, his reference to the President of the United States).

50. (2) It is important for Paul to work with his nurse and establish what he (with appropriate professional input) sees as important personal goals during hospitalization. Issues such as leaving the hospital, where he will be going, and medication compliance should be raised during termination sessions before discharge. Discussion of family system may be asking him to utilize insight that few schizophrenics possess.

51. (3) The eustachian tubes of children are more likely to open inappropriately because the cartilage lining in the tubes is undeveloped.

52. (4) Otitis media and involvement of the middle ear does not cause increased intracranial pressure and bulging fontanelle.

53. (4) Temperature of up to 104° F can be expected in acute suppurative otitis media.

54. (1) The fluid in the middle ear may be gluelike and so viscous and tenacious that even with a patent eustachian tube, the fluid remains in the middle ear.

55. (4) In a normal tympanic membrane, the light reflex is cone shaped and is located in the anterior-inferior quadrant.

56. (3) Leukemia is a complex disease with numerous cell types at varying levels of maturity; there is still much confusion and inconsistency in classifying leukemias.

57. (4) In the leukemic process, immature cells reproduce to such an extent that all other white blood cell forms are deprived of nutrients and crowded out.

58. (4) Infiltration of the marrow by immature blood cells prevents normal development of red blood cells, thrombocytes, and granulocytic white blood cells; therefore, anemia, bleeding tendencies and increased susceptibility to infection result. There is no increase in iron deposition in the liver because red blood cells are not destroyed in greater numbers.

59. (3) Since the child's immune system is depressed, administration of virus, even though attenuated, can cause overwhelming disease.

60. (3) The liver detoxifies and the kidneys excrete the powerful antileukemic drugs, and it is essential for successful treatment that both organs function normally.

61. (2) Because hypothyroidism is characterized by hypercholesterolemia, patients with long-standing thyroid hypofunction are predisposed to coronary arteriosclerosis. Therefore, Lee should be questioned and examined for evidence of coronary insufficiency and congestive heart failure. Lethargy and personality changes occur in hypothyroidism, but tremor (which occurs in hyperthyroidism) and ataxia do not. Constipation, rather than diarrhea, is characteristic of hypothyroidism. Urinary frequency and urgency do not result from thyroid hypofunction, but urinary output can be expected to increase following thyroid replacement therapy owing to elimination of edema fluid.

62. (3) Since lowered metabolic rate is associated with decreased peristalsis, constipation is common in hypothyroidism. Therefore, a high fiber diet with high fluid intake, stool softeners, and daily exercise are needed to prevent constipation and fecal impaction. A low calorie diet is recommended because weight gain is typical in hypothyroidism. The myxedema of hypothyroidism is not the result of hypernatremia, therefore sodium need not be restricted.

63. (4) Since lack of thyroid hormone increases serum cholesterol levels, atherosclerosis and arteriosclerosis are frequently associated with myxedema. Thyroid hormone replacement therapy is begun slowly in myxedema because the hormone increases the rate of cellular metabolism and cellular O_2 demand, thereby increasing cardiac workload. The heart must be given time to adjust to this greater workload. If severe coronary arteriosclerosis exists, the patient may experience angina, which would indicate that the dose of sodium levothyroxine (Synthroid) should be decreased for a time and then slowly increased until euthyroid level is achieved.

64. (3) Because administration of thyroxine facilitates removal of gelled fluid from interstitial spaces, diuresis develops after 2 to 3 days of Synthroid therapy. Although increased physical and mental activity are expected following several days of Synthroid therapy, a decrease, rather than an increase of fatigue should accompany rising serum levels of T_4 and T_3. While it is expected that appetite will increase as the patient returns to the euthyroid state, weight loss—due to diuresis and greater activity—rather than weight gain is expected. While a return to normal levels of physical and mental activity should follow Synthroid administration, nervousness and irritability would indicate too high a dosage of the drug, rather than an expected treatment result.

65. (1) Thyroid hormones interact significantly with other drugs, such as insulin, oral hypoglycemic medications, phenytoin, tricyclic antidepressants, digitalis, and anticoagulants. Failure of the myxedematous patient to take exogenous thyroxine could lead to myxedema coma, a life-threatening emergency. Therefore, Mrs. Perry should wear a Medic Alert tag that indicates she is hypothyroid and specifies her daily dose of Synthroid, in the event that she is injured or critically ill and cannot inform caregivers of her long-term medical problems. Unless Mrs. Perry is found to have concomitant cardiovascular or gastrointestinal disease, there will be no need to restrict fluids, fiber, or exercise after she has achieved euthyroid state.

66. (3) Deposition of uric acid crystals in renal tubules can cause chronic renal failure. Failure of the kidney to remove nitrogenous wastes from the blood results in gradual elevation of serum creatinine (normal level of 1.2 to 1.5 ml/dl). Elevation of the white blood cell count (normal is 5000 to 10,000/mm^3) is a manifestation of the joint inflammation produced by deposition of urate crystals, but the white blood cell count can be expected to return to normal following resolution of the acute arthritic episode. The slight increase in Mr. Pine's hematocrit value (normal is 41 to 53%) and slight elevation of serum glucose level (normal is 70 to 110 mg/dl) may indicate dehydration but do not suggest the complication of gout.

67. (2) During an acute attack of gout, the involved joint is so exquisitely painful that a slight jarring of the bed or the weight of the bed linen on the foot is unbearable. Therefore, a bed cradle should be used to support the upper bed linen. Neither elevation of the foot nor leg abduction would decrease the pain.

68. (1) Although the action of colchicine is not understood, it relieves the pain of gouty arthritis without reducing the level of serum uric acid. Toxic symptoms of the drug result from gastrointestinal irritation and include nausea, vomiting, diarrhea, and abdominal

pain. Usually symptoms of the acute attack have significantly lessened by the time that such toxic symptoms develop (after 12 to 24 hours of drug therapy).

69. (2) Urolithiasis may occur in patients with gout as a result of increased urinary uric acid excretion. To prevent urinary stone formation, fluid intake should be from 2000 to 3000 ml/day. Although exercise fosters weight reduction, which will decrease joint trauma in the obese individual, exercise per se will not prevent complications of gout. Although acute infection may precipitate an attack of gout, immunization against pneumonia and influenza will not prevent complications of gout. Highly spiced foods would have no effect on blood uric acid levels or urinary excretion of uric acid.

70. (4) Because probenecid competes with several drugs for the same tubular excretory mechanism, it can interfere with renal excretion of these drugs and potentiate their effects. This potentiating effect occurs with penicillin, sulfonamides, and indomethacin, but not with digitalis.

71. (4) Separation-individuation issues do not surface in the admission data. Her refusal to eat, her compulsive activity, and her possible distortion of body image ("I would rather be a boy.") are all addressed in the admission data.

72. (1) Nursing staff should not be caught up in the manipulative behavior of the anorexic. All food is to be eaten (adaptive behavior), her excessive physical activity (maladaptive behavior) is to cease, and activities that provide interaction with others (off the unit privileges) are to be encouraged.

73. (1) Lack of interest in school and social withdrawal are usually the first hint to the parent of an adolescent that something is wrong.

74. (1) The nursing care plan would be built around a daily program of behavior modification. Healthy, adaptive behaviors would be rewarded, and non-healthy, maladaptive behaviors would be ignored or penalized.

75. (3) Increased food intake, decreased physical activity done for the purpose of losing weight or prohibiting weight gain, and appropriate initiation of interpersonal interactions are the hoped for outcomes of Patti's hospitalization. The desire is that the healthy behavior will generalize to the home and college environment.

76. (3) A child with chronic illness should be encouraged to maintain a life style that is as normal as possible for his age, such as attending school regularly and doing his share of chores at home. Since infection with resultant increase in metabolism predisposes to sickling crisis, any infection, however minimal, should receive medical attention. A vegetarian diet, which eliminates animal sources of protein, would deprive the child of nutrients needed for growth.

77. (4) Sickling results from deoxygenation and hemoconcentration. Diet and food ingestion have not been identified as causative factors for sickling.

78. (2) There is no cure for sickle cell anemia, so in all probability, he will continue to have these crises. The occurrence of sickling is not related to the age of the patient.

79. (4) Sickledex and blood smear are unreliable or give incomplete results. Electrophoresis provides an accurate definitive picture of the hemoglobin. Mantoux's test is used to identify sensitivity to chemical products of the tuberculosis mycobacterium.

80. (4) Adolescents come to see themselves as distinct individuals after going through preliminary endeavors for identification. The first 3 tasks listed are all tasks that should have been resolved during the middle and late school-age period.

81. (3) In Addison's disease, normal responses to stress are lacking. Infection can precipitate addisonian crisis or hypotensive crisis, which is life threatening. Therefore, the patient with Addison's disease should be protected from contact with visitors or staff members with acute infectious diseases. Since the patient with Addison's disease is anorexic, gifts of food and drink should not be discouraged. By cautioning visitors to avoid upsetting topics and to visit for only brief periods, the nurse can protect Mr. Kent from avoidable emotional upset and fatigue without depriving him of needed support from significant others.

82. (1) Fludrocortisone, a synthetic mineralocorticoid, is given to decrease urinary excretion of sodium, which in turn will conserve body water and increase intravascular fluid vol-

ume. Until this effect is realized, Mr. Kent should increase fluid intake to compensate for previous fluid losses and to increase circulating blood volume and increase blood pressure. Although Mr. Kent is weak and easily fatigued, he need not be confined to bed: he should be supervised when changing position and ambulating, as he is subject to orthostatic hypotension. Until hormone replacement has returned Mr. Kent to normal adrenal functioning, he should be encouraged to rest, and an hourly stir-up regimen would be contraindicated. Mr. Kent is hyponatremic, and sodium must be administered in liberal quantities to correct extracellular fluid depletion.

83. (2) Both hydrocortisone and fludrocortisone will cause sodium and fluid retention and increased potassium excretion, so a steady increase in body weight and a decrease in serum potassium level would indicate the expected result of drug therapy. In Addison's disease, the temperature is subnormal and pulse rate is slow and weak, so with correction of adrenal cortex hypofunction, body temperature should increase to normal and the pulse rate should increase.

84. (2) Profuse diaphoresis and diarrhea cause marked losses of fluid and sodium ion. In the normal individual, there is markedly increased secretion of adrenocorticoid in response to stress, such as infection. Since the patient with Addison's disease cannot increase endogenous supplies of adrenocortical hormones, the doses of exogenous hydrocortisone and fludrocortisone must be increased during acute infection, extremely hot weather, and other similar stresses. Mr. Kent's laboratory test results would indicate that the adrenal cortex insufficiency is a permanent rather than a temporary condition. Since his diagnosis was primary rather than secondary adrenal cortical insufficiency, there is no reason to expect additional endocrine diseases in the future. Androgen replacement is not needed in Addison's disease because androgen is produced by the testes as well as by the adrenal cortex.

85. (4) The patient with Addison's disease should wear a Medic Alert tag indicating diagnosis, physician's name and telephone number, and the following instruction: "I have adrenal insufficiency. In the event of injury, vomiting, or unconsciousness, the hydrocortisone in my pocket (or case) should be injected under my skin, and a physician should be notified." Although the blood glucose level may fall in addisonian crisis, adrenocorticoid hormone rather than oral glucose should be given to correct the condition. Shock, rather than convulsion, is the expected consequence of addisonian crisis.

86. (3) Repeated phlebotomy, with removal of 500 ml of blood on each occasion until the hematocrit value is reduced to 50% or less, will reduce the danger from hypervolemia and hyperviscosity. Immediately following phlebotomy the patient's blood pressure should be checked, and he should be directed to sit up for several minutes before attempting to walk, since orthostatic hypotension frequently develops, and the patient is at risk of falling. Rather than withholding fluid, the patient should be encouraged to drink 500 to 750 ml of water or juice after phlebotomy to restore fluid loss and decrease blood viscosity. The venipuncture wound should be cleaned with antiseptic and covered with a Band-Aid, and Betadine ointment and an occlusive dressing would be unnecessary. There is no reason that blood pressure cannot later be measured in the phlebotomized extremity.

87. (4) Hyperviscosity of the blood in polycythemia predisposes to deep vein thrombosis. Gout may result from overproduction of uric acid associated with breakdown of increased numbers of blood cells per unit of time. Congestive heart failure may result from increased blood volume and hypertension. Diabetes mellitus is not an expected consequence of polycythemia.

88. (2) The patient with polycythemia often suffers severe pruritus due to increased histamine released by excessive granulocyte turnover. Since the pruritus is accentuated by a hot bath and shower, both should be avoided. Although hepatomegaly and splenomegaly are common in polycythemia, there is no reason for the patient to avoid the side-lying position. Forcible foot dorsiflexion may be needed to test for deep vein thrombosis in the lower extremity. If the patient is troubled with headache due to hypervolemia and hypertension, he may be more comfortable with the head of the bed elevated.

89. (4) It is thought that ^{32}P and the chemotherapeutic drugs that will decrease red blood cell formation in primary polycythemia (bisulfan and chlorambucil) may all cause leukemia, so the drugs are used sparingly in treating primary polycythemia. Repeated phlebotomies at 2- to 4-week intervals are used to keep the hematocrit value below 50%.

90. (1) In polycythemia, increased blood viscosity predisposes to intravascular clotting. In order to prevent thrombus formation, Mr. Dwyer should be instructed to remain as physically active as possible, to increase daily fluid intake, and to move about and change position frequently while in bed. Increased protein and iron intake are not needed, as the rate of red blood cell formation is already greater than normal.

91. (3) Behavior therapy is short term, problem oriented, and has a good success rate for these types of disorders. Mr. Williams should be able to drive to work 8 to 10 weeks after therapy is started, with no recurrence of symptoms.

92. (3) Mr. Williams will need to move from the *least* threatening open space to other open spaces as he can tolerate it. The nurse must carefully assess his physical and emotional reactions to these outings.

93. (4) If he is to learn new behavior it would be non-therapeutic to encourage him to ignore the maladaptive behavior he is using. He needs to explore what does not work in a healthy way for him before he can begin to eliminate those behaviors and replace them with adaptive, healthy responses.

94. (4) Of primary importance is his physical and emotional response to being off the unit. If the outing is not well tolerated, a less threatening excursion will be planned for the next time. If this one was non-threatening, and the patient did not experience overwhelming physical and emotional symptoms, an outside experience of greater sophistication can be implemented for the next time.

95. (3) Recent research points to a possible physical etiology for panic disorders (and possibly other anxiety neuroses). Behavior modification theory states that once a symptom is "cured" it will not return nor will it be replaced by some other maladaptive behavior.

Section 4

COMPREHENSIVE EXAMINATION: ANSWERS AND RATIONALES

1. (1) Vaginal bleeding is a symptom of several complications of pregnancy (among them spontaneous abortion, placenta pravia, and abruptio placentae). Pain is associated with bleeding in abruptio placentae, and since this complication is a severe threat to both mother and child, the nurse should determine whether Judy's bleeding is associated with pain in order to establish the probable reason for bleeding. The other questions would not elicit information that could differentiate among the usual reasons for hemorrhage.

2. (3) Since massive blood loss would decrease maternal blood volume and threaten fetal welfare, the nurse should auscultate fetal heart tones and notify the physician of the condition of the fetus before taking a history, examining the patient, palpating the uterus for tone, and performing Leopold's maneuvers.

3. (2) Manipulation of the lower uterine segment may cause profound hemorrhage in the patient with placenta pravia. Therefore, until the patient has been typed and cross matched and blood has been obtained for transfusion, a vaginal examination should not be performed.

4. (3) The double setup is advisable so that either a vaginal delivery or a cesarean delivery can be performed if profuse bleeding is provoked during the vaginal examination. An operating room that is equipped for cesarean delivery would be preferred to the delivery room for the double setup.

5. (3) In threatened abortion the patient in early pregnancy demonstrates vaginal spotting or bleeding, with mild cramping. At this point there is no cervical dilation or passage of tissue. In threatened abortion it is assumed that the process of interrupting pregnancy has begun but that the process may abate with appropriate patient management.

6. (1) Gastric secretions are composed predominantly of sodium, hydrogen, and chloride ions and acidic substances. Excessive vomiting, loss of hydrogen ions, and conservation of bicarbonate ions lead to increased production of sodium bicarbonate. This increase in the buffer base constitutes metabolic alkalosis.

7. (3) Electrolyte balance along with fluid balance is critical because the rate of fluid exchange in the infant is 7 times greater than that of the adult. Because of this rapid exchange and the general immaturity of his systems, Tony is prone to rapidly become acidotic or alkalotic.

8. (1) The normal range of serum sodium level for an infant is 139 to 146 mmol/L and serum chloride level is 98 to 106 mmol/L.

9. (4) Pyloromyotomy is a relatively simple, elective surgical procedure in which an incision is made through the circular muscle fibers of the pylorus down to the submucosa. Therefore, as soon as clear liquids are retained approximately 24 hours post-operatively, formula can be started. The infant is placed on his right side after feedings in order to facilitate emptying of the stomach; the infant's head is elevated slightly to minimize the likelihood of vomiting.

10. (3) A normal infant should be able to hold his head up 45 degrees while lying on his stom-

ach at approximately 2 months. The normal infant is able to roll over at around 4 to 4½ months of age, reaches out for his favorite toy at 4½ to 5 months, and feeds himself a cracker at 5 to 8 months of age.

11. (2) Carbamazepine (Tegretol) is an anticonvulsant that relieves the pain of trigeminal neuralgia by decreasing synaptic transmission within the trigeminal nucleus. It may cause marrow depression with anemia, decreased resistance to infection, and bleeding tendencies. Phenytoin, another drug that is sometimes used to relieve trigeminal neuralgia, causes gingival hypertrophy. Neither tinnitus nor diarrhea is an expected effect of carbamazepine.

12. (4) Pain paroxysms are initiated by skin stimuli over certain trigger points, often the alae nasae, lip, chin, or teeth. Simple touch, pressure, or a cold draft over the trigger point is enough to provoke the pain. Talking or chewing will initiate pain episodes in some patients, and these patients will avoid talking or eating during clusters of these episodes in order to avoid pain, but the nurse should not discourage the patient's eating and talking. Because the pain of trigeminal neuralgia is severe and prolonged, there is some danger of habituation to analgesics. The patient should take such drugs to relieve, not prevent facial pain.

13. (3) Many patients with trigeminal neuralgia are as incapacitated by fear of pain as by the pain episodes themselves. Some patients remain indoors to avoid drafts, withdraw from social intercourse to avoid talking, and lose weight because they avoid eating. The patient should be encouraged to continue all normal activities between attacks and to shun adoption of the sick and disabled role. Trigeminal neuralgia is too uncommon a disorder to attract quacks and bogus remedies. Attacks are initiated by physical stimuli to trigger points rather than by respiratory infection or emotional stress.

14. (2) Brushing the teeth triggers trigeminal neuralgia in some patients, so cotton tipped applicators with a tepid mouthwash should be used to cleanse the mouth of bacteria and debris with a minimum of mechanical stimulation. During periods of frequent attacks the patient may avoid bathing and washing the face at all, so she may need encouragement to carry out even minimal self care activities.

15. (3) Although percutaneous radiofrequency gangliolysis (electrocoagulation of the nerve) is intended only to destroy small pain fibers and to leave the fibers that convey touch sensation intact, incorrect placement of the needle or use of excessive current may destroy touch fibers as well. Therefore, the patient must be tested for sensory deficits so that she can be taught how to protect herself from injury in the event of sensory loss.

16. (4) Since air is sucked through the wound into the pleural space with each descent of the diaphragm, the wound should be sealed immediately to prevent pneumothorax, which can cause collapse of underlying lung tissue and, if massive, mediastinal shift and collapse of the opposite lung. After the wound has been sealed, the patient should be examined thoroughly for evidence of additional wounds. A central venous line should be inserted to obtain blood for typing and cross matching, to monitor the patient for hypovolemia, and to administer intravenous fluids or blood as necessary. The emergency medical technician, police, or accompanying relatives may be able to give information about the caliber of the bullet.

17. (2) Since massive blood loss, pneumothorax, and hemothorax are common following penetrating chest wounds, and since the bullet may have caused injury to the heart and blood vessels as well as to the lung, asphyxia, atelectasis, cardiac tamponade, shock, and heart failure may develop quickly following Marie's injury. Her airway, breathing, and circulation should be assessed so that cardiopulmonary resuscitation can be promptly initiated if respiration or circulation are inadequate to sustain life. A thoracotomy set and water seal–type drainage equipment should be obtained as either or both will be necessary after emergency care has been completed. Greater ventilatory efficiency is possible in the semi-sitting position than in the side-lying position. After chest tubes have been inserted and x-rays have been taken, surgery may be necessary to explore and repair tissue damage caused by the bullet. Eventually, an indwelling catheter and a nasogastric tube should be inserted, but cardiopulmonary assessment and resuscitation have higher priority immediately following Marie's admission to the emergency room.

18. (3) Tension pneumothorax, or accumulation of an increasingly large amount of air in the left pleural space, causes mediastinal structures to shift to the right, so the trachea will be found to deviate to the right when palpated above the suprasternal notch. Observing the degree of movement of the outstretched hands along the lower anterior costal margin would enable the nurse to evaluate chest expansion not mediastinal shift. Identifying the cardiac outline by percussion might give some indication of mediastinal shift, but since heart size and location can be altered by several factors, such information is less useful than evidence of tracheal deviation. The aortic component of the second heart sound normally is heard best in the second right intercostal space along the sternal border.

19. (2) Percussion over an area of pneumothorax yields hyperresonance as a result of the increased air below the plexor finger. Crepitant rales indicate inflammation or congestion of alveoli. Dullness to percussion throughout the lower half of a hemithorax would suggest pleural effusion or hemothorax. "Splitting" of the second cardiac sound, or separation in time of the aortic and pulmonary valve closure, may occur in right bundle branch block and atrial septal defect.

20. (1) The purpose of closed chest drainage is to foster removal of fluid and air from the pleural space during inspiration and to prevent reflux of air or fluid into the pleural space during expiration—thus promoting lung expansion. For the system to work, the glass tube to which the chest catheter is attached must be submerged below the level of liquid in the bottle (water seal), and all connections between catheter, glass tubing, stopper, and bottle must be secured. Marie should be encouraged to deep breathe and cough at frequent intervals to clear the bronchi of secretions and foster lung expansion by forcing air and fluid from the pleural space into the drainage bottle.

21. (3) The conflict area, according to psychoanalytic theory, is resolved by getting sick. The paralyzed arm reduces the anxiety since her fears can no longer be realized.

22. (2) The symptom Rita displays is an unconscious defense mechanism, yet typically the patient with a conversion disorder displays no concern or worry over the dysfunction.

23. (3) The symptom is unconscious, therefore she has no insight into her problem. The symptom serves as a coping mechanism to deal with her stress and anxiety.

24. (3) Since the limb has no organic disease process causing the paralysis, and the arm can be (and probably is) moved when she is unaware, there will be no wasting away.

25. (3) According to Freud, this defense mechanism is operating at an unconscious level.

26. (3) The pregnant uterus compresses pelvic veins, impairing venous return flow to the heart and predisposing to development of varicose veins in the lower extremities. Following major surgery, patients are at risk of hypercoagulability as a result of dehydration and hypovolemic hypotension. Therefore, following cesarean birth, the mother should be checked for signs of thrombophlebitis, among which is a positive Homans' sign that consists of calf pain on dorsiflexion of the foot.

27. (2) Methylergonovine has a vasoconstrictor effect and can cause sudden hypertension if given to a hypertensive patient or a patient with extremely labile blood pressure. Therefore, the drug should not be administered to a patient with a history of pre-eclampsia or eclampsia (pregnancy induced hypertension).

28. (1) The physiological stress of cesarean delivery tends to focus the mother's attention on her own pain and discomfort for a longer period following delivery than a mother who delivers vaginally. The intensive recovery room care required by the mother who undergoes cesarean delivery also delays mother to infant contact, further impeding bonding. Therefore, as soon as the mother feels well enough, the nurse should arrange for the mother to hold and examine her infant, so as to support early and strong emotional bonding between the two.

29. (2) Since the feeding situation provides the basis for the mother-to-child relationship, considerable effort should be directed toward making the feeding experience as pleasant as possible for both. Since pain, fear, and fatigue tend to interfere with the let-down reflex, breast-feeding will be more successful if the mother is comfortable during the procedure. Therefore, the mother should be encouraged to experiment with different positions in order to maximize her own and the infant's pleasure in the situation.

30. (3) Many mothers who undergo cesarean delivery view the inability to deliver their infants vaginally as inadequate maternal role performance. Since impaired self concept would interfere with performance of desired maternal behaviors, the nurse should encourage the mother to explore her feelings about her cesarean delivery. A non-directive interviewing technique would encourage ventilation of feelings, while empty reassurances would inhibit such expression.

31. (3) Clinical manifestations of cerebellar invasion include hypotonia. With increased intracranial pressure, any of the cranial nerves may be involved. After closure of cranial sutures, there is no enlargement of head circumference. Ordinarily there is no edema at this stage of brain tumor development.

32. (2) A lumbar puncture may be done post-operatively to analyze spinal fluid for tumor cells. Generally, pre-operative symptoms such as headaches and neuromuscular symptoms subside after surgery, but in some cases these symptoms are aggravated by surgery. Usually the entire scalp is covered after a craniotomy with a pressure dressing. Ordinarily the child is returned to intensive care for several days or until the child's condition stabilizes.

33. (3) A child between the ages of 2 and 4 years is in the preconceptual or prelogical phase; she is totally incapable of abstraction at this stage. According to Piaget, at this age, the child lacks the concept of conservation or the realization that an object can be changed and brought back to its original shape or condition. In addition, preschoolers judge what they see by the immediate visual clues given them. Therefore, by wrapping a doll's scalp the nurse can give the preschooler concrete and visual clues about her post-operative dressing.

34. (2) Because of post-operative cerebral edema and danger of increased intracranial pressure, fluids are carefully monitored.

35. (4) A lumbar puncture, or insertion of a needle into the subarachnoid space of the spinal cord in the lumbar region, is usually performed following removal of a brain tumor in order to obtain a sample of cerebrospinal fluid to be analyzed for the presence of tumor cells. The procedure, although it is performed under sterile conditions, need not be performed in an operating room and would not be repeated several days in a row. Intrathecal injection of antibiotics would not be performed as a prophylaxis against central nervous system infection.

36. (2) Inadequate treatment of acute suppurative otitis media leads to chronic suppurative otitis media, with tympanic scarring, hearing loss, and cholesteatoma; therefore, the full course of ordered antibiotic should be taken to ensure destruction of all pathogens in the middle ear. Although sterile cotton can be placed loosely in the external auditory canal to absorb drainage, care must be taken not to obstruct the flow of purulent exudate. The canal should not be irrigated, as the irrigating solution would carry purulent material back into the middle ear. Since forceful nose blowing is probably responsible for driving contaminated nasal secretions into the middle ear in the first place, nose blowing should be discouraged.

37. (2) Since forceful expiration while holding the nostrils closed inflates the eustachian tube, this maneuver should be performed several times a day to open the tube and facilitate drainage of secretions from the middle ear. Cotton tipped applicators should never be inserted into the external auditory canal, particularly not in this case, since the tympanic membrane has been ruptured. Warm oil should not be dropped into the external auditory canal because the tympanic membrane is ruptured, and the oil could enter the middle ear. There is no need to keep the head inclined to the right. The pseudoephedrine and Valsalva's maneuver will facilitate drainage of secretions from the ear.

38. (4) Increased pain, hearing loss, and vertigo may indicate pus under pressure in the middle ear, labyrinthitis, or brain abscess; therefore, Ms. Stott should seek medical follow-up if these symptoms develop after 2 to 3 days of treatment. However, the purulent discharge may drain through the external auditory canal for several days following initiation of therapy if the tympanic membrane has ruptured. The infectious process will cause weakness, fatigue, and anorexia for several days. Organisms and toxins in the purulent exudate may irritate the skin of the external auditory canal and pinna, causing itching.

39. (2) Until the rupture in the tympanic membrane has healed, water could flow into the middle ear while swimming or washing the hair, so Ms. Stott should avoid these activities until given approval by her physician. When she is no longer febrile and troubled with vertigo, Ms. Stott should be able to go out-of-doors if warmly dressed and protected against chilling. There is no reason to avoid sleeping on her right side if she is comfortable in that position. The auricle should be cleaned gently with soap and water, not alcohol, using care to keep water from entering the external auditory canal.

40. (2) Chronic otitis media may lead to suppurative labyrinthitis, with tinnitus, deafness, vertigo, vomiting, and nystagmus. Dry mouth is a manifestation of Sjögren's syndrome. Migraine headache results from initial vasoconstriction, followed by dilation of intracranial and extracranial branches of the external carotid artery. Attacks may be provoked by certain foods, emotional excitement, fatigue, and alcohol.

41. (2) The bone demineralization that occurs in multiple myeloma causes hypercalcemia and hypercalciuria, so the patient is predisposed to renal stone formation. To prevent nephrolithiasis, the patient's daily fluid intake should be 3000 to 4000 ml, and he should be encouraged to remain as active as possible to decrease calcium mobilization from bones. Although the patient is susceptible to infection, good hydration and frequent changes of position should prevent pneumonia without need for postural drainage or reverse isolation.

42. (2) Because multiple myeloma is characterized by infiltration of bone marrow by malignant plasma cells, reduction in normal hematopoietic cells in the marrow may result in decreased numbers of circulating platelets (normal number is 150,000 to 350,000/mm^3). Since Mr. Stern's platelets are considerably reduced, he should be observed closely for bleeding tendencies. Although the osteolytic lesions of multiple myeloma often lead to abnormally high serum calcium levels followed by hypercalciuria and osmotic diuresis, these complications are not evident, as Mr. Stern's serum calcium concentration is in the high normal range (normal is 8.5 to 10.5 mg/dl). Although hypercalciuria may cause renal stones and renal failure, Mr. Stern's urine specific gravity shows no loss of concentrating ability (normal urine specific gravity is 1.010 to 1.020). His fasting serum glucose level is within the low normal range (normal is 70 to 115 mg/dl).

43. (4) As a result of weakness and bone demineralization, Mr. Stern is predisposed to falls and pathological fractures. Therefore, although he should be encouraged to walk, he should be accompanied by a relative or a hospital employee while walking and should use a cane or walker to protect against falls. Convulsions are not an anticipated complication; he is not expected to become disoriented; and itching is not a symptom of multiple myeloma; therefore, a padded tongue blade, a Posey's vest, and cloth mitts will not be needed.

44. (3) To prevent renal stones, urinary infection, pneumonia, and skin breakdown, Mr. Stern should change position frequently following surgery. However, until bony healing is complete, his spine will be unstable; therefore, to prevent further damage to the spinal cord, his spine should be kept in perfect alignment at all times, and log rolling should be used when changing his position.

45. (1) Since pain may prevent Mr. Stern from wholehearted involvement in planned therapies, the ordered analgesic should be given promptly and liberally to control pain. Because multiple myeloma is characterized by anemia and wasting, Mr. Stern's energy level will be low, so he should be encouraged to rest or nap on the nursing unit between therapies rather than to repeat his physiotherapy and occupational therapy exercises. By taking full responsibility for bathing, grooming, and dressing Mr. Stern, the nurse would subvert the purpose of the rehabilitation program. Urging him to match another patient's accomplishments exposes him to the possibility of failure and loss of self esteem.

46. (4) The patient with a simple diagnosis of Alzheimer's disease (uncomplicated by another disorder) would not have any psychotic symptoms such as delusions or hallucinations.

47. (4) Information from the recent past may be forgotten, but the patient does not have an organized delusional system.

48. (2) Insight therapy is not appropriate for Margaret. She is past understanding the whys and wherefores of what has happened to her, and insight would not help her to change her behavior. Her behavior is organic in origin.

49. (4) At this stage in the disease process the nurse can encourage Margaret's social interaction, maintaining contact with the here and now, and caring for herself with appropriate supervision.

50. (4) Death occurs 2 to 10 years after the onset, and the age of onset is early (presenile).

51. (3) The most common cause of meningitis is bacteria reaching the brain from a focus of infection elsewhere.

52. (4) Clinical manifestations depend primarily upon the age of the child, the type of organism, and the effectiveness of therapy for the illness that immediately preceded meningitis. The usual immunization program protects the child against diphtheria, pertussis, tetanus, measles, rubella, mumps, and poliomyelitis.

53. (3) The intracranial pressure triggers the pressor response that elevates the blood pressure.

54. (4) There may be some nuchal rigidity, and lying on her side without a pillow and with head slightly elevated would be most comfortable for her.

55. (2) A definitive diagnosis of the cerebral spinal fluid for meningitis shows elevations of pressure, white blood cell count, and protein concentration, and a reduction of glucose concentration.

56. (4) Bacterial valvular vegetations are friable, so they may break free of the valve surface and embolize into the systemic circulation. Removal of a vegetation from a valvular leaflet alters the dynamics of blood flow through the valve, causing an abnormal heart sound or changing the intensity of a murmur formerly present. Therefore, the nurse should auscultate Jan's heart sounds daily to detect new murmurs or changed murmurs and, when these are found, should examine Jan for conjunctival, palatal, buccal, and extremity petechiae, which would be evidence of such embolization. Increase in body weight and abdominal girth could suggest edema formation if congestive heart failure develops as a complication of endocarditis, but the nurse would probably detect earlier symptoms of failure (tachycardia, dyspnea). Increase in calf circumference would suggest thrombophlebitis rather than a complication of endocarditis.

57. (2) In patients with infectious endocarditis the valvular vegetations are friable, so pieces may be broken off and carried by the circulating blood to the brain, lung, liver, spleen, and extremities. An embolus that obstructs a branch of the middle cerebral artery would cause unilateral weakness. Migraine headache results from dilation of branches of the external carotid artery. Petechiae, rather than skin rash, occur in infectious endocarditis. There would be no reason to expect hematemesis in endocarditis.

58. (1) Congestive heart failure is a complication of bacterial endocarditis and results from valve destruction, allergic vasculitis of the coronary vessels, or emboli blocking coronary arteries. To prevent excessive physical exertion while the infectious organisms are being eradicated, the patient should be occupied with quiet diversionary activities. Unless the patient develops congestive heart failure, there will be no need to maintain the patient in Fowler's position or to limit fluid intake. Unless the patient develops pulmonary infection there will be no need for postural drainage.

59. (4) Since the intravenous infusion site, the intravenous needle, and the tubing may become colonized by bacteria and seed infectious organisms into the circulation, the venipuncture site should be rotated every 3 to 4 days and the intravenous needle and tubing should be changed every 24 to 48 hours to reduce the risk of infection. Temperature measurements every 4 hours are advisable to detect symptoms of continuing or recurrent endocardial infection. Liberal fluid intake is needed to reduce risk of renal infection from circulating microorganisms. Unless the patient is febrile or in congestive heart failure, complete bed rest would be unnecessary.

60. (2) The oropharynx, genitourinary tract, and gastrointestinal tract are common portals of entry for the organisms causing infectious endocarditis. Therefore, prophylactic antibiotic therapy should be given for dental procedures, tonsillectomy, bronchoscopy, catheterization, prostate surgery, gallbladder and colon surgery, as well as for cardiac surgery. Unless the patient develops congestive heart failure, there will be no need to limit physical activity or to sleep with the head elevated. Although persons with upper respiratory infections should be avoided, there is no need to avoid all contact with children.

61. (2) Since many of the agents used for general anesthesia cause nausea and vomiting, inhalation anesthesia should not be administered for 6 to 8 hours after the patient has ingested food or liquids. Apart from indicating the amount of physical stress and fatigue that the patient has experienced, the duration of abdominal pain will convey little useful information about his physiological status. His normal defecation pattern will be of little significance until normal bowel function resumes a few days following surgery. Tetanus infection typically occurs in a puncture wound from an object that has been contaminated by a soil organism rather than by one in a surgical wound.

62. (1) Peritonitis or bacterial infection of the peritoneum could result if the ligature on the appendiceal stump should slip loose and bowel contents leak into the peritoneal cavity. The result of infection and inflammation of the peritoneum is transudation of fluid and protein from abdominal blood vessels into the peritoneal cavity, causing distention; hypovolemia and hypoproteinemia, causing decreased blood pressure; reflex acceleration of heart rate in response to falling blood pressure; and decreased depth of respirations in an unconscious effort to decrease abdominal pain.

63. (3) The patient will be taken to the operating room for resuturing of the wound. Until the wound can be closed surgically, the exposed intra-abdominal tissues should be protected from contamination with a sterile dressing and should be protected from drying by soaking the gauze dressing with sterile, normal saline solution. Relieving strain on the suture line is less urgent than preventing contamination of exposed tissues. Manipulation of the gas-filled bowel loop could traumatize the inflamed tissue and cause gangrene or rupture of the bowel. Application of a binder could compress the bowel, causing obstruction or ischemia.

64. (1) In peritonitis extreme temperature elevation, severe abdominal pain, and fluid and electrolyte imbalances combine to cause confusion and disorientation. Therefore, the bed's side rails should be kept elevated to prevent the patient from falling. Restraining the arms often provokes resistance and restlessness in the confused patient; therefore, restraints should be avoided, if possible. Unless wound dehiscence occurs, there will be no need for an abdominal binder; unless the patient has arthritis or lower back pain, there will be no need for a bed board.

65. (4) Appendiceal rupture is followed by chemical and bacterial peritonitis, which results in acute prostration and may be fatal. The popular belief that a "bellyache" is the result of eating the wrong food and should be treated with a laxative is responsible for many cases of appendiceal rupture. The public should be taught that nausea, vomiting, periumbilical pain, or right abdominal pain may signify appendicitis and indicates need for medical attention. Swallowing small seeds, use of rectal suppositories, and straining at stool are not thought to cause appendicitis or appendiceal rupture.

66. (2) Thought disorder, inappropriate affect, fixed delusions, and autistic behavior are part of the psychopathology of schizophrenia. Psychotherapy is not very effective with personality disorders unless it is implemented on an intensive, long-term basis.

67. (2) Long-term hospitalization is the least common and would be used for treatment and rehabilitation. The usual practice is to return him to a more autonomous setting as soon as possible since individuals with the disorder do not usually have problems with day-to-day functioning.

68. (3) Projection is a mental mechanism by which a repressed desire or inclination is disguised as belonging to someone else. Mr. Williamson's accusations that his wife is interested in other men may be a projection of his own unconscious homosexual issues. According to psychoanalytical theory, Freud believed that this coping mechanism may be a defense against such unconscious homosexual issues.

69. (4) Chemotherapy may halt the delusions and make him more amenable to psychotherapy. In order to establish a therapeutic relationship the nurse must monitor feelings about the patient and deal with them in order to approach him with unconditional positive regard and acceptance. Marital therapy would certainly be an important component of the treatment since there are 2 people involved here, i.e., the marital pair.

70. (4) Though this topic will be important as a long-term goal, it would not be an integral part of the initial approach with Mr. Williamson.

71. (4) When Betty's attention shifts from concern for herself and her own needs to concern for her infant's needs, this signals a switch from the taking in phase to the taking hold phase.

72. (4) Applying warm compresses before feeding facilitates the let-down reflex. Cold compresses should be avoided, as they would inhibit the let-down reflex. Pain medication, if taken routinely, would be apt to pass through the breast milk to the baby.

73. (1) Normal breast care would include daily washing with water. No other breast care is required unless cracking or abrasions occur. Because alcohol has a drying effect, cleansing with an alcohol pledget could cause skin fissuring.

74. (4) Stools of the breast-fed infant are generally yellow or greenish yellow and are watery and curdy. They may contain a small amount of mucus. They would not be expected to be either well formed or dark in color.

75. (1) Bromocriptine (Parlodel) inhibits prolactin release by the anterior pituitary gland, thereby restoring ovarian function and inhibiting lactation. The patient who receives bromocriptine should be informed that a side effect of the drug is early resumption of ovulation and menstruation in order that she can institute appropriate contraceptive methods, if desired.

76. (2) Patients with infectious mononucleosis complain of fatigue and lack of energy, and since adolescence is a time of high energy activity, the adolescent's chief complaint usually reflects this persistent fatigue.

77. (3) Infectious mononucleosis is an acute disease that affects lymphoid tissue causing enlarged, tender lymph nodes and enlarged spleen.

78. (4) Adolescents consider their peer group the main source of their support and approval, and in order to maintain psychological equilibrium, above all else, they need to maintain contact with their peers.

79. (3) An adolescent has finally come to see himself as a distinct individual definitely unique and separate from every other individual. Establishing gender role identification and identifying himself as separate from his parents take place earlier during childhood.

80. (1) In infectious mononucleosis a rising titer of 1:160 is considered diagnostic.

81. (2) In typhoid fever, the causative organism invades and ulcerates Peyer's patches in the ileum. The ulcer may erode a blood vessel in the bowel wall, causing hemorrhage, or perforate the bowel wall, causing peritonitis. In some patients perforation is accompanied by a sudden sharp pain that lasts only a few seconds and is followed by abdominal tenderness and rigidity. Chills, fever, and headache are typical symptoms of typhoid fever, as is bradycardia. Lethargy and bowel and bladder incontinence are seen in very toxic typhoid fever victims.

82. (3) Since the *Salmonella typhi* organisms are present in stool and urine, the nurse should wear gown and gloves while handling the patient's excreta or objects contaminated by excreta. Since the organism is not airborne, a mask is not necessary. Simple hand washing would not prevent transfer of the organism to the nurse's uniform and to other individuals. The urban sewage disposal system will remove and kill the causative organism, so chlorinated lime need not be added to excreta before discharge into the hospital plumbing.

83. (4) The patient with typhoid fever is distressed by the odor created by the frequent, watery, large volume stools passed during the acute stage of illness. A room deodorizer, by increasing the attractiveness of the patient's surroundings, will not only add to the patient's comfort, but will probably increase the amount of time spent by the nursing staff at the patient's bedside. The patient will be able to change her position in bed, so a Circolectric bed will not be needed. Tepid sponges, rather than ice bags, should

be used to reduce fever. There is no need for an over-the-bed cradle.

84. (1) As a result of high fever and fluid and electrolyte imbalance, the patient with typhoid fever may become delerious during the acute phase of illness. Hence, the bed's side rails should be kept elevated to prevent falls. The application of restraining sheets is apt to increase agitation in the delirious patient. If the lower bed linen is kept clean and dry and the perianal skin is cleaned and dried following each diarrheal stool, an alternating pressure or flotation mattress will not be needed to prevent decubitus ulcers.

85. (2) As a result of the passage of frequent watery, large volume diarrheal stools, the patient with typhoid fever rapidly becomes dehydrated unless fluid losses are continuously replaced. Oral administration of fruit juice, broth, tea, and water will be effective in replacing fluids unless the patient experiences severe nausea and vomiting. Although hourly administration of milk and cream is not necessary, milk shakes are a good source of high carbohydrate, high protein intake. Although a high caloric intake is advisable in any febrile illness, a high residue diet would be irritating to a patient with acute enteritis. Since most typhoid fever patients can take food and fluids orally, parenteral hyperalimentation would be unnecessary.

86. (3) Although muscles are generally stronger in the morning, if all physical activity was scheduled during the morning the patient would rapidly tire. Similarly, if most physical activity was scheduled for afternoon to take advantage of peak levels of adrenocorticosteroids, the patient would rapidly fatigue. It would be best to alternate activity and rest periods throughout the day and to schedule necessary but demanding activities for 1 to 2 hours following pyridostigmine administration, in order to take advantage of the peak effects of the drug.

87. (4) Severe muscle weakness occurs in cholinergic crisis secondary to overdosing with an anticholinesterase drug (neostigmine or pyridostigmine) owing to a depolarizing block at the neuromuscular junction. Excessive dosing with either drug tends to cause sialorrhea, rather than dry mouth. Neither tinnitus nor tetany is a symptom of pyridostigmine overdosing.

88. (4) In myasthenia gravis symptoms tend to fluctuate in severity. In the event of a sudden severe worsening of symptoms, the greatest danger to the patient is the possibility of respiratory failure. Therefore, the patient should be observed for decreasing respiratory excursions and shortness of breath so as to determine whether respiratory support is needed. Abdominal cramping is a symptom of pyridostigmine overdosing. Myasthenic crisis is characterized by severe muscle weakness rather than by muscle spasms.

89. (2) For the patient with dysphagia, soft semisolid foods are less apt to cause choking and aspiration than are liquids and solid foods. Small pieces of ground meats or shredded vegetables can easily be aspirated.

90. (3) Certain antibiotics, such as neomycin, kanamycin, and gentamycin, cause a block of neuromuscular transmission, which can accentuate the muscle weakness of myasthenia gravis. Therefore, Nan should be instructed to alert all later caregivers to the fact that she has myasthenia gravis and is receiving pyridostigmine therapy.

91. (1) Shirley's main occupation since the age of 17 years has been that of an ill person. It is doubtful that with her symptomatology, her obsession with her bodily functions, and her surgical procedures she has had the time or energy to engage in interpersonal relationships of any depth. As a result her social skills will be minimal.

92. (2) She has utilized physiological conversion to keep her anxiety at a tolerable level.

93. (4) Fugue states typically involve amnesia and a flight away from the site of the anxiety producer. Often, those who are affected run away from home and cannot remember who they are or where they came from.

94. (4) This could be a *long-term* goal after Shirley has made some progress in the other 3 areas. This would be *very* anxiety provoking since she has only lived away from her parents for 2 of her 35 years.

95. (2) Insight therapy is not a good tool for a patient such as Shirley. It is more important for her to learn that her response to anxiety is maladaptive, in that it leads to her dysfunction, and to learn new responses that can lead to better functioning.

Index

Note: This is an index of the Nursing Review Content Outlines.
Numbers followed by a t indicate a table.

Abortion, 8
  categories of, 8
Abruptio placentae, 10–11
  complications of, 11
Abscess, of lung, 139
Acetylsalicylic acid (aspirin), in rheumatoid arthritis, 180
Acid-base balance, 109–110
Acidosis, metabolic, 110, 152
  respiratory, 111
Acrocyanosis, in newborn, 24
Active listening, 223
Active nonspecific immunity, 187
Active transport, 108
Acute lymphocytic leukemia (ALL), 63
Acute myelocytic leukemia (AML), 63
Addison's disease, 136
Adenoma, 130–131
Adolescence, 56–57
  Sullivan's theory of, 222
Adolescent behavior disorders, 228–230
Adulthood, Sullivan's theory of, 222
Affective disorders, 235–239
Afterload, 148
Alcohol abuse, 164, 231–232
Alkalosis, metabolic, 110–111
  respiratory, 111
Alkylating agents, 187
Allergic disorders. *See also* Hypersensitivity.
  asthmatic, 75
Altruism, in groups, 226, 227
Alzheimer's disease, 230
Ambu-bag, 118
Amnesia, psychogenic, 242
Amniocentesis, 7
Amnion, 4
Amniotic fluid, 5
Amphetamines, abuse of, 233
Amputation, 157
Amyotrophic lateral sclerosis, 118–119
Anal stage, 53, 220
Anaphylaxis, 182–183
Anasarca, 149
Anastomosis, esophageal, 159
  of bowel segments, 73, 167
Anemia, in leukemia, 64
  sickle cell, 61
  thalassemic, 62
Anesthesia, 105
Aneurysm, aortic, 155–156
Angina, 146
Angiogram, carotid, 132
Angioplasty, 156
Angle closure glaucoma, 125, 126
Anhedonia, 234
Anions, 108
Anterior cerebral artery disturbance, 119
Antibiotics, anticancer, 187
Antibodies, antitumor, 187
Anticholinergic drugs, 117, 165
Anticholinesterase drugs, 118
Anticoagulants, 153–154
Anticonvulsive drugs, 68, 115
Antidepressants, 117, 237
Antidiuretic hormone (ADH; Vasopressin), 109, 131t
  inappropriate secretion of, 121
Antigen, carcinoembryonic, 186
Antihistamines, 117, 184
Antihypertensive drugs, 151
Anti-inflammatory drugs, 180, 181
Antimetabolites, 187
Antisocial personality, 243
Antispasmodic drugs, 181
Antitumor antibodies, 187
Antiviral drugs, 117
Anxiety, in children, 228–229
  interpersonal theory of, 220
Anxiety disorders, 239–242
  dissociative, 242
  generalized, 239–241
  somatoform, 241–242
Aortic aneurysm, 155–156
Aortogram, 155–156
Aorto-iliac bypass graft, 156–157
Apgar scoring, 22
Arrhythmias, 150
Arteriography, 156
Arteriosclerotic brain syndrome, 230–231
Arteriosclerotic obliterative disease of the lower extremities, 156–157
Arteriovenous fistula, 175
Arthritis, rheumatoid, 180–181
Ascites, 149, 163–164
Aspirin, in rheumatoid arthritis, 180
Assertiveness training, 225
Asthma, bronchial, 141–142
  extrinsic, 141
  in children, 75–76
  intrinsic, 141
Ataxic cerebral palsy, 76
Atelectasis, 25, 139
Athetoid cerebral palsy, 76
Atrial fibrillation, 150
Atrial flutter, 150
Atrioventricular block, 150
Autism, 229
Autoimmune reaction, in Graves's disease, 133
Autonomous bladder, 171
Autonomy, versus shame and doubt stage, 53, 221
Aversion therapy, 224–225
Avoidant personality, 243

Babinski's reflex, 164
Bacille Calmette-Guérin (BCG) vaccine, 187
Balanced traction, 178
Balloon pump, intra-aortic, 152
Barbiturate abuse, 232–233
Basophilic adenoma, 130, 131
Behavior contracting, 225
Behavior modification, 235
Behavior theories, 218–220
Behavior therapy, 224–225
Bicarbonate buffer system, 109
Bilirubin level, 25–26
Billroth procedures, 161
Biofeedback training, 225, 244
Biological deficiencies, in behavior disorders, 219
Biopsy, 185
Bipolar disorders, 238–239
Bladder, areflexive, 122
  autonomous, 171
  cancer of, 172–173
  distention of, 169
  in multiple sclerosis, 116
  neurogenic, 170–171
  paralytic, 171
  reflex, 170–171
  uninhibited, 170–171
Bleeding, gastrointestinal, 163
  in leukemia, 64
  postpartum, 19–20
Blood disorders. *See specific disorders.*
Blood plasma, interstitial fluid shifts and, 113–114
Blood pressure. *See* Hypertension.
Blood transfusion, hypersensitivity reaction to, 183
Body temperature, in newborn, 21, 23
Body weight. *See also* Physical development.
  of newborn, 24
Borderline personality, 243
Bouginage, 159
Boutonniére deformity, 180
Bowel program, 122–123
Bowen, Murray, 226
Bradycardia, sinus, 150
Brain injury, 120–121
Brain syndrome, arteriosclerotic, 230–231
  organic, 230
Brain tumors, in children, 66–67
Braxton Hicks' contractions, 14
Breast, mammography and, 185
  mastitis of, 21
Bronchial asthma, 141–142
Bronchiectasis, 139–141
Bronchitis, chronic, 142–143
Bronchoscopy, 140
Bronchospasm, 141
Bryant's traction, 178
Buck's traction, 178
Buffer system, pH regulation and, 109
Burns, 58–59
  degrees of, 59
Butyrophenones, 117
Bypass grafts, 156–157

Calcium, body fluid levels of, 112
Calculosis, urinary, 171–172
Cancer. *See also* Radiotherapy; Tumor.
  chemotherapy in, 133, 167, 187
  of bladder, 172–173
  of colon, 166–168
  oral, 157–158
Cannabis, abuse of, 233
"Capillary dynamics," 58
Caput succedaneum, 24
Carbonic anhydrase inhibitors, 126
Carcinoembryonic antigen, 186
Cardiac dilation, 148
Cardiac enlargement, 148
Cardiac hypertrophy, 148
Cardiogenic shock, 151–153
Cardiovascular disorders, 146–157
  during pregnancy, 12–13
Carotid angiogram, 132
Cast, application and maintenance of, 177–178
CAT scan, 66, 70, 132, 165
Cataract, 124–125
Cataract lenses, 125
Catatonic schizophrenia, 234
Catecholamines, behavior disorders and, 219
  bipolar disorders and, 238
  depression and, 235
Catharsis, in groups, 226, 227
Catheter, intraventricular, 132
  suprapubic, 170
  Swan-Ganz, 151–153
  urethral, 170
Cations, 108
Cellular hypersensitivity, delayed, 183–184
Cephalhematoma, 24
Cerebral artery disturbance, 119
Cerebral palsy, 76–78
  types of, 76
Cerebrospinal fluid, 133
  detecting drainage of, 121
  in hydrocephalus, 79
Cerebrovascular accident, 119–120
Cervix, 3
  scraping of, 185
Chadwick's sign, 6
Chemotherapy, colon cancer and, 167
  malignant tumor and, 187
  transphenoidal tumor removal and, 133
Chest drainage, 140–141
Cheyne-Stokes respirations, 148
Child(ren). *See also* Infant; Newborns.
  adolescent, 56–57, 222
  asthma in, 75–76
  behavior disorders in, 228–230
  brain tumors in, 66–67
  burns in, 58–59
  cerebral palsy in, 76–78
  cleft lip and palate in, 71–79
  cognitive development of, 52–57
  cystic fibrosis in, 78–79
  fluid and electrolyte disturbances in, 57–58
  gastrointestinal anomalies in, 71
  health maintenance and promotion in, 53–57
  hemophilia in, 62–63
  Hirschsprung's disease in, 72–73
  hydrocephalus in, 79–80
  leukemia in, 63–65
  meningitis in, 65–66
  mental retardation in, 69–70
  neonatal necrotizing enterocolitis in, 73–74
  physical development of, 5–6, 51–57
  pneumonia in, 74–75
  preschool, 54–55
  psychosocial development of, 52–57
  pyloric stenosis in, 72
  renal disorders in, 59–61
  school-age, 55–56
  seizure disorders in, 67–69
  sickle cell anemia in, 61
  tetralogy of Fallot in, 80–81
  β-thalassemia in, 62
  toddler age, 53–54
Childhood behavior disorders, 228–230
Chlorothiazide, 151

Chondrosarcoma, 185
Chorion, 4
Choroiditis, 127
Chromophobe adenoma, 130–131
Chronic obstructive lung disease, 141–143
Chvostek's sign, 135
Chymopapain, 123
Circulatory system, fetal, 5
  in newborn, 23
Circumoral cyanosis, transient, 24
Cirrhosis, 162–164
Claudication, intermittent, 156
Cleft lip and palate, in children, 71–72
Closed chest drainage, 140–141
Closed fracture, 158, 177
Coagulation disorders, in children, 62–63
Cocaine abuse, 233
Cognitive development, of adolescent, 57
  of infant, 52
  of preschooler, 54–55
  of school-age child, 56
  of toddler, 53–54
Cognitive restructuring therapy, 225
Cognitive-behavioral therapy, 225
Cohesive stage, of group, 227
Coitus interruptus, 28
Colectomy, 166
Colitis, ulcerative, 165–166
Colon, cancer of, 166–168
Colonoscopy, 166
Colostomy, 73, 167
Coma, Glasgow coma scale and, 120
  in myxedema, 134
  patient care and, 119–120
Comminuted fracture, 177
Communication barriers, 223–224
Communication theory, 223–224
Compound fracture, 158, 176–177
Compulsive personality, 243
Concrete operations stage, 56
Conditioning, 219–220
Condom, 28
Conflict stage, of group, 227
Confrontation, 223
Congenital glaucoma, 125
Congestive heart failure, 147–150
  pathophysiology of, 148
Conjoint family therapy, 226
Consciousness level, assessment of, 106, 120
Contact allergy, 183–184
Contraceptive methods, 28–29
Contractility, myocardial, 148
Contractions, Braxton Hicks', 14
  induction and control of, 15
Conversion disorder, 241–242
Corneal transplant, 127
Corpus, uterine, 3
Corrective reenactment, in groups, 226, 227
Corticosteroids, 118, 180, 184
Corticotropin releasing factor, 130
Cortisol, 109, 131t. *See also* Glucocorticoid(s).
Coughing, pre-operative instruction in, 104
Coumadin, 153
Counter-transference, 224
Craniotomy, 116
Credé's maneuver, 116
Crutchfield's tongs, 122
Cryoextraction, of cataract, 124
Cushing's disease, 131, 135–136
Cushing's syndrome, 135
Cyanosis, in newborns, 24
  tetralogy of Fallot and, 80–81
Cyclitis, 127
Cystectomy, 173
Cystic fibrosis, 78–79
Cystogram, 169
Cystometrogram, 169
Cystoscopy, 169, 172–173
Cytological examination, 185
Cytolytic reaction, 183
Cytotoxic reaction, 183

Danger signs, during labor, 16
  during pregnancy, 8
Decompression laminectomy, 122
Deep breathing, 179
  pre-operative instruction in, 103
Defense mechanisms, 219
Deformities, in rheumatoid arthritis, 180
Dehydration, in children, 58
Delayed cellular hypersensitivity, 183–184
Delinquent behavior, 229–230
Delirium tremens, 232
Delivery. *See* Labor and delivery.
Denial, 219
Dependent edema, 148
Dependent personality, 243
Depression, 225, 235–238
Desensitization, systematic, 224
Development. *See also* Psychosocial development.
  cognitive, 52–57
  fetal, 5–6
  physical, 5–6, 52–57
  principles of, 51–52
Developmental disorders, 69–70, 76, 228
Diabetes insipidus, 133
Diabetes mellitus, 136–137
  in pregnancy, 13–14, 27
  types of, 136, 137
  White's classification of, 13
Diagnostic and Statistical Manual of Mental Disorders (DSM III), 227–228
Dialysis, 175–176
  peritoneal, 174–175
Diaphragm, contraceptive, 28
Diffusion, 108
Digestive disorders, 157–168
Digitalis, toxicity of, 149
Digoxin, 149
Dilation, cardiac, 148
Disc, intervertebral, 123–124
"Disease" model, of alcohol abuse, 232
Dislocation, 176
Disorganized schizophrenia, 234
Displacement, 219
Disseminated intravascular disease, with abruptio placentae, 11
Dissociative disorders, 242
Diuretics, 149
Dopamine, behavior disorders and, 219, 233
"Dopamine hypothesis," 233
Doppler flow detector, 153
"Double bind" theory, 234
Drainage tubes, postoperative assessment of, 107
Dream interpretation, 224
Drug(s). *See also specific names and types of.*
  in aversion therapy, 225
  in childhood behavior disorders, 230
  in pregnancy, 7
  in schizophrenia, 235
  postoperative administration of, 107
Drug abuse, 231–233
Ductus arteriosus, 5
Ductus venosus, 5
"Dumping syndrome," 161–162

Dyspnea, 141
  nocturnal, paroxysmal, 148
Dystocia, 17–18
Dysuria, 169

Ear disorders, 128–130
Echolalia, 229
Eclampsia, 12
Ectopic pregnancy, 9
Edema, 58, 113
  dependent, 148
  pulmonary, 146, 148, 149–150
Ego, 219
Ego defense mechanisms, 219
Electric shock, in aversion therapy, 225
Electric shock therapy, 235, 237
Electroencephalogram, 115
Electrolyte disturbances. *See* Fluid and electrolyte disorders.
Electromyography, 118–119
Embolism, pulmonary, 144–145
Emotional changes, of pregnancy, 6–7
Emotional problems, 222–227
Emphysema, pulmonary, 143
Empyema, 139
Encephalopathy, hepatic, 164
Endocarditis, rheumatic, 147–148
Endocrine disorders, 130–137
Endometritis, during postpartum period, 20
Enuresis, 170
Eosinophilic adenoma, 130, 131
Epidural block, 105
Epidural hematoma, 120
Epilepsy. *See* Seizure disorders.
Epinephrine, 131t, 152
Epstein's pearls, 24
Esophageal stricture, 158–159
Esophagoscopy, 159
Estrogens, 131t
  osteoporosis and, 182
Exercises, for legs, 104
  isometric, 181
  Kegel, 170
  muscle setting, 179, 181
  range of motion 179, 180
Existential factors, in groups, 226, 227
Exophthalmos, 133–134
External counterpulsation device, 152–153
Extinction, 224
Extracapsular extraction, of cataract, 124
Extracellular volume excess, 58
Extrinsic asthma, 141
Eye care, for newborn, 22
Eye disorders, 124–128

Facial nerve paralysis, 129
Fallopian tubes, 3
Family, 51
Family planning, 27–29
Family therapy, 226, 235
Femoral thrombophlebitis, 20
Femoro-popliteal bypass graft, 156–157
Fertilization, 4
Fetal distress, signs of, 16
Fetal membranes, 4–5
Fetus. *See also* Labor and delivery; Pregnancy.
  assessment of, 16–17
  circulation of, 5
  development of, 5–6
  heart rate of, 16–17

Fibrillation, atrial, 150
  ventricular, 150
Fibrinolytic drugs, 153–154
Fibrosarcoma, 185
Field block anesthesia, 105
Fingers, deformities of, 180
First degree burns, 59
Fistula, arteriovenous, 175
Flexion contractures, 180
Fluid, intake and loss of, 108
  interstitial, shifts of, 113–114
Fluid and electrolyte disorders, 108–114
  in children, 57–58
  patient care with, 110–114
  physiology of, 108–110
Focal seizures, 115
Fontanel, 24
Foramen ovale, 5
Forearm splints, 123
Formal operations stage, 57
Fracture, 176–179
  compound, 158, 176–177
  mandibular, 158
  simple, 158, 177
Free association, 224
Freudian theory, 220–221
Fugue, psychogenic, 242
Fusiform deformity, 180
Fusion, spinal, 122

Gag reflex, 106, 159
Gallop, 148
Gallstones, 164
Gardner-Wells tongs, 122
Gastrectomy, partial, 161
Gastric analysis, 161
Gastric resection, 161–162
Gastrointestinal anomalies, in children, 71
Gastrointestinal bleeding, 163
Gastrointestinal system. *See also* Digestive disorders.
  in newborn, 24
Gastroscopy, 161
General adaptation syndrome, 102
General anesthesia, 105
Generativity versus self absorption stage, 221
Genetic factors, in behavior disorders, 219
Genital stage, 221
Genitalia, female, 3
  male, 4
Genitourinary disorders, 168–176
Genitourinary system, of newborn, 24
Glasgow coma scale, 120
Glaucoma, 125–126
  types of, 125
Glioblastoma, 185
Glomerular filtration, 60, 174
Glomerulonephritis, 60, 173–174
Glucocorticoid(s), 109, 131t
  in Addison's disease, 136
  in Cushing's disease, 135
Gold salts, 180
Goodell's sign, 6
Gout, 179–180
Grafts, of skin, 155
  vascular, 155–157
Grand mal seizures, 114
Graves's disease, 133–134
Group(s), stages of, 227
  types of, 226–227
Group cohesion, 226, 227
Group therapy, 226–227, 235
Growth. *See* Physical development.

Growth hormone releasing factor, 130
Guilt, 240

Hallucinogens, abuse of, 233
Halo brace and jacket, 122
"Hardening of the arteries," 230–231
Harrington's rods, 122
Head, of newborn, 24
Head injury, 120–121
Headache, migraine, 115–116
with adenomas, 131
Health history, pre-operative, 103
Health maintenance, in adolescent, 57
in infant, 53
in preschooler, 55
in school-age child, 56
in toddler, 54
Heart defects, congenital, 80–81
Heart failure, congestive, 147–150
Heart rate, fetal, 16–17
Heart rhythm, abnormal, 148
Hebephrenic schizophrenia, 234
Heberden's nodes, 181
Hegar's sign, 6
Hemangiomas, in newborn, 24
Hemangiosarcoma, 185
Hematoma, epidural, 120
in newborn, 24
subdural, 120
Hematuria, 169
Hemochromatosis, 62
Hemodialysis, 175–176
Hemolytic disease, in newborn, 26–27
Hemophilia, in children, 62–63
Hemorrhage, postpartum, 19–20
Hemorrhoids, 168
Heparin, 153
Hepatic encephalopathy, 164
Hepatitis, alcoholic, acute, 164
viral, 162
Hernia, hiatus, 159–160
Herniated intervertebral disc, 123–124
Hiatus hernia, 159–160
Hierarchies, 224
High output heart failure, 147
Hip replacement, 181–182
Hirschsprung's disease, in children, 72–73
Histrionic personality, 242
Homan's sign, 179
Hormonal control, of fluid and electrolyte balance, 108–109
of menstrual cycle, 4
Hormone(s). *See also specific hormones.*
behavior disorders and, 219
effects of, 131t
hypothalamic, 130
in chemotherapy, 187
steroid, 187
Humanistic theory, 220
Huntington's chorea, 117, 230
Hydatidiform mole, 8–9
Hydralazine, 151
Hydrocephalus, in children, 79–80
types of, 79
Hyperbilirubinemia, 25–26
Hypercalcemia, 112, 134
Hypercapnia, 144
Hyperkalemia, 111–112
Hypermagnesemia, 113
Hyperosmolar disturbances, 110
Hyperparathyroidism, 134–135
Hypersensitivity, 182–184. *See also* Allergic disorders.
general approach to prevention and management of, 184
type I, 182–183
type II, 183
type III, 183
type IV, 183–184
Hypertension, 150–151
pregnancy induced, 11–12
Hyperthyroidism, 133–134
Hypertrophy, cardiac, 148
Hyperventilation, 121
Hypnosis, 242
Hypnotics, abuse of, 232–233
Hypoalbuminemia, 163
Hypocalcemia, 112
Hypochondriasis, 241
Hypokalemia, 111
Hypomagnesemia, 112–113
Hypo-osmolar disturbances, 110
Hypoparathyroidism, 135
Hypopituitarism, 130–133
Hypothalamus, endocrine disorders and, 130
Hypothermia, anesthetic, 105
Hypothermia blanket, 121
Hypothyroidism, 134
Hypovolemic shock, 151–153
Hypoxia, acute, 144

Id, 219
Identification, 219
Identity versus role diffusion stage, 221
Ileostomy, 166
Imitative behaviors, in groups, 226, 227
Immobility, complications of, 179
Immune complex reaction, 183
Immune response, inadequate, 184–188
Immunity, nonspecific, active, 187
Immunological disorders, 182–188
Immunologically active lymphocytes, 187
Immunosuppressive drugs, 176, 180, 183
Immunotherapy, 187–188
active, 187
passive, 187–188
Impacted fracture, 177
Implantation, of fertilized egg, 4
Incontinence, 170
Industry versus inferiority stage, 55, 221
Infancy, Sullivan's theory of, 222
Infant, 52–53. *See also* Newborns.
Infection(s), in leukemia, 64
in newborn, 22, 27
puerperal, 20
urinary, 171
Infiltration anesthesia, 105
Informal groups, 226
Informed consent, facilitating, 103
Initial phase, of group, 227
Initiative versus guilt stage, 54, 221
Insulin, diabetes mellitus and, 131t, 136, 137
Integrity versus despair stage, 221–222
Intensive care unit, surgical, 106
Interdisciplinary theory, 220
Intermittent claudication, 156
Interpersonal learning, in groups, 226, 227
Interpersonal theory, 220
Interstitial fluid shifts, 113–114
Intervertebral disc, herniated, 123–124
Intimacy versus isolation stage, 221
Intoxication, 231
Intra-aortic balloon pump, 152

Intracapsular extraction, of cataract, 124
Intracranial pressure, head injury and, 120, 121
  transphenoidal tumor removal and, 132
Intra-uterine devices (IUDs), 28–29
Intravascular disease, with abruptio placentae, 11
Intravenous anesthesia, 105
Intravenous infusions, postoperative assessment of, 107
Intravenous pyelogram, 168
Intraventricular catheter, 132
Intrinsic asthma, 141
Introjection, 219
Intuitive phase, 54, 55
I.Q., in mental retardation, 69–70
Iridectomy, peripheral, 126
Iritis, 127
Isolation, 219
Isometric exercises, 181
Isoproterenol (Isuprel), 152
Isotonic disturbances, 110
Isuprel, 152

Jaundice, in newborn, 23, 26
Joint replacement, 181–182
Juvenile era, Sullivan's theory of, 222

Kegel exercises, 170
Keratitis, 126–127
Kidney. *See under* Renal.

Labor, dysfunctional, 17
Labor and delivery, 14–18. *See also* Fetus; Pregnancy.
  complications of, 17–18
  danger signs during, 16
  fetal assessment during, 16–17
  induction and control of uterine contractions and, 15
  mechanism of, 15
  nursing care during, 15
  nursing care immediately following, 16
  premature, 18
  signs of impending labor and, 14–15
  signs of true labor and, 15
  stages and phases of, 15
  terminology of, 14
Labyrinthine irritation, 129
Lactogenic hormone. *See* Prolactin inhibiting factor.
Laminectomy, decompression, 122
  posterior, 123–124
Laser beam surgery, with retinal detachment, 128
Latency stage, 220–221
Latent content, 224
Learned helplessness theory, 235
Learning, 219
  in groups, 226, 227
Left-sided heart failure, 147, 148
Leg exercises, pre-operative instruction in, 104
Leiomyosarcoma, 185
Lens implantation, intra-ocular, 124
Lethality Scale, 237–238
Leukemia, in children, 63–65
Leukoplakia, 157
LeVeen's peritoneojugular shunt, 164
Levophed, 131t, 152
Lightning, 14
Lip, cleft, 71–72
Listening, active, 223
Lithium carbonate, 239
Lobectomy, 140
Lochia flow, 18
Log rolling technique, 123
Lou Gehrig's disease, 118–119
Low output heart failure, 147
Lung abscess, 139
Lung disease, obstructive, chronic, 141–143
Lupus erythematosus, 183
Luteinizing hormone releasing factor, 130
Lymphocytes, immunologically active, 187
Lymphosarcoma, 185

Magnesium, body fluid levels of, 112–113
Malignant meningioma, 185
Malignant tumor, 184–188. *See also* Cancer.
  types of, 185
Mammography, 185
Mandibular fracture, 158
Mania, 238
Manic-depressive illness, 238–239
Manifest content, 224
Manipulation, of dislocation, 176
"Master gland," 130
Mastitis, during postpartum period, 21
Mastoidectomy, 129
Mastoiditis, 129
Meconium, 24
Medical-biological model of behavior, 219
Megacolon, in children, 72–73
Ménière's disease, 129–130
Meningioma, malignant, 185
Meningitis, in children, 65–66
Menstrual cycle, 4
Menstrual phase, of menstrual cycle, 4
Mental retardation, 69–70, 76
Metabolic acidosis, 110, 152
Metabolic alkalosis, 110–111
Micturition reflex, 170–171
Middle cerebral artery disturbance, 119
Migraine, common, 115–116
Milia, in newborn, 24
Milieu therapy, 226, 235
"Milk leg," 20
Miotic drugs, 125–126, 127
Modeling, 225
Mole, hydatidiform, 8–9
Mongolian spots, in newborn, 24
Monoamine oxidase inhibitors (MAO inhibitors), 237
Moral theory, of alcohol abuse, 232
Motor paralytic bladder, 171
Mucopolysaccharide deposition, 134
Multiple myeloma, 185
Multiple personalities, 242
Multiple sclerosis, 116
Muscle relaxants, anesthesia and, 105
Muscle setting exercises, 179, 181
Musculoskeletal disorders, 176–182
Myasthenia gravis, 117–118
Myeloma, multiple, 185
Myocardial contractility, 148
Myocardial infarction, 146–147
Myocarditis, rheumatic, 147
Myringotomy, 129
Myxedema, 134
  pretibial, 133–134

Nagele's rule, 7
Narcissistic personality, 242
Narrow angle glaucoma, 125, 126
Neonatal necrotizing enterocolitis (NEC), 73–74
Nephrotic syndrome, 60
Neuralgia, trigeminal, 116

Neuroendocrine regulation. *See* Hormonal control.
Neurogenic bladder, 170–171
Neurogenic shock, 151–153
Neurological assessment, with head injury, 120–121
Neurological disorders, 114–124
Neurotic behavior, 241
Neurotransmitters, behavior disorders and, 219
Newborns, 21–27
  abnormal presentations and positions of, 17–18
  body temperature of, 23
  diseases affecting, 25–27
  gastrointestinal system of, 24
  genitourinary system of, 24
  head of, 24
  immediate postdelivery care of, 16
  neurological system of, 25
  normal, 21–23
  nursing management of, 22–23
  physical characteristics of, 23–25
  respiratory status of, 23
  skin of, 24
  weight of, 24
Nocturia, 169
Nocturnal dyspnea, paroxysmal, 148
Nodules, subcutaneous, 180
Norepinephrine (Levophed), 131t, 152
Nutritional guidelines, during pregnancy, 7

Obliterative disease, arteriosclerotic, of lower extremities, 156–157
Obsessive-compulsive disorder, 240
Oedipal stage, 54
Oliguria, 169
Open angle glaucoma, 125–126
Open fracture, 158, 176–177
Operant conditioning, 219
Oral cancer, 157–158
Oral contraceptives, 28
Oral dependent stage, 52, 220
Organic brain syndrome (OBS), 230
Organic mental disorder, 230–231
Orientation stage, of group, 227
Oropharyngeal airway, postoperative assessment for, 106
Orthopnea, 148
Osmolality, 108
Osmotic pressure, 108
Osteoarthritis, 181–182
Osteogenic sarcoma, 185
Osteoporosis, 182
Otitis media, 128–129
Otosclerosis, 129
Ovaries, 3
Oxygen administration, 138–139

Pain, psychogenic, 241
  with genitourinary disorders, 169
Palate, cleft, 71–72
Pancreatic pseudocyst, 165
Pancreatitis, 164–165
Panhypopituitarism, 133
Panic attacks, 240
Papanicolaou's smear, 185
Paracentesis, 163–164
Paralytic bladder, 171
Paralytic ileus, 139
Paranoid personality, 242
Paranoid schizophrenia, 234
Parataxic mode, 220, 222
Parathormone, 131t
  in hyperparathyroidism, 134
  in hypoparathyroidism, 135
Parkinson's disease, 116–117
Paroxysmal nocturnal dyspnea, 148
Partial seizures, 114–115
Passive-aggressive personality, 243
Peptic ulcer, 160–162
Pericarditis, rheumatic, 147
Peri-operative care, 102
Peritoneal dialysis, 174–175
Peritoneojugular shunt, 164
Person centered therapy, 224
Personality, multiple, 242
Personality disorders, 228, 242–244
  ineffective coping and, 243–244
  types of, 242–243
Petit mal seizures, 114
pH, of body fluids, 109–110
Phallic stage, 220
Pharyngeal reflex, 106, 159
Phenothiazines, 117, 235
Phlebography, 153
Phlebothrombosis, 153
Phobic disorder, 240–241
Phosphate buffer system, 109
Physical development, of adolescent, 56–57
  of fetus, 5–6
  of infant, 52
  of preschooler, 54
  of school-age child, 55
  of toddler, 53
Pituitary gland, 130
  tumor of, 136
Placenta, 5
Placenta previa, 9–10
Plant alkaloids, 187
Plasma, interstitial fluid shifts and, 113–114
Pleural effusion, 139
Pleurisy, 138
Pneumonectomy, 140
Pneumonia, 138–139
  bacterial, 74
  complications of, 139
  in children, 74–75
  lobar, 138
  tuberculous, 145
  viral, 74
Polyps, rectosigmoid, 167
Postpartum period, 18–21
  complications during, 19–21
  emotional care during, 19
  nursing management during, 19
  physiology during, 18
Potassium, body fluid levels of, 111–112
Preadolescent era, Sullivan's theory of, 222
Preconceptual phase, 53, 54–55
Preeclampsia, 11–12
Pregnancy. *See also* Family planning; Fetus; Labor and delivery.
  abortion and, 8
  cardiovascular disease during, 12–13
  common discomforts during, 7–8
  complications of, 7–12
  danger signals during, 8
  diabetes in, 13–14
  diagnosis of, 7
  drug use during, 7
  ectopic, 9
  emotional changes of, 6–7
  high risk, 12–14
  maternal changes during, 6
  nutritional guidelines during, 7
  physiology of, 4–7
  prenatal care during, 7
  prolonged, 18
  tubal, 9
Pregnancy induced hypertension (PIH), 11–12

Pregroup stage, 227
Preload, 148
Premature labor and delivery, 18
Prenatal care, 7
Preoperational stage, 54–55
Pre-operative nursing care, 103–104
Preschooler, 54–55
Pressure ventilator, 144
Projection, 219
Prolactin inhibiting factor, 130
Proliferative phase, of menstrual cycle, 4
Protein buffer system, 109
Prototaxic mode, 220, 222
Pseudocyst, pancreatic, 165
Psychiatric disorders, therapeutic interventions in, 222–227
Psychoanalytic theory, 219, 224
Psychodynamic theory, of alcohol abuse, 232
Psychogenic amnesia and fugue, 242
Psychogenic pain disorder, 241
Psychomotor retardation, in depression, 236, 238
Psychomotor seizures, 115
Psychosocial development, Eriksonian theory of, 221–222
  Freudian theory of, 220–221
  of adolescent, 57
  of infants, 52
  of preschooler, 54
  of school-age child, 55–56
  of toddler, 53
    Sullivanian theory of, 222
Psychosocial model of behavior, 219–220
Psychosomatic disorders, 244
Psychotherapy, group, 227
  individual, 240, 241
Puerperal infection, 20
Puerperium. *See* Postpartum period.
Pulmonary edema, 146–150
Pulmonary embolism, 144–145
Pulmonary emphysema, 143
Pulmonary stenosis, in tetralogy of Fallot, 80–81
Pulmonary tuberculosis, 145–146
Punishment, 224–225
  fear of, 240
Pupil reactivity, with head injury, 120–121
Pyelogram, intravenous, 168
Pyloric stenosis, in children, 72
Pyloroplasty, 161

Radical excision, 186
Radiography. *See* CAT scan; X-rays.
Radioisotopes, 134, 186
Radiotherapy, bladder cancer and, 172–173
  colon cancer and, 167–168
  external, 186
  interstitial, 186
  pituitary tumor and, 136
  malignant tumor and, 186–187
  following transphenoidal tumor removal, 133
Range of motion exercises, 179, 180
Rational emotive therapy (RET), 225
Rationalization, 219
Reaction formation, 219, 240
Recovery room, 106
  patient assessment in, 106–107
Rectoperineal resection, 167
Rectosigmoid polyps, 167
Reflex(es), Babinski's, 164
  bladder, 122
  gag, 106, 159
  micturition, 170–171
  in newborn, 25
  pharyngeal, 106, 159
Reflex bladder, 170–171
Reflux, vesicoureteral, 169
Regional anesthesia, 105
Regression, 219
Reinforcement, 219–220, 224
  positive, 225
Relaxation training, 224
Renal disorders, in children, 59–61
Renal failure, 174–176
Renal regulation, of pH, 110
Renal transplantation, 176
Renin, 109
Rephrasing, 223
Repression, 219
Reproductive organs, female, 3, 4, 18–21, 24
  male, 4, 24
  of infant, 24
Reserpine, 151
Resistance, analysis of, 224
Respiration(s), Cheyne-Stokes, 148
  in newborn, 22
Respiratory acidosis, 111
Respiratory alkalosis, 111
Respiratory disorders, 137–146. *See also specific disorders.*
Respiratory distress syndrome, 25
Respiratory failure, 143–144
Respiratory regulation, of pH, 109–110
Respiratory system, in newborn, 22, 23
Respondent conditioning, 219
Response shaping, 225
Restatement, 224
Retinal detachment, 127–128
Rh incompatibility, 26
Rhabdomyosarcoma, 185
Rheumatic endocarditis, 147–148
Rheumatic fever, 147
Rheumatic myocarditis, 147
Rheumatic pericarditis, 147
Rheumatoid arthritis, 180–181
Rhinorrhea, 120
Rhizotomy, 116
Rhythm method, 28
Right-sided heart failure, 147, 148–149
Romberg's test, 67
Running traction, 178

"Sacral sparing," 121
Saphenous vein ligation and stripping, 154
Sarcoma, osteogenic, 185
Schizoaffective disorder, 234
Schizoid personality, 242
Schizophrenia, 233–235
  types of, 234
"Schizophrenogenic" parents, 233
Schizotypal personality, 242
School-age child, 55–56
Scleral buckling, with retinal detachment, 128
Sclerosing solution, 154
Sclerosis, lateral, amyotrophic, 118–119
  multiple, 116
Second degree burns, 59
Secondary glaucoma, 125
Secretagogue, 161
Secretory phase, of menstrual cycle, 4
Sedatives, abuse of, 232–233
Seizure(s), generalized, 68
  grand mal, 114
  partial, 68, 114–115
  petit mal, 114
  psychomotor, 115

Seizure disorders, 114–115
  in children, 67–69, 76
Self stimulation, in autism, 229
Self-care instruction, pre-operative, 103–104
Sengstaken's tube, 163
Sensitivity training groups, 227
Sensorimotor stage, 52, 53
Sensory paralytic bladder, 171
Sepsis, in newborn, 27
Serotonin, behavior disorders and, 219
Serum analysis, for carcinoembryonic antigen, 186
Serum electrolyte levels, 58
Shock, 139, 146, 151–153, 164
  spinal, 121–122, 171
  types of, 151–153
Sickle cell anemia, 61
Sigmoidoscope, 167
Silence, utilizing, 223
Simple fracture, 158, 177
Sinus bradycardia, 150
Sinus tachycardia, 150
Skeletal traction, 122, 178, 179
Skin, of newborn, 24
Skin color, postoperative assessment of, 106–107
Skin grafting, 155
Skin traction, 178
Sleep deprivation, in behavior disorders, 219
Social interaction, in groups, 226, 227
Sociocultural theory, 220
Sodium, water volume and, 110–113
Sodium nitroprusside, 152
Somatoform disorders, 241–242
Spastic cerebral palsy, 76
Spermicides, 28
Sphincter of Oddi, 164, 165
Spinal block, 105
Spinal cord injury, 121–123
Spinal fusion, 122
  posterior, 123–124
Spinal shock, 121–122, 171
Splenomegaly, 62
Splints, forearm, 123
Stapedectomy, 129
Status asthmaticus, 141–142
Sterilization, 29
Straight traction, 178
Stress, depression and, 235–236
Stress incontinence, 170
Stricture, esophageal, 158–159
Structured family therapy, 226
Structuring, 223
Stryker's boots, 123
Stryker's frame, 122, 123
Subarachnoid screw, 121, 132
Subcutaneous nodules, 180
Subdural hematoma, 120
Subinvolution, uterine, 21
Subluxation, 176
Substance abuse, 231–233
Sucralfate, 160
Suicide, 237–238
Superego, 219
Suprapubic catheterization, 170
Surfactant, in newborn's lungs, 23
Surgery. *See also specific procedures.*
  effect on patient, 102–103
  evening before, 104
  for aortic aneurysm, 155–156
  for cataract removal, 124–125
  for cirrhosis, 163
  for corneal transplant, 127
  for esophageal stricture, 159
  for glaucoma, 126
  for hemorrhoids, 168
Surgery (*Continued*)
  for hiatus hernia, 159–160
  for Hirschsprung's disease, 73
  for hyperpituitarism, 132–133
  for mastoiditis, 129
  for Ménière's disease, 130
  for oral cancer, 158
  for pancreatic pseudocyst drainage, 165
  for retinal detachment, 128
  for tumor removal, 135, 136, 186–188
  morning of, 104
  patient care during, 105–108
  reasons for, 102
Surgical consent, 103
Surgical intensive care unit, 106
Suspension traction, 178
Swan neck deformity, 180
Swan-Ganz catheter, 151–153
Sympathomimetics, 152, 183
Syndrome of inappropriate antidiuretic hormone secretion, 121
Syntaxic mode, 220, 222
Systematic desensitization, 224
Systemic lupus erythematosus, 183

T_3. *See* Triiodothyronine.
T_4. *See* Thyroxin.
Tachycardia, 148, 150
Tachypnea, 148
Taraxein, behavior disorders and, 219
Termination phase, of group, 227
Testes, 4
Tetralogy of Fallot, in children, 80–81
β-Thalassemia, in children, 62
Therapeutic groups, 227
Therapeutic interventions, in psychiatric disorders, 222–227
Third degree burns, 59
"Third spacing," of body fluids, 114
Thrombophlebitis, 153–154
  during postpartum period, 20–21
Thymectomy, 118
Thyroid tumors, 186
Thyroidectomy, 134
Thyrotropin releasing hormone, 130
Thyroxin (T_4), 131t
  hypersecretion of, 133
"Time out," 238
Toddler, 53–54
Token economies, 225, 235
Tolerance, 231
Topical anesthesia, 105
Touch, with schizophrenic patients, 234
Tourniquet, in anaphylaxis, 182
  in pulmonary edema, 149–150
Tracheobronchitis, acute, 137
Traction, application and maintenance of, 178–179
  types of, 178
Tranquilizers, minor, 240, 244
Transference, analysis of, 224
Transient circumoral cyanosis, 24
Transient ischemic attack, 119
Transplant rejection, 184
Transport, active, 108
Traumatic head injury, 120–121
Trigeminal neuralgia, 116
Triiodothyronine (T_3), 131t
  hypersecretion of, 133
Trocar, 170
Trousseau's sign, 135
Trust versus mistrust stage, 52, 221
Tubal pregnancy, 9

Tuberculosis, pulmonary, 145–146
Tuberculous pneumonia, 145
Tumor, adrenal, 136
  in colon cancer, 167
  in hypopituitarism, 130
  malignant, 184–188
  of brain, 66–67
  oral, 158
  parathyroid, 135
  thyroid, 186
Turning, pre-operative instruction in, 104

Ulcer, peptic, 160–162
Ulcerative colitis, 165–166
Ultrasonic Doppler flow detector, 153
Ultrasonography, 7, 155–156, 165, 169, 185–186
Umbilical cord, 5
  care of, 22
  prolapsed, 18
Undifferentiated schizophrenia, 234
Undoing, 219
Universality, of groups, 226, 227
Unsocialized disturbance of conduct, 228
Urethral blockage, 170
Urethral catheterization, 170
Urethritis, 171
Urgency incontinence, 170
Urinary calculosis, 171–172
Urinary frequency, 169
Urinary hesitancy, 169
Urinary incontinence, 170
Urinary retention, 169–170
Urinary tract infection, 171
Urinary urgency, 169, 170
Urine, acidifying, 122, 171
Urine culture, 168
Urine sensitivity test, 168
Uterus, 3
  postpartum complications of, 19–21
Uveitis, 127

Vagina, 3
Vagotomy, 161–162
Valsalva's maneuver, 129
Varicose veins, 154–155
Vascular disturbances, 151–157
  abruptio placentae and, 11
Vascular graft, 155–156
Vasectomy, 29
Vasoactive drugs, 152, 163
Vasogenic shock, 151–153
Vaso-occlusive crisis, in sickle cell anemia, 61
Vasopressin. *See* Antidiuretic hormone.
Veins, varicose, 154–155
Ventilators, 121, 144
Ventricular fibrillation, 150
Vertebrobasilar disturbance, 119
Vesicoureteral reflux, 169
Viral hepatitis, 162
Visual field examination, 132
Vital signs, postoperative assessment of, 106
Vitamin(s), in behavior disorders, 219
  in cirrhosis, 163
Volume ventilator, 144

Warfarin (Coumadin), 153
Water volume, sodium and, 110–113
White's classification, of diabetes, 13
Withdrawal, from drugs and alcohol, 231
  in children, 228–229
  in schizophrenia, 234
Working phase, of group, 227
Wound dressing, postoperative assessment of, 107

Xeroradiography, 185
X-rays. *See also* CAT scan.
  diagnosis of pregnancy and, 7
  in epilepsy, 115
  in osteoarthritis, 181
  of breast, 185
  of colon, 166–167
  of malignant tumors, 185
  of urinary tract, 168
  upper gastrointestinal, 161